Principles and Methods of
Adapted Physical Education and Recreation

Principles and Methods of

Adapted Physical Education and Recreation

DAVID AUXTER, Ed.D.

Professor of Developmental Education,
Slippery Rock University,
Slippery Rock, Pennsylvania

JEAN PYFER, P.E.D.

Chairman of Physical Education,
Texas Woman's University,
Denton, Texas

FIFTH EDITION

with 300 illustrations

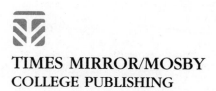

TIMES MIRROR/MOSBY
COLLEGE PUBLISHING

ST. LOUIS   TORONTO   SANTA CLARA   1985

Editor   Nancy K. Roberson
Developmental editor   Michelle A. Turenne
Project editor   Marjorie L. Sanson
Manuscript editor   Laura Kaye McNeive
Designer   Diane M. Beasley
Production   Margaret B. Bridenbaugh

Cover photo by Stewart Halperin taken at the
International Games for the Disabled.

FIFTH EDITION

Copyright © 1985 by Times Mirror/Mosby College Publishing

A division of The C.V. Mosby Company
11830 Westline Industrial Drive
St. Louis, Missouri 63146

Previous editions copyrighted 1969, 1973, 1977, 1981

Printed in the United States of America

Library of Congress Cataloging in Publication Data

Auxter, David.
    Principles and methods of adapted physical
education and recreation.

    Rev. ed. of: Principles and methods of adapted
physical education and recreation / Walter C. Crowe,
David Auxter, Jean Pyfer. 4th ed. 1981.
    Includes bibliographies and index.
    1. Physical education for handicapped children—Study
and teaching—United States. 2. Handicapped children—
United States—Recreation. I. Pyfer, Jean. II. Crowe,
Walter C. Principles and methods of adapted physical
education and recreation. III. Title.
GV443.A98   1985   371.9′044   84-22642
ISBN 0-8016-0378-1

C/VH/VH   9 8 7 6 5 4 3 2 1 02/C/228

Preface

Physical education for handicapped persons is undergoing many changes as a result of refined interpretations of Public Law 94-142. This has an impact on the teaching of motor skills to exceptional children. Consequently, the fifth edition of *Principles and Methods of Adapted Physical Education and Recreation* reflects these changes, the most dramatic of which is the instructional process that physical education teachers should provide for their handicapped students. We stress a process approach in which the unique needs of each child are determined through the integration of appropriate assessment, programming, and implementation procedures. It provides information about processes the physical education teacher should perform to enable all handicapped children to learn. This is in contrast to previous approaches that are descriptive of the handicapping conditions and physical activity, but are void of processes that link motor needs to activity at unique ability levels. Litigation concerning the nature of service in physical education for the handicapped has prompted the endorsement of revolutionary techniques and procedures that can maximize motor development of the handicapped.

This edition also describes the procedures for conducting individualized education programs, which are in accord with the latest United States Department of Education regulations for IEPs. The ongoing interpretation of Public Law 94-142 will continue to have a major impact on the conduction of physical education programs for the handicapped.

EDUCATIONAL APPROACHES

Two major alternatives for the implementation of IEPs for the handicapped are emerging. One is a developmental (bottom, up) approach, in which deficiencies are determined by measuring against normal development. If developmental prerequisites are found to be deficient, programming is then implemented to fulfill them. The other is a functional assessment of relevant motor skills for self-sufficiency. When using this approach the educator asks the question, "What do handicapped individuals need to attain self-sufficient motor behaviors in natural community environments?" If the specific motor skills needed cannot be developed, the question to ask is, "What prerequisites must be mastered to enable the acquisition of functional motor skills?" Thus the top, down approach begins with determination of specific skills that need to be developed and then a probe down through the needed prerequisites (the task-specific approach). The bottom, up approach considers a variety of prerequisites to determine which ones are deficient and then programs to correct those conditions. Chapters 1 through 6 provide a sound foundation for understanding the types and purposes of assessment that can be employed to conduct both of these approaches required by IEPs.

DEVELOPMENT OF THE FIFTH EDITION

A variety of sources contributed to the revision of the fifth edition. Litigation in federal courts clarified instructional procedures that should be implemented in IEPs. U.S. Department of Education regulations introduced new concepts for conducting adapted physical education, which we have incorporated.

Furthermore, comments and criticisms from users of the fourth edition were carefully considered for this revision. A panel of reviewers currently teaching adapted physical education were selected to assess whether the revised manuscript met the needs of the instructors and their students. There was close scrutiny of the book to verify that content was appropriate for training modern physical educators and that it applied to physical education settings in the real world.

Research was conducted to determine existing content taught to physical educators and new developments in the field of physical education. The research confirmed a shift in approach. The traditional categorical approach describes handicapping conditions, which suggested that nonspecific modifications to physical tasks have moved to a process-oriented skill development approach. This approach is geared toward enabling handicapped children to gain meaningful motor skills for participation in regular classes and the community, which enhances self-sufficiency in community environments.

This edition, therefore, comprises a major restructuring that offers methods and techniques commensurate with the state of the art for delivering physical education programs to handicapped persons.

Despite the restructuring, the text has strong coverage of the nature of handicapping conditions, curriculum content in physical education, and the organization and administration of such a program. The understanding of these concepts is still an important aspect of the design and implementation of physical education programs for the handicapped. Thus we continue to emphasize including the handicapped in physical activity while developing motor skills that contribute to self-sufficient life in the school and community.

ORGANIZATION

The organization of the fifth edition has been modified from the previous edition. Parts One and Two describe the nature of physical education services and instructional processes for facilitating motor development of the handicapped. Part Three describes handicapping conditions and ways of modifying physical activity to enable participation in activity. The final section includes techniques and procedures for the organization and administration of the total physical education program for the handicapped.

The fifth edition of *Principles and Methods of Adapted Physical Education and Recreation* is intended to synthesize each chapter into a process that enables implementation of IEPs for handicapped children. However, almost any chapter can be taken out of sequence and studied as a self-contained unit. Since each instructor has particular topic preference, the structure is comprehensive but flexible. Furthermore, each chapter has clear subdivisions to help the instructor decide the breadth of coverage to fit specific time parameters of parts of a given chapter. Thus the book can be made flexible for instructors with respect to the time they have to cover material and the detail that is desired for presentation of any topic.

An Organizational Alternative

Although we have arranged the chapters in a sequence that we believe is a logical progression of topics, we recognize that there are other orders in which chapters may be effectively presented. Therefore the following alternatives are offered:

1. Chapters 5, 6, and 7 provide practical suggestions for pinpointing students' motor development needs, for tying evaluation results to what is taught in the curriculum,

and for designing an educational environment conducive to learning. Chapter 2, which focuses on the specific mandates required by Public Law 94-142, could be combined with Chapters 5 through 7 and studied after covering the specific disabilities described in Chapters 9 through 18.

2. Chapters 19 through 22, covering organization, administration, equipment, and facilities, can be taught as a unit at either the beginning or the end of the course.

CONTENT

The individualized education program outlined in Public Law 94-142 requires instruction through objectives. This allows the results from research and demonstration from the behavioral sciences to be incorporated into the instructional system. Chapter 7 provides future teachers with techniques for bringing about changes in pupils to achieve the objectives through control of the learning environment.

The ultimate objective of the physical education program for the handicapped is the use of motor skills to enable adaptation to social life, community living, and the recreational environment. The fifth edition places emphasis on games and sports as a microsociety where social characteristics can be developed and generalized to subsocieties in natural living environments.

Another important new feature is emphasis on the multidisciplinary approach. Chapter 19 discusses this aspect of physical education as it relates to the human delivery system. Interdisciplinary interaction is a theme that is interwoven throughout various chapters of the book. It is expressed in Chapter 1 within the context of service to the handicapped and in Chapter 2 in reference to the various services that provide input for the IEP. It is also discussed in Chapter 5 under assessment of common developmental delays, in Chapter 13, since cooperation is needed with the medical profession to design physical education programs, and in Chapter 21, which discusses organization and administration support. Further-

more, the fifth edition has been updated in every area and includes references to the most recent literature.

NEW TO THIS EDITION

A number of other changes have also been made in the fifth edition:

1. A comparison is made between a task-specific, functional assessment, programming approach and a developmental approach.

2. Chapter 1, Educating the Disabled, has been updated to inform the reader of the latest developments in litigation for the handicapped and results from research and demonstration related to facilitating development of motor skills of the handicapped.

3. Chapter 2, The Individualized Education Program, has been updated to conform to the latest Department of Education regulations on the IEP.

4. Chapter 4 describes the types and purposes of assessment. It provides sufficient information so that physical education teachers can appropriately use a general developmental approach or a task-specific, functional assessment, programming approach.

5. Chapter 5 provides information on how to assess developmental motor delays of handicapped children.

6. Chapter 6 synthesizes procedures for integrating assessment and programming. Appropriately applied, this information enables implementation of an instructional process that meets the measured needs of each child.

7. Chapter 7 provides information from research and demonstration on what teachers can do with the learner to enhance positive learning through the IEP and control disruptive behavior so that handicapped children can learn.

8. Chapter 8 has been revised to provide information that supports wellness programs for the handicapped.

9. Chapter 9, Psychosocial Development, provides information on how general social characteristics can be achieved through participation in sports and games and how they may generalize to social settings outside of formal physical education instruction.

10. New Chapter 11 provides in-depth treatment of specific learning disabilities.

11. Chapter 13, Orthopedic Handicapping Conditions, has been revised and includes extensive sections on the care of the physically handicapped who must wear braces or are in wheelchairs. It also contains a new section on computerized movements for paralyzed muscles, providing the most current information available.

12. There is a new section on methodological procedures for working with the deaf-blind in Chapter 14, Hearing Impairments.

13. In Chapter 16, specific postural activities have been designed which link muscles that afflict postural with activity conditions. This enables assessment and programming to be integrated and leads to meaningful conduction of postural programming.

14. New training systems for developing physical fitness have been added to Chapter 17, Physical Development.

15. Chapter 18, Other Conditions, has been updated to include anemia, diet and its effect on the menstrual period, and programming for the diabetic student.

16. Chapter 21, Program Organization and Administration, has been completely revised to improve readability and make the organization and administration of programs more practical.

17. Chapter 22, Facilities and Equipment, has been expanded to include equipment that is applicable to a wide variety of activities and handicapping conditions.

18. Two appendices provide tests and activities for specific developmental delays.

In conclusion, the fifth edition has included current literature on best practices in physical education for the handicapped and has made revision in light of extensive review from users of the textbook and others in the field of motor development and physical activity for the handicapped.

PEDAGOGICAL AIDS

Unique to this text, color is introduced in this edition to increase visual appeal and to contrast concepts and topics. The illustration program includes all new photographs and completely revised line art, which incorporates the second color.

Many learning aids are offered to help the student master the material. The mission of each chapter is clearly defined with a list of Objectives to help orient the students to the main topics to be covered. A Chapter Summary reviews the main topics covered. Review Questions also appear at the end of each chapter, which provide assistance when studying for exams or for class discussion. Support is provided for the instructor with a list of Student Activities. Complete and current References and Suggested Readings appear at the end of each chapter and offer sources for further exploration of the subject matter. A comprehensive Glossary at the end of the text facilitates quick reference to terminology.

INSTRUCTOR'S MANUAL

A comprehensive manual has been developed with this edition to assist the professor using this text. Lecture preparation and student understanding are enhanced when the complete teaching package is employed. For each chapter of the text the instructor's manual includes the following:

1. Suggested lecture outlines to assist in classroom preparation

2. Major concepts, highlighted for each chapter

3. Helpful teaching suggestions, designed to enhance students' understanding of the major concepts and issues

4. Tests for each chapter, including matching, corrected true-false, listing, and essay questions

5. Six appendices including:
   a. Test answers
   b. Annotated bibliography
   c. Annotated film bibliography
   d. National organizations serving the handicapped
   e. Equipment and facility suppliers
   f. Transparency masters

ACKNOWLEDGMENTS

Many persons have contributed their efforts in the preparation of the fifth edition. We wish to acknowledge Lee Ann Gills, Sue Rooney, Marian Talbert, Sandy Schleiffers, Ron Davis, and Jim Van Dyke for preparation of the manuscript; Eugenia Kriebel of International Goal Ball for the Blind, Karrin Mancuso and Tom Songster of Special Olympics, Greta Stash of the Children's Rehabilitation Center, Toni Roberts of the Verland Foundation, and Ann Hull of Achievement Products Incorporated for their efforts to solicit illustrations; Dick McCandless, Steve Hetrick, Dave Martin, Colleen Mulrooney, Jim Yarger, and Kim Oren for their photographic skills. Also, we wish to acknowledge the American Red Cross, the Joseph P. Kennedy Foundation, Achievement Products Incorporated, Western Pennsylvania Special Olympics, and Childcraft Education Corporation for contributions of photographs.

We would also like to express our sincere appreciation to the publisher's reviewers for their critical reading of the manuscript for the fifth edition. Their numerous suggestions for improvement greatly influenced the final draft.

Leon E. Johnson, Ed.D.
University of Missouri at Columbia

Luke E. Kelly, Ph.D.
Michigan State University

Robert A. Rider, Ph.D.
Florida State University

Christine F. Summerford, P.E.D.
San Francisco State University

Robert Wiegand, Ph.D.
West Virginia University

Finally, we wish to extend our appreciation to Michelle Turenne and Marjorie Sanson of Times Mirror/Mosby College Publishing for their outstanding work as editors of this book.

David Auxter
Jean Pyfer

Contents

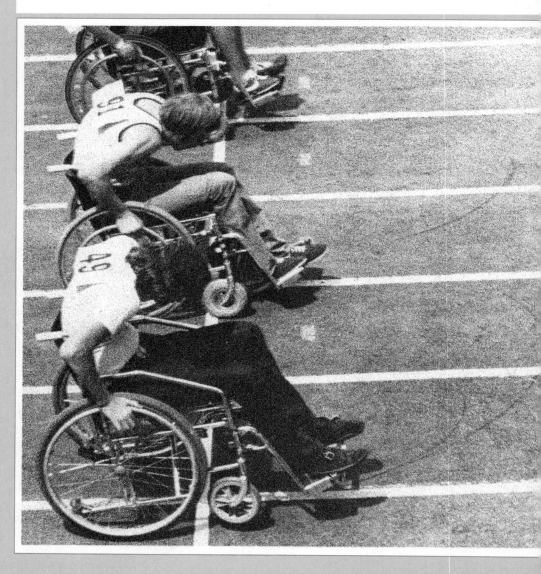

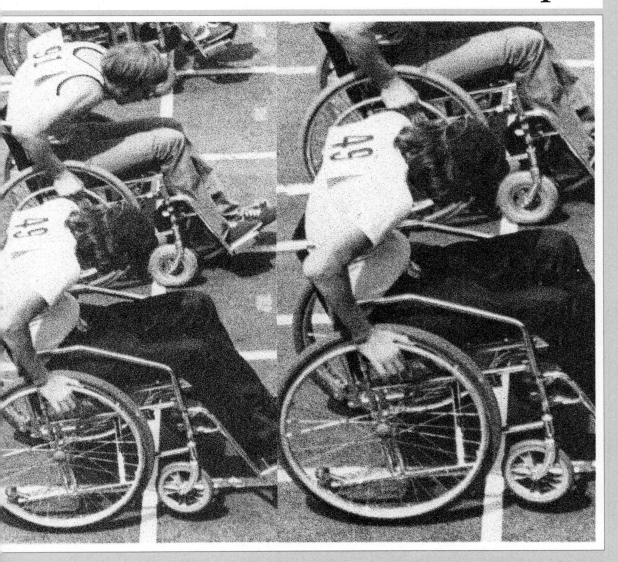

In this section we have provided a historical overview of societal attitudes toward individuals with disabilities. In the 1980s the United States is still attempting to implement the commitment to protecting individual and civil rights of persons with disabilities mandated by legislation of the 1970s. The mandates and detailed procedures to follow for compliance with the laws are presented in this section. Effective teaching methods and types of assessment to meet specific needs are discussed.

CHAPTER 1

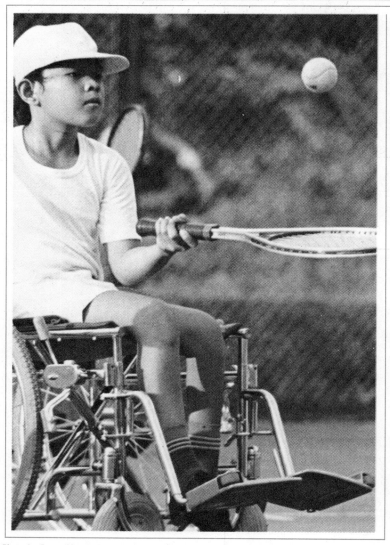

Photo by Bruce Haase; Peter Burwash International.

Educating the Disabled

OBJECTIVES

♦ Understand the nature and prevalence of handicapping conditions.

♦ Know the history of services to the handicapped.

♦ Understand the impact of legislation for provision of physical education services to the handicapped.

♦ Understand the effects of handicapping conditions as they relate to social forces during school and postschool years.

♦ Understand the role of the physical teacher within the context of a generic human delivery system.

Physical education teachers instruct children with a variety of handicapping conditions in many different instructional settings. The mission of the physical education teacher is to promote the development of motor skills and abilities so that children can live healthful and productive lives and engage in recreational and sport activities of their choosing. This chapter concerns the nature of handicapping conditions, the benefits of the physical education program, and the idea of a service delivery system in physical education for the handicapped.

INCIDENCE

The exact incidence of handicapped children in the public schools is not known. One point of view is that traditional estimates are too high. However, other educators believe that the number of children who need assistance with special education is unrealistically low. Kaufman[10] indicates that if schools identify these children as those whom they do not have the money and personnel to serve, they run the risk of court action. Under such circumstances schools might choose to avoid identifying children with mild handicaps.

Actually it is estimated that 12% of the total school-age population from birth to age 22 are handicapped.[19] Kennedy and Danielson[12] reported less than the expected 12% were being served as of 1977-1978, and French and Jansma[8] indicate a drop in the number of handicapped children being served in all categories of handicapping conditions. Thus the identification of handicapped children may vary among school districts.

The incidence of handicapped children in the public schools does not represent the magnitude of the need of persons who can benefit from special physical activity designed to accommodate the needs of individuals. In addition to those conditions outlined in the Education for All Handicapped Children Act of 1975 (P.L. 94-142), other special needs may qualify a child for special physical education considerations.

In a given year nearly 467 million acute (short-term) illnesses and injuries occur in our population. Approximately 68 million persons are injured annually, and more than three times as many have colds, sinus infections, influenza, and other respiratory tract diseases. Furthermore, accidents are responsible for an estimated 10.2 million disabling injuries per year. Of this number, 380,000 prove to be permanent impairments.[6] Paralysis, orthopedic disorders, hearing defects, speech defects, and heart disease also represented a considerable number of those conditions reported.

The number of individuals with multiple disabilities also is increasing. The reasons are many, but the primary ones seem to be the higher rate of survival among infants born prematurely and advanced techniques of medical science that are keeping children with one or more disabilities alive.

HISTORICAL IMPLICATIONS

Early History

In highly developed countries the current level of concern for the well-being of the individual has evolved gradually over thousands of years. One characteristic of the typical early primitive cultures was their preoccupation with survival. Historians speculate that members of many early primitive societies who were unable to contribute to their own care were either put to death, allowed to succumb in a hostile environment, or forced to suffer a low social status. In some societies persons displaying obvious behavioral deviations were considered from converse points of view: either filled with evil or touched by divine powers.

Humanitarianism

Great social and cultural progress occurred during the Renaissance. The seed of social consciousness had been planted. From this time on a genuine concern for the individual developed, giving each person dignity. With a desire for social reform came a multitude of movements to improve life. Reforms dealing with peace, prison conditions, poverty, and insanity were organized, and many social and moral problems were attacked in the first decade of the nineteenth century.

During the latter part of the nineteenth century and the early part of the twentieth century, emphasis was placed on development of instructional methodology to educate intellectually handicapped persons. This work had a significant impact on modern pedagogy. The Montessori approach was developed for work with the mentally retarded during the early part of the twentieth century. This was a didactic system in which learners used sequential materials that could accommodate the ability levels of each child. The Montessori approach was a forerunner of individualized instructional programming, which is widely used at present.

World War I was a period of greatly advanced medical and surgical techniques designed to ameliorate many physically disabling conditions. In addition, individuals were restored to usefulness by vocational and workshop programs. During the interim between World War I and World War II state and federal legislation was enacted to promote vocational rehabilitation for both civilians and the military disabled. The Smith-Sears Act of 1918 and the National Civilian Vocational Rehabilitation Act of 1920 were the forerunners of the Social Security Act of 1935 and the Vocational Rehabilitation Act of 1943, which provided the handicapped both physical and vocational rehabilitation.

With World War II came thousands of ill and incapacitated service personnel. Means were employed to restore them to function as useful and productive members of society. Physical medicine became a new medical specialty. Many services heretofore considered hospital services became autonomous ancillary medical fields. The paramedical specialties of physical therapy, occupational therapy, and corrective therapy considerably decreased the recovery time of many patients.

However the main impetus for aiding the dis-

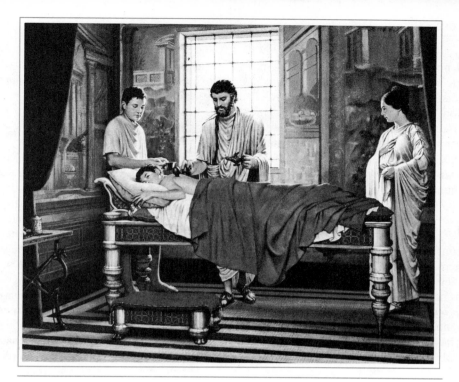

FIGURE 1-1
Galen treating an ill child by cupping.
(Courtesy Parke, Davis, & Co., Detroit.)

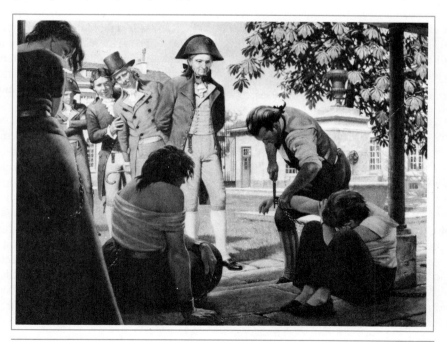

FIGURE 1-2
Pinel unchains the insane.
(Courtesy Parke, Davis, & Co., Detroit.)

abled did not occur until early in the twentieth century and as late as the early 1960s for the mentally retarded and the emotionally disturbed. The contributions of figures such as President Franklin D. Roosevelt, supporting the fight against crippling diseases such as poliomyelitis, and the Kennedy family, working to help the mentally retarded, can hardly be overlooked when discussing the humanitarian concerns in the United States.

Physical Activity

The relationship of physical activity to functional development and well-being has long been valued. In 460 BC Hippocrates used exercise to strengthen muscles and aid rehabilitation. Galen (30 BC) recommended specific exercises for muscle tonus, and Erasistratus advocated walking for dropsy. The fundamental value of the exercise was the physical well-being of the individual achieved through specific exercise regimens.

After World War II an emerging philosophy was social participation in sports and games. Such activity provided an opportunity to meet social-recreational needs as well as promote physical and organic development. In 1952 the Committee on Adapted Physical Education adopted the following resolution to accommodate handicapped children in physical education programs[1]:

It consisted of a diversified program of developmental activities, games, sports, and rhythms suited to the interests, capacities, and limitations of students with disabilities who may not safely or successfully engage in unrestricted participation in the vigorous activities of the general education program.

The evolution of instructional and behavioral technologies enabled maximization of the motor skill potential of handicapped persons. Consider the work of Gold,[9] who trained another teacher to teach a person who was legally blind and deaf, physically handicapped, and mentally retarded (IQ of 28) to assemble a complex 16-part Bendix bicycle coaster brake in 20 trials.

The technology Gold used in the motor task of the bicycle brake assembly is equally effective in the development of other physical and motor tasks. Recent advancements in applied behavioral analysis and research and demonstration for developing motor skills for the handicapped promise exciting work in the future.

DEFINITIONS OF HANDICAPPING CONDITIONS

Handicapped persons are grouped according to common characteristics. A name is then ascribed to each group. The term *developmental disabilities* represents all handicaps collectively. Although each state or authority may have differing definitions of developmental disability or specific handicaps, this text is concerned with current federal definitions.

The Rehabilitation, Comprehensive Service, and Developmental Disabilities Amendment of 1978 defines developmental disabilities as a severe chronic disability of a person that:

- Is attributable to a mental or physical impairment or combination of mental and physical impairments
- Is manifested before the person attains age 22
- Is likely to continue indefinitely
- Results in substantial functional limitations in three or more of the following areas of major life activity: self-care, receptive and expressive language, learning, mobility, self-direction, capacity for independent living, and economic self-sufficiency
- Reflects the person's need for a combination and sequence of special, interdisciplinary, or generic care, treatment, or other services that are lifelong or of extended duration and are individually planned and coordinated

The scope of special education for the exceptional child is broad. Programs of instruction can be offered in a number of places, depending on the needs of the child. Special education is available in hospitals and special residential and day schools as well as in home instruction and special classes for the handicapped within the regular schools. However, the majority of handicapped students attend regular schools.

The concern of all persons is that every handicapped individual should have the opportunity to reach full potential through an individualized education program.

PHYSICAL EDUCATION FOR THE HANDICAPPED

Handicapped persons engage in physical activity that is administered by many different types of personnel and carried out in a variety of settings. Following are some of the terms associated with personnel who administer physical activity to the handicapped:

adapted physical education Modification of traditional physical activities to enable the handicapped to participate safely, successfully, and with satisfaction

corrective physical education Activity designed to habilitate or rehabilitate deficiencies in posture or mechanical alignment of the body

remedial physical education Activity designed to habilitate or rehabilitate functional motor movements and develop physical and motor prerequisites for functional skills

New Definition of Physical Education

There is and has been a traditional curriculum common to most physical education programs. For the most part physical education activities include participation in sports and development of sufficient physical fitness to accomplish the activities of daily living.

Traditionally, good teaching implies accommodation of the individual needs of the learner to enable successful participation. Special accommodations are made in the teaching of skills, and adaptations are made to include children in sport activity and group games. Physical education for the handicapped was specifically defined in P.L. 94-142. It included all of the previous definitions mentioned but was simply stated. We have accepted the following P.L. 94-142 definition for use in this textbook[19]:

1. The term means the development of:
   a. Physical and motor fitness

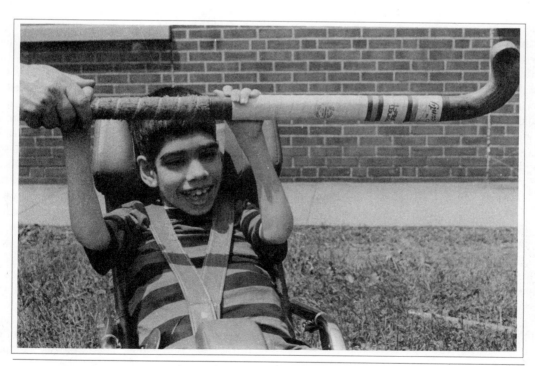

FIGURE 1-3
This child has a multiple disability. He is physically handicapped and mentally retarded.
(*Courtesy Slippery Rock University Laboratory School for Exceptional Children.*)

  b. Fundamental motor skills and patterns
  c. Skills in aquatics, dance, and individual and group games and sports (including intramural and lifetime sports)
2. The term includes special physical education, adapted physical education, movement education, and motor development.

The two essential components of physical education for the handicapped are teaching the defined curricula of physical education and conducting an individualized program for the handicapped child.

Benefits of Physical Education for the Handicapped

When a child is identified as handicapped, it serves notice to educators and parents that the child risks becoming dependent on others for social living skills. The physical educator can make a major contribution to reduce this risk and facilitate independent living in the following ways:

♦ Develop recreational motor skills for independent functioning in the community.
♦ Develop physical fitness for maintenance of health.
♦ Develop ambulatory skills to master mobility in domestic and community environments.
♦ Develop physical and motor prerequisites to self-help skills required for independent living.
♦ Develop physical and motor prerequisites to vocational skills required for independent living.
♦ Develop prerequisite motor skills necessary for participation in self-fulfilling social activity.

The physical education program is a vital part of the total education program, which is designed to maximize the potential for self-sufficient living in the community.

Scope of Physical Education for the Handicapped

Public policy requires that handicapped children be provided with physical education. The scope regulations (development of physical and motor fitness, fundamental motor patterns and skills, and team and lifetime sport skills). The incorporation of physical education into P.L. 94-142 has led to many opportunities for services to handicapped children, such as the following:

♦ Teaching motor skills to all handicapped children, who will use these skills in recreational environments in the community
♦ Teaching the handicapped to generalize skills obtained in instructional settings into the community[4]
♦ Helping to develop the fundamental motor skills, such as walking for persons with impaired ambulation
♦ Developing prerequisite physical and motor fitness for the severely involved so they may develop self-help skills, such as feeding and dressing
♦ Being involved directly and meaningfully with severely and profoundly handicapped persons, for whom the primary education program is motor

Clearly, the physical education program is vital to every handicapped person. Often the need for physical education bears a direct relationship to the severity of the handicap. Profoundly mentally retarded persons often have an educational program of development of ambulation skills, self-care skills, and communication. The physical education profession is needed to develop the fundamental skills of ambulation and the physical and motor prerequisites for the self-help skills. Those handicapped persons who are mentally impaired often rely on recreational motor skills for their leisure.

Physical Education: an Integral Part of Special Education

The content and purposes of physical education were well known long before the evolution of the instructional procedures that have been identified with effective intervention systems for handicapped children. However, individualized formats

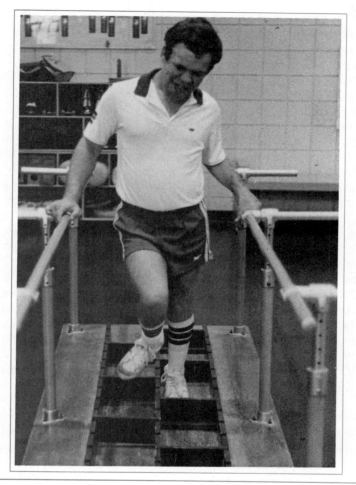

FIGURE 1-4
A handicapped person in a therapeutic program to restore walking function.
(Courtesy Verland Foundation, Sewickley, Pa.)

of instruction have added new meaning to the physical education profession. The focus of physical education for the handicapped has had the following benefits for the physical education profession:

1. It has enabled an identifiable body of content that is the physical education curriculum (defined by federal law), developed out of a substantial history and tradition.
2. It now has unique integrity with the recognized procedure and products associated with special education (specially designed instruction to meet unique needs as set forth in the individualized education program).
3. The integrated disciplines of special and physical education rely on accurate language to meet public policy demands.

The inclusion of physical education as an integral part of special education, as a matter of public policy, has made adapted physical education a unique discipline.

Coordination of Services

The mission of physical education for the handicapped is to improve their quality of life. However, for physical education programs to be of greatest benefit, they must be carried over into daily leisure activities in the community after school. This requires coordination of services and resources in the home, school, and other community agencies.

Parents often mediate for children with school and community. For them to maximize opportunities for their children they need to know specifically the benefits and the skills that are developed in school physical education programs and opportunities in the community where these acquired skills can be expressed. Therefore physical education teachers and parents of handicapped children should meet frequently to plan and revise the planning for handicapped children so that the school programs meet the children's need for participation in the community.

LEGISLATION FOR THE HANDICAPPED

Equal educational opportunity is an accepted philosophical principle of our society. Two federal laws codified the education and services for the handicapped: the Rehabilitation Act of 1973 (P.L. 93-112) and the Education for All Handicapped Children Act of 1975 (P.L. 94-142). An integral part of both acts was the opportunity for handicapped persons to take part in an environment that was the least restrictive to their personal liberty.

Rehabilitation Act of 1973

The Rehabilitation Act of 1973 is considered civil rights legislation for the handicapped. The most far-reaching part of the act is Section 504. It states that "no qualified handicapped individual . . . shall be excluded from participation or denied the benefits . . . under any program receiving federal financial assistance."[18] This clause brought up the question of possible differential treatment of the handicapped within existing programs. Statements in subsequent regulations

dealt specifically with "nonacademic and extracurricular activities," including physical education (Section 84, 37).

Education for All Handicapped Children Act

The Education for All Handicapped Children Act of 1975 sought to provide all handicapped children individual education programs that, to the greatest extent possible, would make them self-sufficient and independent of government assistance. Physical education was the only mentioned curriculum. Also contained within the regulations was mention of equal opportunity in intramural and interscholastic competition to the same extent as the nonhandicapped enjoyed.[21]

Accommodation of Individual Difference

Each handicapped child should have an individualized physical education program. The activities of the program should promote the acquisition of a skill, and each activity should begin at the child's present level of ability and progress in a sequence of small steps. It is also expected that aids be introduced and the environment modified to enable successful participation. Tasks that meet the needs of the specific learner should be selected, and the length of participation on the tasks should be commensurate with the amount of self-sufficiency the child needs to develop.

For example, consider a young severely handicapped child who has difficulty sitting erect because of insufficient abdominal strength. Sit-ups might be selected as an activity to strengthen the muscles. The angle of inclination of a board on which the child does the sit-ups can make the task more or less difficult. (The angle of the board reflects the angle of the child's body, with his back against the board.) If the board is flat on the floor (180°), the task is of considerable difficulty. If the board is perpendicular to the floor (90°), the degree of difficulty is diminished to zero. Alteration of the position of the board between 180° and 90° enables a sequence of difficulty. The variance of the distance of the movement and the length of the lever arm on which gravity acts pro-

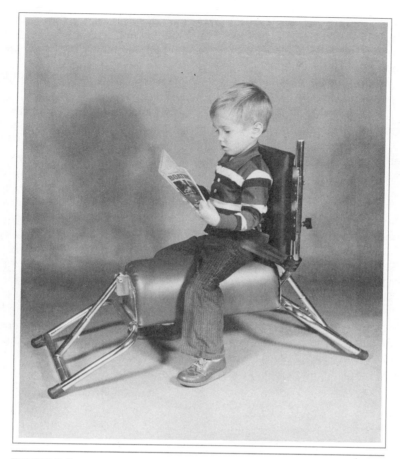

FIGURE 1-5
A child uses a leg spreader to develop flexibility prerequisites for ambulation.
(Courtesy Achievement Products Incorporated.)

vide a sequence that can accommodate a wide range of abilities. The student might participate in this activity for 5 minutes out of each physical education period to develop this specific muscle group, so beneficial to this particular child.

Concepts from Legislation

Three primary concepts that have emerged from legislation have implications for the conduction of physical education for the handicapped: (1) school personnel must spell out achievable objectives in detail and be held accountable for subsequent evaluation; (2) parents must be fully in-

formed of the nature of the programs in which their children participate; and (3) the education should take place in the most integrated setting, with normal children in regular class, if possible. Each of these components of the educational delivery system requires the focus to be on the individual needs and learning of children with specific handicaps.

Intramurals and Interscholastic Sports

Handicapped children need the same opportunities for participation in intramurals and interscholastic sport activities as do nonhandicapped children. Furthermore, these opportunities ideally are provided in the most integrated setting. However, provisions should be made to separate the handicapped from normal children during participation "when it is necessary to ensure the health and safety of the students, or to take into account their interest."[18] The central theme of the provision of equal opportunity in intramural and interscholastic participation for the handicapped is that of "reasonable accommodation" for these learners (Section 84.46).[18]

Due Process

When a person's civil rights are violated, he is entitled to due process (the right to be heard in a formal hearing). Due process complaints under P.L. 94-142 are usually filed to resolve the content or procedures employed in conduction of the individualized education program or placement in an appropriate setting. A hearing may also be possible through an Office of Civil Rights (OCR) complaint under Section 504. Lack of opportunity for participation in intramural and interscholastic activities would most likely be addressed through the OCR forum. Due process is a safeguard for achieving the goal of quality and equal educational opportunity for all handicapped children.

Least Restrictive Environment
Legal Precedents

Handicapped persons historically have been segregated in isolated settings. These segregated settings have hospital-like characteristics and are removed from the daily activity of a normal community. At one time it was believed that if sufficient numbers of persons who have special problems were in one place, they could be better served because management would be easier. However, beginning in the early part of the century legal precedents were set for what is known as the doctrine of the *least restrictive environment* (14th amendment of the U.S. Constitution; right to liberty issue). Confinement to an institution massively curtails one's liberty, which also occurs when decisions about one's welfare are made by others. Such infringements exist when others decide when one will arise in the morning, when one goes to bed in the evening, when and

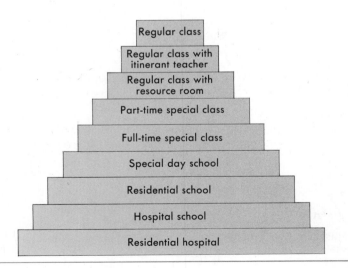

FIGURE 1-6
A continuum of lesser restrictive environments. The most restrictive is at the bottom and the least restrictive at the top. The teacher develops behaviors through the IEP that move the child to the least restrictive environment as soon as possible.

what one will eat, where one will live, where one will toilet and wash, if and where one can work, when one can work, and what one will do. It is decided what health services will be provided and when and where, and the extent of those provisions. There often is little recreation; when there is, the restrictions surrounding it are extensive. Clearly, institutionalized living is in many instances incarceration with no crime committed by the incarcerated.

Brown v. the Board of Education of Topeka in 1954 was the landmark case in which segregation of the races in our public schools was challenged. Separate but equal education was declared unequal. Other litigation based on the least restrictive environment principle is as follows:

♦ *Wolf v. the Legislature of Utah (1954):* The court ruled that segregation into special classes developed a "sense of inferiority and not belonging" and "could plague motivation for educational purposes," and "has the tendency to retard the educational, emotional, and mental development" of the children involved.

♦ *Mills v. the Board of Education (1972):* The court ruled that emotionally disturbed children had a right to education and should be placed in as normal a setting as possible, one in which little interference with the educational process would be likely to occur.

♦ *Hairston v. Drosick (1976):* The court conducted an extensive investigation of denial of unconditional inclusion of a handicapped child in regular classes and concluded the following[10]:

There are a great number of other spina bifida children throughout the State of West Virginia who are attending public schools in the regular classroom situation, the great majority of which have more severe disabilities than the plaintiff child Trina Hairston, including children having body braces, shunts, Cunningham clips, and ostomies, and requiring the use of walkers and confinement to wheelchairs. The needless exclusion of these children and other children who are able to function adequately from the regular classroom situation would be a great disservice to these children. . . . A major goal of the educational process is the socialization process that takes place in the regular classroom, with the resulting capability to interact in a social way with one's peers. It is therefore imperative that every child receive an education with his or her peers insofar as it is at all possible. This conclusion is further enforced by the critical importance of education in this society.

Such legal procedents, together with other legislation, led to the Education for All Handicapped Children Act of 1975, in which the concept of appropriate placement in the least restrictive environment was firmly established. Testimony by social scientists, which indicated that segregation and restriction of children from culturally relevant social learning experiences was undesirable, convinced Congress of such worth. Senator Stafford of Vermont made the following points before Congress[16]:

For far too long handicapped children have been denied access to the regular school system because of an inability to climb the steps to the schoolhouse door, and not for any other reason. This has led to segregated classes for those children with physical handicaps. This is an isolation that is in many cases unnecessary. It is an isolation for the handicapped child and for the "normal" child as well. The sooner we are able to bring the two together, the more likely that the attitudes of each toward one another will change for the better. . . . I firmly believe that if we are to teach all of our children to love and understand each other, we must give them every opportunity to see what "different" children are like. . . . If we allow and, indeed, encourage handicapped children and nonhandicapped children to be educated together as early as possible, their attitudes toward each other in later life will not be such obstacles to overcome. A child who goes to school every day with another child who is confined to a wheelchair will understand far better in later life the limitations and abilities of such an individual when he or she is asked to work with, or is in a position to hire, such an individual.

Social integration of the handicapped is a matter of public policy. Procedures should be taken to ensure that to the maximum extent appropriate handicapped children are educated with children who are not handicapped[16] and that they be moved to special classes and programs only when a regular class, plus special services, cannot meet their needs. The fundamental premise of integration of the handicapped in the schools is that it prepares handicapped children and non-handicapped children for life in a world in which they must live and work with one another.

Brown and co-workers[5] address the reasons surrounding improved learning that schooling severely handicapped children with nonhandicapped children provides. For the most part these benefits reflect those of the integration concept proposed by Congress. They maintain the following position[4]:

Long-term heterogeneous interactions between severely handicapped and nonhandicapped students facilitate the development of the skills, attitudes, and values that will prepare both groups to be sharing, participating, contributing members of complex, postschool communities. Stated another way, separate education is not equal education. . . . Segregated service delivery models have at least the following disadvantages:
  1. Exposure to nonhandicapped student models is absent or minimal.
  2. Severely handicapped students tend to learn "handicapped" skills, attitudes, and values.
  3. Teachers tend to strive for the resolution of handicapping problems at the expense of developing functional community-referenced skills.
  4. Most comparisons between students are made in relation to degrees of handicap rather than to criteria of nonhandicapped performance.
  5. Lack of exposure to severely handicapped students limits the probability that the skills, attitudes, and values of nonhandicapped students will become more constructive, tolerant, and appropriate.
Certainly, it is possible that interaction may not take place even if severely handicapped students are in the physical presence of nonhandicapped students. However, unless severely handicapped and nonhandicapped students occupy the same space, interaction is impossible. . . . In the future, severely handicapped students, upon the completion of formal schooling, will live in public, minimally segregated, heterogeneous communities, where they will constantly interact with nonhandicapped citizens. Thus, the educational experience should be representative and help prepare both severely handicapped students and nonhandicapped students to function adaptively in integrated communities.

Fundamental Concepts of Least Restrictive Environment

Despite legal support for the principle of least restrictive environment (integration of the handicapped with nonhandicapped), school placement of children with specific handicaps will be argued in informal discussions and formal hearings. The following points are critical to the concepts of least restrictive environment:

- ◆ The placement of handicapped children must be flexible and reevaluated. Appropriate action should be taken on the reevaluation.
- ◆ The desirable placement goal is movement of the child to less restrictive environments where it is possible to participate in normal community and school activities with normal children.
- ◆ Eventual placement of the handicapped in less restrictive, more normalizing environments requires individual programs so that they can learn skills which allow for participation with normal children in normal settings.

ACCOMMODATING THE HANDICAPPED IN INTEGRATED SETTINGS

Many argue that teaching children with heterogeneous learning characteristics is impractical; however, growing numbers of educators take exception to that position. Initiatives were taken by the United States Office of Education in the 1960s and 1970s to encourage innovative ways to accommodate individual differences. Programmed instruction had proved to be extremely productive in the development of knowledge and skills for all persons, the handicapped included. With considerable federal investment, learning research laboratories developed systems for individualization of *all* children. Materials are now available that enable all children to participate at their current level of educational performance.[21,22] Certain training programs for physical education teachers, as a matter of course, prepare their teachers to conduct the individualized education program for all children, either handicapped or not in the regular class.[2,21]

Prerequisite to the conduction of physical education skills with individualized formats are (1) prearranged written physical education skills with

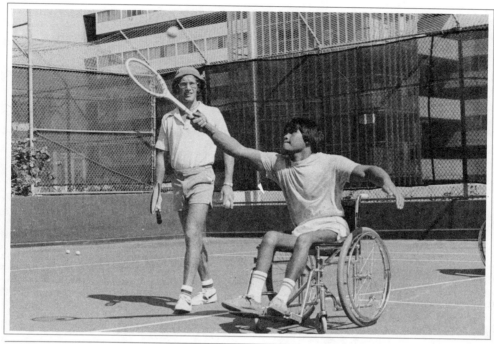

FIGURE 1-7
Handicapped persons can learn tennis skills so they can participate in this recreational activity in the community.
(Photo by Bruce Haase; courtesy Peter Burwash International.)

written objectives and (2) a training system that enables learners to direct and evaluate their own learning. Handicapped learners at mental age 6 are usually able to convert stick figures into objective performance.[14,23] We want to emphasize that such individualized instruction for accommodation of individual differences applies only to the development of skills for each individual. Play in group games requires procedures for modification of tasks, rules, and the environment to enable accommodation in group play. Descriptions of procedures for modification of specific handicapping conditions for specific types of tasks are included in subsequent chapters.

Successful teaching of handicapped individuals in regular classes requires teaching skills which enable the accommodation of heterogeneous groups through individualization of instruction. It also requires teachers who can modify rules, environments, and tasks to promote meaningful play among the handicapped and nonhandicapped.

LEAST RESTRICTIVE ALTERNATIVE

It is accepted public policy that there should be a continuum of alternate placements to meet the needs of the handicapped in the least restrictive environment. Handicapped children have a wide range of physical education needs. A recognized continuum of educational settings with services may be matched with a specific child at a *specific* point in time. Children should be moved from more to less restrictive environments as their needs warrant. Through the application of the individualized education program the abilities of handicapped children should change. These changes should be directed toward advanced placements on the continuum. Progress of children advancing on a continuum of least restrictive alternatives

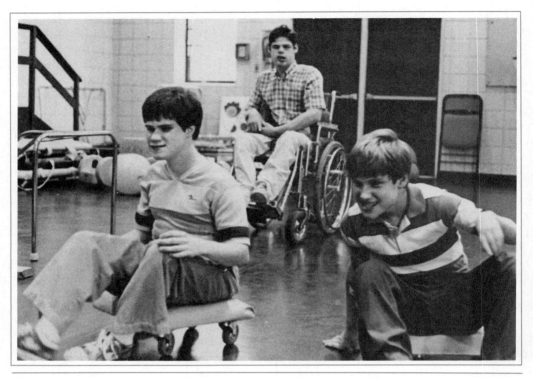

FIGURE 1-8
Intramural activity for the severely handicapped can be adapted to competitive tasks and in environ-
ments where there are few options for activity.
(Courtesy Verland Foundation, Sewickly, Pa.)

requires (1) periodic review of educational progress, (2) frequent assessment of what least restrictive environment means for a particular child
at a particular time, and (3) possible modifications in the type of delivery of services that may
produce optimum progress in the future.[7] Fig. 1-6
shows a *cascade system* of least restrictive environments available to the handicapped.

MOST APPROPRIATE PLACEMENT

Handicapped children should be placed in a setting that most appropriately meets their physical
education needs. Clearly, handicapped children
should not be placed in regular classes if it is not
in their best interest. Appropriate placement requires consideration of several variables, such as
the characteristics of the regular class teacher,
the nature of the activity the child is to perform,
and available support services.

Needs of the Child

Handicapped children have physical, social, and
emotional needs that are to be met in physical
education class. To accomplish this the following
four conditions should be met:

1. The instructional level of activity should be
   commensurate with the ability level of the
   child. Some form of individualized instruction should be provided.
2. Activities should be modified to accommodate individual differences in group games.
3. The social environment should be such that
   it can promote interaction (see Chapter 6).
4. Activities should enable participation rather
   than spectatorship.

Teacher Qualities

The characteristics of classes that restrict individual liberties for free association with peers vary. Teachers may possess different skills for accommodation of individual differences when teaching specific content. Teacher attitudes toward acceptance of handicapped children in their class and their ability to accommodate handicapped children are considerations for appropriate placement.

Nature of the Activity

Some activities enable accommodation of differences more so than others. Individual sport skills such as tumbling and gymnastics do not depend on the performance or ability of others. Skill development in sports is not particularly difficult to individualize in a regular physical education class. The application of these sport skills in competition is much more difficult. The nature of the activity and ability of the teacher to implement participation in the activity are relevant to the placement of the handicapped child in a regular class.

Handicapped children should be placed in an environment where they may participate successfully and safely.

COMMUNITY-BASED PROGRAMMING

Handicapped children risk becoming dependent on society. The mission of physical education programs for the handicapped is to contribute to the greatest extent possible to their independent living in their community. This requires that physical educational programming be extended beyond the traditional school day and instructional setting. A relationship should be established between skills learned by students in instructional environments and the application of those skills to natural environments in the community. Such programming in physical education starts with the needs of the student for successful participation in physical activity in neighborhood and recreational centers and opportunities in the community. This requires mutual relationships between handicapped students and the total com-

munity environment, both physical and social. For further information about community-based approaches in the education for the handicapped refer to the work of Brown[4] and Wilcox and Bellamy.[24]

NORMALIZATION

Normalization "means making available to the handicapped patterns and conditions of everyday life which are as close as possible to the norms and patterns of the mainstream of society."[12] For this to occur, society's view of the handicapped must be consistent with the following conditions:

- They must be perceived by society as human beings, not as subhuman (vegetables, animals, etc.).
- They must be perceived by society as possessing a legal and constitutional identity (due process of law for involuntary institutionalization and equal opportunity in education, housing, employment).
- They must be viewed as persons who can adapt to their environment and acquire skills for as long as they live.
- They must be provided opportunity by society to take full advantage of their culture.
- Services must be provided by trained personnel with technical competence in education and habilitation.
- The human services which care for the handicapped and provide opportunity for skill development must be valued and well understood by society.
- The handicapped must be provided opportunities to play valued roles and lead valued lives in our culture.

In the past, many handicapped persons have been considered social deviants. Wolfensberger[25] indicates that a person may be regarded as deviant if some characteristic or attribute is judged different by others who consider the characteristic or attribute important and who value this difference negatively. An overt and negatively valued characteristic that is associated with a deviance is a *stigma*. For instance, members of ethnic minorities, persons with cosmetic disfigurements,

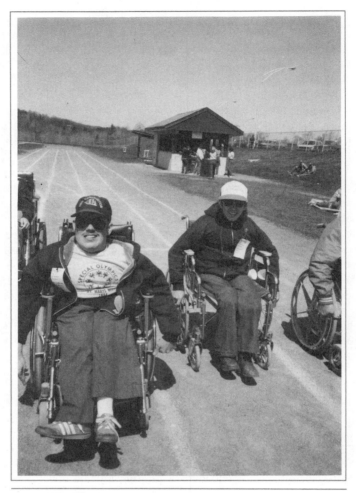

FIGURE 1-9
Some children may need to participate in handicapped-only activity.
(Courtesy Karrin Mancuso, Western Pennsylvania Special Olympics.)

dwarfs, and children with handicapping conditions have been considered deviant.

Deviance is a social perception. It is not characteristic of a person but rather of an observer's values as they pertain to social norms.[25] When a person is perceived as deviant or is stereotyped, as is the case with many handicapped children, he or she is prescribed to a role that carries great expectancies by the nonhandicapped. Furthermore, most of these social perceptions clearly reflect prejudices that have little relationship to reality. As Wolfensberger indicates, the lack of objective verification is not a crucial element in the shaping of a social judgment or social policy.

EDUCATIONAL ACCOUNTABILITY FOR THE HANDICAPPED

When applied to the teaching process, the concept of accountability means that a particular pro-

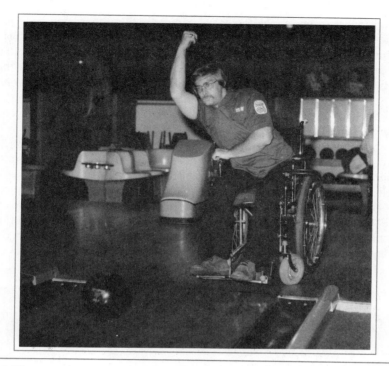

FIGURE 1-10

A self-sufficient handicapped person participates in community recreation bowling. *(Courtesy Daryl Pfister, American Wheelchair Bowling Association.)*

gram, method, or intervention can be demonstrated to cause a significant positive change in one or more behaviors.[17] It is accepted policy that written records be maintained on each handicapped student to document specific progress toward preestablished goals and objectives. Technical procedures for the appropriate selection of objectives for specific learners have been developed.[3,9] Once these specific meaningful behaviors have been defined, it is than possible to apply accepted behavioral principles to develop them with this sophisticated technology.

Coordination of Delivery of Services

There has been considerable emphasis on the belief that programs for the handicapped should be of an interdisciplinary nature. However, according to Stone,[17] problems have existed in the delivery of services within the system. Professionals within the system have taken on the roles, functions, and goals of each other. This has happened because of inadequate planning or coordination and without consideration of the effectiveness of the various professionals in their new roles. As a result we have homogenized professionals who no longer have defined expertise and programs that are less than desirable. Although Stone was not addressing physical education specifically, his view may well relate to the coordination of physical education and the related services (therapies). Role confusion can lead to duplication of services in some programs and voids in others, which result in a lack of comprehensive programming for handicapped children.

Public policymakers have assigned educational functions to those who are to provide direct services and those who provide indirect services. Direct services are those such as physical education that teach curricula sanctioned by school boards. Related services help handicapped children gain benefits from the intended outcomes of the direct services (such as physical therapy, occupational therapy, and recreational therapy).

The Concept of Related Services

Before a related service such as physical therapy, occupational therapy, or recreational therapy can be implemented in the curriculum, it should be determined whether the limitations of that particular child are such that direct services (physical education) cannot effectively deal with the child's educational problem. A related service should be provided when a child cannot make the expected progress in skill development in physical education. For instance, if it is decided that a handi-

capped child does not have the prerequisite strength of a specific muscle group to acquire a sport skill and that the physical educator cannot rectify the problem, a physical therapist may be called on to provide a related service. The physical therapist designs a program for the specific muscle group to establish prerequisite strength; then the child can acquire the skills to be taught by the physical educator. The physical therapist's plan should include measurement of developmental progress in terms of the strength of the specific muscle group. In addition, the physical therapist and those who plan for the related service should indicate the dates of initiation of services, the dates of termination of services, and the duration of the training. However, the development of the skill to be taught in the physical

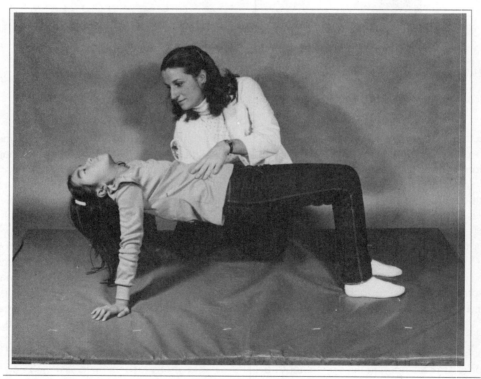

FIGURE 1-11
An occupational therapist provides a related service in a safe environment with a mat.
(Courtesy Achievement Products Incorporated.)

education class is the responsibility of the physical educator. The development of the physical prerequisites (of a pathological nature) to a skill is the responsibility of the related service provider. Such a procedure streamlines services, with greater emphasis on the education of the child, and upgrades the quality of instruction.

SUMMARY

Concern for the needs of disabled individuals surfaced during the Renaissance; however, social reforms directed toward improving the quality of life for the disabled did not begin until the nineteenth century. World Wars I and II provided the impetus to develop rehabilitation programs to improve the function of disabled persons. Focus on upgrading the opportunities for mentally retarded individuals became a reality in the 1960s. A national effort to provide school and community services for all handicapped persons began with the Rehabilitation Act of 1973 and the Education for All Handicapped Children Act of 1975. These two pieces of legislation mandated appropriate physical education programs and opportunities to participate in intramurals and interscholastic sports for handicapped citizens of school age.

Physical education for the handicapped is a comprehensive service delivery system designed to identify problems of children in physical and motor fitness, fundamental motor patterns and skills, and sport skills and games. Services include assessment, individualized education programming, and coordination of activities with related resources and services. These services may be delivered by specialists who possess skills to conduct instruction for the handicapped in regular or handicapped only classes. Special physical education may serve both handicapped and nonhandicapped children. Specially designed physical education also may occur in any setting on the least restrictive alternative continuum.

An estimated 10% to 20% of the total school-age population at sometime during their education will perform inadequately on physical education tasks. Many of these children are handicapped and need an individualized education program in physical education. The physical education program should develop physical and motor fitness, fundamental motor patterns and skills, and skill development that enables participation in team and lifetime sports. The physical education curriculum and teachers must be able to service children with sensory, physical, mental, and social-emotional handicaps. The services should be provided for handicapped children in environments where they have an opportunity to engage in culturally relevant learning experiences with their peers. This would be the regular class if possible. However, each handicapped child must be placed in the school environment that is most appropriate for the specific child. The physical educator must coordinate the services with the special education teacher, related services, school administrators, and parents. All parties are cooperatively involved with the physical education program for the handicapped child.

REVIEW QUESTIONS

1. What are the three most prevalent handicapping conditions?
2. What is a historical theme in services for the handicapped?
3. What is a legal definition of physical education?
4. What are some benefits of a physical education program for handicapped children?
5. Describe the purposes of the Rehabilitation Act of 1973 and the Education for All Handicapped Children Act.
6. What are the entitlements of the handicapped for intramural and interscholastic sports under federal legislation?
7. What is the difference between least restrictive environment and least restrictive alternative?
8. Can you describe a "cascade of systems of least restrictive environments"?
9. What is community-based physical education programming?
10. Describe some principles of normalization.
11. What is a related service? What is the relationship of a related service to a direct service?
12. Why is physical education an integral part of special education?
13. What are some of the roles and tasks of physical education teachers of the handicapped?

STUDENT ACTIVITIES

1. Interview a handicapped person or the teacher or parent of a handicapped person to determine enjoyable physical activities.
2. Provide physical activity for a child with a specific handicapping condition. Indicate your feelings before and after the teaching experience.
3. Select two environments where services for the handicapped are delivered. One environment should be more restrictive than the other. Describe the differences between the two environments.
4. Identify two or three skills of a handicapped child that would assist self-sufficient living in the community where the child lives.
5. Visit and interview a physical education teacher of the handicapped. Survey the tasks that are performed while the teacher conducts the class.
6. Interview some handicapped students of different ages to determine their interests.

REFERENCES

1. American Association of Health, Physical Education, and Recreation: Guiding principles for adapted physical education, J. Health Phys. Ed. Rec. April 1952, p. 15.
2. Auxter, D.M.: Integration of the mentally retarded training programs, J. Health Phys. Ed. Rec. Sept. 1970, pp. 61-62.
3. Bellamy T., Peterson, L., and Close, D.: Habilitation of the severely and profoundly retarded: illustrations of competence, Educ. Train. Ment. Retard. **10**(3):174-186, 1975.
4. Brown, L., et al.: A strategy for developing chronological age appropriate and functional curricular content for severely handicapped adolescents and young adults, J. Spec. Educ. **13**:81-90, 1979.
5. Brown, L., et al.: Toward the realization of the least restrictive educational environments for severely handicapped students, Position paper, University of Wisconsin-Madison, Grant no. OEG 0-73-6137, U.S. Department of Education, Office of Special Education, 1977.
6. Carroll, C., and Miller, D.: Health: the science of human adaptation, Dubuque, Iowa, 1982, William C. Brown and Co., Publishers.
7. Cratty, B.J.: Adapted physical education for handicapped children and youth, Denver, 1980, Love Publishing Co.
8. French, R.W., and Jansma, P.: Special physical education, Columbus, Ohio, 1982, Charles E. Merrill Publishing Co.
9. Gold, M.: Task analysis: a statement and example using acquisition and production of complex assembly task by the retarded blind, Urbana-Champaign, Ill. 1975, Institute for Child Behavior and Development, University of Illinois.
10. *Hairston vs. Drosick*, 423 F. Suppl., 180 (S.D. W. Va., 1976).
11. Kaufman, J.M.: Characteristics of children's behavior disorders, ed. 2, Columbus, Ohio, 1981, Charles E. Merrill Publishing Co.
12. Kennedy, M.M., and Danielson, L.C.: Where are unserved handicapped children? Educ. Train. Ment. Retard. **13**:408-413, 1978.
13. Nirje, B.: The normalization principle. In Kugel, R.B. and Shearer, F., editors: Changing patterns in residential services for the mentally retarded, Washington D.C., 1976, Presidents Committee on Mental Retardation.
14. Runac, M.: Acquisition of motor awareness related tasks between kindergarten and primary mentally retarded children through individually prescribed instruction, Master's thesis, Slippery Rock State College, 1971.

15. Sherrill, C.: Adapted physical education and recreation, ed. 3, Dubuque, Iowa, 1985, William C. Brown Co., Publishers.
16. Stafford, J.: Congress. Rec. **121**:10961, 1975.
17. Stone, A.: Mental health and law: a system in transition, Washington D.C., 1976, U.S. Department of Health, Education, and Welfare.
18. U.S. Department of Health, Education, and Welfare: Regulations for the Rehabilitation Act of 1973, Fed. Reg. **42**:22676-22702, 1977.
19. U.S. 94th Congress: Public Law 94-142, Nov. 29, 1975.
20. Weigand, R.: A comparison of acquisition of basketball dribbling skills among normal and socially maladjusted boys ages twelve to thirteen through the use of an individually prescribed system, Master's thesis, Slippery Rock College, 1972.
21. Weigand, R., and Hawkins, A.: Program to prepare physical educators to instruct West Virginia's handicapped children, Morgantown, W.Va., 1982, West Virginia University, Sponsored by the USDE (Office of Special Education) Grant no. G008200529.
22. Wessel, J.: Fundamental skills, Northbrook, Ill., 1976, Hubbard Press.
23. White, C.: Acquisition of lateral balance between trainable mentally retarded children and kindergarten children in an individually prescribed instructional program, Unpublished master's thesis, Slippery Rock State College, 1972.
24. Wilcox, B., and Bellamy, G.: Design of high school programs for severely handicapped students, Baltimore, 1982, Paul H. Brookes Publishing Co.
25. Wolfensberger, W.: Principles of normalization, Toronto, 1972, National Institute on Mental Retardation.

SUGGESTED READINGS

Lewis, R., and Doorlag, D.H.: Teaching special students in the mainstream, Columbus, Ohio, 1983, Charles E. Merrill Publishing Co.

Seaman, J.A., and DePauw, K.P.: The new adapted physical education: a development approach, Palo Alto, Calif. 1982, Mayfield Publishing Co.

Sherrill, C.: Adapted physical education and recreation, ed. 3, Dubuque, Iowa, 1985, William C. Brown Co., Publishers.

Wolfensberger, W.: Principles of normalization, Toronto, 1972, National Institute on Mental Retardation.

CHAPTER 2

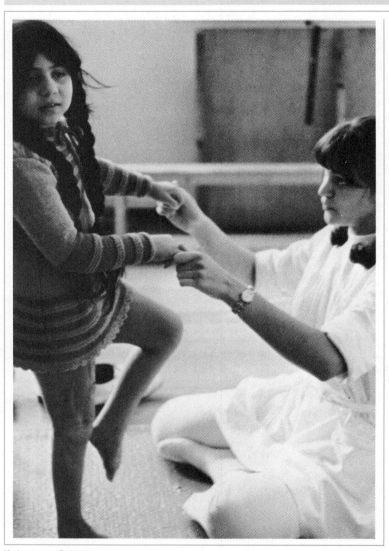

H. Armstrong Roberts

The Individualized Education Program

OBJECTIVES

◆ Understand the purpose of the individualized education program (IEP).

◆ Understand the construction of goals and objectives of the IEP.

◆ Understand the appropriate use of objectives through implementation of task analysis and programmed instruction.

◆ Understand the relationship of an instructional plan to the IEP.

The individualized education program (IEP) required by P.L. 94-142 represents the culmination of a long-standing position in American education. Proponents of individualization of instruction have included designers of computer-assisted instruction and those interested in mastery learning and applied behavioral analysis. The heterogeneous characteristics of handicapped children made individualization of instruction a necessity. While early efforts consisted of individualizing services on the basis of categorical labels, the focus has moved to designing instruction for each child regardless of handicap or categorical designation.

Professionals at various levels of administrative authority may perceive the purpose of the IEP differently. It may be viewed as (1) a set of statements guiding instructional strategies, (2) an educational strategy for which resources must be committed, or (3) a legal document indicating a school's (district's) commitment to handicapped children. This chapter provides physical educators with an understanding necessary to imple-ment IEPs from the perspective of day-to-day class activities.

VALUE OF THE IEPs

IEPs are useful to handicapped students, parents, teachers, and society in the following ways:

Handicapped students: IEPs are personal and fair. The handicapped student is not entirely like others nor entirely different. The IEP acknowledges special needs and confirms that no part of the physical education will be neglected.

Parents: It ensures the parents a voice in planning services and instructional content.

Society: The IEP is a useful document to ensure to the greatest extent possible that education contributes to the self-sufficiency of the student and hence less dependency on societal resources.

Teachers: It provides accessible and current data; it is a tool that links supportive expertise. The IEP is the basis for day-to-day lesson planning.[3] It keeps student and teacher on target because the predicted outcome is in clear view to both. The IEP also promises support for redesigning the instructional plan.

CONTENT OF THE IEP

Public policy requires that several components be included in the IEP: (1) annual goals, (2) short-term instructional objectives, (3) present levels of educational performance, (4) specific educational services to be provided, (5) extent to which each child will be able to participate in regular physical education programs, (6) projected date for initiation and anticipated duration of such services, and (7) criteria and evaluation procedures for determining whether instructional objectives are being achieved.

The IEP process ideally should be divided into two stages: (1) the development of a total service plan and (2) the development of the individualized instructional program. The total service plan is the end product of the IEP committee's work, and the individualized instructional program includes those instructional tasks taught by the teacher.

Process of the Individualized Instructional Program

The product of the process of the individualized instructional program is objective data, which focus on the learning of motor and physical skills. The three interrelated components of the process of the individualized instructional program are the goals, present levels of educational performance, and short-term instructional objectives. Goals are measurable, observable, broad instructional tasks that are achieved over time. It is essential that they are well defined so that they can be broken down and converted into observable and measurable short-term instructional objectives, which are the intermediate steps to goal acquisition. The present levels of educational performance define the existing limits of performance at a given point in time on which the short-term objectives are developed.

Fig. 2-1 shows the relationship of goals, objectives, and present levels of educational performance as they interface with sequential learning tasks on an instructional time frame.

It must be pointed out that if no specific goals are formulated, then the rest of the program fails. No short-term objectives can be developed and

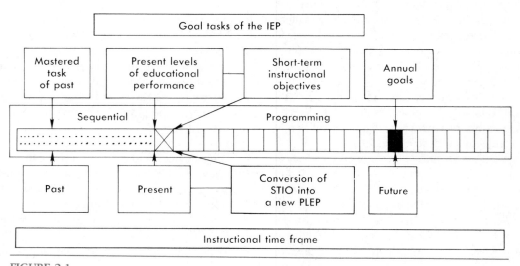

FIGURE 2-1
A description of the instructional components of the IEP.

no sequence of learning that can be measured is on a continuum toward goals, and consequently no determination of present levels of educational performance results. If the small steps (short-term instructional objectives leading to the goal) are too large or are improperly sequenced, then the experiences will be a punishing failure.[5] If the steps can already be demonstrated by the student, there can be no learning. Children do not need to relearn things they already can do. Thus the programmed instruction task analysis of the behaviors to be taught provides the structure and opportunity for application of the individualized instructional process.

Goals of the IEP

Characteristics of goals. Goals are statements that describe what a handicapped child should be able to accomplish over a specified time. There should be a direct relationship between the goal, the present level of educational performance (written in measurable objective terms), and the short-term instructional objectives. An-

nual goals should be reviewed any time during the year as the need indicates.[3] Examples of appropriate and inappropriate goals are listed in Table 2-1. There are arguments as to how precise goals need be. The more specific the goals, however, the easier it is to judge the effectiveness of the program. Martin[5] makes the following comments about the characteristics of quality goals:

1. There must *be* goals. — Actions not related to any goal cannot be judged as either worthwhile or pointless.

2. They must be concrete. — They must be actual and realizable.

3. They must be visible. — There must be no dispute about whether they are being obtained.

4. They must be objectively stated. — Administrators, students, and parents all can use the same language and agree on results and subsequently decisions made as to whether the goal was achieved.

5. Each goal can be divided into a sequence of tasks. — Without subtasks there can be no measure of progress. Evaluation would have to wait until the terminal goal was reached, with no feedback provided.

6. There must be a measure for successful completion of the task. — No comparisons can be made to measure progress of change.

7. The goal must bear a reasonable relationship as to why the person is in special education. — Either the persons are aquiring skills to return to normative levels in regular class, or they are being prepared for self-sufficient living in specific natural environments.

8. Goals should be individualized. — Grouping must come after a goal has been postulated, not before.

TABLE 2-1
Acceptable and unacceptable goals and objectives through evaluation of appropriate criteria and conditions

Action	Condition	Criterion
Acceptable objectives		
Run	1 mile	In 5 minutes 30 seconds
Walk	A balance beam 4 inches wide, heel to toe, eyes closed, and hands on hips	For 8 feet
Swim	Using the American crawl in a 25-yard pool for 50 yards	In 35 seconds
Unacceptable objectives		
Run		As fast as you can
Walk	On a balance beam	Without falling off
Swim		The length of the pool

There are two aspects of learning motor tasks that can be incorporated into an IEP. One is the acquisition of correct execution of form of the skill, and the other is improved performance of the skill. Task analysis is used to express goals, objectives, and present levels of educational performance in the acquisition of the form of a skill. The box below shows a task analysis of running a mile, which was designed for the Special Olympics curriculum. All prerequisite behavioral components of the form and strategy are marked with an *X*. These behaviors are within the repertoire of the learner. This constitutes the present level of educational performance. All unmastered components of the task analysis of acquisition of form are short-term instructional objectives. Achievement of all of the unmastered objectives constitutes acquisition of the goal. This is the sum total of all form components and strategies necessary to run a mile. Improved performance would require that the learner better his time for running a mile. This requires measurable ongoing performance of student participation in the mile run.

Goals	Present Level of Performance	Objectives
Run the mile in 8 minutes	8 minutes and 30 seconds	8:25, 8:20, 8:15, 8:10, 8:05

Shaping is used to communicate the instructional process of the IEP. The best performance to date might be 8 minutes and 30 seconds (present level of performance). The goal might be 8 minutes, and the short-term institutional objectives are times between 8 minutes and 8 minutes and 30 seconds. The setup on the left indicates the relationship of the components of the instructional process of the IEP.

Decisions for goal selection. A child, by public policy, must demonstrate an adverse performance on physical education tasks before that child is considered handicapped in physical education. Once adverse performance in physical education is determined, a decision should be made as to whether the purpose of the special physical education is to facilitate development of skills for unrestricted participation and normative functioning, or whether it serves to plan for specific education and training for independence in specific community environments. All handicapped children, including the moderately and severely handicapped, need to be trained for self-

---

COGNITIVE ACQUISITION OF SOUND RUNNING STRATEGY WHILE PARTICIPATING IN THE 1-MILE DISTANCE EVENT (SPECIAL OLYMPICS RULES): TASK ANALYSIS

X   1. Assume a crouched starting position.
X   2. Move on the command to start.
X   3. Demonstrate a steady running pace if more than four paces from the runner ahead.
      4. Stay close to the inside of the track.
X   5. Run to the right of the runner ahead to pass.
      6. Increase arm action to lengthen the stride while passing.
X   7. Listen for approaching runners and take longer strides to increase the distance from them.
      8. Gradually accelerate during the final lap and try to sprint the last 100 meters.

   X = Behaviors mastered and present level of performance. All behaviors unmarked are short-term objectives. Acquisition of all of the behaviors represents attainment of a goal.

   A modification of the Special Olympics Track and Field Sports Skills Instructional Program provides a data base for measuring acquisition of running strategies while participating in the mile distance event. Data to indicate present levels of performance, goals, and objectives require a record of specific components mastered. When all short-term objectives are satisfied, the goal of sound running strategy will be achieved.

The Joseph P. Kennedy, Jr. Foundation; accredited by Special Olympics, Inc. for the Benefit of Mentally Retarded Citizens.

sufficiency. Two proposed approaches for achieving this end are the developmental model and the community-based ecological (task-specific) model described by Brown and associates.[2]

Developmental Model	Community-Based Ecological Model
1. Goals are selected from developmental sequences or longitudinal sequences.	1. Goals are selected from tasks of adult life and broken down to present level.
2. Each step in the developmental sequence is prerequisite to the next.	2. Teach what is necessary, not what is next.
3. The developmental level of the child determines the next goals (the concept of readiness).	3. The next environment the individual functions in will indicate the goals.
4. Simple behaviors can be elaborated into more complex forms.	4. Design functional alternatives to participation in normal activities.
5. Goals portray the characteristics of those of a young age.[7]	

Value judgments assume critical importance in the selection of possible physical education goals for the IEP. Goals that are achieved should enhance performance and participation for independence in daily living. Curricula designed for universal audiences may serve higher functioning children, but not the severely handicapped. With these students, local referenced goals that are functional in the student's own community should be targets of instruction.

Brown and co-workers[2] advocate an analysis of each individual's various environments to inventory skills necessary for successful participation. The skills physical educators should focus on are community recreational activity and the motor skills needed for independent living. The environments where these skills can be used are at school, in the home, and in the community. The goals of the IEP should reflect the activities of nonhandicapped peers. The identification of these goals can be accomplished in a number of ways:

- Direct observation of peers and adults without handicaps.
- Expert interviews with persons knowledgeable about the community.
- Determine the important activities of peers who live independently.
- Logical analysis of needs.
- Studies of handicapped persons well adjusted in the community.

The individualization of goals implies that two broad sets of decisions have been made independently for each pupil. The individualization of the goal affects, in essence, both the content and sequential rate at which instruction is presented. The scheduled instruction is a function of the student progress. Individualization is not synonymous with personal attention but rather denotes student by student selection of goals and flexibility in how they are taught.

Short-Term Instructional Objectives

Short-term instructional objectives are "measurable intermediate steps between present levels of educational performance and the annual goals."[10] Because the present levels of performance are observable and measurable and all components of the IEP instructional process are related, the goals and objectives also should be observable and measurable. They are "the cornerstone of the individual education program."[8]

Objectives occur at different levels of curricular development and must be appropriate for the ability level of a specifically diagnosed individual. They require an assessment of the learner's capabilities. In the event that mastery of a specific behavior is not possible, the question is asked: What prerequisites are needed for this individual to achieve mastery of this task? This question, once answered, is restated until the student's present level of performance is determined and the appropriate instructional objective is determined. A sequence of prerequisite activities thus provides a chain of instructional events that leads the learner from lower to higher levels of mastery within the instructional content. The use of this instructional process requires that detailed records be kept on each learner so that the responsible personnel can determine the student's position in a learning activity sequence. The mastery of one objective is the prerequisite that gives rise to a more complex objective, making development progressive.

In the shaping process that uses programmed instruction to formulate objectives, hierarchies enable measurement of learner progress. A hierarchy is a continuum of ordered activities in which a task of lesser difficulty is prerequisite to acquisition of a task of greater difficulty. Progress from one task to another in a hierarchy serves as a measure of student development and answers three vital, educationally relevant questions: (1) What is the student's present level of educational performance? (2) What short-term instructional objectives should be provided to extend the present level of educational performance for development? (3) How much development has already occurred? Task analysis is a valuable tool for the development of instructional hierarchies.

The instructional objective must incorporate four concepts: (1) it must possess an action; (2) it must establish conditions under which actions occur; (3) it must establish a criterion for mastery of a specific task; and (4) it must lie outside the child's present level of educational performance.

Present Levels of Educational Performance

Present levels of educational performance can be determined through testing, by completing a task analysis and observing what components the student can do, or by determining where on a hierarchy a student is performing. Until the present levels of performance are determined, decisions about what activities a student should participate in cannot be made. Present levels of performance provide the foundation for a unique instructional plan and indicate to all concerned (including parents and child) that this program is truly individually designed.[3] Some argue that the present level of performance is the demonstrated functioning level on a series of tasks that lead to a goal. Others argue for areas selected for the program being "described in relation to the student's total school functioning."[6] These authors agree with the first premise. Decisions about specific ways to determine present levels of educational performance are found in Chapters 4 and 6.

Specific Educational Services to be Rendered

In the broadest sense the specific educational services to be rendered means what professional services (for example, remedial reading, speech therapy) will be made available to the student. In a stricter sense specific educational services has been interpreted to mean what activities (such as aerobic activities, weight-lifting) the student will engage in. This latter example relates directly to the instructional plan that will be used to achieve the goals and objectives included on the IEP. Every activity selected should contribute toward reaching specific objectives.

There are at least two phases of the learning process that can be incorporated into the IEP. One is the skill acquisition phase, and the other is the performance phase. Skill acquisition involves learning the techniques of executing the skill. Performance is concerned with how high one can jump, how fast one can run, or how far one can throw. For a student in the skill acquisition stage, activities that relate directly to learning the actual skill are chosen. If the student has learned the skill but needs to improve performance, then activities that lead to achieving that goal are selected.

The box on pp. 31 and 32 is an example of a task-specific instructional plan that includes both skill acquisition and performance objectives as well as the sequence of activities that should be used to achieve those objectives. Several activities that can be used to reach specific goals are enumerated in Chapter 6.

Related Services

Related services help the handicapped child to benefit from the IEP. If there are goals on the IEP that the physical educator cannot fulfill, related

GOALS, SHORT-TERM OBJECTIVES, AND PRESENT LEVELS OF EDUCATION PERFORMANCE OF AN INDIVIDUALIZED PHYSICAL EDUCATION PROGRAM

Goals, Sports Skills, and Team Games	Present Levels of Performance	Short-Term Objectives
Perform the track and field skills of the Special Olympics (SSIP)	Relay exchange, sprinting, and high jump	Throw and distance running*
Perform the soccer skills of the Special Olympics (SSIP)	Soccer kick and trap	Soccer pass and dribble*
Perform the basketball skills of the Special Olympics (SSIP)	Pass and dribble	Shooting and guarding*
Perform the volleyball skills of the Special Olympics (SSIP)	Set and bump	Spike and serve*
Perform and gymnastic skills of the Special Olympics (SSIP Task Analysis)	Forward roll and side roll	Headstand and backward roll*
Physical and Motor Fitness		
Run a mile in 8 minutes	8 minutes and 45 seconds	8:40, 8:35, 8:30, 8:25, 8:20, 8:15, 8:10, 8:05
Perform a military press with 70 pounds, 10 repetitions	60 pounds, 7 repetitions	60 pounds/10 repetitions, 65 pounds/10 repetitions
Perform 30 bent-knee sit-ups	18 bent-knee sit-ups	20 repetitions, 22 repetitions, 25 repetitions, 27 repetitions, 29 repetitions
Balance on a 3/4-inch stick for 10 seconds	1-inch stick for 5 seconds	10 feet on a 1-inch stick, 5 feet on a 3/4-inch stick
With the knees straight, bend forward and touch the tips of the fingers to the floor	5 inches from the floor	4 inches, 3 inches, 2 inches, 1 inch
Perform a vertical jump to 7 inches	A height of 4 inches	to 5 inches, 6 inches
Fundamental Motor Pattern		
Skip 30 feet in 15 seconds	20 seconds	19 feet, 18 feet, 17 feet, 16 feet
Run 60 feet in 5 seconds	50 feet	
Fundamental Motor Skills		
Throw a 4-inch ball so it hits a 12 × 12 inch target from a distance of 20 feet	From a distance of 7 feet	8, 9, 10, 11, 12, 13, 14, 15, 16, 17, 18, 19, 20
Bounce an 8-inch ball and travel a distance of 30 feet in 6 seconds	23 feet with an 8-inch ball	24, 25, 26, 27, 28, 29, 30
Kick an 8-inch ball into a 6 × 2 foot target from a distance of 20 feet five times in a row	From 10 feet into a 6 × 2 foot target	11, 12, 13, 14, 15, 16, 17, 18

*Indicates a need for further specification of objectives from Special Olympics (SSIP) curricula.

Continued.

INSTRUCTIONAL PLAN THAT COMES FROM THE IEP*

Acquisition Objectives: Throw	Acquisition Objectives: Mile Strategies
Throws ball straight.*	Assumes crouched starting position.*
Throws ball behind restraining line.*	Moves on command to start.*
Throws ball at 45° trajectory.	Steady running pace.*
Throws ball with cross-lateral pattern.	Stays close to inside of track.
Uses stutter-step approach.*	Runs to right of runner to pass.*
	Increases arm action and stride to pass.
	Listens for approaching runners, takes longer strides.*
	Accelerates and sprints during last 100 meters.

*Mastered short-term instructional objectives or present levels; unmarked behaviors are instructional objectives for the instructional plan. Based on the Special Olympics (SSIP).

PERFORMANCE OBJECTIVES

Action	Conditions	Criteria*
Run a mile	With attained strategies	~~8:40~~, ~~8:35~~, ~~8:30~~, ~~8:25~~, 8:20, 8:15, 8:10, 8:05, 8:00
Throw a ball	4 inches into a 12 × 12 inch target with attained form	~~8'~~, ~~9'~~, ~~10'~~, ~~11'~~, ~~12'~~, 13', 14', 15', 16', 17', 18', 19', 20' five out of five times
Sit-ups	Knees bent	~~19~~, ~~20~~, ~~21~~, ~~22~~, ~~23~~, ~~24~~, 25, 26, 27, 28, 29, 30 (repetitions)
Bounce a ball	8 inches while traveling	~~23~~, ~~24~~, ~~25~~, ~~26~~, 27, 28, 29, 30 (feet)
Balance	On a 1 inch stick	~~5~~, ~~6~~, ~~7~~, 8, 9, 10 (seconds)

*Mastered short-term objectives or present levels; the next unmarked number is the target objective of the instructional plan.

services (occupational and physical therapy) may be called on for assistance. These services should focus on offsetting or reducing the problems resulting from the child's handicap that interfere with learning and physical education performance in school.[8] For instance, for a handicapped child with a recurring hip dislocation that prevents participation in physical education, the physical therapist might treat the condition until a transfer of programming to the physical educator is feasible. Or for a child who lacks some equilibrium reflexes, the physical educator might contact either an occupational or physical therapist for help in selecting appropriate activities to facilitate development of those reflexes. The length of time that is required for the related service to produce the result should be specified. Duration limitations gauge the effectiveness of the service.

Participation in Regular Physical Education

The individual education program for each handicapped child must include a statement of "the extent to which the child will be able to participate in regular (physical) education programs."[8] One

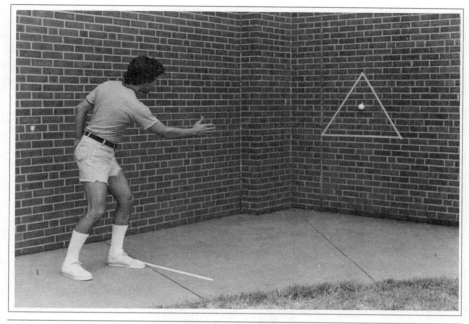

FIGURE 2-2
This person is a measured distance from a target of measured size. Structure can be provided to the activity so the task is individualized to the ability level of the performer. Both skill and performance levels can be measured.

way of meeting this requirement is to indicate the percent of time the child will be spending in the regular education program with nonhandicapped students. Another way is to list the specific regular (physical) education classes the child will be attending.[8]

The Role of the Physical Education Teacher

The regular physical education teacher has new responsibilities for the conduction of IEPs for handicapped pupils:

Whenever a handicapped child is placed in a regular classroom, the responsibility of the regular educator for that child is the same as for any other child in the classroom. Because all children differ with respect to amount of learning, rate of learning, and learning style, modifications in methodology, curriculum, or environment are often necessary for both nonhandicapped and handicapped children. Special education, which involves significant modifications in methodology, curriculum, or environment may also be delivered to some handicapped children in regular classrooms. Whenever this arrangement is specified in the child's IEP, the development of such specially designed instruction is the responsibility of special educators. Regular educators are responsible for assisting the child in carrying out the program. Overall classroom management also continues to be the responsibility of the regular teacher.[1]

Regular educators have any or all of the following duties with respect to handicapped children[1]:

1. Identification of possible handicapping conditions
2. Referrals of children for evaluation and placement
3. Data-gathering
4. Assisting handicapped children with special equipment
5. Participation in developing IEPs
6. Sharing information with parents
7. Integrating handicapped children and nonhandicapped children in the school environment.

Handicapped children are to receive an individual physical education program to meet their

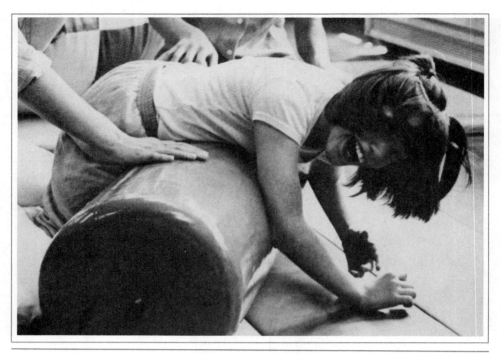

FIGURE 2-3
A child receives related services in which a protector-extensor thrust is facilitated by an occupational therapist.
(Courtesy The Children's Rehabilitation Center, Butler, Pa.)

unique physical education needs. The program includes annual goals, present levels of educational performance, and short-term instructional objectives. Furthermore, there should be a full preevaluation of their physical education needs. The unique physical education needs of handicapped children are determined by identifying discrepancies between existing levels of performance and minimum standards on physical education tasks set by local school districts. Therefore the *physical educator* determines what will be on the IEP by assessing children on tasks from the regular curriculum. Once a task deficiency is noted, goals are set for remediation of the deficiency, present levels are determined, and short-term objectives are postulated. The physical educator is the *only* person who knows the curriculum tasks to carry out this mission and should be the primary author of the short-term objectives of

an individual physical education program. The physical educator knows how each child functions on curriculum tasks implemented in their class.

When a child is placed in special physical education, it should be determined why he or she is there. If participation in a special physical education program can remediate the adverse physical education performance and get the child back in a regular unrestricted class, that is the reason for placement. If it is judged that the child will not acquire skills to enable return to the regular physical education class, specific goals that relate directly to independent functioning in natural community environments should be incorporated into the individual physical education program. Provisions should be made to generalize motor skills attained through instruction to domestic and community recreational settings.

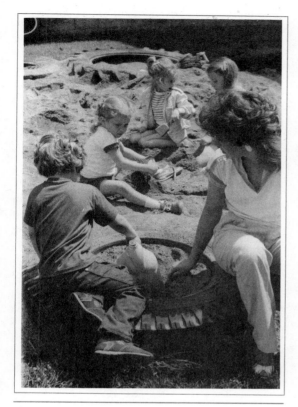

FIGURE 2-4
Children at play in an integrated setting.

Projection Dates for Initiating IEPs and Reaching Goals

All IEPs must include a date when services should begin and an anticipated date when goals will be reached. Whenever possible, delays in beginning a program should be avoided. The sooner the handicapped student can begin to receive program services, the greater the progress that can be expected. Well-coordinated programs move students in and out of class assignments with minimal disruptions. Established policies and procedures should facilitate appropriate placement within a short period after needs have been identified and the IEP is written and approved.

Perhaps the most difficult task when writing an IEP is determining when each student will reach his or her specific goals. Every person is unique. Learning pace, motivation level, present performance level, and severity of the handicapping condition all affect performance progress. Often it is not until the physical educator has worked with a student that it becomes possible to estimate how much progress to expect. The law does not mandate that goals be reached within the specified time, but that progress toward those goals be demonstrated. The alert physical educator will monitor progress closely and modify the instructional plan when it becomes evident that objectives are not being reached.

Evaluation of the IEP

Evaluation is an important aspect of the IEP process. The level of success or failure of learner progress may hinge on evaluation procedures and decisions based on information from the IEP. Well-designed and well-implemented evaluation systems are important for successful IEPs. If there is no evaluation component, necessary modifications to prior IEPs will not be made and new, more appropriate, goals will not be implemented. The student will not receive full potential benefits.

Independent of legal issues, data suggest that IEPs fulfilling the conditions delineated in the regulations are judged to be more useful programmatically than are incomplete IEPs.[4] The Department of Education[8] regulations are a workable model to increase the effectiveness of improving student learning. The requirements for concrete goals and sequenced tasks to which there can be feedback regarding progress provide the essential framework for an efficient delivery system.

The IEP requirements represent minimum components of a truly individualizing and functional education program. Performance criteria and methodology are IEP components that were deleted from initial regulations. The completed IEP becomes the standard for evaluating the effectiveness of educational efforts during the implementation period.

SOME PROBLEMS WITH IMPLEMENTING IEPs

The potential for maximizing educational benefits for handicapped children through the IEP process is great. However there have been problems with IEP implementation. Specific problems and suggested solutions follow.

1. The regular physical educators fail to test students to identify those persons whose performance is adversely affected (criteria for determining the handicapping condition).[9]

   Local school districts should set minimum standards for physical education curriculum tasks.
   This has not been done. There is no basis for determining adverse educational performance. School districts or states need to design curricula with standards so that adverse educational performance can be determined. Furthermore, measurement for the most part is not an integral part of the physical education instructional delivery system. Measurement needs to be incorporated into the curriculum, data collected by teachers, and judgments made from the data as to which children are having problems.

2. School districts fail to include short-term instructional objectives before the child is placed in special physical education.[8]

   Short-term instructional objectives are behaviors taught by the teacher that relate to goals (physical education). Therefore teachers need to be involved in developing the goals. If they are not involved, they may not know how to structure the short-term instructional objectives that will support the goals.

3. School districts are writing IEPs with goals and objectives that bear little relation to the teacher's instructional plans.[8]

   Schools often do not write goals that can be broken down into behaviors that can be incorporated into instructional plans. Also, some teachers cannot make an instructional

plan and implement it so that it relates to the goals of the IEP. The problem can be partially solved by training personnel to write clearer goals and to make instructional plans that support the goals.

4. Educators fear they will be held accountable if the child fails to achieve the goals of the IEPs. The IEP is not a performance contract.[8]

   This problem requires education of teachers by supervisory personnel. A sound data base will indicate progress of children in physical education. Goals are calculated guesses of the degree to which learning takes place. They give instruction direction.

Thus the physical educator assesses handicapped children in the physical education curriculum. The physical educator develops an individual physical education program from the needs assessment, implements the IEP, and records data on the progress of objectives achieved and goals met. If a child does not progress in the physical education component of the IEP, related services may be secured to help the child benefit from the individual physical education program. Thus the physical educator must be an active participant in the development of the individual physical education program.

SUMMARY

The process of designing individual education programs in physical education for the handicapped is a basic component of effective programming. The nature of the program will depend on the intended outcomes for specific handicapped children. The goal for mildly handicapped children may be alleviating deficits so they may participate in regular class as a non-handicapped person. The purpose of the IEP for young, severely handicapped persons may be to promote developmental functioning; however, self-sufficiency in their community is the desired outcome for older individuals.

Appropriate IEPs necessitate ongoing assessment of the attainment of short-term objectives of the IEP, which takes place in both the IEP and the instructional daily plan of the teacher. IEPs for severely handicapped persons should focus on use of functional facilitations or adaptations so the children may participate in age-appropriate activities. IEPs for the severely handicapped should also emphasize goals and objectives that represent discrepancies between existing motor skills and those needed for self-sufficiency in the community. The IEP is a link between the student and the demands of his or her environment. The mildly handicapped should be prepared for environments where they have options similar to those of the nonhandicapped. The IEP for the severely handicapped student is a link between instruction and the demands of the community, and is an important element in the transition from school to adult independent life in specified environments.

REVIEW QUESTIONS

1. What are the components of the IEP that bear directly on teacher implementation?
2. Describe the interrelationships of goals, objectives, and present levels of performance in the documentation of a child's educational progress.
3. What tests are performed to determine whether a child is handicapped in physical education?
4. What are the characteristics of community-based goals for an IEP?
5. What is the difference between selecting goals for a developmental model and those for a community-based model?

STUDENT ACTIVITIES

1. Visit a parent of a handicapped child to determine what motor skills they would like developed through the IEP.
2. Interview a parent or teacher of a handicapped person or an administrator who has exercised due process rights because of an inappropriate IEP. Indicate the issues of the hearing.
3. Construct some goals of an IEP. Perform objectives that are relevant to those goals.
4. Make an instructional plan for a child to achieve the objectives of the IEP.
5. Task-analyze some motor skills to be taught so that each behavior is a short-term instructional objective of the total performance of the task.
6. Prepare a sequence of objectives that will indicate educational progress on the IEP.

7. Interview a parent who has attended an IEP conference. Describe the events of the meeting and perceptions of those involved.
8. Study the IEP. Identify types of assessment that were used to construct and implement the IEP.
9. Study the goals of a hypothetical or real IEP for constructional effectiveness. Indicate its strengths and weaknesses.
10. Make an IEP for a real or imaginary handicapped child.
11. Conduct the instructional process of the IEP and produce a data base from objectives mastered.

REFERENCES

1. Barresi, J., and Mack, J.: Responsibilities of regular classroom teachers for handicapped students. In ERIC fact sheet, Reston, Va., 1979, ERIC Clearinghouse on Handicapped and Gifted Children.
2. Brown, L., et al.: A strategy for developing chronological age appropriate and functional curricular content for severely handicapped adolescents and young adults, J. Spec. Educ. 13:81-90, 1979.
3. Fiscus, E.D., and Nandell, C.: Developing individual education programs, St. Paul, Minn., 1983, West Publishing Co.
4. Maher, C.: Training special service teams to develop IEPs, Except. Child. 47:206-211, 1980.
5. Martin, R.: Legal challenges to behavioral modification: trends in schools, corrections, and mental health, Champaign, Ill., 1979, Research Press.
6. Schmitt, I.: Procedures to guarantee an individual education program for each handicapped student, Bismarck, N.D., 1978, Department of Public Instruction.
7. Seaman, J., and Depauw, K.: The new adapted physical education, Palo Alto, Calif., 1982, Mayfield Publishing Co.
8. U.S. Department of Education: Assistance to states for education of handicapped children: interpretation of the individual education program, Fed. Reg. Jan. 19, 1981.
9. U.S. General Accounting Office: Report to Congress, Feb. 5, 1981.
10. Wilcox, B., and Bellamy, G.: Design of high school programs for severely handicapped students, Baltimore, 1982, Paul H. Brookes Publishing Co.

SUGGESTED READINGS

Fiscus, E.D., and Mandell, C.: Developing individual programs, St. Paul, Minn., 1983, West Publishing Co.
U.S. Department of Education: Assistance to states for education of handicapped children: interpretation of the individual education program, Fed. Reg. Jan. 19, 1981.
Wilcox, B., and Bellamy, G.: Design of high school programs for severely handicapped students, Baltimore, 1982, Paul H. Brookes Publishing Co.

CHAPTER 3

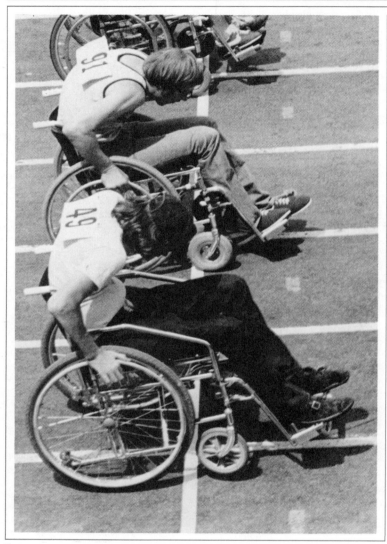

H. Armstrong Roberts

Developmental Versus Specific Adapted Physical Education

OBJECTIVES

♦ Know the difference between a general ability and a specific motor skill.

♦ Understand the purpose of making a functional adaptation to a specific skill.

♦ Understand the purpose of developing general abilities that are prerequisites to motor skills.

♦ Understand the difference in purpose between task analysis of functional skills for independence and development of general abilities.

♦ Understand appropriate application of developmental and task-specific approaches and their differences.

♦ Understand a classification system of sensory inputs and general and motor-specific abilities.

Sensory inputs and general abilities are prerequisites to performance of specific motor skills. Some sensory inputs are vestibular, kinesthetic, and tactile. Some general abilities are flexibility, strength, endurance, and hand-eye coordination. That these factors are prerequisites to specific skills has been validated through clinical practice and proposed in theories of how the individual grows and develops. Some have also been revealed through statistical factor analysis.

A continuing task of educational research is to categorize, through scientific measurement, prerequisites that are common to all individuals. Such research provides objective agreement among educators as to what general needs are. Then educators can maximize development of specific functional skills of the physical education curriculum.

Basic inputs, abilities, and the development of specific sport skills are interrelated. General abilities are constructed from sensory input signals. The quality of the input signal and the genetic makeup and readiness of the individual determine the integrity of the ability structure that results. That general ability structure affects a person's potential for performing specific skills because general abilities are prerequisite to specific skills. A well-developed broad base of ability prerequisites enables more efficient acquisition of and higher levels of performance in a variety of specfic motor skills. Therefore input information, general abilities, and efficient acquisition of specific skills are inseparable.

General abilities give rise to the acquisition of higher ordered specific motor skills in normal children. It is important to identify basic input

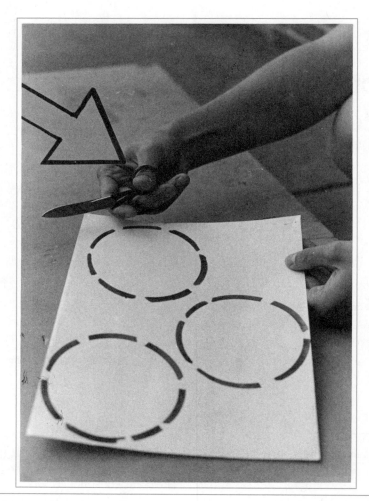

FIGURE 3-1
Kinesthetic and tactile inputs are required to use scissors as well as considerable hand-eye coordination for precise cutting.

functions and abilities of each handicapped child and help them acquire building blocks for specific lifetime leisure skills. It is essential that a viable structure of general abilities be developed on which essential motor skills for self-sufficiency can be built. Only through increased knowledge about the relationships between sensory inputs, general abilities, and specific functional motor skills required for independent living will educators arrive at appropriate instructional objectives to meet the unique motor needs of handicapped children.

Just as there are abilities that can be generalized to all children, each pupil possesses a special profile of abilities. This uniqueness demands specially designed instruction to meet the needs of each handicapped child.

Physical educators who teach handicapped individuals agree that their primary goal is to facilitate development of purposeful skills for each stu-

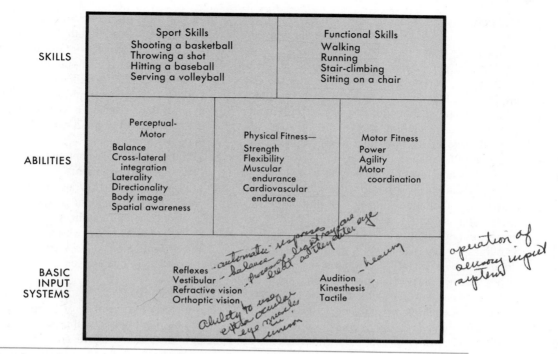

FIGURE 3-2
Levels of motor learning.

dent. There are, however, a variety of different approaches to programming from which physical educators can select. They range from general physical education activities believed to benefit all children, regardless of degree of function, to developmentally sequenced activities that serve as building blocks of motor development, to activities that enhance very specific skills.

Which approach a physical educator selects depends on the age of the students, the teacher's knowledge of motor development and ability to accurately assess and interpret motor performance levels, and the goals the teacher is attempting to achieve in the physical education program.

LEVELS OF FUNCTION

The ultimate goal of physical education for handicapped children is to equip them with motor skills that contribute to independent living. To plan these programs systematically, it is desirable to distinguish clearly the levels of function that contribute to acquisition of the many specific sport skills.

Each of three levels makes a unique contribution to independent functioning: (1) basic input functions, (2) general abilities, and (3) specific skills (Fig 3-2). The physical educator who understands the interrelatedness of these levels and can select intervention activities to facilitate functioning at any given level, depending on a student's needs, will realize success. Those who do not understand the interrelatedness of each level or who ignore the prerequisites will not be successful in helping students reach their full capabilities.

Basic input functions depend on the integrity and operation of the sensory input systems. These systems include primitive and equilibrium reflexes, the vestibular system, refractive and orthoptic vision, audition, and the tactile and kinesthetic systems. Before information can reach the central nervous system for processing, these systems must be intact and operational. The physical educator who automatically assumes these systems are functioning and that adequate stimulation is reaching the central nervous system disregards an important component of purposeful movement.

The second level of functioning is made up of abilities. Like basic input functions, these prerequisites enhance the acquisition of skill. If the sensory input systems are functioning, abilities develop concurrently with movement experiences. Abilities prerequisite to skills include the perceptual-motor, physical, and cognitive categories. They are not as readily forgotten and are maintained longer than are skills. Examples of perceptual-motor abilities are balance, cross-lateral integration, laterality, directionality, body image, and spatial awareness. Physical fitness prerequisites are strength, flexibility, muscular endurance, and cardiovascular endurance. Motor fitness requires agility and motor coordination.

The uppermost level of functioning is skill. Skills are motor behaviors that are either specific to a sport or specific to functional living. Examples of skills are shooting a basketball, serving a tennis ball, climbing stairs, and sitting down in a chair. Proficiency at skills is usually developed through repetitious practice of the skill itself. Many activities associated with individual and team sports that require practice are skills. However, skills can also be nonspecific general tasks, such as walking or running, that are practiced through repetition to the point that proficiency is achieved.

FACILITATING SKILL DEVELOPMENT

Handicapped children often have difficulty learning chronologically age-appropriate skills for sports and games. When deficits in skills become apparent, curriculum decisions and instructional strategies must be made. Both single and combination strategies can be employed:

♦ Provide no specific intervention to alleviate the problem and hope that children will "grow out" of the deficit.
♦ Provide a general physical education program that is believed to benefit all children and hope the handicapped students will benefit from it.
♦ Make functional adaptations that enable immediate participation.
♦ Teach the prerequisites specific to the skill and make functional adaptations while the student is learning the specific skill.
♦ Test to determine which prerequisites are deficient; then select activities to facilitate function in those areas.

No Intervention

Fortunately, the number of people who believe children, if left alone, will grow out of motor deficits is decreasing. However, that position is still voiced by some. Observation of the number of adults, both normal and handicapped, who demonstrate lack of motor skills should be enough to silence the advocates of "no intervention needed." Longitudinal studies of children with delayed motor development are extremely scarce. In a 1980 study Vinzant[2] followed-up on children who had been tested in the University of Kansas Perceptual-Motor Clinic and were found to have sensory input and general ability deficits. However, because of uncontrollable circumstances (such as living too far from the clinic to bring children for intervention, no available transportation, lack of interest), the children did not receive an intervention program specific to their needs. Eight children who had been tested 1 to 2 years earlier were located and retested using the original battery of tests. In every case the children demonstrated the same deficits (except in the reflex area) that had been identified during the original testing sessions. It can be concluded that waiting for a child to grow out of motor delays may indeed be a very long wait.

General Physical Education Program Intervention

There are physical educators who believe that the only stimulus children need to develop motor skills is a variety of interesting activities to keep them moving. The failure of these programs to promote motor development is documented in the studies that report improvement in self-concept but no motor ability gain. Self-concept is important, but if the goal of the program is improved motor skill, it would appear that a different intervention strategy is needed in these cases.

Functional Adaptations

Functional adaptations are modifications such as using an assistive device, changing the demands of the task, or changing the rules to permit students with handicapping conditions to participate. Making functional adaptations in accord with a handicapped child's needs may enable immediate participation in age-appropriate activities selected to enhance specific skills. Following is a list of functional adaptations for children with a deficit:

- Blind children can receive auditory or tactual clues to help them locate objects or position their bodies in the activity area.
- The blind read through touch and can be instructed in appropriate movement patterns through manual kinesthetic guidance (that is, the instructor manually moves the student through the correct pattern) or verbal instructions.
- Deaf children can learn to read lips or learn signing so that they understand the instructions for an activity.
- Physically handicapped children may have to use crutches to enable them to move.
- An asthmatic child may be permitted to play goalie in a soccer game, which requires smaller cardiovascular demands than the running positions.
- Rules may be simplified to accommodate the retarded child's limited comprehension level but still permit participation in a vigorous activity.

In these examples functional adaptations are necessary for the handicapped student to participate in chronologically age-appropriate physical education activities. The approach is useful when the only motor prerequisites lacking are those which are a result of the student's disabling condition or mainstreaming the student to promote social interaction is being done in addition to the adapted physical education program.

Task-Specific: Top, Down

Teaching the skill directly is known as the task-specific approach. Advocates of this approach believe handicapped individuals should be taught functional skills necessary for ultimately independent function in natural environments. This point of view also specifies skill development for specific environments and requires generalization and adaptation to a variety of environments.

The task-specific approach is a "top, down" strategy. When using this approach to assess the students' repertoires, the educator can determine which motor skills are present and which are yet to be taught. Once the skills to be taught are determined, they are prioritized, task analyses of the specific skills to be taught are completed, each skill is evaluated to determine which component parts are missing, and the specific missing components are taught using the direct teaching method. If inefficient movements are found, the teacher investigates the ability components for deficits. If problems are found at the ability level, specific sensory input systems believed to contribute to the deficits at the ability level are tested. When deficiencies are found, activities are selected to promote development at the lowest level first.

The task-specific approach may be the most realistic and expedient type to use with severely handicapped individuals, but it may be inappropriate for higher functioning handicapped children. The essential question to ask when trying to decide whether to use this approach is: "How much time is available?" Facilitating basic input systems and abilities prior to teaching specific skills takes time, perhaps years. Also, there is evidence that children under the age of 12 years respond more readily than do older individuals. When the handicapped individual is older and severely involved and there is a limited amount of time available to develop functional skills needed to live in a natural environment, the task-specific approach may be the best intervention strategy.

Developmental Approach: Bottom, Up

younger child

Motor development is a progressive process. For each of us to learn to move efficiently, we must first be able to take environmental information into the central nervous system. Then it must be processed or integrated so that it can be used to direct movement patterns and skills. Only after the information is received and processed can the brain direct the muscles to work. If anything goes wrong before the information reaches the muscles, movement is inefficient or nonexistent. Advocates of the developmental approach believe that before selecting activities for a child who is deficient in motor skills, one must test to determine which prerequisites are lacking. Only then can the developmentalist make curriculum and intervention decisions.

The developmental approach can be considered a "bottom, up" strategy (Fig. 3-2). That is, some developmentalists will begin by evaluating each of the sensory input systems and then testing the ability components to determine which deficits are in evidence. Once the deficits are identified, activities that promote functioning of each sensory input system found to be lacking are selected. The rationale is to progress to activities that facilitate development of the ability components. Only after each of these building blocks is in place will the developmentalist attempt to teach the specific sport or functional skills.

McLaughlin[1] documented the value of the approach when she followed-up on learning-disabled children who had received this type of evaluation and intervention at the University of Kansas Perceptual-Motor Clinic. Prior to intervention the children demonstrated varied sensory input and ability deficits. One to 2 years after the

deficits had been eliminated and the children released from the clinic program, every child was demonstrating age-appropriate motor skills.

It should be apparent that the developmental approach is not only time consuming, but also requires extensive knowledge of sensory input systems's function and ability level developmental trends. Fortunately for individuals lacking the knowledge base, some available models suggest both testing techniques and intervention strategies for the teacher. Those models are discussed in detail in Chapter 6.

When attempting to determine whether to use a "bottom, up" approach in the adapted physical education program, the teacher must again ask; "How much time is available?" The younger the child and the more time available to the teacher, the more appropriate it is to use this strategy.

Combining Approaches

Note that when using either top, down task-specific or bottom, up developmental approaches considerable individual attention to each child is necessary. That is, for those approaches to be effective, the teacher must work with small groups of children with similar problems or on a one-to-one basis. Children involved in such intensive learning environments often do not have an opportunity to interact with their peers in regular physical education classes. Separating the handicapped children from their normal peers fosters the labeling of children as "different" and inhibits social interactions necessary for sound development. One way to overcome the perils of separation is to permit the handicapped child to engage in physical activity with peers in addition to receiving individual attention in an adapted physical education class.

This approach is workable if functional adaptations are made while the child is engaging in the regular physical education class. This combination of interventions will work if either an indirect method of teaching is used with a movement education or problem-solving program or when direct teaching methods are employed. During direct teaching the standard functional adaptations such as those enumerated earlier can be used. Regardless of whether the teacher selects an indirect or direct teaching method, it is important to remember that all children must experience success when interacting with their peers. Successful interaction with others is necessary for the development of a healthy, positive self-concept. As teachers we must be sensitive to promoting the overall growth of our students.

INCIDENTAL VERSUS PLANNED LEARNING

Most individuals learn from everyday interaction with the environment. This is particularly true if the environment is varied and the learner possesses all the prerequisites needed to convert en-

vironmental stimulation, (that is, fully functioning sensory input systems, certain ability traits, and possibly some skills). This is known as *incidental learning*. The more ready an individual is (that is, the more developed cognitive and motor functions are), the more that can be gained from interaction with the environment. Conversely, the fewer the number of developed prerequisites, the less a person gains from environmental exchanges.

The handicapped individual is often denied opportunities to interact with varied environments. This is a hindrance because for the central nervous system to develop normally, a wide variety of stimulation is necessary. Thus attempts to protect these children from interaction with the environment often delay their development. Be-

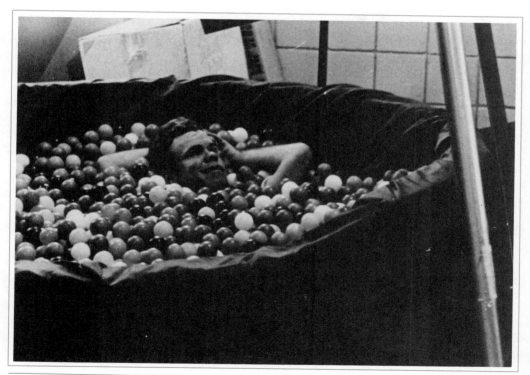

FIGURE 3-3
Handicapped person develops basic input functions of tactile perception.
(Courtesy Verland Foundation, Sewickley, Pa.)

cause of these delays, handicapped learners do not always gain as much from incidental learning as do their normal counterparts.

Teachers of handicapped children must be particularly sensitive to the needs of their students. Until a teacher determines the needs of students, appropriate intervention strategies cannot be planned. The adapted physical education teacher must ensure that each student's motor learning improves. The general approach of providing a wide variety of activities to all their students gives no assurance that motor learning will result. It is true that the children may have fun and could possibly gain some physical fitness from their activity; however, the students will not make the same gains as would be possible if carefully planned intervention strategies were used.

Inherent in the use of a task-specific (top, down) approach and a developmental (bottom, up) approach is assurance that motor performance will improve. Techniques for facilitating motor learning are described in Chapter 6.

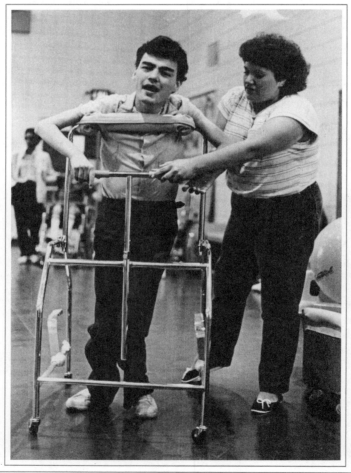

FIGURE 3-4
Children with severe physical handicaps are often denied opportunity for normal interaction in their environment and require programming.
(Courtesy Verland Foundation, Sewickley, Pa.)

SUMMARY

Maximizing performance on the many specific skills of the physical education curriculum is the unique role of the adapted physical educator. Handicapped individuals often possess limited motor skills. Thus the physical educator must determine which skills are needed and select appropriate intervention strategies to ensure that learning occurs. Teaching specific skills, fostering developmental sequences, and employing functional adaptations are three acceptable intervention strategies. Time available, age and readiness level of the learner, and capability of the adapted physical education teacher dictate which intervention strategy to use.

REVIEW QUESTIONS

1. What is the relationship between specific functional motor skills and general ability prerequisites to these skills?
2. What are some examples of making functional adaptations for age-appropriate motor skills, and what are arguments for and against such functional adaptations?
3. What are some of the general abilities of a physical-motor and perceptual-motor structure?
4. Describe functional levels of prerequisites to specific skills.
5. What are some strategies and options for teaching chronologically age-appropriate motor skills to handicapped children?
6. What are the differences between a "bottom, up" (developmental) and "top, down" (task-specific) approach?
7. What value is there to combining a bottom, up approach with a top, down approach?
8. Name two sensory input systems, two general abilities, and two specific skills.
9. What is meant by *incidental learning?* Why are some handicapped children unable to learn as much through incidental learning as children who have no handicapping conditions?

STUDENT ACTIVITIES

1. Talk with adapted physical education teachers about how they determine what objectives and activities to use with their handicapped students. Try to decide whether the teachers are using a "top, down," "bottom, up," or combination of these two approaches.
2. Observe a mainstreamed physical education class. Make a list of the functional adaptations used during the class. Select the two adaptations you believe aided the children most and tell why those adaptations were so helpful.
3. List the ways in which a top, down testing and teaching approach would differ from a bottom, up testing and teaching approach.

REFERENCES

1. McLaughlin, E.: Follow-up study on children remediated for perceptual-motor dysfunction at the University of Kansas perceptual-motor clinic, Eugene, 1980, University of Kansas.
2. Vinzant, D.: Follow-up study on children tested but not remediated for perceptual-motor dysfunction, Unpublished master's thesis, 1982, University of Kansas.

SUGGESTED READINGS

Brown, L., et al.: A strategy for developing chronological age appropriate and functional curricular content for severely handicapped adolescents and young adults, J. Spec. Educ. **13:**81-90, 1979.
Gold, M.: Task analysis: a statement and example using acquisition and production of a complex assembly task by the retarded blind, Urbana-Champaign, Ill., 1975, University of Illinois Institute for Child Behavior and Development.
Seaman, J.A., and DePauw, K.: The new adapted physical education, Palo Alto, Calif., 1982, Mayfield Publishing Co.
Snell, M.: Teaching the severely handicapped, Columbus, Ohio, 1982, Charles E. Merrill Publishing Co.
Wilcox, B., and Bellamy, G.T.: Design of high school programs for severely handicapped students, Baltimore, 1982, Paul H. Brookes Publishing Co.

CHAPTER 4

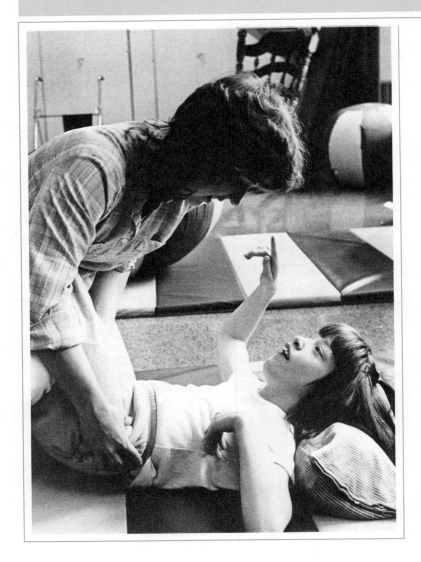

Types and Purposes
of Assessment

OBJECTIVES

♦ Know the different types of assessment.

♦ Know the different purposes of assessment.

♦ Provide examples of each of the different types of assessment.

♦ Know when to use the different types of assessment to achieve a specific outcome.

There has been a distinct shift during the 1970s and 1980s from using tests to classify, accept, or reject students to assessment tailored to meet the instructional needs of children. Traditionally, normative-referenced standardized tests have been used to determine how a child was performing in relation to other children of the same age and sex. Often such test results were used to predict the success a child might achieve in school. When test results were used in this manner, above average normative-referenced test performance levels tended to be perceived by teachers as desirable objectives in and of themselves. Unfortunately, this usage often distorted the true purpose of education, particularly the education of students with handicapping conditions.

The court decision in *Armstrong v. Kline* in 1979[1] emphasized that the educational aim for handicapped individuals is to provide instruction that helps them develop physical and motor skills that will contribute to self-sufficient and independent living. Thus adequate physical education assessment for the handicapped child requires use of test items that will assist in the design of appropriate educational environments and instructional procedures for the child. This latter perspective of assessment requires us to challenge traditional uses of testing and seek new and different ways of determining performance levels. As Haring[9] said, we must begin to think of assessment as measurement of individual performance at any time to determine status in cumulative skill or knowledge.

ASSESSMENT TOOLS

There are several forms of assessment. Each can contribute in some way to enhancing our selection of appropriate educational environments and instructional procedures for the handicapped individual. These include standardized normative-referenced tests, criterion-referenced tests, domain-referenced tests, content-referenced tests, community-based assessments, surveys and inventories, and treatment-referenced assessments. (See Chapter 6 for specific examples of each type of assessment.)

49

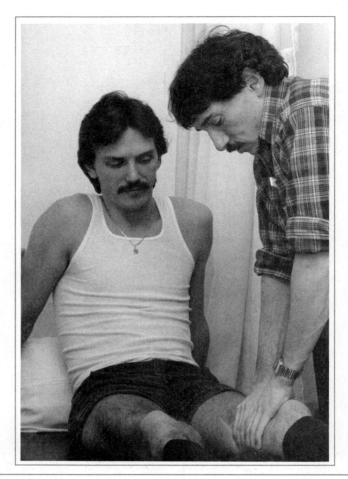

FIGURE 4-1
Assessment with manual muscle testing techniques.
(Courtesy H. Armstrong Roberts.)

Standardized Normative-Referenced Tests

Definition

Normative-referenced tests are administered under similar conditions (standardized) to a large number of people (sampling population). Most often the sampling population includes both sexes, who vary in age and performance levels but do not demonstrate any handicapping condi-

tion. The scores (norms) achieved by the sampling population are placed on a continuum from high to low and are classified according to percentiles, age equivalencies, and stanines. Scores of individuals who later use the test are compared with the norms to determine which percentile, age, or stanine level the scores match. (See Table 4-1.)

Normative - referenced

TABLE 4-1
Norms for the standing long jump in the AAHPERD physical fitness test

Percentile Rank	Test Scores (Meters)*			Percentile Rank
	11 Years	12 Years	13 Years	
100th	2.56	2.26	2.59	100th
95th	1.87	1.98	2.15	95th
90th	1.82	1.90	2.08	90th
85th	1.77	1.85	2.03	85th
80th	1.75	1.82	1.95	80th
75th	1.70	1.80	1.90	75th
70th	1.67	1.75	1.87	70th
65th	1.67	1.72	1.82	65th
60th	1.65	1.70	1.82	60th
55th	1.62	1.67	1.77	55th
50th	1.57	1.65	1.75	50th
45th	1.57	1.62	1.70	45th
40th	1.52	1.60	1.67	40th
35th	1.49	1.57	1.65	35th
30th	1.47	1.54	1.60	30th
25th	1.42	1.52	1.57	25th
20th	1.39	1.47	1.52	20th
15th	1.34	1.44	1.47	15th
10th	1.29	1.37	1.39	10th
5th	1.21	1.26	1.32	5th
0	0.91	0.96	0.99	0

From the American Alliance for Health, Physical Education, Recreation and Dance, Reston, Va.
*To convert to centimeters, move the decimal point two places to the right (1.95 m = 195 cm).

Purpose

The purpose of the normative-referenced test is to permit comparison of an individual's performance level with the performance of the sampling population. P.L. 94-142 requires that one criterion for determining whether an individual is handicapped is the administration of clinical tests by medical or psychological personnel. Most often a clinical handicap is interpreted to mean that the child performs below average on a standardized normative-referenced test; that is, his or her scores are found to fall significantly below the mean.

Comments

There is considerable discussion in the literature concerning the value and use of normative-refer-

enced assessment. The controversy focuses on the use made of the test results. When the test results are used to limit the educational opportunities available to students, protests appear justified; however, when the results can be used to facilitate appropriate placement and enhance program planning, information from normative-referenced tests is perceived more favorably.

Hively, Hofmeister, and Reichle are three educators who voice alarm at the misuse of normative-referenced testing. Hively accurately claims that "to a large extent, our contemporary educational culture has been dominated by the image of norm-referenced testing. Many of us are wearing norm-referenced blinders."[10] Hofmeister[11] feels that many teachers have identified the ethical and curriculum support problems of norm-referenced testing. According to him, potential problems of normative-referenced testing consist of the following:

- Evaluation procedures are often administered, controlled, and developed by personnel outside the school and classroom.
- When results of such evaluations are sent directly to superiors, there is some uneasiness about how the results will be used.
- The curriculum may be controlled by the test rather than by the needs of the children.

Reichle[15] expressed other concerns and limitations of standardized normative-referenced tests. Some of these follow:

- They do not address or directly examine behaviors in the instructional program.
- They do not recommend or reflect a scope and sequence of behaviors to be trained.
- There are limits in the translation of the results of the tests into instructional objectives.
- They limit options in formats for application of results to heterogeneous groups such as the handicapped.
- As a rule they do not relate to the critical skills in the learner's environment.

When normative test results are used to label students as competent (within average performance) or incompetent (below average performance) or are not tied to the curriculum taught, concerns about their use are justified. However, when these test results are used to enhance the quality of education planning for a student, their usefulness becomes more apparent.

Pyfer[14] proposed two benefits that can be derived from normative-referenced test results: (1) if a child's test results show the learner to be below average, the child must be provided with appropriate intervention; and (2) normative-referenced test results used in conjunction with criterion- and domain-referenced test results can provide an overall profile of a child's developmental level, which enables more accurate selection of an appropriate intervention strategy.

A common complaint voiced by physical educators working in the schools is that school administrators interpret P.L. 94-142 as a mainstreaming law for the subjects physical education, art, and music. That is to say, often an administrative decision is made that the least restrictive environment for students with handicapping conditions is placement into regular physical education, art, and music classes. In reality the need for special education (classroom and physical education) must be determined on the basis of standardized test results. Hence it can be justifiably argued that the child with an assessed clinical handicap who performs significantly below average on a standardized normative-referenced test does indeed qualify for some type of special physical education intervention. The type and extent of the intervention cannot be determined by the standardized normative-referenced test results. Additional testing would be required to pinpoint the extent of the learner's limitation and determine which type of intervention is appropriate.

The type of additional testing necessary depends primarily on the age and types of performance problems evidenced by the child. Young children who demonstrate balance problems need to be tested further to determine whether underlying deficiencies such as abnormal reflex development or delayed vestibular functioning are causing the balance problem. Children with poor catching and kicking skills need to be screened for depth perception function. Older children with cardiovascular endurance deficits need to be examined for cardiovascular abnormalities before an intervention program is developed. The standardized normative test results provide clues about what type of motor behavior the child is having difficulty with. Additional types of testing are useful in pinpointing more precisely the reason the child is performing poorly on the standardized normative-referenced test (Table 4-2).

Again, the use of normative-referenced standardized test results solely to label a child incompetent and not to improve the instructional program has little or no value in education. Such test results do have value when used to determine

TABLE 4-2

Normative data expressed in percentiles on perceptual items of a basic motor ability test for 7-year-old boys

Percentiles	Bead Stringing	Target Throwing			Marble Transfer		
		Right Hand	Left Hand	Total	Right Hand	Left Hand	Total
100	15	12	10	22	20	21	41
90	14	12	8	20	19	20	39
80	12	11	7	18	18	16	34
70	11	10	7	17	16	16	32
60	10	9	6	15	14	13	27
50	9	9	5	14	13	12	25
40	7	8	5	13	11	10	21
30	6	7	5	12	10	10	20
20	5	6	5	11	9	8	17
10	3	6	5	11	8	7	15

From Arnheim, D.D., and Sinclair, W.A.: The clumsy child, ed. 2, St. Louis, 1979, The C.V. Mosby Co.

whether a child has an assessed clinical handicap. Once it has been determined that a child qualifies for special physical education, tests that can be related to the curriculum taught in the physical education program should be selected. Federal regulations require adverse physical education performance to be present before a child qualifies for special intervention strategies to be used. The adverse performance can be eliminated if appropriate educational programming is implemented. The more severe the performance deficits, the greater the need for in-depth probing for the cause of the deficiencies. (See also Chapter 6.)

Criterion-Referenced Tests

Definition

Donlon[4] defines criterion-referenced testing in two ways. One is the classic concept derived from use in learning research. The criterion is an arbitrarily established level of mastery that represents an educational goal. The score simply indicates whether an individual has demonstrated performance above, at, or below the criterion level. How far away from the goal a person performed is not considered. Criterion-referenced tests also demonstrate the level of consistency of performance. Measure of consistency is often used when constructing instructional objectives, for example, to hit a target of specific size *three times in a row* or make *7 out of 10 foul shots.* When criterion testing is designed in this manner, it is usually tied to established levels of mastery in curriculum content.

Criterion-referenced assessment is useful for instructional purposes when it meets other conditions. Glaser[8] indicates that a criterion-referenced test is deliberately constructed to give scores that tell what kinds of behaviors individuals can demonstrate. This definition implies classes of behaviors that define different achievement levels and their important nuances. Nitko[13] says that the obtained score must be capable of expressing objectively and meaningfully the individual's performance characteristics in these classes of behavior.

The demands of a criterion-referenced test must be achievable in the context of an instructional program and the behaviors assessed must be teachable.[15] Following are examples of criterion-referenced statements:

1. Throw a 4-inch ball a distance of 20 feet so that it hits a 2 × 2-foot target five out of five times.

2. Perform a military press with a 70-pound weight for 10 repetitions.
3. Run a mile in 6 minutes and 15 seconds.
4. Swim a distance of 25 yards in 30 seconds.
5. Play 30 minutes of volleyball without a rule violation.

Purpose

Criterion-referenced tests are used to determine whether instructional content in the physical education class has been mastered. These tests are derived for the most part from arbitrary judgments concerning what each instructor or school district wants to teach or what students are to learn. Logic must be applied to match assessments with behavior that children are expected to display in natural environments. For instance, if one is teaching throwing so that a child can play softball, a logical criterion-referenced test might be to accurately throw a ball a distance equal to that between third and first base after fielding the ball.

Criterion-referenced assessment involves instructional items and the prerequisite skills contained within a curriculum. Well-structured criterion-referenced assessment should make it possible to generate individual prescriptions for each child that include prerequisite behaviors and subtasks stated in behavioral terms.

Comments

As mentioned before, criterion-referenced assessment should be constructed so that meeting the performance standard prepares individuals to perform in natural environments (that is, daily life settings in the community). With this type of assessment it is possible, and often desirable, for testing itself to take place in natural environments. For instance, if an instructor wants to determine whether a student knows how to bowl, the subtasks required to accomplish an effective bowling ball delivery are written out in proper sequence, and the student's performance is observed while he executes delivery on a bowling lane.

Criterion test items may be selected through the process of logical thought or derived from normative-referenced tests. As was mentioned earlier, when normative-referenced tests are used for this purpose, there must be a cutoff standard below which the student is declared handicapped or said to demonstrate adverse performance. This cutoff point could become one of the criterion-referenced test items. When criterion test items are used in this way, they become the performance level a child must achieve to be moved out of the "handicapped" category.

However, criterion-referenced assessment reaches its full potential only when integrated into the day-by-day functioning so that it is not perceived by the student as an artificial, testing activity.[8] It is valuable for individualizing instruction and monitoring instructional goals.

Domain-Referenced Tests

Definition

Domain-referenced testing involves the measure of a general ability. To do this, one usually tests a specific behavior and then makes inferences about a student's general capability. For instance, if a student cannot walk a balance beam heel-to-toe for its entire length, it might be said that she lacks dynamic balance. Usually several domains are sampled in one test. The outcome of domain-referenced assessment is a student profile of general abilities believed to be important for success in a physical education program.

There is disagreement among professionals about what is included in specific domains as well as about terminology associated with each domain. Some of the physical fitness domains are muscular strength, cardiovascular endurance, muscular endurance, and flexibility. Hypothesized domains for motor fitness are power, motor speed, speed of limb movement, static and dynamic balance, fundamental locomotor skill, and gross body agility. Perceptual-motor domains are spatial orientation, body image and differentiation, ocular control, form perception, perception of position in space, perceptual constancy, tactile discrimination, visual closure, memory, and oth-

TABLE 4-3
Domain-referenced physical fitness test*

Domain	Name of Test	Performance Measure
Extent of flexibility	Sit and reach test	Inches (plus or minus) from the toes
Dynamic flexibility	Bend, straighten, and twist test	Repetitions over time
Static strength	Grip strength hand dynamometer	Pounds of force applied to the dynamometer
Dynamic strength	Chin-ups	Repetitions
Explosive strength	Two-footed standing broad jump	Distance in feet and inches
Trunk strength	Bent-leg sit-ups	Repetitions over time
Stamina	12-minute run	Distance traveled in 12 minutes
Gross body coordination	Rope jump (24-inch rope)	Number of successful jumps in a specified number of trials
Gross body equilibrium	Balance stick test	Number of seconds balance is held on a stick of a specified width

*This domain-referenced test is based on the factor analysis found in Fleishman, E.A.: Structure and measurement of physical fitness, Englewood Cliffs, N.J., 1965, Prentice-Hall, Inc.

ers. (See also Chapter 6.) Table 4-3 represents a domain-referenced physical fitness test.

Purpose

Domain-referenced tests provide information about abilities that are prerequisites to specific skills. If children have learning problems that adversely affect mastery of specific skills, it is helpful to identify the specific abilities that might alleviate the learning problems. Once deficient domains have been identified, activities are selected to strengthen the domains of weakness and are administered. For instance, if a child lacks enough arm strength to support body weight, it is not possible for him to perform a handstand. It is also unlikely that this child would have sufficient strength to perform many other gymnastic activities. Programming specific activities to strengthen the arms may generalize into facilitating the learning of all skills for which arm strength is prerequisite.

Or, consider a child who cannot walk up a staircase effectively because of a lack of balance. Among other prerequisites to walking up stairs is standing on one foot, raising it at least 9 inches,

and placing it on the stair tread. Failure to maintain balance at this level of proficiency impedes normal stair-climbing. Thus domain-referenced testing provides a general overview of the abilities and aptitudes that constitute many skills found in physical education curricula.

Transfer and *generalization* are the underlying assumptions in domain-referenced testing. The central thrust of domain-referenced testing is to define concrete domains of competence and to demonstrate transfer from immediate goals in domains to specific skill activities. As competencies in the domains are acquired, one should see corresponding increases in actual physical education skills.

Comments

Normative-referenced and non–criterion-referenced test batteries are often constructed to measure domains. However, the generalization of performance on a domain-referenced test to performance on skills is a subject of debate. This is particularly the case in perceptual-motor training. There could be several reasons why identifying weaknesses in perceptual-motor domains and then attempting to ameliorate those weaknesses through training do not result in generalization to physical skills. One obvious problem is the assumption that each perceptual-motor domain measures a discrete entity. That is to say, there is evidence to suggest that each of the several domains in the perceptual-motor classification is constructed from other pieces of information. For instance, a study reported by Werbel[16] demonstrated that children who evidence body image and differentiation problems also evidence balance and posture delays. It could be that if a student tests low in body image and differentiation, the true source of the problem could actually be poor balance or other basic abilities.

A second problem with perceptual-motor domains is their failure to be validated by factor analytic studies. In 1983 Pyfer reported on an analysis of a battery of tests administered to 126 children referred for testing because of suspected perceptual-motor problems. The analysis yielded the following factors: (1) hand control and static balance, (2) visual-motor control, (3) social classification, (4) age of parents, (5) hand speed, and (6) reflex development. In the future, through careful research, the commonly accepted perceptual-motor domains may prove to be more theoretical than real constructs.

It is also important to realize that the ability or lack of ability of a learner to generalize may also affect the success of using this form of diagnostic remedial approach to facilitate specific skills. Arguments are made that only by teaching specific skills through programmed instruction will perceptual, physical, and motor domains represented in the skill develop. For instance, in the example of the child who was unable to walk up stairs because of the inability to balance on one foot, the criterion needed to climb the stairs might be to raise the foot 9 inches from the floor (an additional inch is needed to clear an 8-inch stair tread). This behavior could be shaped by having the child practice placing the foot on objects that were ½ inch to 9 inches high. Increments of step sizes could be matched to the learner's ability. It must, however, be remembered that before using the shaping method, the teacher must ascertain that the learner has reached the prerequisite stages of development (that is, has adequate vestibular and depth perception development) to permit the shaping to be effective.

If the learner demonstrates prerequisite stages of development, the application of the shaping procedure would do two things. It would guarantee the attainment of prerequisites for a functional skill of stair-climbing and at the same time develop the balancing domain, which could be generalized to other skills that require balance. Under these circumstances domain-referenced testing and criterion-referenced testing would coexist. There would be measurement over the domain of balance without setting a criterion for it, but a criterion would be set for attainment of a specific functional skill (stair-climbing).

Domains can be validated only by showing that training in them facilitates learning of other valued skills. Hofmeister[11] says that professionals should represent themselves fairly to practitioners in education. He points out that virtually no existing data support the use of predicting performance in specific skills from domain-referenced tests, and that criterion-referenced instruments developed along this approach must still be considered unvalidated. Until the time that such validation occurs, perhaps task analytic approaches specifying specific domains and criterion performance within the context of the skill is the plausible approach.

Content-Referenced Tests

To this point we have discussed normative-referenced, criterion-referenced, and domain-referenced testing. Each has a different purpose. Normative-referenced assessment determines deficiencies according to normal groups. Domain-referenced assessment specifies strengths and weaknesses of general abilities related to motor skills to be acquired. Criterion-referenced assessments, for the most part, determine what pupils can and cannot do in the instructional content of the curriculum. Baker[2] stated that most objectives do not present sufficient information regarding how a teacher should alter instruction to improve learning. Content-referenced assessment attempts to remedy this.

Definition

Content-referenced assessment is the process of determining where on a continuum or a hierarchy a person is performing. Elley's[5] descriptions indicate that to determine an individual's status a behavioral hierarchy is needed. More simply, content-referenced assessment entails developing a series of small learning steps (or pieces of information), placing them in a hierarchy, and then determining where in this sequence a person is performing.

Purpose

Content-referenced testing is used to determine which short-range objectives leading to a behavioral goal a student can perform. It does not compare children with others, but rather ascertains how close a student is to realizing a behavioral goal. As French and Jansma[6] indicate, this process enables the physical educator to provide an individual pupil with instructional activity based on the first short-range objective (in a sequence) the pupil was not able to demonstrate. A pupil's progress from one developmentally sequenced short-term objective to the next in the sequence eventually leads to the acquisition of a major or terminal motor skill. It is easy to understand how this process fits into the IEP process: content-referenced assessment focuses on narrow and specific elements of behavior that lead to goals. In content-referenced testing the teacher always knows the next objective because the objectives are arranged in a hierarchy of easier to more difficult (complex) tasks before any testing or teaching takes place.

Following is a hierarchy of balance objectives. The action of each objective is to stand on one foot, and the criterion for each objective is 5 seconds. A standard condition for all objectives is for the heel of the free leg to be as high as the supporting knee. The tasks are made more difficult by altering the conditions of the sequence of objectives. Conditions of objectives are altered so hierarchies are expressed for each set of conditions. The conditions that are altered are variations of eye position, arm position, and placement of the foot.

Action: Balance on one foot.

Standard condition: Raise the heel of the free leg as high as the supporting knee.

CONDITIONS	CRITERION
1. Eyes anywhere, arms at sides, foot flat	For 5 seconds
2. Eyes anywhere, arms in front, foot flat	For 5 seconds
3. Eyes up, arms at sides, foot flat	For 5 seconds
4. Eyes up, arms in front, foot flat	For 5 seconds
5. Eyes anywhere, arms at sides, heel raised 2 inches	For 5 seconds
6. Eyes anywhere, arms in front, heel raised 2 inches	For 5 seconds
7. Eyes closed, arms at sides, foot flat	For 5 seconds
8. Eyes up, arms at sides, heel raised 2 inches	For 5 seconds
9. Eyes up, arms in front, heel raised 2 inches	For 5 seconds
10. Eyes closed, arms in front, foot flat	For 5 seconds
11. Eyes closed, arms at sides, heel raised 2 inches	For 5 seconds
12. Eyes closed, arms in front, heel raised 2 inches	For 5 seconds

The balance sequence begins with an objective in which the teacher can specify the positions of the eyes, arms, and free heel. The criterion (5 seconds) for each objective remains the same; however, the difficulty of the task is increased from easy to difficult as the positions of the eyes, arms, and heel of the supporting foot are changed. Each objective in the hierarchy becomes the balance content that is to be taught. Placement of the learner within the hierarchy could represent content-referenced testing. The placement would indicate what the learner could and could not do in that sequence of activities.

Although the series of tasks may not be a true hierarchy, altering the conditions forms a hierarchy from simple to more difficult. The tasks are graded in difficulty because (1) standing on the ball of the foot is more difficult than standing with the foot flat, (2) balancing with the eyes closed is more difficult than balancing with the eyes open, and (3) arm placement in front of the body demands greater balance than if they are placed at the sides. The conditions are simply altered to make the task more or less difficult. Criteria for exit from the program can be made by the teacher, depending on how much balance the learner needs to perform sports (or functional) skills satisfactorily.

To content-reference assess an individual in this sequence, one might have the student attempt to perform the odd-numbered objectives in the sequence until he was unable to perform an objective. When a step in the hierarchy is missed, digress one step back and test. The last mastered task would be the present level of educational performance. Once it is determined where in the continuum the learner is functioning, the learner begins at that point and progresses through the sequence at his own rate until the educational goal is reached.[6]

I CAN

Up to this point our discussion of content-referenced testing has concerned analyzing the components of a task that must be mastered to perform the main task and determining what an individual can and cannot do on a hierarchical continuum of activities. There are other ways to incorporate criterion levels of achievement into content-referenced testing. The I CAN[17] series is an example of this combination. In that series of activities the task analysis of the sit-up (and other activities) addresses not only the proper form, but also higher levels of proficiency. For example, skill levels 3 and 4 require sequentially more repetitions with appropriate age and sex criteria. Thus for this specific skill I CAN has embodied content-referenced testing through task analysis

of the behavior and criterion-referenced testing by increasing the number of repetitions while meeting age- and sex-appropriate criteria (Fig. 4-2).

The arrangement of any given step in the hierarchical sequence can be controlled by the teacher. Ensuring that each step in the sequence is appropriate for the specific learner is the teacher's responsibility. Entering criterion levels of performance in the sequence is an additional check on student progress.

The sit-up and balance tasks focus on a sequence that is inherent in the task being assessed. That is, the balancing task focuses on different aspects of balancing on one foot, and the sit-up task includes graduated sit-ups. In each of these examples it is assumed that the learner possesses all of the prerequisite components necessary to achieve at least the simplest step in the sequence. It should be pointed out that this is not always true when dealing with learners who have handicapping conditions. In some cases underlying prerequisites, such as vestibular development or depth perception, may be deficient. If a student is having difficulty realizing success with sequential steps in a hierarchy, the teacher may have to determine whether lower level components are functioning satisfactorily. This type of probing is another form of content-referenced testing. For example, if the task is to balance on one foot with eyes open, hands on hips, and the free leg bent 90 degrees for 5 seconds, and if the learner cannot execute the task according to the criteria, the teacher can either (1) administer a balance test to determine whether the learner demonstrates a vestibular delay, or (2) administer a cover test to determine whether orthoptic visual problems (depth perception difficulties) could be interfering with the learner's ability to use the eyes to help maintain balance.

This can be considered a deep probing content-referenced assessment. If a vestibular development delay or an orthoptic problem is found, these prerequisite components should be corrected by knowledgeable professionals before the learner can be expected to perform the task to

I CAN

PERFORMANCE OBJECTIVE:
TO DEMONSTRATE A FUNCTIONAL LEVEL OF
ABDOMINAL STRENGTH AND ENDURANCE

SKILL LEVELS	FOCAL POINTS FOR ACTIVITY
1. To perform a bent leg sit-up with assistance.	Given a verbal request, a demonstration, and physical assistance (complete assistance through entire movement), the student can perform a bent leg sit-up 2 out of 3 times, without resistance, in this manner: a. Starting position on back with knees flexed 90 degrees, feet flat on floor, arms clasped behind neck, partner holding ankles b. Curl up by tucking chin and lifting trunk, touching elbows to knees c. Return to starting position by uncurling trunk and lowering head in a controlled movement.
2. To perform a bent leg sit-up with partial assistance. 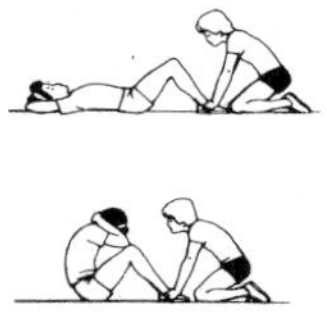	Given a verbal request, a demonstration, and partial assistance (support student's trunk as he sits up), the student can perform a bent leg sit-up 2 out of 3 times in this manner: a. Independently assume starting position on back with knees flexed 90 degrees, feet flat on floor, arms clasped behind neck, partner holding ankles b. Initiate curl-up by tucking chin and lifting trunk; complete curl-up by touching elbows to knees c. Independently return to starting position by uncurling trunk and lowering head in a controlled movement.

I CAN

PERFORMANCE OBJECTIVE:
TO DEMONSTRATE A FUNCTIONAL LEVEL OF
ABDOMINAL STRENGTH AND ENDURANCE

SKILL LEVELS	FOCAL POINTS FOR ACTIVITY
3. To perform a bent leg sit-up without assistance. 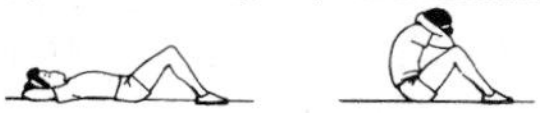	Given a verbal request and a demonstration, the student can perform two consecutive bent leg sit-ups without assistance by curling up and lifting the trunk, touching the elbows to the knees, and returning in a controlled fashion to the starting position.
4. To demonstrate an appropriate level of abdominal endurance and strength.	Given a verbal request, a demonstration, and a command to "start" and "stop," the student can demonstrate consecutive bent leg sit-ups in this manner: a. Start and stop on command b. Meet the minimal performance criteria for individual's age and sex. (See table 1.)
5. To maintain an appropriate level of abdominal endurance and strength through activity participation.	Given the ability to perform the bent leg sit-up at the appropriate age and sex criteria (see Table 1), the student can maintain that criteria over a 12-week period.

FIGURE 4-2
The I CAN program provides a task analysis (focal points for activity) and tests performance at the appropriate age and sex criteria.
(From I CAN Primary Skills, Janet A. Wessel, Director. Reprinted with permission of the publisher, Hubbard.)

TABLE 4-4
Components tested by five domain-referenced tests

	Purdue PMS	Bayley	Stott	Bruininks-Oseretsky	Basic Motor Ability Test
Strength	X	X		X	
Flexibility	X				X
Endurance					
Agility				X	
Power					
Balance	X	X	X	X	X
Speed			X	X	
Vision	X	X			
Eye-hand coordination			X		X
Kinesthetic awareness	X				
Tactile discrimination	X		X	X	
Rhythm	X				
Gross motor	X	X	X	X	X
Fine motor		X	X	X	X

standard. Table 4-4 includes tests that can be used to probe for suspected underlying deficiencies.

Comments

The advantages of activity sequences that are prerequisite to content-referenced assessment consist of the following:

1. Sequences identify what skills learners do and do not perform and what skills are to be taught next.
2. Sequences eliminate the need for the concept of readiness.
3. The teacher never waits for a learner to be ready to learn a given skill, but begins to teach the prerequisite skills specified in the skill sequence.
4. Skill sequences make individualization of instruction easier.

With content-referenced assessment, testing becomes an integral part of the educational process.[8] To accommodate the handicapped learner, the increments in the learning continuum must be small. When this sequence of steps is used, it provides information to the students and teachers about how a student is progressing toward a goal and can provide clues to selection of appropriate teaching strategies.

Programmed instruction or task analysis (see Chapter 6) is an essential prerequisite of content assessment because it permits each task to be treated as a test of competence. Achieving each step in the sequence reinforces the learner's belief in personal competence and provides incentive to continue to try. Programmed instruction becomes programmed testing, and the outcome of each test is used to make an instructional decision. If the learner reaches the next step in the sequence, the teaching strategy is continued. If the learner fails to achieve the next step, the teaching strategy is modified to better facilitate the learner's success. It should be kept in mind that using this procedure to test and teach will prove successful only if the programmed instruction or task analysis contains every step necessary to accomplish the goal. Inadequate or poorly sequenced steps will lead to learner and teacher frustration.

When programmed instruction or task analysis is in use, each behavior becomes an objective

CONTENT TASK ANALYSIS OF A SOFTBALL THROW

1. Demonstrate the correct grip 100% of the time.
   a. Select a softball.
   b. Hold the ball with the first and second fingers spread on top, thumb under the ball and the third and fourth fingers on the side.
   c. Grasp the ball with the fingertips.
2. Demonstrate the proper step pattern for throwing the softball 3 out of 5 times.
   a. Identify the restraining line.
   b. Take a side step with the left foot.
   c. Follow with a shorter side step with the right foot.
3. Demonstrate the proper throwing technique and form 3 out of 5 times.
   a. Grip ball correctly.
   b. Bend rear knee.
   c. Rotate hips and pivot left foot, turning body to the right.
   d. Bring right arm back with the ball behind the right ear and bent right elbow leading (in front of) hand.
   e. Bend left elbow and point it at a 45-degree angle.
   f. Step straight ahead with the left foot.
   g. Keep the right hip back and low and the right arm bent with the ball behind the ear and the elbow leading.

   h. Start the throwing motion by pushing down hard with the right foot.
   i. Straighten the right knee and rotate the hips, shifting the weight to the left foot.
   j. Keep the upper body in line with the direction of throw and the eyes focused on the target.
   k. Whip the left arm to the rear, increasing the speed of the right arm.
   l. Extend the right arm fully forward. completing the release by snapping the wrist and releasing the ball at a 45 degree angle.
   m. Follow through by bringing the hand completely down and the right foot forward to the front restraining line.
4. Throw a softball on command 3 out of 5 times.
   a. Assume READY position between the front and back restraining lines with feet apart.
   b. Point the shoulder of the nonthrowing arm towards the restraining line.
   c. Focus eyes in the direction of the throw.
   d. Remain behind the front restraining line.
   e. Throw the softball on command.
   f. Execute smooth integration of skill sequence.

Permission for the Special Olympics Sports Skills Instructional Program provided by Special Olympics, created by The Joseph P. Kennedy, Jr. Foundation. Authorized and accredited by Special Olympics, Inc., for the Benefit of Mentally Retarded Citizens.

and learning principles can be applied to teaching because there is precise definition of what is to be learned. When content-referenced testing is a part of the education process, there is provision for open measures that are public. They are precisely repeatable and mutually understandable so that all concerned parties know where students are in their education development and how far they must go to achieve measurable educational goals.[7] Content-referenced tests may be more practical and appropriate than other tests because they reflect what is actually being taught on a daily basis and focus on raw data that reflect a pupil's precise performance.

Assessing Specific Sports Skills

Two basic forms associated with content-referenced testing are task analysis of specific instructional content that has not yet been mastered and improvement of skill proficiency after it is performed in some manner. In motor skills the development of form and increased levels of proficiency usually occur at the same time. Both forms of assessment make instructional decisions for a specific learner easier.

The task analyses for the Special Olympics sports curriculum are examples of breaking a skill into teachable components. While the specific skill is taught, assessments can be made to determine which specific components can and cannot be done by a learner. In the softball throw 19 observable components are listed. Using the task analysis of the throw to teach from involves content-referenced assessment because there is a direct relationship between assessment and the end result of the instruction. This might also be considered criterion-referenced testing because a standard of mastery could be set for all 19 components of the task (see box on p. 61).

Community-Based Assessment

Handicapped persons are often perceived as being dependent on others, including government, for the duration of their life. The purpose of special education and physical education is to alleviate continued dependence on others. If, through testing, it is determined that a student is on the borderline between normal and below-normal functioning, special education can help the individual move into the range of normal functioning. Educational remedies should be directed toward raising the student's ability to perform curriculum tasks adequately. If, on the other hand, the student is judged to be so deficient in ability that she is unable to compete on an equal basis in a normal adult society, then the education of that student should focus on more practical things. Probably the most practical approach is to develop their ability to function in specific community living environments. Toward this end, community-based assessments should be provided for moderately to severely handicapped students. Following is a list of community-based behaviors from which assessments can be made to determine which needs are to be developed that lead toward independent participation. Behaviors

that are deficient can be content referenced through task analysis and programmed instructional procedures.

1. Participates in recreational swimming at the Ford City Y.M.C.A.
2. Bowls once a week at the Ford City Bowlo-drome.
3. Participates at Smith's Miniature Golf complex at least five times during the summer.
4. Jogs 10 miles per week.
5. Participates in a church summer league softball program.
6. Participates in the Ford City volleyball recreation program during December through February.

Definition

Community-based assessments are strategies for defining what skills and knowledge an individual will need to function adequately in a community environment. The process for conducting a community-based assessment is aptly described by Brown and co-workers.[3] The steps suggested follow:

1. Delineate the most relevant and functional least restrictive current and subsequent school and nonschool environments.
2. Analyze these environments and divide them into subenvironments (school, home, neighborhood, playground, etc.).
3. Designate some of the most relevant and functional activities that occur in these environments.
4. Determine the skills needed to participate in the activities and describe possible adaptations that allow participation.
5. Design and implement instructional programs to teach students the skills necessary for participation in chronologically age-appropriate activities in the natural environments.

Purpose

The community-based assessment and the IEP should define which skills are mastered and which are not. When environments are changed, new skills are needed for adaptation. There should be a match between skill functionality and instructional tasks. This lowers the risk of requiring unnecessary steps in the generalization process.

Comments

Brown[3] uses the term *ecological inventory* to describe a checklist of the behaviors that the student should learn to become self-sufficient in the natural environment. Learner performance is studied across a variety of tasks that occur throughout the day.[15] The community-based assessment provides detailed information on how the behaviors are to be performed by the individual. Once these behaviors are defined to the extent that they can be subjected to either task analysis or programmed instruction, either content- or criterion-referenced testing and programming can be applied to facilitate development. The analysis of the functional skills will identify missing prerequisites. Objectives on the IEP should be related to those functional activities.

Community-based assessment and programming are based on the principle of partial participation. Whatever the learners *can* do, they do. Only the amount of assistance needed to function successfully in a natural environment is provided. Adaptations to help persons accommodate to the environment are (1) personal assistance, (2) adapted materials and devices, (3) adapted social environments, and (4) skill sequences.

Other Types of Assessment Instruments
Inventories

Inventory assessments are composed of checklists of tasks to be accomplished. Usually they are not in sequential order, and there is little or no functional relationship between the tasks. Even though the activities are not behaviorally stated, they are nevertheless useful.

One of the most prevalent checklists used is the one to determine acquired swimming skill (see box on this page). Two problems arise from the use of such checklists. First, it is possible that the student could master all of the tasks and still

---

SWIMMING CHECKLIST

1. Splash water.
2. Wash face with water.
3. Move down steps into water.
4. Wade in water.
5. Move backward in water.
6. Place nose in water.
7. Submerge head in water.
8. Blow ping-pong ball across pool.
9. With mouth in water, blow bubbles.
10. Jump while in water.
11. Squat underwater.
12. With hands on steps, bring legs up to floating position.
13. With hands on steps, kick fast.
14. While held in prone position, recover.
15. Retrieve objects from 2 feet of water.
16. Roll over from a prone float position.
17. Prone glide and recover.

---

not be able to swim. Second, one may be able to swim but not be proficient in many of the subtasks. Checklists are inventories of characteristics and provide a guide for selection of activities, but they are not objectives. Thus programmed instruction or task analysis as it relates to the task to be learned must still be done. One cannot determine specific behavioral performance in natural environments from checklists.

Formative Assessment

Many physical education sport skills are taught in a specified form. Once the desirable form is decided on, the sport skill is divided into observable portions. These portions or elements are often called *coaching points*. The formative assessment is similar to, but different from, classic task analysis. For instance, in classic task analysis of tying a shoe, all of the many steps in the task must be mastered before the shoe can be tied. However, in throwing a ball the ball may be propelled by a novice even though the form of the task is not exactly the way the instructor wants it. Usually, there are two ways of assessing a physical skill performance. One is the formative assessment, which is used to determine if a student replicated a desired form. The other is content-referenced assessment, which generally measures skill proficiency on a continuum of speed, distance, number of repetitions, and so on. In throwing a ball, accuracy and distance of the throw would be measured if one were using content-referenced assessment.

Treatment-Referenced Testing

According to Donlon,[4] treatment-referenced tests are designed to determine which teaching strategy would be most successful with a given student. When using treatment-referenced tests,

TABLE 4-5
A practical summary for selection of appropriate test types

Test Type	Purpose	When to Use	Examples
Standardized norm referenced	To determine status compared with normal population	To compare the results of programs between school districts	AAHPERD Physical Fitness Test
Criterion referenced	To establish a standard of performance at which point instruction can be discontinued	To set standards for curriculum content in the instructional setting	I CAN materials that indicate performance standards of skills
Domain referenced	To study the ability characteristics of physical, motor, and perceptual structures	To determine weakness in ability structures for remedial purposes	Fleishman and Rarick physical fitness tests
Content referenced	To determine placement in a hierarchical sequence to adapt instruction to the ability of the learner	When teaching physical education tasks of the curriculum	Usually developed by teachers for specific skill and specific age group; few such tests in physical education; Special Olympics and I CAN task analyses
Community-based assessment	To identify behaviors that lead to self-sufficiency in the community	When children will not return to regular class and instruction is linked with self-sufficiency in the community	Developed by teachers through study of community; then converting behaviors to content-referenced assessment
Inventories	To identify behaviors that have and have not been achieved	To determine tasks for instructional purposes	Gymnastics and swimming checklists; American Red Cross swimming checklist
Treatment referenced	To determine appropriate instructional strategies that maximize learning	When instructional strategies are not working	Few in physical education; most in area of reading
Surveys	To determine area for which content-referenced testing must be developed	When there are many complex problems that may relate to physical, motor, or perceptual deficiency	Postural assessment with New York State Physical Fitness Test Survey

careful study is made of antecedents and consequences that bring about desired changes. This assessment form results from recognition that learners are different, and thus different intervention strategies may have to be used. If one strategy does not work, more information is gathered and another treatment form is tried. This approach is often used to control disruptive behavior or bring about positive cognitive change in people with learning disabilities.

Tests with Multiple Characteristics

Assessment instruments do not always fit neatly into the specific classification system that has been described so far. Rather, instruments may possess characteristics of several different types of tests. Furthermore, a specific test may be used for more than one purpose.

There are several assessment instruments available in the physical education literature. Many of these tests are commercial domain-referenced tests with norms (see Chapter 6). Table 4-5 indicates the names of several tests, domains covered by each test, and whether the tests can be used for placement, programming, or both.

Milani-Comparetti Development Chart. This chart is a norm-referenced assessment instrument for determining achievement of motor milestones. It is domain referenced in that it classifies the maturation of reflexes (evoked responses) and postural control as they lead to active locomotion. The comprehensiveness of definitive domains found in the Milani-Comparetti chart is limited (Fig. 4-3).

Developmental checklists. Whereas the items in the Milani-Comparetti chart are for the most part arranged in prerequisite order (for example, lying down precedes sitting, sitting precedes standing), not all developmental checklists are placed in that order. The developmental checklist of walking behavior on the right,[16] for example, can be used primarily for assessing normative-referenced attainment of specific skills. When these checklists are used as criterion assessments, specific programs can be designed from them. Once a specific behavior on the checklist is achieved to criterion, that specific program is discontinued.

A diagnostic normative-referenced checklist is shown below.

Assessing developmental stages of a specific skill. Two types of normative-referenced, developmental checklists of motor behaviors have been described. The first included chronologically sequenced behaviors in which one behavior is prerequisite to the other. The second encompassed specific skills that mature at specific chronological ages. Some specific skills progress through stages of development. Each development stage is descriptive in nature and represents a step toward a mature locomotor behavior. Assessments can be made by comparing the performance of the learner against the known stages of development of the pattern. Developmental lag on that specific pattern can be determined. Descriptions of the stages in acquiring the ability to throw appear in Fig. 4-4.

Text continued on p. 71.

A DEVELOPMENTAL CHECKLIST OF WALKING BEHAVIORS

WALKING BEHAVIORS	NORMATIVE DEVELOPMENT
Stands alone	13 months
Walks alone	14 months
Walks sideways	16.5 months
Walks backward	16.9 months
Runs flat footed (no support phase)	18 months
Transfers weight from heel to toe	24 months
Walks with one foot on beam 2 1/2 inches wide and 4 inches high	27.6 months
Walks on tiptoes	31 months
Walks a 1 inch line for 10 feet	37 months
Walks a circular path 21 1/2 feet without stepping off	45 months
Walks on a 4-inch × 8-foot balance beam	56 months

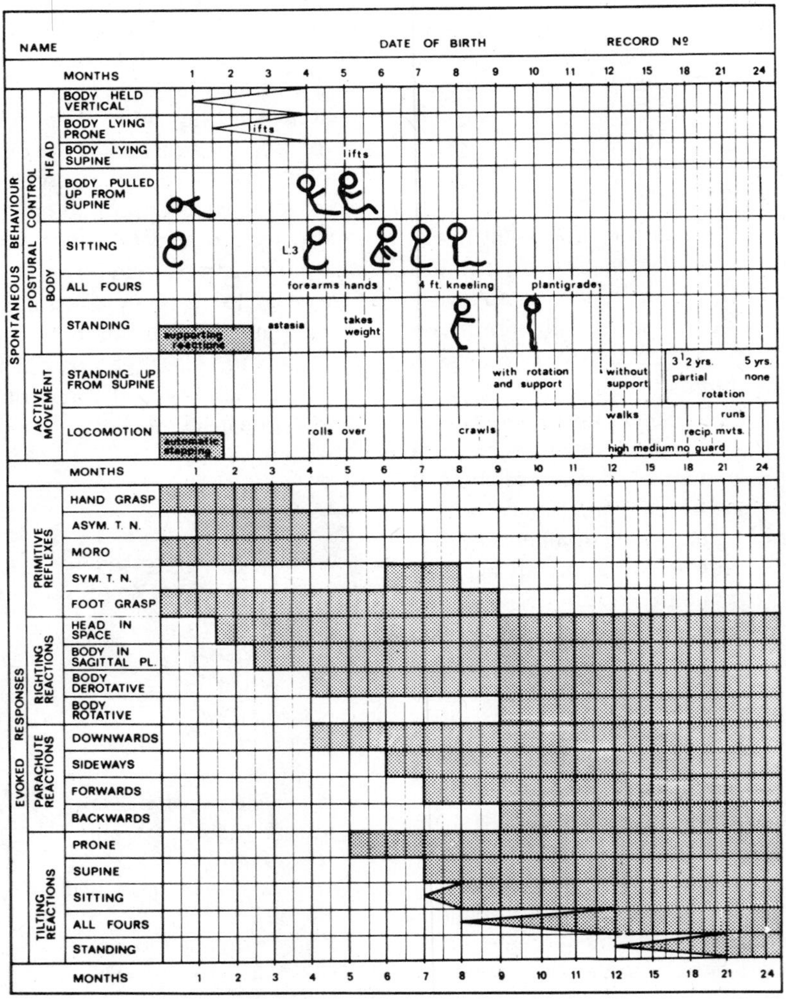

FIGURE 4-3
The Milani-Comparetti Developmental Chart.
(Reproduced with permission of The Association for the Severely Handicapped.)

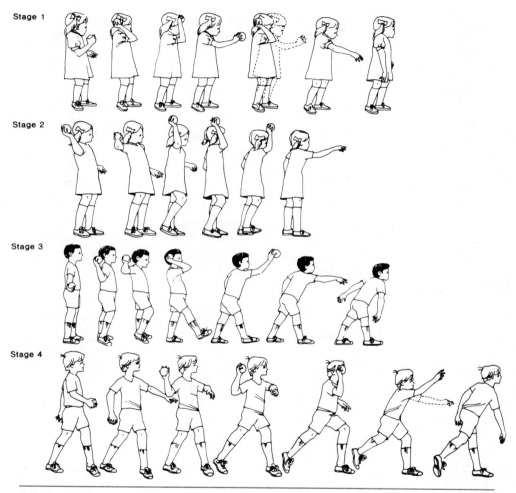

FIGURE 4-4
Developmental stages of throwing.
(Redrawn from Sherrill, C.: Adapted physical education and recreation, ed. 2, Dubuque, Iowa; © 1981 by William C. Brown Publishers.)

ANATOMICAL FUNCTIONAL CONTENT-REFERENCED CHECKLIST FOR WALKING

Directions: (1) Study the four phases of the walk (heel strike, midstance, push-off, and midswing). Study the child to see if the walking pattern fits in column I (normal and mature). (2) Determine behaviorally the deficit related to a specific phase at a specific anatomical location. (3) When a behavioral deficit has been determined anatomically and in a specific phase of the pattern, pair it with column III to determine potential weak muscles, which may contribute to deficient walking. The initial survey to determine specific muscles that need programmed instructional objectives is complete. Integrated programming would involve (a) matching activity with muscles to be developed, (b) constructing a sequence of objectives that develop the activity, and (c) matching task differently to ability level of the learner. This assessment system assesses *only* strength deficits related to walking.

I: Mature, Normal Walking Pattern	II: Immature, Pathological Walking Pattern	III: Weak Muscles that may Contribute to Deficit
Phase 1: Heel Strike		
1. Pelvis has slight anterior rotation.	Pelvis has posterior rotation.	Back extensors and flexors
2. Heel strike knee is extended.	Knee is locked in hyperextension.	Knee extensors and flexors
3. Heel strike foot at right angle to leg.	Heel strike foot placed flat on floor with slapping.	Ankle dorsiflexors
4. Heel strike leg is in vertical alignment with pelvis.	Heel strike leg is in abduction at the hip.	Hip abductors
5. Plantar surface of forefoot of heel strike leg is visible.	Plantar surface of heel strike leg is not visible.	Ankle dorsiflexors
6. Head and trunk vertical.	Head and trunk tip to support leg; pelvis tilts upward on the swing leg side.	Hip abductors of the support leg side
Phase 2: Midstance		
7. Pelvis is tilted slightly downward on the side of the swing leg.	Exaggerated downward tilt of the pelvis on the swing leg side.	Hip abductors of the support side
8. Support leg is in slight lateral rotation.	Exaggerated outward rotation of the hip on the support leg side.	Hip abductors, medial rotators, knee extensors, and foot evertors of the support side leg
9. Toes of support foot are in direction of travel.	Toes of the support foot turn out; toes of the support foot turn in.	Foot invertors and evertors

ANATOMICAL FUNCTIONAL CONTENT-REFERENCED CHECKLIST FOR WALKING—cont'd

Phase 3: Push-off

10. Support leg is slightly rotated laterally.	Support leg is in exaggerated lateral rotation.	Hip and knee extensors of the support leg
11. Slight anterior rotation of the pelvis.	Exaggerated anterior rotation of the pelvis.	Abdominals and hip extensors
12. Push-off ankle is plantar-flexed.	Push-off ankle has limited plantar flexion.	Ankle plantar flexors
13. Toes of the push-off ankle are hyperextended.	Toes are straight.	Ankle plantar flexors
14. Plantar surface of foot at mid-push-off is visible.	Plantar surface of foot at mid-push-off is not visible.	Ankle plantar flexors, hip and knee extensors

Phase 4: Midswing

15. Swing foot is at right angle to the leg.	Toes of swing foot drag on the floor.	Hip and knee flexors and ankle dorsiflexors
16. Hip and knees of the swing foot are flexed (toes clear floor).	Exaggerated hip and knee flexion of the forefoot of swing leg is dropped.	Ankle dorsiflexors
17. Pelvis has very slight anterior rotation.	Pelvis has posterior rotation.	Back extensors and hip flexors
18. Head and trunk are vertical.	Trunk is displaced to support leg; pelvis is lifted on swing leg side.	Hip and knee flexors and ankle dorsiflexors
19. Swing leg is in vertical alignment with the pelvis and has slight medial rotation at the hip.	Swing leg is laterally rotated at the hip.	Hip medial rotators
20. Swing foot is at right angle to the leg with slight eversion.	Forefoot of the swing leg is dropped (eversion is not available).	Ankle dorsiflexors and foot evertors

MOTOR DEVELOPMENT CHECKLIST

Name _____   Examiner _____
Birthdate _____ Sex _____   Date _____

Category	Special Notes and Remarks		
Static balance	___does not attempt tasks	___heel-toe stand, 5 secs balance on preferred foot, arms hung relaxed at sides __ __ __ __ __5 secs	___heel-toe stand, eyes closed, 5 secs balance on preferred foot, arms hung relaxed at sides, eyes closed __ __ __ __ __10 secs ___5 secs __ __ __ __ __10 secs
Hopping reflex	___no response ___no righting of head, ___trunk no step in direction of push ___right ___left ___forward ___backward	___head and body right themselves ___step or hop in direction of push, ___right ___left ___forward ___backward	
Running pattern	___loses balance ___almost ___twists trunk ___leans excessively ___jerky, uneven rhythm	___elbows away from body in arm swing ___limited arm swing ___short strides	___full arm swing in opposition with legs ___elbows near body in swing ___even flow and rhythm
Jumping pattern	___loses balance on landing ___no use of arms ___twists or bends sideways	___arms at side for balance ___legs bent throughout jump	___arms back as legs bend ___arms swing up as legs extend ___lands softly with control
Throwing pattern	___pushing or shoving object ___loss of balance ___almost	___body shifts weight from back to front without stepping	___steps forward with same foot as throwing arm ___steps forward with foot opposite throwing arm
Catching pattern	___loses balance ___almost ___shies away ___traps or scoops	___arms stiff in front of body	___arms bent at sides of body ___arms "give" as catch ___uses hands
Kicking pattern	___misses ___off center	___arms at sides or out to sides ___uses from knee down to kick	___kicks "through" ball ___arm opposition ___uses full leg to kick ___can kick with either foot

Courtesy Beverly Hyde.

Checklists. Content-referenced assessments for a top, down approach may be designed to test deficiencies in both performance and abilities related to a skill. Specific motor skills are task analyzed into observable components, and both desirable and undesirable behaviors are included. Content assessment can be made by observing performance of the skill. This type of assessment is unique because the teacher checks off not only what efficient components of the skill the performer demonstrates, but also the errors demonstrated (see box on pp. 68 and 69).

Hyde[12] developed a similar instrument for screening kindergarten children for developmental delays (see box on p. 70).

Such checklists are useful for screening one student or a whole class of students prior to beginning a unit of instruction. Through the use of the checklist the teacher can determine which tasks a student can already execute and which tasks need to be taught.

Behavioral checklists that indicate abnormal behavior are also widely used (see box on left).

The Special Olympics curriculum sport skill guides require extensive application of different forms of assessment. These include content (task analysis and performance) and criterion (mastery of all parts of the content task analysis) assessments. The curriculum sport skill guides also have a checklist of performance of skills. Worthy of note is that the checklists require assessment of the skills as they are performed in competition. The items included in the checklists are behavioral outcomes of either the component parts of the task or the measure of performance.

As a rule, behavioral checklists assess a series of behaviors that may be found in a physical education curriculum. Once it has been determined whether a student can perform the tasks on the checklist, items that cannot be performed can be broken down and organized for content-referenced testing (see middle columns, pp. 68-69).

Surveys. Postural screening is an example of a survey assessment. The objective of the postural survey is to identify postural misalignments. A widely used postural survey chart is presented in Fig. 4-5.

Once the postural screening is completed, further procedures are required before appropriate intervention activities can be initiated. Steps in the follow-up procedure include:

1. Identify the muscles that are too tight and those which are weak and causing the postural misalignment.
2. Select activities that will strengthen the weakened muscles and stretch the tight muscles.
3. Construct a behavioral intervention program for the specific task.
4. Grade the exercises (content-reference the task) so that you begin the intervention program at a reasonable level for that specific learner (see Chapter 6 for more detailed procedures).

CHECKLIST OF ABNORMAL BEHAVIOR

1. Talks out
2. Does not follow directions
3. Limited range of interests
4. Self-stimulating behavior
5. Self-abusive
6. Hyperactive
7. Inattentive

CHECKLIST OF GYMNASTIC SKILLS

1. Stork stand
2. Cartwheel
3. Roundoff
4. Forward roll
5. Backward roll
6. Tip-up
7. Headstand
8. Inchworm
9. Log roll
10. Front scale

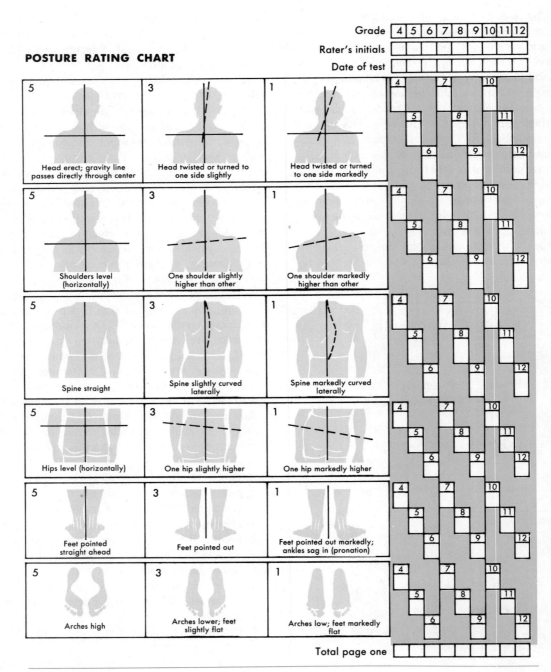

FIGURE 4-5
New York State postural survey.
(Courtesy New York State Education Department.)

This specific survey is also a form of normative-referenced assessment. In Fig. 4-5 the figures in the left column represent the norm, or the desired posture. The figures in the middle and right columns represent deviations from the norm.

USING ASSESSMENT TO CLASSIFY

Assessment is sometimes used to classify performers so that competition between individuals is as equal as possible. To classify competitors, performance in the skill is observed to determine what the athlete is capable of doing. Once the abilities of the performers are determined, those with similar capabilities compete against one another. A running classification for physically handicapped performers follows:

1. Move a wheelchair forward continuously a distance of 10 yards.
2. Move a wheelchair forward continuously a distance of 30 yards.
3. Move a wheelchair continuously up a 10-degree incline that is a length of 10 yards.
4. Move a walker continuously a distance of 10 yards.
5. Move a walker continuously a distance of 30 yards.
6. Move with crutches a distance of 10 yards.
7. Move with crutches a distance of 25 yards.
8. Move with a cane continuously a distance of 15 yards.
9. Move with a cane continuously a distance of 30 yards.
10. Move independently over a distance of 10 yards.
11. Move independently a distance of 30 yards.
12. Run a distance of 30 yards (flight phase).

SUMMARY

Three fundamental purposes of testing are (1) comparing performance of an individual to a normal population, (2) determining appropriate teaching content, and (3) adapting instruction to the ability level of the individual learner. Standardized normative-referenced assessment is used for determining status of an individual in a normal group, that is, it can help determine developmental lag on a specific test item. In some cases this type of test is used for instructional grouping. Domain-referenced and criterion-referenced assessments indicate what needs to be taught. Domain-referenced assessment identifies deficient physical, motor, or perceptual characteristics, and criterion-referenced tests indicate what skills in the curriculum need to be taught to encourage mastery. Checklists usually do not have criterion measures but provide a rough guide for skills and subskills that are to be taught to master large areas of the curriculum. Surveys are useful in determining areas of intended emphasis in the physical education curriculum. Community-based assessment refers to behaviors identified from ecological study that relate to self-sufficiency for more severely handicapped children.

The two types of assessment used in daily instruction of curriculum tasks to handicapped children are content-referenced and treatment-referenced assessment. Content-referenced assessment involves ongoing study of the learning in the instructional content so that it is adapted to the ability level of the learner. Treatment-referenced assessment enables formation of a hypothesis of instructional strategies to facilitate learning. All types of assessment do not fall into these neat categories. Most of the assessment techniques need to be employed to conduct efficient individualized physical education programs for the handicapped.

REVIEW QUESTIONS

1. What is the difference between a content- and normative-referenced test?
2. When would one use a normative-referenced test? A content-referenced test?
3. What are some potential problems of normative-referenced tests?
4. What is the purpose of a domain-referenced test?
5. What are professional concerns with the use of domain-referenced tests?
6. Activity sequences are prerequisite to content-referenced tests. What advantages do content-referenced tests have for direct instruction?
7. What is a community-based test and when should it be used?
8. What are the purposes of treatment-referenced tests?
9. How does a developmental checklist differ from a content-referenced checklist?
10. What are the purposes of surveys?
11. What are the purposes of assessment?
12. Give two examples of each of the following types of tests: (a) standardized normative-referenced, (b) criterion-referenced, (c) domain-referenced, and (d) content-referenced.
13. When is it appropriate to use each of the following types of tests: (a) standardized normative-referenced, (b) criterion-referenced, (c) domain-referenced, and (d) content-referenced.

STUDENT ACTIVITIES

1. Identify 10 assessment tools. Analyze each one and try to classify the assessment instrument.
2. Set up a physical fitness program. Explain how you would incorporate standardized norm-referenced tests, criterion-referenced assessment, domain-referenced assessment, and content-referenced assessment.
3. Study some data bases of handicapped children (hypothetical if need be) and indicate the types of assessments that were used to gather the data.
4. Observe teachers assessing learners. Indicate the types of assessment used.
5. Make an assessment of a child or another student using a test item from a norm-referenced test, a criterion-referenced test, a domain-referenced test, a community-based assessment, an inventory, and a survey.
6. Interview a teacher of adapted physical education. Find out what types of tests the person uses to evaluate handicapped students and why these tests are used. Ask to see a copy of these tests. Determine what type of test (normative-referenced, criterion-referenced, domain-referenced, and/or content-referenced) each is.
7. Compare and contrast normative- and criterion-referenced tests. How are they similar? How do they differ?
8. Make a list of behaviors a handicapped person would need to master to bowl successfully in your community.

REFERENCES

1. *Armstrong vs. Kline*. United States District Court for the Eastern District of Pennsylvania Civil Action, 1979.
2. Baker, E.: Beyond objectives: domain-referenced tests for evaluation and instructional improvement, Educ. Tech. **14**(6):10-16, 1974.
3. Brown, L., et al.: A strategy for developing chronological-age-appropriate and functional curricular content for severely handicapped adolescents and young adults, J. Spec. Educ. **13**:81-90, 1979.
4. Donlon, T.: Referencing test scores: introductory concepts. In Hively, W., and Reynolds, M., editors: Domain-referenced testing in special education, Reston, Va., 1975, The Council for Exceptional Children.
5. Elley, W.: The development of a set for content-referenced tests of reading, 1971, New Zealand Council of Educational Research.
6. French, R., and Jansma, P.: Special physical education, Columbus, Ohio, 1982, Charles E. Merrill Publishing Co.
7. Gay, L., Educational evaluation and measurement, Columbus, Ohio, 1980, Charles E. Merrill Publishing Co.
8. Glaser, R.: Educational psychology and education, Am. Psychol. **28**:7, 1973.
9. Haring, N.G.: Developing effective individualized educational programs for severely handicapped children and youth, Columbus, Ohio, 1977, Special Press.
10. Hively, W., and Reynolds, M.: Domain-refereced testing in special education, Reston, Va., 1975, The Council for Exceptional Children.
11. Hofmeister, A.: Integrating criterion-referenced testing and instruction. In Hively, W., and Reynolds, M., editors: Domain-referenced testing in special education, Reston, Va., 1975, The Council for Exceptional Children.
12. Hyde, B.J.: A motor development checklist of selected categories for kindergarten children, Unpublished thesis, University of Kansas, 1980.
13. Nitko, A.J.: Problems in the development of criterion-referenced tests: the IPI experience, Unpublished working paper, University of Pittsburgh, 1975.
14. Pyfer, J.L.: Criteria for placement in physical education experiences, Except. Educ. Quart. **3**(1):10-16, 1982.
15. Reichle, J., et al.: Curricula for the severely handicapped: components and evaluation criteria. In Wilcox, B., and York, R., editors: Quality education for the severely handicapped, Washington, D.C., 1980, U.S. Department of Education, Office of Special Education.
16. Werbel, V.J: Reflex dysfunction, Unpublished thesis, University of Kansas, 1975.
17. Wessel, J.: Body management, Glenview, Ill., 1976, Hubbard Press.

SUGGESTED READINGS

Hively W. and Reynolds, M., Domain-referenced testing in special education, Reston, Va., 1975, The Council for Exceptional Children.

Reichle, J., Williams, W., Vogelsberg, T., and Williams, F., Curricula for the severely handicapped: components and evaluation criteria, In B. Wilcox and R. York, (Eds.) Quality education for the severely handicapped, Washington D.C., U.S. Department of Education, Office of Special Education, 1980.

Wilcox, B. and Bellamy, G.T., Design of high school programs for severely handicapped students, Baltimore, Md., 1982, Paul H. Brookes Publishing Co.

PART TWO

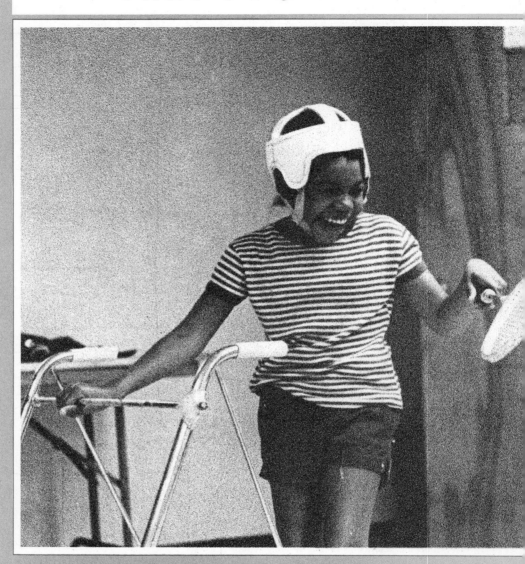

Key Knowledge and Techniques

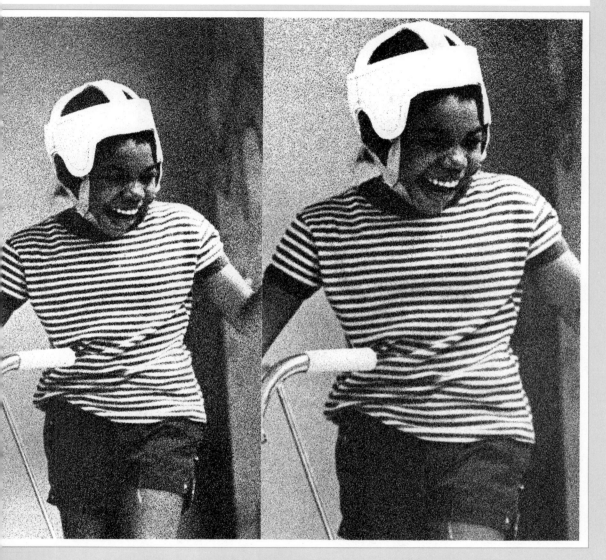

We agree that the types of specific physical and motor problems learners demonstrate are common to many children rather than characteristic of given types of disabilities. In this section specific clues for determining each individual's present level of educational functioning, regardless of disability, and precise programming techniques are described. The need for developing healthful ways to deal with stress and suggestions for doing so are detailed in Chapter 8.

CHAPTER 5

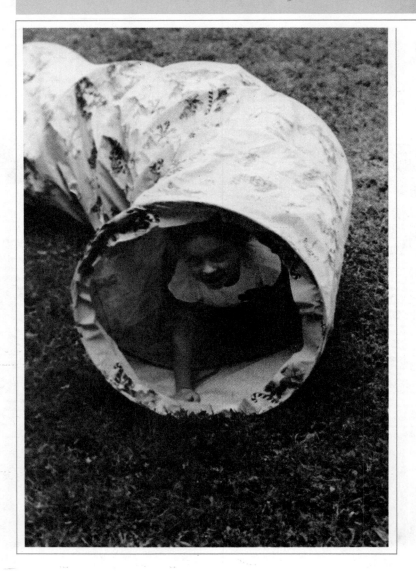

Common Developmental Delays

OBJECTIVES

♦ Know what developmental delay means.

♦ Know the two criteria for determining whether a child is handicapped.

♦ Know what adverse physical education and performance means.

♦ Know the expected outcome of placement in each of the physical education settings.

♦ Know specific examples of clues to developmental delays.

Developmental delays are retarded or arrested stages of performance that hinder a child's ability to be successful at a task. The term *developmental* means one in a series of increasingly complex steps that normal children achieve. The term *delay* means that the child performs at a lower step or stage than do other children of the same age. The terms together imply that through proper programming it should be possible for the child to increase performance ability. The ultimate goal is for instructional programming to be so precise that eventually a child overcomes all developmental delays and performs to age-appropriate standards in all tasks. Such levels of achievement are not always possible; however, the knowledgeable physical education teacher who is skillful at identifying developmental delays and then selecting appropriate activities to facilitate development can expect dramatic improvement in students' performance abilities.

ADVERSE PHYSICAL EDUCATION PERFORMANCE

There are two criteria for determining whether a child is handicapped: psychological or medical verification that a handicap exists and adverse performance in the physical education class. Unless a child has been identified in the preschool years or has an obvious sensory, physical, motor, mental, or emotional impairment, that child is not judged as having adverse performance in a physical education class unless he demonstrates below average standards in the regular class. When a child's performance level is below the performance standard of the majority of children in the regular class, he is said to demonstrate *adverse physical education performance*. Regardless of the type of disability a child has, he does not qualify for an IEP in physical education unless adverse performance is identified.

Children who are classified as educable mentally retarded, learning disabled, partially sighted, having impaired hearing, health impaired, or emotionally disturbed may demonstrate adverse physical education performance early in the formal schooling years. They are identified through observation or measurement standards set for normal children of the same age. Acceptable standards for passing are set by each school district. More severely handicapped individuals have usually been identified prior to entering school.

Regardless of when the adverse performance is identified it is necessary to determine what skills the individual must acquire to eliminate adverse performance. The type of physical education class the child is placed in depends on the severity of the problem.

All handicapped children must take their physical education in the least restrictive environment. If it is determined that the goals specified on the IEP can be reached in the regular physical education class, that is where the child is placed. If it is determined that the person would be more likely to develop motor skills needed to eventually function effectively in a regular physical education class in a more personalized setting, that person could be placed in a self-contained adapated physical education class until those goals are reached. Moderately to severely handicapped persons whose goals are to develop self-help skills that will contribute to self-sufficiency in a restricted number of community and domestic environments may be permanently placed in the self-contained adapted physical education class. The important point is that placement is to be based on the individual student's needs. Wholesale placement of students with handicapping conditions into regular physical education classes *does not* satisfy the least restrictive environment requirement. What environment is least restrictive depends on the individual's needs and hence the goals set for that person. *Least restrictive* implies that progress toward goals can be realized. If a student is not making progress toward specific goals, the environment may be too restrictive. Progress should be carefully monitored to ensure that the educational environment is permitting progress to occur.

To design appropriate physical education programs for handicapped students, behaviors that contribute to adverse educational performance must be identified and plans formulated to improve the motor functioning of each student. This chapter includes examples of physical, sensory, perceptual, and social development delays that may contribute to adverse motor performance and clues to identifying such delays.

SYSTEMS AFFECTED BY DEVELOPMENTAL DELAYS

Vestibular System

The vestibular receiving mechanism is located in the inner ear. As the body moves, sensory impulses from the vestibular system are sent to the cerebellum and to the brainstem. From these two areas, information about the position of the head is sent to the extraocular muscles of the eye, to the somatosensory strip in the cerebral cortex, to the stomach, and down the spinal cord. Accurate information from this mechnism is needed to help position the eyes and to maintain static and dynamic balance. When maturation of the system is delayed, students may demonstrate the following problems:

1. Inability to balance on one foot (particularly with the eyes closed)
2. Inability to walk a balance beam without watching the feet
3. Inability to walk heel to toe
4. Inefficient walking and running patterns
5. Delays in ability to hop and to skip

Visual System

Both refractive and orthoptic vision are important for efficient motor performance. Refractive vision is the process by which the light rays are bent as they enter the eyes. When light rays are bent precisely, vision is sharpest and clearest. Individuals who have poor refractive vision are said to be nearsighted (myopic) or farsighted (hyperopic) or have astigmatism. The following problems are demonstrated by children with refractive visual problems:

1. Tendency to squint
2. Tendency to rub the eyes frequently
3. Redness of the eyes

Orthoptic vision refers to the ability to use the extraocular muscles of the eyes in unison. When the extraocular muscles are balanced, images entering each eye strike each retina at precisely the same point so that the images transmitted to the visual center of the brain match. The closer the match of the images from the eye, the better the depth perception. The greater the discrepancy between the two images that reach the visual center, the poorer the depth perception. Clues to orthoptic problems (poor depth perception) follow:

1. Turning the head when catching a ball
2. Inability to catch a ball or a tendency to scoop the ball into the arms
3. Tendency to kick a ball off center or miss it entirely
4. Persisting to ascend and descend stairs one at a time
5. Avoidance of climbing apparatus

Kinesthetic System

Information from the kinesthetic receptors informs the central nervous system about the position of the limbs in space. As these joint receptors fire, sensory impulses are sent to the brain and are recorded as spatial maps. As the kinesthetic system becomes more developed, judgment about the rate, amount, and amplitude of motion needed to perform a task improves. Refined movement is not possible without kinesthetic awareness. Possible signs of developmental delays of the kinesthetic system are:

1. Inability to move a body part on command without assistance
2. No awareness of the position of body parts in space
3. Messy handwriting
4. Poor skill in sports that require a "touch," such as putting a golf ball, basketball shooting, and bowling

Tactile System

A well-functioning tactile system is needed for an individual to know where the body ends and space begins, and to be able to tactually discriminate between pressure, texture, and size. Children who are tactile defensive are believed to have difficulty processesing sensory input from tactile receptors. Behaviors demonstrated by the tactile-defensive child include:

1. Low tolerance for touch (unless the person doing the touching is in the visual field of the student)

2. Avoidance of activities requiring prolonged touch, such as wrestling or hugging
3. Avoidance of toweling down after a shower or bath unless it is done in a vigorous fashion
4. Tendency to curl fingers and toes when creeping

Reflexes

Reflexes are innate responses that all normal children develop (Table 5-1). Reflexes that affect movement are of interest to the physical educator because students whose reflex maturation is delayed have inefficient movement patterns. In general, there is a series of reflexes that should appear and disappear during the first year of life. These early (primitive) reflexes are layered over by (integrated into) voluntary movement patterns. As a child begins to experience movement, a different set of reflexes appears. These later automatic patterns are equilibrium reflexes. They help maintain upright posture.

A child would be considered developmentally delayed in reflex development if any of the following conditions existed:

1. The primitive reflexes do not appear during the first year of life.
2. The primitive reflexes appear at the normal time but do not disappear by the end of the first year.
3. The equilibrium reflexes do not appear by the end of the first year of life.
4. Equilibrium reflexes do not persist throughout life.

Primitive Reflexes

The *crossed extension* reflex facilitates extension of a flexed leg when the opposite leg is flexed. It enables a child to creep and eventually walk. Unless the reflex becomes integrated into the movement repertoire of a child, its presence interferes with voluntary movements, such as the two-footed jump (one leg tends to extend when the other is flexed).

Tonic labyrinthine reflexes (supine and prone) help to maintain trunk extension when the child

TABLE 5-1
Primitive and equilibrium reflex development

Reflex	Age	Age Inhibited	Effect on Movement Patterns
Primitive reflexes			
Flexor withdrawal	Birth	2 months	Uncontrolled flexion of leg when pressure is applied to sole of foot
Extensor thrust	Birth	2 months	Uncontrolled extension of leg when pressure is applied to sole of foot
Crossed extension 1	Birth	2 months	Uncontrolled extension of flexed leg when opposite leg is suddenly flexed
Crossed extension 2	Birth	2 months	Leg adducts and internally rotates, and foot plantar flexes when opposite leg is tapped medially at level of knee (scissor gait)
Asymmetrical tonic neck	Birth	4-6 months	Extension of arm and leg on face side or increase in extension tone; flexion of arm and leg on skull side or increase in flexor tone when head is turned
Symmetrical tonic neck 1	Birth	4-6 months	Arms flex or flexor tone dominates; legs extend or extensor tone dominates when head is ventroflexed while child is in quadruped position
Symmetrical tonic neck 2	Birth	4-6 months	Arms extend or extensor tone dominates; legs flex or flexor tone dominates when head is dorsiflexed while child is in quadruped position
Tonic labyrinthine, supine position	Birth	4 months	Extensor tone dominates when child is in supine position
Tonic labyrinthine, prone position	Birth	4 months	Flexor tone dominates in arms, hips, and legs when child is in prone position
Positive supporting reaction	Birth	4 months	Increase in extensor tone in legs when sudden pressure is applied to both feet simultaneously
Negative supporting reaction	Birth	4 months	Marked increase in flexor tone in legs when sudden pressure is applied to both feet simultaneously
Neck righting	Birth	6 months	Body rotated as a whole in the same direction the head is turned
Landau reflex	6 months	3 years	Spine, arms, and legs extend when head is dorsiflexed while child is held in supine position; spine, arms, and legs flex when head is ventroflexed while child is held in supine position
Equilibrium reflexes			
Body righting	6 months	Throughout life	When child is in supine position and initiates full body roll, there is segmented rotation of the body (i.e., head turns, then shoulders, then pelvis)
Labyrinthine righting 1	2 months	Throughout life	When child is blindfolded and held in prone position, head raises to a point where child's face is vertical
Labyrinthine righting 2	6 months	Throughout life	When child is blindfolded and held in supine position, head raises to a point where face is vertical
Labyrinthine righting 3	6-8 months	Throughout life	When child is blindfolded and held in an upright position and is suddenly tilted right, head does not right iself to an upright position
Labyrinthine righting 4	6-8 months	Throughout life	Same as labyrinthine righting 3, but child is tilted to left
Optical righting 1	2 months	Throughout life	Same as labyrinthine righting 1, but child is not blindfolded

Data from Fiorentino, M.R.: Reflex testing methods for evaluating C.N.S. development, Springfield, Ill., 1970, Charles C Thomas, Publishers.

TABLE 5-1
Primitive and equilibrium reflex development—cont'd

Reflex	Age	Age Inhibited	Effect on Movement Patterns
Equilibrium reflexes—cont'd			
Optical righting 2	6 months	Throughout life	Same as labyrinthine righting 2, but child is not blindfolded
Optical righting 3	6-9 months	Throughout life	Same as labyrinthine righting 3, but child is not blindfolded
Optical righting 4	6-8 months	Throughout life	Same as labyrinthine righting 4, but child is not blindfolded
Amphibian reaction	6 months	Throughout life	While child is in prone position with legs extended and arms extended overhead, flexion of arm, hip, and knee on same side can be elicited when pelvis on that side is lifted
Protective extensor thrust	6 months	Throughout life	While child is held by pelvis and is extended in air, arms extended when the child's head is moved suddenly toward the floor
Equilibrium-supine position	6 months	Throughout life	While child is supine on a tiltboard with arms and legs suspended, if the board is suddenly tilted to one side, there is righting of the head and thorax and abduction and extension of the arm and leg on the raised side
Equilibrium-prone position	6 months	Throughout life	Same as equilibrium-supine, except child is prone on tiltboard
Equilibrium-quadruped position	8 months	Throughout life	While child balance on all fours if suddenly tilted to one side, righting of head and thorax and abduction extension of arm and leg occur on raised side
Equilibrium-sitting position	10-12 months	Throughout life	While child is seated on chair, if pulled or tilted to one side, righting of head and thorax and abduction-extension of arm and leg occur on raised side (side opposite pull)
Equilibrium-kneeling position	15 months	Throughout life	While child kneels on both knees, if suddenly pulled to one side, righting of the head and thorax and abduction-extension of the arm and leg occur on the raised side
Hopping 1	15-18 months	Throughout life	While child is standing upright, if moved to the left or right, head and thorax right and child hops sideways to maintain balance
Hopping 2	15-18 months	Throughout life	While child is standing upright if moved forward, head and thorax right and child hops forward to maintain balance
Hopping 3	15-18 months	Throughout life	While child is standing upright, if moved backward, head and thorax right and child hops backward to maintain balance
Dorsiflexion	15-18 months	Throughout life	While child is standing upright, if tilted backward, head and thorax right and feet dorsiflex
See-saw	15 months	Throughout life	While child stands on one foot, another person holds arm and free foot on same side; when arm is pulled forward and laterally, head and thorax right and held leg abducts and extends
Simian position	15-18 months	Throughout life	While child squats down, if tilted to one side, head and thorax right and arm and leg on raised side abduct and extend

is supine and trunk flexion when prone. If either of these reflexes does not become integrated, the following movement problems will be exhibited:

1. Supine
   a. Difficulty doing sit-ups
   b. A tendency to extend the trunk during the backward roll
   c. Rolling over on side when trying to rise from a back-lying position

2. Prone
   a. Difficulty doing a full push-up
   b. Inability to extend body fully when lying belly down on a scooter

The *positive support* reflex causes the legs to extend and the feet to plantar flex when the child is standing. Clues to its presence are apparent if there is an inability to bend the knees when attempting to jump or no "give" at the knees and hips on landing.

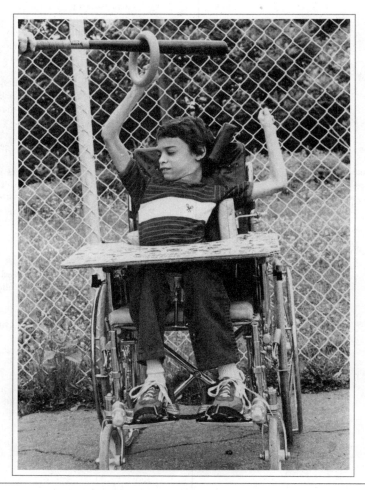

FIGURE 5-1
A residual asymmetrical tonic neck reflex is elicited as a child attempts to reach for a ring on the end of a bat.
(Courtesy Verland Foundation, Sewickley, Pa.)

When the *negative support* reflex is present, there is flexion of the knees when pressure is removed from the feet. Inability to inhibit the expression of the reflex causes the following problems:

1. During vertical jumps, the legs will bend as soon as the weight is taken off the feet; hence, explosive power is lost.
2. Inability to maintain extension of the legs while bouncing on a trampoline.

Presence of the *asymmetrical tonic neck* reflex enables extension of the arm on the face side and flexion of the arm on the skull side when the head is turned. Positioning the arms in this fashion when the head is turned is often referred to as the *classic fencer's position.* Early in life it serves to direct the child's visual attention toward the extended hand. If it persists beyond the tenth month of life, it interferes with bringing the hands to the midline when the head is turned and thus prevents turning the head while creeping and throwing and catching a ball.

By means of the *symmetrical tonic neck* reflex the upper limbs tend to flex and the lower limbs extend during ventroflexion of the head. If the head is dorsiflexed, the upper limbs extend and the lower limbs flex. If this reflex does not become fully integrated within the first year of life, the child will demonstrate the following:

1. Instead of using a cross pattern creep, the child will "bunny hop" both knees up to the hands.
2. If, while creeping, the child lowers the head, the arms will tend to collapse.
3. If, while creeping, the child lifts the head to look around, movement of the limbs ceases.

Equilibrium Reflexes

The *protective extensor thrust* causes immediate extension of the arms when the head and upper body are tipped suddenly forward. The purpose of the reflex is to protect the head and body during a fall. The reflex is used during handsprings and vaulting. If the reflex does not emerge, the child will tend to hit the head when falling.

Presence of the *body righting* reflex enables segmental rotation of the trunk and hips when the head is turned. As a result of this segmental turning children can maintain good postural alignment and maintenance of body positions. Without it, for example, when doing a log roll, the child will tend to turn the knees, then the hips, and then the shoulders.

Labyrinthine and *optical righting reactions* cause the head to move to an upright position when the body is suddenly tipped. Once the head rights itself, the body follows. Thus, these reflexes help us to maintain an upright posture during a quick change of position. Without these reflexes the child will fall down often during running and dodging games and even tends to avoid vigorous running games.

Like the labyrinthine and righting reactions, the other equilibrium reactions help us to maintain an upright position when the center of gravity is suddenly moved beyond the base of support. If the equilibrium reactions are not fully developed, children fall down often, fall off chairs, and avoid vigorous running games.

EFFECTS ON SPECIFIC PHYSIOLOGICAL, COGNITIVE, AND SOCIAL AREAS
Hearing

The ability to hear enables us to orient ourselves by means of sound. Hearing is usually screened in most school systems. Occasionally, however, hearing problems are first detected in physical education settings. Evidence that hearing problems may exist include the following:

1. Inattention to verbal instructions
2. Repeatedly being out of position or failing to respond to instructions called out by the team members or the teacher
3. Equilibrium problems (This is particularly evident when the child has a history of ear infections or nerve deafness is present.)

Laterality

Laterality is an awareness of the difference between the two sides of the body. Children who have not developed laterality very often demonstrate balance problems on one or both sides. Delays in the development of laterality may be indicated by the following types of behavior:

1. Avoiding use of one side of the body
2. Walking sideways in one direction better than the other
3. Using one extremity more often than the other
4. Lacking a fully established hand preference

Spatial Relations

Spatial relations concerns the ability to perceive the position of objects in space, particularly as they relate to the position of the body. Problems may be indicated by:

1. Inability to move under objects without hitting them or ducking way below the object
2. Consistently swinging a bat too high or low when attempting to hit a pitched ball
3. Inability to maintain an appropriate body position in relation to moving objects
4. Inability to position the hands accurately to catch a ball

Visual-Motor Control

Visual-motor control includes the ability to fixate on and to visually track moving objects as well as the ability to match visual input with appropriate motor response. Observed deficiencies might include:

1. Failure to visually locate an object in space
2. Failure to visually track a softball when attempting to hit it
3. Failure to visually track a fly ball or ground ball
4. Failure to keep a place when reading
5. Difficulty using scissors or tying shoelaces
6. Poor foot-eye coordination
7. Messy handwriting

Cross-Lateral Integration

Cross-lateral integration is the ability to coordinate use of both sides of the body. It normally follows the development of balance and laterality. A child who has not developed cross-lateral integration by age 8 years is said to have a *midline*

problem because there is difficulty using the hands efficiently at and across the center of the body. Teachers will note the following problems demonstrated by a child with a midline problem:

1. Difficulty using both hands to catch a ball
2. Tendency of eyes to jump when trying to visually track an object that is moving from one side of the body to the other
3. Inability to master a front crawl stroke with breathing while trying to swim
4. Inability to hop rhythmically from one foot to the other
5. Tendency to move the paper to one side of the body when doing paper and pencil tasks

Walking

Walking is critical for independent living in domestic and community life. There is also an esthetic value attached to the way one walks. Many handicapped persons demonstrate walking gaits that deviate from the norm to such an extent that it readily points out their difference from others. Atypical gaits are easily detected; however, the specific cause of the deficit requires careful observation. A list of deficiencies common to abnormal walking gaits that may indicate developmental delays follows:

1. Toeing-in when the foot is placed
2. Toeing-out when the foot is placed
3. Shuffling gait
4. Exceedingly slow walk
5. Placing the feet far apart (wide base)
6. Arrhythmical gait (the time between each cycle varies)
7. Excessive forward lean, which gives the appearance of falling forward, with the feet moving at uneven rates to catch up
8. Placing the foot flat on the ground rather than using a heel-to-toe sequence
9. Attending to the feet while walking rather than looking straight ahead
10. Asymmetrical gait (different amounts of time, space, and force are used on the right and left sides of the body)

Any of the gait deficiencies may be observed in the general population; however, some gait patterns have specific characteristics and are associated with specific diseases and neurological impairment. A description of some abnormal gait patterns follows:

scissors gait Legs are flexed and adducted at the hips, causing them to alternately cross in front of each other. The weight of the body is taken primarily on the toes. This gait is common in children who have spastic cerebral palsy.

hemiplegic gait Both arms and legs on the same side of the body are rigid and swing from the hip joint in a semicircle. The individual achieves this action by leaning to the affected side and holding the arm rigid.

festination gait The individual walks with a forward leaning posture and short shuffling steps that begin slowly and become progressively more rapid. This type of gait is associated with Parkinson's disease.

shuffling gait The foot is not lifted off the ground but is shuffled along. Lack of balance or strength in the hip flexors may account in part for the gait problem.

staggering gait An uneven gait with which the person has difficulty walking a straight line. It may be associated with alcoholism or brain tumor.

waddling gait The child locks the knee in a straight position and shifts the weight over the leg (so that it becomes a sort of crutch) and then twists the trunk so the opposite foot advances.

tabetic gait The individual has a wide base, shuffles, tends to slap the feet, and watches the ground. This is similar to the shuffling gait. Balance or impaired visual perception may contribute to this type of abnormal gait.

steppage gait This gait is characterized by slapping the feet to the floor and letting the toes drag. Knee action is higher than normal.

Trendelenburg gait Each time the weight is transferred to the affected side, the body leans to the nonaffected side.

Leaping

Leaping involves taking off from one foot into a flight phase and then landing on the opposite foot. Leaps can be forward or backward. Prerequisite activity to the leap is stepping down from an obstacle at a specified height. This stepping down teaches the child how to land by taking the weight on the opposite foot. Stepping down behavior can be initiated at approximately 24 months. Behaviors that may indicate delayed leaping ability are sliding the feet along the floor instead of including a flight phase and taking off from one foot and then landing on both feet.

Hopping

Hopping is taking off from one foot into a flight phase and landing on the same foot. The ability to hop occurs at about age 4 years and becomes increasingly more refined up through approximately 8 years of age. Indications of an immature hop follow:

1. Holding the free (nonhopping) leg bent in front of the body
2. Excessive use of the arms to help lift the body
3. Frequently touching the free foot to the floor to help maintain balance
4. A limited flight phase

Galloping

A gallop is actually a leap, followed by a small step on the trailing foot, followed by another leap. Approximately 90% of all children should be able to gallop by age 4 years. Two errors that are observed in the gallop are lack of a flight phase and an uneven shift of weight from one gallop to the next.

Sliding

The slide uses the same pattern as the gallop, but the slide is done sideways. Common errors are rotation of the head, trunk, or pelvis in the direction of the slide and not leading with the shoulders.

Running

Running is a functional skill that relates to many school and community activities. It differs from a walk in having a flight phase. It demands more balance than walking, because of the landing aspect after the flight phase, and requires explosive strength of the hip and knee extensors. If the necessary strength of those muscles is not available, the individual will have difficulty running. Obvious development delays that can be observed when a child is running are as follows:

1. Flat-footed run
2. Inadequate knee lift
3. No extension at the knee (runs with knees bent)

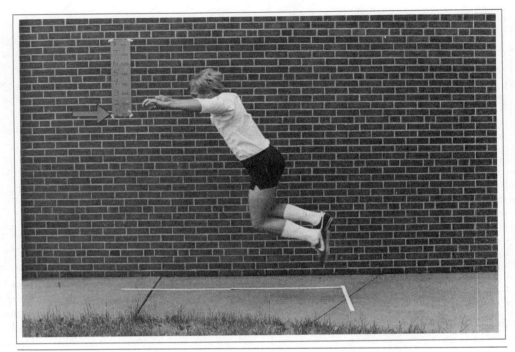

FIGURE 5-2
A jump involves taking off from two feet simultaneously and landing on both feet.

4. Arms swing across the chest, causing excessive rotation of the trunk
5. Little opposition of the arm and leg on opposite sides of the body
6. Failure to lean forward
7. Failure to understand the concept of speed

Throwing

Throwing is the ability to project an object through space. Like many of the basic locomotor patterns, throwing ability progresses from a very rudimentary action to a highly refined motion. It is helpful to know the actions that characterize each stage in the development of throwing. Individuals who have not yet developed a mature throwing pattern display some of the following behaviors:

1. Will not step forward on the foot opposite the throwing arm

2. Little weight transfer from one foot to the other
3. Little hip and spinal rotation
4. Does not release ball at a 45-degree angle to the ground for optimum trajectory
5. Little follow-though

Ascending and Descending Stairs

The mature pattern for ascending and descending a staircase involves a foot-over-foot action that enables the individual to alternately place the feet on every other stair tread. Most 3-year-olds can demonstrate a mature ascending pattern, but the mature descending pattern is not evidenced until 1 year later. Common faults observed in the immature patterns follow:

Faults in ascending
1. Marking time pattern (steps on every tread with each foot)

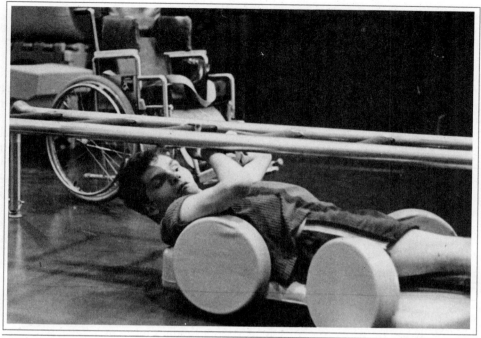

FIGURE 5-3
A child pulls himself with his hands on a horizontal ladder while lying on the back of a scooter. Motor planning is involved in deciding when to reach and pull with each arm and when to lift the head without striking the horizontal ladder.
(Courtesy Verland Foundation, Sewickley, Pa.)

2. Using the handrail
3. Watching the feet
4. Leaning forward from the hips
Faults in descending
1. Marking time pattern
2. Using the handrail
3. Leaning forward or backward
4. Looking down and watching the steps

Motor Planning

Motor planning involves the ability to organize information in sequential segments and then carry out the plan in a smooth and integrated fashion. The ability to plan motor acts of increasing complexity requires practice and neurological maturation. Developmental delays can be observed as children perform specific series of tasks. Some

limitations that might represent developmental delays are listed:
1. Ability to vocalize the steps in the series but not demonstrate the steps
2. Slow and deliberate movement
3. Aborted movement; movement is begun but is uncertain and not fluent (hesitant)
4. Inability to clap in rhythm or perform a rhythmical pattern

Differentiation and Integration

One of the accepted principles of development is that gross random movements gradually become refined. Isolated movements of body parts become possible, and eventually partial patterns emerge and become integrated to permit purposive movements. When differentiation or integration does not develop, certain delay patterns can be observed:

1. Extraneous movements when attempting to execute a skill or motor pattern
2. Inability to isolate one body part for use
3. Traces of primitive reflexes during movement
4. Inability to smoothly coordinate both sides of the body during movements that require reciprocal action
5. Poor co-contraction of the agonist and antagonist muscles that move the limb (movement is jerky)
6. Overflow of movement to parts of the body other than those needed for the action

Discrimination

Discrimination is the cognitive ability to detect variations between sensory stimuli. Until a person is able to discriminate visual, auditory, vestibular, kinesthetic, and tactile sensory inputs, it will not be possible to fully use the sensory information. Some symptoms which may indicate developmental delays in sensory utilization follow:

1. Inability to discriminate different sounds from one another
2. Inability to detect variations in pitch, volume, or rhythm
3. Inability to differentiate between pressures applied to or by the body
4. Inability to differentiate the rate, speed, and direction the body is moving
5. Inability to perceive the size and shape of objects
6. Inability to perceive simultaneous stimuli

Attention

Attention to an instructional task is necessary for learning to take place. Developmental delays in motor functions may be a result of inattention to the learning task. Some observable behaviors that may be associated with inattentiveness follow:

1. Short attention span
2. Hyperactivity such that attention is not focused on the task

3. Attention to irrelevant stimuli
4. Inability to be aroused to a state of attentiveness

Memory

Memory is the length of time that information can be retained. There are many types of memory. Short-term and long-term memory exists for each of the senses and for combinations of the different senses. Some developmental delays that may relate to memory are:

1. Inability to follow complex directions
2. Inability to recall visual and auditory sequences and spatial relations
3. Repetition of the same errors because of an inability to use vestibular and kinesthetic feedback from motor tasks

Sensory Processing

To process sensory information efficiently after the sensory receptor fires, the resulting sensory impulse must move over the appropriate neurons to a precise receiving point in the central nervous system. Once the impulse arrives at its destination, it is combined with other types of sensory impulses and projected to other areas for immediate use and also for storage. Should the flow of the sensory impulse be interrupted or greatly increased at any point along the way, processing problems result. Even casual observation reveals that some people overreact (are hyperresponsive) and some people underreact (are hyporesponsive) to sensory stimulation. Thus hyperactive children have a difficult time integrating information. On the other hand, the hyporesponsive child does not appear to receive the information and as a result fails to respond or responds inappropriately. Some problems demonstrated by children who have sensory processing impairments are listed below:

1. Aversive reaction to sound or touch
2. Self-stimulation behaviors such as swinging, spinning, or rocking
3. Avoidance of swinging and spinning
4. Desire to touch objects

5. Self-abusive behaviors such as scratching self or banging head or body against objects
6. Inability to imitate movement of others
7. Inability to identify where a body part has been touched

General Motor Coordination

Normally, as a child gets older, general motor coordination improves; however, any developmental delays of the conditions described earlier in this chapter can contribute to an overall delay of general motor coordination. When any or all of the following coordination problems are apparent, the physical educator should probe through the contributing components to determine what is causing the general coordination problem(s).

1. Inability to hop
2. Awkward gait
3. Uneven or hesitant movements
4. Inability to maintain balance in a squatting position
5. Poor coordination of both sides of the body
6. Difficulty in weight transfer during throwing or gymnastic tasks
7. Difficulty using both feet equally when jumping
8. Rapid and inappropriate movement
9. Failure to synchronize opposite arm and leg while walking and running

Posture

Some posture problems make body structures mechanically ineffective. Such conditions may impair the health of the individual at a future date besides contributing to inefficient movement. Some observable postural deficits follow:

1. Body slump because of inadequate strength of the antigravity muscles that right the body
2. One shoulder lower than the other
3. Tight hamstrings causing contractures of the knees
4. Toeing-out or toeing-in
5. Hollow back (lordosis)

Physical Fitness

Strength, flexibility, and endurance are prerequisites for fundamental motor patterns and skills as well as a number of sport skills. Some clues to specific physical fitness insufficiencies follow:

1. Frequent rests from activity
2. Inability to climb up or over objects
3. Inability to support the body weight with the arms
4. Failure to make an all-out effort during running games
5. Overweight

Social Delays

Children participate in physical and motor activity within a social context. Simple social behavior involves only oneself; successful complex social behavior requires strict adherence to rules and standards when interacting with others. Games and play activities are done in microsocieties with varying degrees of rules and social standards of conduct. Children who have difficulty interacting with their peers in game situations often do so because they feel inadequate and fear failure. The following types of social behaviors are clues that a child may feel inadequate, and indeed may have motor deficiencies:

1. Usually plays with younger children
2. Whenever possible, avoids playing with same-age peers
3. Picks a quarrel or argues frequently during a game
4. Wants to play a different game than that selected by the group
5. Has a narrow range of interests
6. Withdraws from teachers
7. Will not persist at practicing a task

SUMMARY

Assessment of delays in educational performance is an essential condition to determine whether a child meets one criterion for being handicapped. One of the methods for determining developmental delays is through testing with standardized normative-referenced domain tests. The results from domain-referenced tests provide information about delays of specific abilities that relate to a broad spectrum of skills. Developmental delays can also be determined through content-referenced testing and observation of fundamental motor patterns and skills and sport skills.

The physical educator can observe clues to developmental delays while formally testing children or while watching them at play or in class. The identification of developmental delays provides the information needed to develop appropriate educational intervention programs.

REVIEW QUESTIONS

1. What is a developmental delay?
2. What are the two criteria for determining whether a child is handicapped?
3. What are some possible developmental delays involving the sensory input system (vestibular, visual, kinesthetic, and tactile)?
4. Can you describe the behavior for three reflexes when they are positive? When they are negative?
5. What are some common problems with children who have developmental delays in walking?
6. What are common developmental delays involving locomotor skills such as leaping, hopping, galloping, and running?
7. What are some problems a child might have in class if there were developmental delays in cognitive areas such as discrimination, attention, memory, and sensory processing?
8. What are some common developmental delays that would indicate general motor incoordination?

STUDENT ACTIVITIES

1. Select and administer a test to some students to determine if any have developmental delays.
2. Simulate activity that would portray developmental delays in the vestibular, visual, kinesthetic, and tactile systems. Have a partner attempt to identify the delays.
3. Assess some handicapped children and identify developmental delays in laterality, spatial relations, visual-motor control, and cross-lateral integration.
4. Assess some handicapped children and indicate developmental delays in walking patterns.
5. Simulate deficiencies on the tasks of leaping, hopping, galloping, running, and throwing. See if a partner can identify the deficiency.
6. Perform an activity and simulate a potential developmental delay in motor planning, differentiation and integration of behavior, discrimination, attention, and memory. A partner should attempt to identify the problem.

Each do two —

Try to know what each condition is indicative of: e.g. Can't track a ball etc — visual problem

SUGGESTED READINGS

Ayres, A.J.: Sensory integration and learning disorders, Los Angeles, 1972, Western Psychological Services.

Corbin, C.: A textbook of motor development, ed. 2, Dubuque, Iowa, 1980, William C. Brown & Co., Publishers.

Fiorientino, M.R.: Reflex testing methods for evaluating C.N.S. development, ed. 2, Springfield, Ill., 1970, Charles C Thomas, Publishers.

Kephart, N.C. Slow learner in the classroom, Columbus, Ohio, 1971, Charles E. Merrill Publishing Co.

Knobloch, H., and Pasamanick, B., editors: Developmental diagnosis, ed.3, New York, 1974, Harper & Row, Publishers.

Seaman, J.A.: The new adapted physical education: a developmental approach, Palo Alto, Calif., 1982, Mayfield Publishing Co.

Sherrill, C.: Adapted physical education and recreation, ed. 3, Dubuque, Iowa 1985, William C. Brown & Co., Publishers.

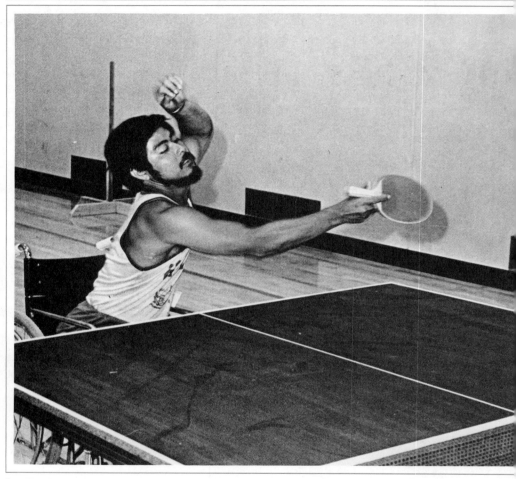

CHAPTER 6

Curt Beamer; courtesy Paralyzed Veterans of America: Sports 'n Spokes Magazine.

Integrating Evaluation and Programming

OBJECTIVES

♦ Know how to determine the unique physical education needs through content- and normative-referenced assessment procedures.

♦ Know how to determine present levels of physical education performance from task analyses.

♦ Understand how to construct an instructional objective and alter conditions and criteria to accommodate the present level of ability and plot progress of acquisition of higher ordered objectives.

♦ Understand the theory and practical application of hierarchical behavioral programs and standard teaching sequences.

A statement often voiced by educators is that educational settings must be structured to meet the unique needs of the student. In the past such a phrase has represented a desire more than a reality; however, current diagnostic and instructional procedures have been so refined that unique educational needs can be met through precise measures. As a result of these improved techniques both school personnel and parents are able to determine whether a child is truly progressing through the specific tasks included in the IEP.

A unique physical education need can be identified through evaluation of a student's performance. If there is a discrepancy between a child's performance level and a normative standard on a test, and if that discrepancy represents a developmental delay, then it can be said that the child has a unique need. Needs may be expressed through skill requirements (shooting a basketball, serving a tennis ball, climbing stairs), through do-

mains of abilities (strength, flexibility, hand-eye coordination), or by sensory input functions (vestibular, kinesthetic, visual). Progress on skills, abilities, and sensory input functions is evidence that unique needs are being met.

It should be pointed out that a need does not necessarily have to represent a deficit. Rather, it may be a skill that a child is interested in developing further. Very often when a skill is identified, continued participation in that skill enhances the individual's satisfaction. Physical skills can be developed further through participation in intramural and interscholastic competition and can provide opportunity for participation in the community.

DETERMINING UNIQUE NEEDS

The first step in determining a unique need is to identify the present level of educational performance. We identify present level of educational performance by testing. This crucial step requires skill in selecting the appropriate instrument and then understanding what the test measures.

Very often in physical education teachers select domain- or criterion-referenced tests because they are designed to differentiate between abilities and the skills measured by those instruments. That is, the test is designed to measure physical fitness, perceptual-motor performance, coordination, or perhaps locomotor skills. These types of tests also describe how the student being tested compares with other children or a standard of performance, but that information might not be useful in preparing a program for the child. We are not implying that these tests are never helpful. But it is important to keep in mind that the information gained from such tests simply provides a profile of the student, which is limited to the abilities and skills measured by the test. What is needed in addition is information about the status of the components that make up or contribute to each task being tested. Until the functional level of the components that contribute to the ability or skill is known, we cannot determine what is causing the performance deficiency.

The entire process can be compared with that of starting a car's engine. We know that when we turn the ignition key, the criterion for success is that the engine start. If the engine does not start, we must determine what is preventing the performance of the engine and correct the condition before the car can be driven. Someone has to evaluate the components or parts that contribute to starting the engine (battery, spark plugs, wiring, starter, etc.). Once the faulty part is found and replaced or corrected, the engine should start. In the same way, when our students do not perform to expected standards, we must analyze the various components to determine which ones are faulty and then correct those components before the child is able to function at normal levels.

The procedures a teacher should follow to determine and meet unique needs of students are as follows:

1. Select a criterion- or domain-referenced test that measures the skills and abilities you are interested in evaluating.

2. Administer the test.
3. Study the results to determine which skills and abilities are deficient.
4. Analyze each area found to be deficient to determine the components that contribute to the ability or skill.
5. Once the underdeveloped components are identified, establish goals and objectives that are specific to these components.
6. Select activities that contribue to progress toward these goals and objectives.
7. Develop a teaching sequence that permits objective monitoring of progress.

Selecting Criterion- and Domain-Referenced Tests

Several tests and what is measured by each are presented in Chapter 4; additional sources are listed in Table 6-1. Review these tests before deciding which one to use. Keep in mind the age and comprehension level of your students as well as what areas you believe are important to evaluate. The greater the number of abilities and skills measured by a test, the broader the student profile you are able to develop from the results. Teachers who select 6- to 10-item tests because little time is required to administer the test gain limited information about the capabilities of their students. At the other extreme, educators who spend much of their time administering a great number of tests may end up with a great overall profile of each child but have little time left for programming activities that will help the child develop. A balance between developing a useful profile and time spent administering the test must be found.

Administering the Test

Specific procedures for administering tests are discussed in Chapter 4. Some practical considerations to keep in mind include the following:

1. How a child performs a task can often be more informative than whether the child is successful with the movement. Watch for extraneous arm, trunk, or leg movements and unusual head positioning as the child performs.

TABLE 6-1
Selected motor tests

Test	Source	Population	Motor Components	Norms
Adapted Physical Education Manual	Kansas State Dept. of Education Kansas State Education Bldg. 120 E. 10th St. Topeka, KS 66612 (free)	Normal, moderately, and mildly retarded, learning disabled, emotionally disturbed; ages 4-12 years	Strength, endurance, flexibility, basic locomotor skills, ocular control, body awareness, laterality, directionality, bilateral integration, spatial awareness, coordination, agility, balance	Percentiles and discrete scores
Assessment of Individual Motor Skills	Education Service Center Region XIII 7703 N. Lamar Austin, TX 78752 (free)	Normal, retarded learning disabled, emotionally disturbed; ages 3-12 years	Posture, gait, strength, flexibility, reflexes, balance, laterality, body awareness, spatial awareness, basic locomotor skills, balance, ocular-motor, fine motor, hand-eye, and foot-eye coordination	Percentiles and discrete scores
Bruininks-Oseretsky Test of Motor Proficiency	American Guidance Services Publishers' Bldg. Circle Pines, MN 55014 (approx. $160)	Normal, retarded, and learning disabled; ages 4½-14½ years	Speed and agility, balance, bilateral coordination, strength, fine motor, response speed, hand-eye coordination, and upper limb speed and dexterity	Percentiles and age-equivalent scores
Marianne Frostig Developmental Test of Visual Perception	Stoelting Co. 1350 S. Kostner Ave. Chicago, IL 60623 (approx. $20)	Normal, retarded, learning disabled, deaf; ages 4-8 years	Eye-motor coordination, figure-ground, constancy of shape, position in space, and spatial relationships	Standard scores and age-equivalency scores for normal
Motor Free Visual Perception Test	Western Psychological Services 12031 Wilshire Blvd. Los Angeles, CA 90025 (approx. $30)	Normal, learning disabled, motor impaired, physically handicapped, and mentally retarded; ages 5-7 years	Spatial relationships, visual discrimination, figure-ground, visual closure, and visual memory	Standard scores
Purdue Perceptual Motor Survey	Charles E. Merrill Publishing Co. 936 Eastwind Dr. Westerville, OH 43081 (approx. $20)	Normal, learning disabled, mildly retarded, emotionally disturbed; ages 6-10 years	Balance and posture, body image and differentiation, perceptual-motor match, ocular control, and form perception	Discrete scores
Quick Neurological Screening Tests	Stoelting Co. 1350 S. Kostner Ave. Chicago, IL 60623 (approx. $25)	Normal and learning disabled; ages 5-17 years	Auditory, visual, fine motor, hand-eye coordination, ocular control, balance, laterality, and locomotor skills	Discrete scores

Continued.

TABLE 6-1
Selected motor tests—cont'd

Test	Source	Population	Motor Components	Norms
Reflex Testing Methods for Evaluating Central Nervous System Development	Charles C Thomas, Publisher 2600 S. First St. Springfield, IL 62717 (approx. $20)	Normal, learning disabled, mentally retarded, emotionally disturbed; ages 6 months-12 years	14 primitive and 22 equilibrium reflexes	Subjective evaluation
Riley Motor Problems Inventory	Western Psychological Services 12031 Wilshire Blvd. Los Angeles, CA 90025 (approx. $20)	Normal or children with speech, reading, and/or learning disorders; ages 4-9 years	Oral-motor tasks, fine-motor tasks, balance, and locomotor skills	Discrete scores
Southern California Sensory Integration Tests	Western Psychological Services 12031 Wilshire Blvd. Los Angeles, CA 90025 (approx. $130)	Normal, learning disabled, or mildly retarded; ages 4-10 years	Space visualization, figure-ground, position in space, design copying, motor accuracy, kinesthesia, tactile, coordination, laterality, balance, vestibular	Standard scores

2. Keep the testing conditions as comfortable as possible. Children perform better when the surroundings are free from distractions, the evaluator is relaxed and reinforcing, and the lighting and temperature are comfortable.
3. Test when a child is fresh. Midmorning and midafternoon are better times to test than early morning, just before lunch, or late in the day.
4. Keep the number of observers to a minimum. Children with handicaps are often hesitant about performing in front of peers or parents. When they are insecure about their ability to perform, they will try too hard or fail to give their best effort if people are watching them.
5. Repeat trials when you think the child might be able to perform adequately if given more time or is less tense. If a child is having difficulty with a given task, go on to easier tasks until she regains some confidence. Then go back to a task that was failed earlier.
6. Observe the child on different days if possible. Children are just like adults—they have their good days and their bad days. If the testing can be spread over 2 or 3 days, the child will have the opportunity to show different performance levels.
7. Gather information about what is going on in the child's life. Children who have just suffered a trauma, are excited about an upcoming event, or have been removed from their favorite activity for the testing session will not perform to their best levels.
8. Limit testing time to reasonable periods. Children will perform best for a period of 30 to 60 minutes. If the time is too brief, the child does not have time to get warmed up and into the procedure. If you go beyond 1 hour of testing time, fatigue and distractibility often interfere with performance.

A sensitive evaluator keeps the child's best interests in mind at all times. Focusing on the test rather than the child distorts test results and gives an inaccurate picture of the child's true capabilities.

Studying the Results for Deficit Areas

Once you have the test results in hand, it is important to analyze them as soon as possible. The shorter the time lapse between administering and interpreting the results, the easier it is to remember how the student performed individual tasks in the test. When interpreting the test results, usually any total or subtest score that falls beyond one standard deviation below the mean or below the 25th percentile or 1 year below the performance expected for the age of the child is considered a

TABLE 6-2
Task analyses and educational performance

Type of Task Analysis	Type of Task	Examples
Content analysis of discrete tasks	Discrete tasks broken down into the many parts that make up the entire task	Feeding, dressing, layup shot in basketball, square dancing
Content analysis of continuous skills	Identifying errors in continuous patterns	Running, jumping, walking, throwing
Prerequisite analysis	Prerequisite components that contribute to a motor behavior are identified	Any skill

deficit area. But do not rely on those scores alone. Poor performance on individual tasks is a clue to deficit areas. If a child does well on push-ups but poorly on sit-ups, we cannot conclude that strength is adequate. Rather, we note that sit-up ability is a very definite unique need. Make a list of the test items performed below expectations for that age group.

Analyzing Deficit Areas

After determining areas or tasks that appear to be deficient, it is necessary to ascertain how far below the desired level of performance the child is functioning on each task. That is, it is necessary to determine what the present level of educational performance is on each task. Until it is known at what level the child is functioning, progress on activity programming cannot proceed. For a program to be effective, intervention must begin at the level the child is functioning and build up from there. Task analysis is a useful "top, down" technique for determining what components contribute to the task and which of these is deficient.

"Top, Down" Approach

There are several types of task analysis from which present levels of educational performance can be determined. The types and their descriptions are listed in Table 6-2.

Content analysis of discrete tasks involves breaking the task down into the variety of parts that make up the task. For instance, to be able to execute a layup shot in basketball, the individual must be able to perform each of the following parts: (1) bounce a basketball with one hand, (2) bounce a basketball at waist height with one hand, (3) run while bouncing a basketball at waist height, (4) take a short step and jump vertically off the foot opposite the shooting hand, (5) time the jump to occur just before the body reaches the area under the basket, (6) release the ball at the top of the jump, (7) direct the ball to a point on the backboard that will permit the ball to rebound from the backboard into the basket, and (8) control the body when coming down from the jump.

To determine which part of the task is contributing to the student's inability to perform the layup, the student should be observed executing the entire movement. When the deficient parts are found, the educator knows that part must be corrected to improve the student's performance on the task.

Content analysis of continuous skills requires the ability to observe one pattern to determine if any mechanically inefficient movements are occurring. To be able to analyze patterns, the teacher must be familiar with the ideal, or the mechanically efficient pattern. Once the mature pattern is firmly in mind, the teacher can observe the student executing the pattern and identify which components are being executed incorrectly. The box on p. 100 is an example of how content analysis can be used to determine mechanical insufficiencies.

Prerequisite task analysis is a process of probing into each of the underlying components that

STANDING LONG JUMP

IMMATURE PATTERN	MATURE PATTERN
Preliminary Crouch	
1. Little crouch	1. Crouch with at least 90° (hips and knees)
2. Trunk upright	2. Trunk parallel to ground
3. Arms: no backward swing prior to takeoff	3. Arms swing up as weight is shifted forward
Takeoff	
4. Simultaneous extension of hips and knees	4. Successive extension of hips, knees, and ankles
5. Takeoff more than 45°	5. Takeoff at 45°
6. Uncoordinated swing of arms and legs	6. Arms in straight line with body at takeoff
7. Incomplete knee and hip extension	7. Flexion at hip and knees
Flight	
8. Incomplete knee extension at end of flight	8. Knees extended at end of flight
Landing	
9. Toes or balls of feet contact the ground before heel	9. Heels hit first
10. Incomplete spinal and hip flexion at moment of contact	10. Immediate giving in to gravity
11. Center of gravity too far back at moment of impact	11. Center of gravity enables recovery of body over base
12. Hands touch the ground	12. Arms reach forward and up to assist in maintaining balance

From Sherrill, C.: Adapted physical education and recreation, ed. 3, Dubuque, Iowa. Copyright 1985 by William C. Brown Publishers.

contribute to ability to perform a task and attempting to determine which of the prerequisites are lacking. An example of using prerequisite task analysis to determine which components contribute to stair climbing appears in the box on p. 101.

When probing for prerequisite deficiencies, whole tests, parts of tests, or single test items can be administered to determine which components are deficient. The box on pp. 102 and 103 includes specific suggestions of tests and observations that can be used to probe for prerequisite deficiencies.

Severely handicapped persons are often nonambulatory, and locomotor skills such as running, hopping, skipping, galloping, and leaping are beyond their capabilities. For these individuals to gain greater independence, they must develop a means of locomotion that is within their capabilities. Since one cannot observe their locomotor pattern to determine their present level of performance, an alternative method of assessing their performance capability is required. An anatomical task analysis that evaluates prerequisites to the locomotor pattern is an appropriate alternative method of assessing their performance level.

An anatomical task analysis involves evaluating the function level of the joints and muscles that contribute to the pattern. If a person cannot walk, an anatomical analysis might include evaluation

STAIR CLIMBING	
Task Components	**Contributing Prerequisites**
Raise foot the height of the step (9")	Balance, flexor strength in knee and hip
Place the foot on at least half the tread	Depth perception, kinesthetic perception, and spatial relations
Straighten the leg placed on the tread	Extensor strength in hip and knee
Raise the trailing leg so that advancing two steps is possible	Dynamic balance and bilateral coordination

of the range of motion at the hip, knee, and ankle as well as strength and endurance of the muscles used to hold the body erect and move the legs. It is common for a child to have a deficient gait as a result of loss of range of motion in the ankle, knee, or hip.

If a child cannot perform any part of a movement pattern or skill with direct instruction, an attempt should be made to identify prerequisite deficiencies. If any such deficiencies are determined, activities should be selected to facilitate development in that specific area.

"Bottom, Up" Approach

The task analysis procedures described thus far can be considered a "top, down" approach for determining present level of educational performance. Some educators prefer one of two types of "bottom, up" approaches, such as simple hierarchies to determine developmental level. The other method is to complete a comprehensive evaluation and then arrange the test results in an elaborate hierarchy of basic components, abilities, and skills.

A hierarchy is a continuum of ordered activities in which a task of a lower order and of lesser difficulty is prerequisite to acquisition of a task of greater difficulty. In a hierarchy similar tasks are arranged in order from simple to more difficult. The sequence selected usually follows the developmental progress of normal children. Progress from one task to another in the hierarchy serves as a measure of student development and answers three vital and relevant questions: (1) How much development has already occurred? (2) What is the student's present level of educational performance? (3) What short-term instructional objective should be provided to extend the present level of educational performance or development?

Identification of hierarchies of motor development tasks enables identification of the present level of performance. If a child is following a normal developmental sequence and cannot perform a task in the hierarchy, it should not be possible to perform a higher level task. If a person can perform a task in the hierarchy, he should be ready to learn the next task in the sequence.

Simple hierarchies can be determined by observing the process of normal motor development. For example, cephalocaudal development represents a hierarchy of behaviors. A child progresses from head-raising in a prone position, to sitting, to kneeling, and then to standing erect. Obviously there is a hierarchy of muscular development that parallels the development of these behaviors. The following information shows the relationship of development of the musculature and the motor behaviors that lead to the ability to stand.

Motor Behavior	**Muscular Development**
Head-raising (prone)	Cervical and thoracic areas of the spinal column
Sitting	Thoracic and lumbar portions of the spinal column
Kneeling	Extensors of the hips
Standing	Extensors of the knees and ankles

Placement of a child's performance on a sequence of hierarchically arranged tasks indicates the limits of capability and tells the teacher what

TESTING FOR PREREQUISITE DEFICIENCIES

I. Basic level
  A. Reflex abnormalities: administer some or an entire reflex of tests (Fiorentio's Reflex Testing Methods for Evaluating CNS Development, Milani-Comparetti Developmental Chart, Barnes, Crutchfield, and Heriza's Reflex Evaluation, Bobath's Reflex Evaluation)
  B. Tactile deficiencies
    1. Localization of single points of stimulation to hands and cheeks compared with localization of double points of stimulation to hands, to cheeks, to hand and cheek on same side of the body and opposite sides of the body (Southern California Sensory Integration Tests)
    2. Aversion to being touched that is expressed verbally or physically
    3. Response to tactile praise
    4. Excessive signs of fidgeting or discomfort when seated
  C. Vestibular delays
    1. Postrotatory nystagmus test: nystagmus should be approximately half as long as the spinning time (Southern California Postrotatory Nystagmus Test)
    2. Compare ability to balance on one foot with eyes open and eyes closed (ability to balance with eyes open but not with eyes closed may indicate vestibular delay). (Bruininks-Oseretsky Test of Motor Proficiency and Southern California Sensory Integration Tests)
    3. Changing constancy board performance (deQuiros and Schrager)
    4. Caloric tests given by physicians
  D. Visual problems
    1. Refractive: Snellen chart
    2. Orthoptic (depth perception)
      a. Cover test: single and alternating
      b. Stereo Fly Test
      c. Convergence/divergence (Purdue Perceptual-Motor Survey)
      d. Biopter
      e. Figure-ground subtest score (Frostig Developmental Test of Visual Perception)
  E. Kinesthetic deficiencies
    1. Finger-to-nose test (Bruininks-Oseretsky Test of Motor Proficiency)
    2. Overflow while performing "angels in the snow" (Purdue Perceptual-Motor Survey)
    3. Imitation of movement (Purdue Perceptual-Motor Survey)
  F. Auditory deficiencies
    1. Directions need to be repeated
    2. Auditory distractibility
    3. Difficulty remembering directions or performing verbal commands in proper sequence
II. Domains of abilities
  A. Static balance delays
    1. Marked discrepancy between ability to balance on either foot
    2. Marked decrease in ability to balance as the base of support is narrowed (Bruininks-Oseretsky Test of Motor Proficiency)
  B. Dynamic balance problems
    1. Trouble with directional movements (forward, backward, sideways) on the low balance beam (Purdue Perceptual-Motor Survey)
    2. Inability to walk heel-to-toe (Bruininks-Oseretsky Test of Motor Proficiency)
  C. Body image delays
    1. Identification of body parts: note errors and/or hesitancy when locating body parts (Purdue Perceptual-Motor Survey)
    2. Self-drawing: note maturity of drawing for age, inclusion of detail for age, and any body parts omitted from the drawing (Goodenough-Harris)

TESTING FOR PREREQUISITE DEFICIENCIES—cont'd

D. Cross-lateral integration delays
1. Any indication of midline jump when visually tracking (Purdue Perceptual-Motor Survey)
2. Lack of arm/leg opposition when throwing (Bruininks-Oseretsky Test of Motor Proficiency)
3. Difficulty coordinating tapping on opposite sides of the body (Bruininks-Oseretsky Test of Motor Proficiency)
4. Difficulty isolating movements on opposite sides of the body while performing "angels in the snow" (Purdue Perceptual-Motor Survey)
5. Avoidance of midline crossing during desk activities
E. Spatial awareness delays
1. Difficulty walking backward (Bruininks-Oseretsky Test of Motor Proficiency and Purdue Perceptual-Motor Survey)
2. Crowding letters together when printing words
3. Drawing forms by connecting dots (Frostig Developmental Test of Visual Perception, Southern California Sensory Integration Tests)
4. Obstacle course: difficulty moving over, under, or through objects (Purdue Perceptual-Motor Survey)
5. Position in space subtest score (Frostig Developmental Test of Visual Perception)
6. Organization of drawn geometric forms (Purdue Perceptual-Motor Survey)
7. Space visualization subtest (Southern California Sensory Integration Tests)
F. Form perception and constancy delays
1. Accuracy when reproducing geometric forms (Purdue Perceptual-Motor Survey and Bruininks-Oseretsky Test of Motor Proficiency)
2. Manual form perception (Southern California Sensory Integration Tests)
G. Strength insufficiencies
1. Static (absolute) strength: a brief maximum contraction measured by a dynamometer or tensiometer
2. Explosive: muscular contraction through range of motion measured by machines such as Cybex, Orthrotron, long jump, or jump and reach
3. Dynamic: repeated isotonic contractions usually measured by functional tests such as sit-ups or push-ups (total number possible with no time limit)
H. Endurance insufficiencies
1. Muscular: ability to engage in repeated muscular contractions in a given period of time; usually any dynamic strength test (sit-ups or push-ups) that measures number of repetitions within a given period of time (Bruininks-Oseretsky Test of Motor Proficiency)
2. Cardiovascular: an individual's capacity to use oxygen during physical activity, tested one of several ways
   a. Vital capacity (V_{O_2} test)
   b. Compare resting and working heart rate (Harvard Step Test or bicycle ergometer)
   c. Distance covered in a set amount of time (9-minute run)
   d. Time needed to cover a set distance (300-yard, 600-yard, or mile run)
I. Flexibility: range of motion limitations
1. Functional tests such as the sit and reach
2. Goniometer
3. Flexometer
J. Agility: inability to change direction in space, measured with functional tests such as obstacle run or shuttle run
K. Excessive body fat: caliper measurements
L. Speed: 30- or 50-yard dash

the child can and cannot do. Such knowledge will assist in selection of appropriate annual and short-term goals.

Comprehensive hierarchies include whole sets of sensory input functions, reflexes, abilities, and skills that are believed to be related to one another. Many of the theories of perceptual-motor development include models of comprehensive hierarchies. An even more comprehensive hierarchy could be developed if all the theories were interwoven so that every basic level component was tied to all of the abilities, and those in turn were tied to all the skills. That model has not yet been developed and tested; however, if an evaluator wanted to look at each of these levels of function, the following approach might be used.

Select a series of tests that measure a wide range of performance, for example, a reflex test, the Bruininks-Oseretsky Test of Motor Proficiency, the Purdue Perceptual-Motor Survey, the Frostig Developmental Test of Visual Perception, a postrotatory nystagmus test, and a tactile perception test. After all the tests are administered, arrange individual test items or subtest scores as follows:

A. Basic level
   1. Reflex test results
   2. Vision test results
   3. Vestibular test results
   4. Kinesthetic test results
   5. Tactile test results
B. Ability test results
   1. Balance
      a. Static balance
      b. Dynamic balance
   2. Perceptual-motor
      a. Body image
      b. Cross-lateral integration
      c. Spatial awareness
      d. Form perception and constancy
   3. Physical fitness
      a. Strength
      b. Endurance
      c. Flexibility
      d. Agility
      e. Body fat
      f. Speed
C. Skills
   1. Basic locomotor
   2. Fine motor

After test items are arranged, study the results while looking for deficiencies at the basic or ability levels. If deficien-

cies are determined, select activities to facilitate development at the lowest level found to be deficient. For example, if abnormal reflexes, vestibular delays, balance problems, strength deficiencies, and locomotor skill problems are identified, choose activities that correct the reflex and vestibular problems first. Once those deficiencies are corrected, you can concentrate on improving the balance and strength delays. After the child is performing at expected levels for age in balance and strength, implement activities to improve the locomotor problems.

It should be evident that using both a comprehensive evaluation and programming from the basic level up is time consuming. There is, however, evidence that this approach is effective in eventually eliminating skill deficiencies.

Regardless of whether a "top, down" task analysis or a "bottom, up" hierarchical sequence is conducted, once specific deficits have been identified the teacher is ready to select goals and objectives and begin appropriate intervention.

ESTABLISHING GOALS AND OBJECTIVES
Long-range Goals

Once the physical educator has determined what the present level of educational performance is, long-range goals can be developed. Goals are specific target behaviors that the child should be able to demonstrate after instruction has been given. Goals are usually written annually because in most school systems the life of an IEP is 1 year.

Goals should be written in behavioral terms that are measurable and reflect an improvement over the present level of educational performance. For instance, if through testing it is determined that a 10-year-old child functions at the 7-year 6-month level in relation to hand-eye coordination (as measured by a specific test), a reasonable annual goal could be: "Johnny will demonstrate hand-eye coordination (on the Jones test) at the 9-year 6-month level by May 15." If Mary scores at the 5th percentile in physical fitness as measured by the AAHPERD Health-Related Physical Fitness Test, an appropriate annual goal could read: "By May 15 Mary will score at the 15th percentile in all areas measured by the AAHPERD Health-Related Physical Fitness Test." This directs attention toward improvement on a test that may not directly relate to functional skills for self-sufficiency.

School personnel, parents, and (when appropriate) the handicapped student should agree on annual goals based on the evaluation at the beginning of the school year. Everyone is then clear about what behaviors the physical education program is concerned with. It is not mandatory that the student reach each annual goal; however, goals are necessary before the steps leading to the goals (the short-term objectives) can be selected. That is, before we can decide how to get where we are going, we must know what our destination is.

Short-term Objectives

The annual goal is a specific, predetermined learning experience that, if mastered, extends a child's present level of performance. There is an intricate balance between present level of performance, goals, and objectives. Because goals are specific to the needs of each handicapped student, any given individual can have a series of goals that represent different levels of performance in each of the curriculum areas.

Before selecting goals for a learner the teacher must determine at what level the student is performing. When a student demonstrates an inability to perform a specific behavior, the teacher must determine what prerequisites are needed for the individual to achieve mastery of the task. Until this question is fully answered, it is restated until the student's present level of performance is discovered. Then a reasonable long-range goal is stated. The short-term objectives follow; they represent increasingly difficult steps leading from present level of performance to each annual goal. It is necessary to keep detailed records on each learner to monitor where the child is performing in the learning sequence. The mastery of one objective is prerequisite to the next complex or more difficult objective.

In addition to the hierarchical linkage between the present level of performance, the annual goals, and each of the short-term objectives, the annual goals and short-term objectives must incorporate four concepts: (1) possess an action (what?), (2) establish conditions under which the action should occur (how?), (3) establish a crite-

---

GENERAL OBJECTIVE: DEVELOP THE ELBOW EXTENSORS AND ARM FLEXORS WITH PUSH-UP ACTIVITY

Specification of Conditions	Rationale
1. Straighten back and hips to 180 degrees.	Bending either part of body reduces length of resistance arm and decreases degree of difficulty of task.
2. Place hands shoulder width apart on floor.	Spreading hands wider than shoulder width increases difficulty of task.
3. Tuck chin against sternum.	Raising head while performing tends to bend the back and shorten resistance arm.
4. Touch forehead to floor.	Touching forehead indicates starting and ending position of push-up.
5. Straighten arms to 180 degrees.	Straightening arms indicates degree of movement of arms (will count as one repetition).
6. Support weight on hyperextended toes, which rest on floor.	Supporting weight indicates the point of the fulcrum to control length of resistance arm.

rion for mastery of a specific task (at what level?), and (4) lie outside the child's present level of educational performance.

The Action Concept

The action portion of the instructional objective indicates *what* the learner will do when performing the task. It is important that the action be stated in verb form, such as throw, strike, kick, sit up, or serve a volleyball.

Conditions

The conditions under which the action should occur describe *how* the learner is to perform at the task. It is important to be explicit. Changing the conditions makes a task easy or more difficult, inefficient or efficient, simple or more complex. Examples of conditions are: "With eyes closed and nonsupporting leg bent to 90 degrees, the student will . . . ." "From a prone position the learner will . . . ." "Keeping the back straight and arms at the side of the body the student will . . . ."

Statements of conditions are particularly necessary to ensure appropriate *levels* of difficulty in developmental sequences that lead to long-range goals. If the conditions are not specified, it is impossible to determine what the true capability of a student is and what activities are needed to advance the developmental level. If the conditions are not precise, it is unclear how the student is to perform the task, and once again the *value* of the objective is lost. The conditions for performing a push-up and the rationales for specifying these conditions are presented in the box on p. 105.

Acceptable and Unacceptable Instructional Objectives

There are three essential features to sound instructional objectives: (1) there must be justification that the objectives are relevant to the learner; (2) objectives must possess the capability of being reproduced when implemented by independent instructors; and (3) there must be agreement on what is to be taught and when it has

TABLE 6-3
Acceptable and unacceptable objectives

Action	Condition	Criterion
Acceptable Objectives		
Run	1 mile	In 5 minutes 30 seconds
Walk	A balance beam 4 inches wide, heel to toe, eyes closed, and hands on hips	For 8 feet
Swim	Using the American crawl in a 25-yard pool for 50 yards	In 35 seconds
Unacceptable Objectives		
Run		As fast as you can
Walk	On a balance beam	Without falling off
Swim		To the end of the pool

been mastered by the student. When behaviors are stated in the form of objectives, behavioral principles for facilitating learning can be applied (see Chapter 7). Examples of acceptable and unacceptable objectives are presented in Table 6-3.

The acceptable objectives include what, how, and at what level the behaviors are to be performed. The unacceptable objectives fail for several reasons, as discussed below:

1. Run as fast as you can.
   Conditions: The condition, distance, or environmental arrangements such as hurdles or nature of the course are not specified.
   Criterion: Neither an objective, measurable distance nor a specified time has been included in the objective. "As fast as you can" is subjective. The students may believe they are running as fast as they can, but the teacher may have a different opinion.

2. Walk a balance beam without falling off.
   Conditions: The width of the balance beam, the position of the arms, and where the eyes

are positioned make the task more or less difficult. None of these is specified.

Criterion: The distance to be traveled or distance over time is not specified.

3. Swim to the end of the pool.

Conditions: The type of stroke is not specified.

Criterion: Swimming pools are different lengths. It is unclear what exact distance the student is to swim.

MEASURING TASK PERFORMANCE

Measurement is an integral part of instruction for handicapped children. It enables adapted physical education teachers to secure information needed to make precise instructional decisions for skill development. Three different types of measures may be used to assess present levels of performance and develop objectives: ratio, interval, and ordinal measures. The definition of each of these three types of measures and an example of each follow:

Types of Measures	Examples
Ratio: a common unit of measure between each score and a true zero point	Number of repetitions of a task
Interval: a common unit of measure but no true zero point	Developmental quotients such as IQ
Ordinal: a specialized order or rank that does not have a common unit of measure but can be hierarchically ordered	Class ranking or scores in a shifting criterion program
Nominal: a word or statement that represents a value	Par in golf, which falls into one of two categories. Par was achieved or it was not.

Criterion for Mastery

The criterion for mastery of a task is the standard at which the task should be performed. Being able to perform the task to criterion level indicates mastery of the task and hence pupil prog-

ress. Reaching criterion serves notice that one prerequisite in a series has been mastered and that the student is ready to begin working toward the next step. Measures for task mastery can take several forms:

- Number of repetitions (10 repetitions)—ratio
- Number of repetitions over time (20 repetitions in 15 seconds)—ratio
- Distance traveled (8 feet on a balance beam without stepping off)—ratio
- Distance traveled over time (200 yards in 25 seconds)—ratio
- Number of successive trials without a miss (4 times in a row)—ratio
- Specified number of successful responses in a block of trials (3 out of 5)—ratio
- Number of degrees of movement (flexibility in degrees of movement from starting to ending positions)—ratio
- Mastery of all the stated conditions of the task—nominal

The intent of the instructional process is to add new behaviors to present levels of performance. Therefore, instructional objectives are not valid unless they are directed toward the acquisition of behaviors beyond what a learner is capable of doing. That is why teachers assess each learner on a continuum of activities to determine present level of performance *before* instructional objectives are selected.

SELECTING ACTIVITIES AND INSTRUCTIONAL STRATEGIES

Once a child's present level of performance has been determined and objectives have been selected and sequenced, the teacher can determine which instructional strategies to use. Physical educators have traditionally included exercises, individual stunts and tumbling, games, sports, rhythmic activities, and gymnastics in their curricula. Often these activities are selected according to teacher bias. More recently, particularly since the mandates of P.L. 94-142 became effective, greater care is being exercised by teachers in selecting activities to include in their programs. Activities should be selected on the basis of what they can contribute to the instructional objectives of the students.

Activities

Once the evaluation of the learner's needs has been carefully completed and the behavioral objectives clearly stated, the physical educator is ready to select activities that will enable the student to progress. The three most important factors to keep in mind when selecting activities are (1) appropriateness for the specific objectives, (2) adequate practice time to ensure that learning will occur, and (3) modification of the activity to make it increasingly more difficult.

The following list presents activities and suggestions on ways to vary them. The suggested activities can be used with any child (whether retarded, learning disabled, deaf, or otherwise handicapped) who demonstrates specific needs. More general suggestions for adapting games, sports, stunts, tumbling, and rhythms is found in later chapters.

1. Vestibular stimulation
   - Log rolls (number to be completed)
   - Spin self while sitting or lying on a scooter (amount of time)
   - Teeter-totter (amount of time)
   - Bounce on a trampoline while sitting, kneeling, or standing (number of bounces or amount of time)
   - Swing (amount of time)
   - Ride down a ramp on a scooter with head up and arms and legs extended (number of times)
2. Reflex development
   a. Inhibit positive support reaction (activities requiring landing on both feet and simultaneously flexing hips, knees, and ankles)
      - Jumping on tires, air mats, trampoline, truck tire tubes (amount of time or number of bounces)
      - Bunny hop (length of time or number of hops)
      - Jump rope (length of time or number of jumps)
   b. Inhibit tonic labyrinthine supine (ability to hold flexed position while supine is developed when child practices lifting head against gravity)
      - Egg rolls (length of time)
      - Lie on back on scooter and hold chin close to chest while moving scooter using hands and feet (distance to be traveled)
      - Practice rocking forward and back while wrapping arms around bent legs and holding self in tight ball (length of time or number of rocks)
   c. Inhibit tonic labyrinthine prone (ability to hold body in extension while prone is developed when child practices lifting head against gravity)
      - Wheelbarrow walk with partner with head up (distance to be traveled)
      - Scooter relays in prone position with head up (distance to be traveled)
      - Scooter tag (length of time)
      - Propels self with hands while prone on a scooter with head up (distance to be traveled or length of time)
   d. Facilitate equilibrium reflexes
      - Tug of war (length of time)
      - Bouncing on air mat (length of time or number of bounces)
      - Crack the whip (length of time)
      - Scooter relays while sitting or lying on scooter and being pushed or pulled by a partner (distance to be traveled)
3. Kinesthetic development (increased pressure on joints)
   - Tug of war (length of time)
   - Wearing wrist or ankle weights while playing (amount of weight and length of time)
   - Propel self with hands or feet while sitting or lying on a scooter (distance to travel or length of time)
   - Balancing on "points" during movement exploration activities (length of time)
   - Push a large cage ball with hands or feet (distance ball is to travel or amount of playing time)
4. Motor planning
   - Number of motor activities in a sequence
   - Throw a ball in the air and touch body parts (greater number of parts that can be touched during the period the ball is tossed and caught)
   - Moving through an obstacle course blindfolded (amount of time)
   - Speed with which angels in the snow can be played (number of errors over 10 trials)
   - Move to the beat of a drum (errors in 10 moves)
5. Space and form perception
   - Movement through different size hoops
   - Navigating a maze where there is less space for movement and traveling greater distances over a time frame than previously
   - Reproduction of mirror image moves (number of moves over time without error)
   - Duplicating pegboard patterns (time to completion and errors)
   - Dropping clothespins into containers (size of opening and greater number in a block of trials)

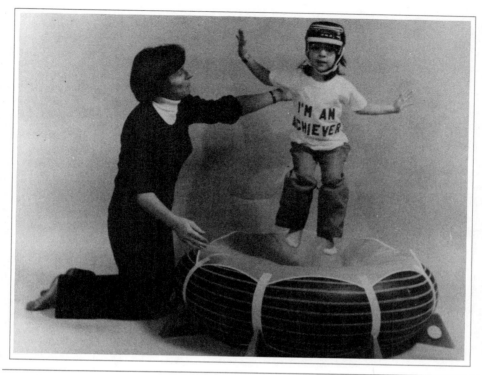

FIGURE 6-1
Bouncing on an inner tube trampoline stimulates the vestibular mechanism.
(Courtesy Achievement Products, Incorporated.)

6. Ocular tracking
  - Following a ball on a trough (repetitions without error)
  - Hitting a swinging ball with a bat (increased number of hits in a block of trials)
7. Flexibility (range of motion)
  - Increase the range of motion in degrees in all joints in all directions
8. Head control
  - Prone position (height the chin can be moved from the floor or table)
  - Sitting (raise head from different position)
  - Start the head in a position where the person can be successful
  - Head righted for time (endurance)
  - Pull child from supine to sitting (start the pull where there is no head lag)
9. Rolling over (stimulus: place an object in reach of the child; use an auditory signal to elicit the response)
  - Roll a specified number of revolutions (start on side; roll 90 degrees; increase a degree at a time)
  - Roll (inches of deviation from a straight line)
  - Roll up an incline (number of revolutions over time)
10. Crawling
  - Pattern (without, bilateral, homolateral, cross-lateral)
  - Distance over time
  - Over obstacles (distance over time)
11. Creeping:
  Action: Four point; move forward on hands and knees
  Sequence
  - Creep (for distance)
  - Creep (distance over time)
  - Creep (over a predetermined obstacle course)
12. Sitting (trunk righted with buttocks as base of support; head up)
  - Size of the base (long sit, cross sit, hands for support when sitting)
  - Length of time that one can sit
  - Sitting on different objects (floor, chair, other objects)

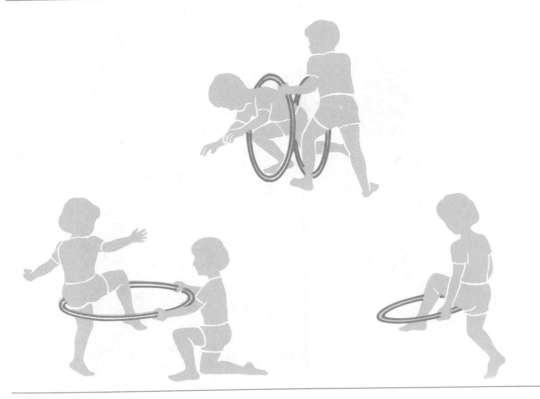

FIGURE 6-2
Activities that may develop an understanding of spatial relationships.

13. Kneeling
    - Amount of support (two hands, one hand, no hands)
    - Movement (distance over time)
    - Length of time in a kneel/standing position
14. Standing
    - Amount of support (two hands, one hand, no hands)
    - Length of time to stand
    - Stand and reach (how high tips of the fingers are from ground)
15. Walking
    - Distance
    - Distance over time
    - Number of steps over a specified distance
    - Amount of support (hand support on a rail, number of hand supports over a specified distance)
    - Width of the pathway of travel
16. Stair-climbing
    - Height of the step
    - Alternate versus mark-time pattern
    - Rate of stair-climbing
    - Number of steps
    - Size of the pathway of travel
17. Hand-eye coordination
    - Place object in a box (size of object, size of box, number of placements over time)
    - Block stacking (number that can be stacked)
    - String beads (number strung over time)
    - Placing pegs in holes (number placed over time)
    - Pick up tiny objects (number secured over time)
18. Walking
    - Up and down inclines (slope of the incline)
    - Walk on footprints (distance and placement of prints and number of steps over time)
    - Walking through an obstacle course (number of seconds to travel the course)
19. Running
    - Distance over time
    - Run backward (distance over time)
    - Run up incline (distance over time)
    - Run a maze (distance over time)

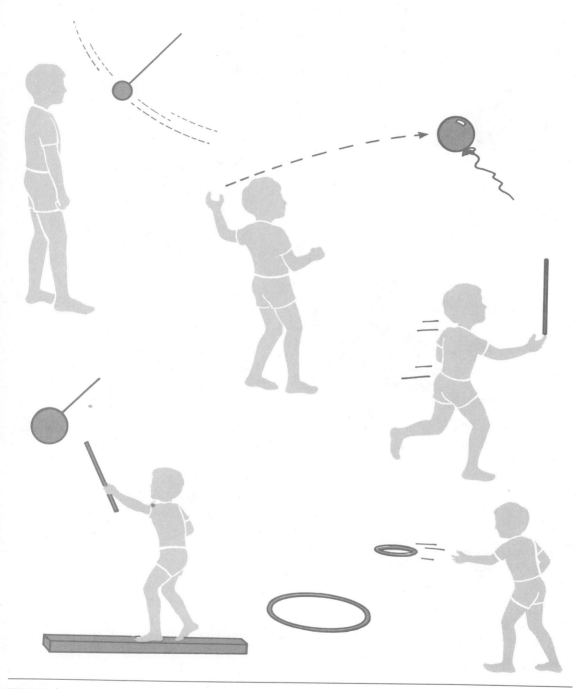

FIGURE 6-3
Activities that contribute to the development of visual systems.

Continued.

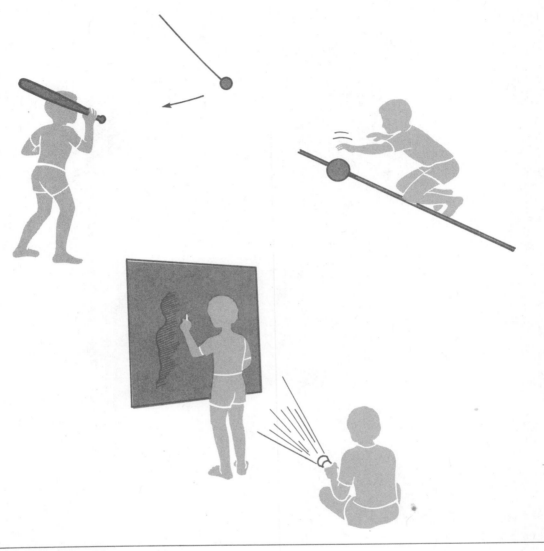

FIGURE 6-3—cont'd
Activities that contribute to the development of visual systems.

20. Jumping
    - Distance of jump
    - Distance and height of jump
    - Distance in a series of three jumps
    - Distance of jump from a raised platform
    - Jump and reach (height)
    - Rope jumping (repetitions over time, number of jumps without a miss, length of rope)

21. Hopping
    - One hop for distance
    - Two hops for distance
    - Nonpreferred and preferred
    - Hop through an obstacle course (distance over time)

22. Sliding (number of slides, repetitions over time; see side straddle test)

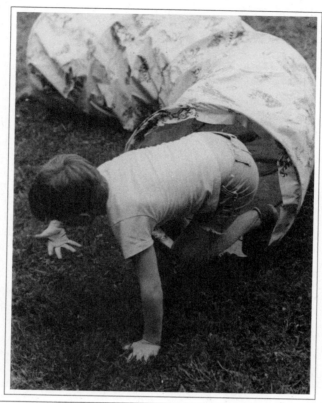

FIGURE 6-4
A child must have spatial relationship abilities to fit the body through the circular tunnel.

23. Stretching
   • Reach over head on wall (inches from ground)
   • Bend at waist (distance in inches fingertips are from the floor or are below floor level; stand on object if fingertips touch floor)
   • Stretch backward (distance chin is from wall)
24. Twist and turn
   • Bend at waist, touch floor, straighten, twist, and touch target shoulder height in rear (repetitions over time)
   • Twist trunk laterally, twist 180 degrees in opposite direction (repetitions over time)
25. Pushing
   • Push-ups (repetitions)
   • Push-ups (repetitions over time)
   • Propel self forward on scooter board (distance over time, distance in one thrust, distance in three thrusts)
26. Pulling
   • Chin-up (repetitions)

   • Rope climb (distance over time)
   • Pull an object attached to a rope (weight of object, distance over time)
27. Galloping (same foot leads on each step)
   • Number of gallops over a specified distance
   • Number of gallops it takes to get to a specified distance
   • Distance traveled in a number of specified gallops
   • Width of a path in which one can gallop
28. Skipping (alternate step-hop action with each foot; weight shifts forward with step; arms move in opposition)
   • Number of skips without error
   • Distance traveled with a specified number of skips
   • Number of skips to travel a specified distance
   • Number of skips in rhythm to music
29. Leaping (push forward with support leg and catch with opposite leg; alternate arm action during leap)
   • Distance one can leap
   • Height one can leap

30. Rolling a ball
    - Position (sit, kneel, stand, run)
    - Toward a target (varies in size)
    - With two hands versus one hand
    - Roll the ball for distance
    - Vary the size of the ball (the bigger, the more difficult)
31. Throwing
    - Size of ball (the bigger, the more difficult)
    - Pattern (underhand, side arm, overarm)
    - Distance
    - Throw for a moving versus a stationary target
    - Nature of the object (beanbag versus ball)
32. Bouncing a ball
    - Two hands versus one hand
    - Small ball more difficult than large ball
    - Continuous bounce more difficult than single bounce
    - Walk and bounce more difficult than stand and bounce
    - Dribbling around cones more difficult than no constraints on dribble
    - Bouncing ball low more difficult than high
    - More dribbles more difficult than fewer dribbles
33. Catching
    - Positions (standing, sitting)
    - Adjustment of hands to the ball (chest high is easiest)
    - Large balls easier to catch than small balls
    - Catching from a shorter distance easier than from a farther distance
    - The higher the ball, the more difficult to catch
    - The farther the player must run, the more difficult
    - Catching while moving more difficult than catching when standing
34. Making striking activities more or less difficult
    - Body position (sit, kneel, stand, moving)
    - Size of object
    - Size of implement (bat, wider bat, paddle)
    - Speed of object (suspended, thrown from greater distance, and speeds)
    - Accuracy of hit (at different size targets)
    - Position of object (greater deviations from shoulder level and across middle of plate)
    - Holding the implement (two hands or one)
35. Making kicking activities more or less difficult
    - Contact of foot with object (arch, toe, instep)
    - Foot (preferred versus nonpreferred foot)
    - Kick the ball a greater distance
    - Kick the ball more accurately
    - Kick the ball while it approaches at varying speeds
    - Kick the ball while it travels at different positions in space
    - Kick the ball while (standing versus running)
    - Dribbling a ball

- Receiving a pass
- Making a pass
36. Bending
    - Direction (forward, backward, sideways, rotation)
    - Body part (trunk, shoulder, hip)
    - Rate of speed

Instructional Strategies

Instructional strategies are the ways to arrange an educational environment so that maximum learning will take place. Factors that affect the type of instructional strategy selected include levels of performance demonstrated by individual students in the class, age of the learners, comprehension levels of the students, class size, and number of people available to assist the teacher. An instructional strategy that meets the needs of a wide range of learners and can be delivered by a limited number of personnel is more valuable for ensuring that individual needs are met than is a strategy that presumes homogeneous grouping. For handicapped learners with heterogeneous needs an instructional strategy that promotes individualized learning is not only desirable, but absolutely necessary.

Individualization of instruction can be realized through the use of programmed instruction. The major goals of programmed instruction are to promote students' ability to direct their own learning and to develop a communication system between the student and teacher that enables them to become independent of each other. The teacher's primary goals are to guide and manage instruction according to the student's individual needs and learning characteristics. The programmed instruction approach enables a teacher to cope with heterogeneous groups of children and to accommodate large numbers of children in the same class without sacrificing instructional efficiency.

To implement such a program, however, three major factors must be taken into consideration: (1) programming must be constructed on the basis of scientific principles[1]; (2) learners must be trained in specific behaviors[2]; and (3) learning principles must be applied through the use of programmed curricula.

The most expeditious way to manage an aver-

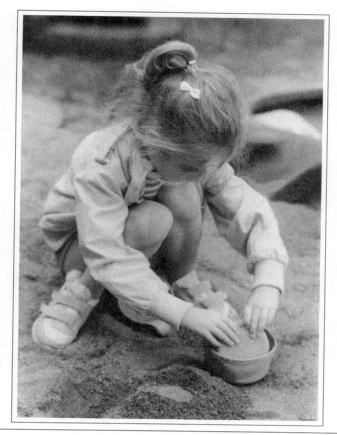

FIGURE 6-5
Tipping a bowl of sand into another container aids development of the visual system.

age size class in a public school, using the individualized developmental approach, is by means of instructional objectives that shift learning conditions to create developmental task sequences. Prearranged instructional objectives take the form of self-instructional and self-evaluative programs appropriate for typical and atypical children. However, for the child who cannot self-instruct and self-evaluate, task analysis and pattern analysis will facilitate development. A child functioning at a low level, like a child who strives to reach upper limits of development for competitive purposes, needs special types of programming and thus specific attention by instructors when the teacher-student ratio is low. Self-instructional and self-evaluative materials composed of prearranged objectives help students to develop skills at their own rates.

Principles of Programmed Instruction

An adapted list of characteristics for programmed instruction has been suggested by Lindvall and Bolvin[3]:

1. Definition of the objectives the students are expected to achieve must be clear and specific.
2. Objectives must be stated in behavioral terms.
3. Objectives must lead to behaviors that are carefully analyzed and sequenced in a hierarchical order so that each behavior builds on the objectives immediately pre-

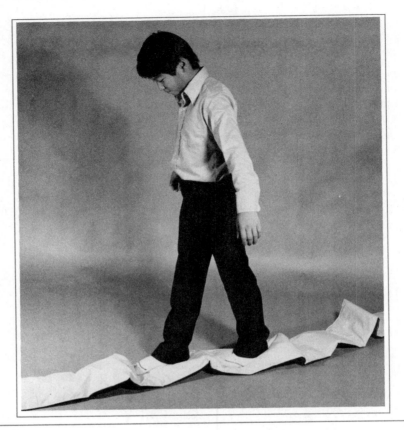

FIGURE 6-6
If the child moves the left arm so it is opposite the right leg, he is performing cross-lateral walking. *(Courtesy Achievement Products, Incorporated.)*

ceding and is prerequisite to those which follow.

4. Instructional content of a program must consist of a sequence of learning tasks through which a student can proceed with little outside help and must provide a series of small increments in learning that enable the student to proceed from a condition of lack of command of behavior to a condition of command of behavior.

5. A program must permit the student to begin at the present ability level and allow him or her to move upward from that point.

6. A program must allow each student to pro-

ceed independently of other students and learn at a rate best suited to his or her own abilities and interests.

7. A program must require active involvement and response on the part of the student at each step along the learning sequence.

8. A program must provide immediate feedback to the student concerning the adequacy of his or her performance.

9. A program must be subjected to continuous study by those responsible for it and should be regularly modified in light of available evidence concerning the student's performance.

10. A program must accommodate the ability range of many students, thus enabling continuous progress.

These principles can be applied when a hierarchical behavioral program is designed for each child. When using a hierarchical teaching sequence, a single task is broken down into small steps that are then arranged in order of difficulty. Pupils enter the sequence at their present level of performance and then advance at their own rate through the sequence. This sequencing of steps can be used for basic input systems abilities and skills. As children master one level of performance, they move on to the next. It is essential that the steps be arranged in a hierarchy or it will not be possible for the students to progress from simple to more difficult levels of performance.

Progressively more difficult performance standards are built in to the program by shifting either the conditions under which the task must be performed or the criteria for success. Condition shifting alters the conditions surrounding performance of the task. For example, in bowling, conditions such as the performer's distance from the pins, the distance apart that the pins are set, and the size of the ball can be changed to make the task more or less difficult. Criterion shifting alters the level of acceptable performance by increasing the number of repetitions, the distance traveled, the speed, or the range of motion needed to accomplish the task. Examples of shifting criterion measures are building strength by increasing the number of repetitions or amount of weight lifted, building cardiovascular endurance by increasing the distance run, and building flexibility by increasing the range of motion at a specific joint.

Once the teacher has decided whether to use a criterion- or condition-shifting program (or a combination of both), the teaching sequence should be decided on. There are several different strategies for developing standard teaching sequences. A standard procedure often used is as follows:

1. Select a behavior that needs to be developed (identify a long-range goal).
2. Identify a way to measure the behavior objectively.

3. Select the conditions or criteria that will be used to make the task more difficult.
4. Write your short-term objectives.
5. Arrange the short-term objectives in a hierarchy from simple to difficult.
6. Identify the materials or equipment that will be needed in the teaching sequence.

Examples of two teaching sequences—one using a shifting criterion and one using a shifting condition—are found in the box on pp. 118 and 119. These examples focus on specific skills. The same type of teaching sequence can be developed for basic levels and for abilities. When programming to develop basic levels, such as vestibular function, activities believed to facilitate that system are selected and arranged in a hierarchy. For example, the teacher may decide to use activities such as rolling, turning, or spinning to stimulate the vestibular system. A technique for determining whether the activities have been useful for activating the system could be duration of nystagmus immediately after the activity. A sequence of short-term objectives might be 3 seconds of nystagmus after 30 seconds of spinning, 3 seconds of nystagmus following 25 seconds of spinning, 3 seconds of nystagmus after 20 seconds of spinning, and so on until the child demonstrates nystagmus for half the spinning time (that is, 3 seconds of nystagmus after 6 seconds of spinning). The next step in the sequence would be to increase the amount of time nystagmus is demonstrated (that is, 5 seconds of nystagmus following 30 seconds of spinning). The sequence is continued until the child reaches the normally expected duration of nystagmus (10 seconds of nystagmus after 20 seconds of turning at a speed of 180 degrees per second.)

When programming for abilities, the same format is used. If the need to develop cross-lateral integration has been identified, an objective measure of this ability would be decided on such as percent of time the student uses the right hand to pick up objects on the left side of the body. A criterion- or condition-shifting sequence would be constructed, and activities to promote the behavior would be selected.

Whenever possible, the teaching strategy

The system requires only that the teacher note the child's progress using the following symbols: × = the steps (activities) in the standard teaching sequence that can be mastered by the student, in this case step nos. 1, 2, 3, and 4; / = immediate short-term instruction objective, in this case no. 5;* = goal, in this case no. 18. All behaviors between the present level (/) and the goal (*) are potential objectives (6 to 18).

11.1.35 Walks unsupported (step no.): 1̶ 2̶ 3̶ 4̶ 5̶ 6 7 8 9 10 11 12 13 14 15 16 17 18* 19 20 21 22 23 24 25 26

Two-footed standing broad jump

Type of program: Shifting criterion
Conditions
   1. Both feet remain behind restraining line before takeoff.
   2. Takeoff from two feet.
   3. Land on two feet.
   4. Measure from the restraining line to the tip of the toe of the least advanced foot.
Measurement: Distance in inches.

Two-footed standing broad jump (inches)	60	62	64	6̶6̶	6̶8̶	7̶0̶	7̶2̶	74	76	78	80	82*	84
Date mastered				9/7	9/21	10/5							

The scoring procedure of the ongoing development of the person would be explained as follows. The program that the child is participating in is the two-footed standing broad jump. The child began the program at an initial performance level of 66 inches on September 7 and increased performance by 4 inches between September 7 and October 5. Thus the present level of educational performance is 70 inches (note the last number with an X over it). The child will attempt to jump a distance of 72 inches (immediate short-term objective) until he or she masters that distance. The child will continue to progress toward the goal, which is 82 inches (note the asterisk). It is a mistake in the applications of learning principles to ask the child to jump the 82 inches when it is known that the goal far exceeds the present level of educational performance. Unreasonable instructional demands from the learner by the teacher violate the principle of learning in small steps, which guarantees success for the child.

The same procedure could be used when teaching a child to throw a ball for accuracy. In the following example, a shifting condition program is used. For instance, two hierarchies that are known in throwing for accuracy are the size of the target and the distance between the thrower and the target. Thus a standard teaching sequence might be similar to the following sequence of potential objectives: demonstrate the ability to throw a 4-inch ball a distance of _____ feet and hit a target that is _____ feet square five out of five times.

Throwing for accuracy

Type of program: Shifting condition
Conditions
   1. Remain behind the restraining line at all times.
   2. Complete an overhand throw (ball released above the shoulder).
   3. If the ball hits any part of the target, it is a successful throw.

STANDARD TEACHING SEQUENCE—cont'd

The previous information would be contained in a curriculum book. However, the specific standard teaching sequence would be placed on a bulletin board at the performance area in the gymnasium. This would enable the performer to read his or her own instructional objective. The measurement of the performer's placement in the standard teaching sequence would be indicated on the prescription sheet.

Criterion for mastery: Three successful hits out of three.

DISTANCE OF THROW	SIZE OF TARGET	DISTANCE OF THROW	SIZE OF TARGET
1. 6'	3' square	10. 18'	2' square
2. 9'	3' square	11. 21'	2' square
3. 12'	3' square	12. 24'	2' square
4. 15'	3' square	13. 27'	2' square
5. 18'	3' square	14. 30'	2' square
6. 21'	3' square	15. 21'	1' square
7. 24'	3' square	16. 24'	1' square
8. 27'	3' square	17. 27'	1' square
9. 30'	3' square	18. 30'	1' square

STUDENT RECORDING SHEET

The steps of the standard teaching sequence can be reduced and tasks can be added that are more or less complex as the situation requires.

Throwing for accuracy (step No.)	1̶	2̶	3̶	4̶	5̶	6	7	8	9	10	11	12	13	14*	15	16	17	18
Date mastered																		

should be as self-directed as possible. If children are not able to read written instructions, pictures or figures that represent the action to be performed should be included in the lesson.

Values of Preplanned Activities

The preplanned activities from task analysis and programmed instruction enable adequate monitoring for a handicapped child's progress throughout the school year because of the specificity of what is to be taught.[8] Furthermore, preplanned activities enable the parent to take part in the process.[4] There are several distinct ways in which preplanned activities help children learn. Programmed instructional objectives function as follows:

♦ They assist teachers with evaluation of the curriculum so that it may be revised to facilitate the child's learning at a subsequent time.

♦ They structure behavior so that there are interrelationships between activities. This facilitates development.

♦ They can introduce scientific validity to curriculum materials. This enhances accountability and assists refinement of measures that indicate the child's educational progress.

♦ They enable employment of procedures that

indicate limits of the child's current functioning on a specific task.

♦ They provide opportunities for the child to become a self-directed learner and to have an IEP in the regular class without undue attention.

♦ They enable a comparison between where the child is in the sequence and where the child should be based on chronological age expectancies.

♦ They provide information about the strengths and weaknesses of the child so that relevant instructional decisions can be made to meet unique needs.

♦ They enable communication with the parents so that instructional programming may be continued in the home.

♦ They free the teacher from curriculum construction so that he or she can manage individualized instruction.

♦ They facilitate the monitoring of the instructional delivery system.

♦ They enable evaluation of instructional technique through knowledge of measurable learning outcomes.

♦ They enable the child to progress continuously when the instructional setting is changed and facilitate the coordination of efforts between the physical educator and those who provide related services.

♦ They guide the revision process when changes are made in the IEP.

♦ They expedite the attainment of goals of the IEP.

♦ They assist with appropriate allocation of responsibility, time, facilities, and other resources among professionals.

♦ They enable placement of the handicapped child in a regular class where he or she can work independently on the IEP.

♦ They enable the systematic application of principles of learning to behavioral analysis.

REPORTING THE RESULTS TO PARENTS

Parents should always be informed of their children's educational performance levels and the goals and objectives of the school curricula. P.L. 94-142 requires that the parents be apprised of the educational status of their children and approve the IEP that has been designed for them. When the procedures described in this chapter are followed by the teacher and the information shared with the parents, there will be no question about the educational process. Parents may question whether appropriate goals have been selected for their children; but usually, when evaluation results and the importance of their child achieving as normal a performance level as possible are explained, parents agree with the professional educator's opinion.

It is important to point out to the parents their child's specific deficiencies and how those deficiencies interfere with the child's functional ability. Wherever possible, basic level and ability deficiencies should be linked to skill performance. That is, the educator should explain not only what deficits exist, but how those deficits relate to the child's present and future levels of performance ability. Once parents understand these relationships, they usually endorse the school's efforts on behalf of their children. In addition to pointing out a child's deficiencies, it is important to tell the parent about areas of strength their child has demonstrated. Parents of handicapped children need to hear positive reports as frequently as possible. Do not overlook that need.

SUMMARY

Present levels of educational performance are the functional capabilities of a student along a developmental continuum at a particular point in time. Determining present levels of performance is necessary before goals and objectives for the student can be determined. Standardized normative- and criterion-referenced tests may be helpful in deciding whether a child is in need of a specialized program; however, content-referenced assessment such as task analysis or hierarchical analysis is necessary to determine the precise levels at which a student is functioning. Once a student's levels of functioning are determined, goals and objectives are agreed on and activities that lead to their attainment are selected. A teaching sequence that permits ongoing measurement is designed. Shifting criterion and condition programs that are carefully sequenced enables constant measurement of progress. All this information and the importance of this process should be explained to parents.

REVIEW QUESTIONS

1. How are unique needs in physical education determined?
2. How are present levels of performance determined through administration of domain-referenced standardized tests?
3. How does one determine a present level of educational performance through task analysis of a skill that is to be taught to a student?
4. What is a prerequisite analysis and how is it used to determine present levels of performance for a child?
5. Provide examples of hierarchies in tasks that can increase or decrease difficulty of the task.
6. What are the types of measures that can be incorporated into the instructional process? Provide examples of each.
7. Describe the interrelationships of the components of the instructional process of the IEP.
8. Construct an instructional objective.
9. Provide an example of a deficient prerequisite that can be observed in a specific sport skill.
10. What is the difference between determining a present level of performance during skill acquisition and during the performance phase?
11. Evaluate the constructional effectiveness of a behavioral shaping program.
12. Find your present level of performance in a hierarchical behavioral shaping program.
13. What are the different types of behavioral programs in which present levels can be determined?
14. Describe a standard teaching sequence/hierarchical behavioral program.
15. How can behavioral programs of abilities be used with the top, down and bottom, up approaches?
16. How can one determine a present level of performance in a cardiovascular fitness program?
17. How does one determine the fitness level in the Cooper Aerobic Program?
18. How are present levels of performance determined on social behaviors?

STUDENT ACTIVITIES

1. Use a combination of normative-referenced and content-referenced data to develop an individualized program of activities to meet the unique needs of a hypothetical child.
2. With a hypothetical data base from domain-referenced tests that have norms, determine the specific activities that would constitute a physical education program.
3. Perform a task analysis of a sport skill.
4. Assess a real or hypothetical learner who has a deficient teachable component of a task-analyzed skill.
5. Use a hierarchical behavioral program to instruct a student and plot his progress.
6. Plot the progress of a learner in the acquisition phase of a skill that has been task analyzed.
7. Write an exercise prescription from present levels of performance for a person in a cardiovascular fitness program.

REFERENCES

1. Bellamy, T., Peterson, L., and Close, D.: Habilitation of the severely and profoundly retarded: illustrations of competence, Educ. Train. Ment. Retard. **10**(3):174-186, 1975.
2. Gold, M.: Task analysis: a statement and example using acquisition and production of a complex task by the retarded blind, University of Illinois at Urbana-Champaign, 1975, Institute for Child Behavior and Development.
3. Lindvall, C.M., and Bolvin, J.D.: Programmed instruction in the schools: an application of programming principles in individually prescribed instruction, Sixty-sixth Yearbook of the National Society of the Study of Education, Chicago, 1967, University of Chicago Press.

SUGGESTED READINGS

Bellamy, T.: Habilitation for the severely handicapped, Baltimore, Md., 1979, Paul H. Brookes Publishing Co.
Gold, M.: Did I say that? Champaign, Ill., 1983, Research Press.
Mager, R.: Preparing instructional objectives, ed. 2, Belmont, Calif., 1975, Fearon Publishers.
Snell, M.: Educating severely handicapped children, Columbus, Ohio, 1983, Charles E. Merrill Publishing Co.
Taber, J., Glasser, R., and Schaefer, H.: Learning and programmed instruction, Reading, Mass., 1965, Addison-Wesley Publishing Co.

CHAPTER 7

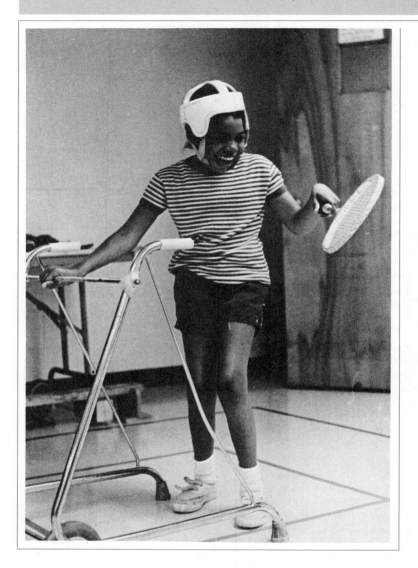

Facilitating Learning

OBJECTIVES

♦ Know how to use "bottom, up" and "top, down" teaching techniques in connection with the areas of growth and development, generalization process, control of sensory inputs, nature of activity and quality of experience, training regimens, motivating children, and managing the instructional environment.

♦ Know the procedures for planned behavioral intervention.

♦ Know how to collect data when observing behaviors.

♦ Know a variety of positive intervention strategies.

♦ Know how to eliminate behaviors using positive and negative methods.

♦ Know how to construct a contingency management program.

♦ Know how to apply principles of learning to instructional objectives.

The benefit of physical education programs can be maximized if acceptable principles of learning and development are applied to instruction. Teachers of handicapped children bear the responsibility for ensuring that learning takes place. In the past, teachers often were assigned to handicapped children on the basis of tolerance or because they enjoyed working with children with disabilities. The physical education programs that teachers designed often focused on the children's enjoyment of them. If the children appeared to be having a good time, the teacher was judged to be effective. Since the advent of P.L. 94-142, the qualifications for teachers of handicapped learners have changed dramatically. Now these teachers not only must enjoy their work, but they must also be masterful at designing educational environments that promote maximum learning.

Teachers of handicapped learners must be able to test children, interpret test results, write appropriate long-range goals and short-term objectives that lead to those goals, and apply principles of learning, development, and behavioral strategies that contribute to classroom learning. In addition to these skills, the teacher provides patterns of behavior for the child to copy. From their teachers, immature children learn how the environment works and how persons cope with changing environments.

These teachers must be emotionally stable, flexible, and empathetic toward atypical behavior while encouraging learning. To best understand what the handicapped child is experiencing, teachers must be sensitive enough to perceive the importance of even the slightest change in the child's behavior. This degree of understanding provides a medium through which a child may better understand his or her own behavior and then modify it. This is no easy task. Being in contact with anxiety-provoking persons often stretches the teacher's emotional capacities.

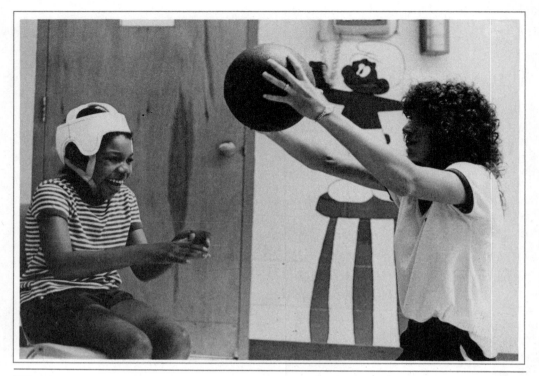

FIGURE 7-1
An instructor uses behavioral techniques to communicate with a handicapped child. *(Courtesy Verland Foundation, Inc.)*

Some of the behaviors that teachers often tolerate are implied rejection from the child and conflicting demands from the child, which range from demanding that immediate needs be met to severe withdrawal, aggressive tactics, and immature behavior.

Teachers who work with normally developing children may be unaccustomed to the many behaviors demonstrated by handicapped students. To succeed, teachers must understand and accept the behavior patterns of atypical children while designing and implementing programs that ensure learning progress. The best defense a teacher has is knowledge of what is occurring coupled with teaching and behavioral strategies to move the child beyond present levels of educational performance.

PRINCIPLES OF DEVELOPMENT

There are several universally accepted principles of development, which are based on the study of normal children. These principles are generally independent of child-rearing practices and cultural influences and are valuable aids to understanding the motor sequences through which a child should pass. Although these rules cannot be used categorically, the principles do provide guidelines in programming for handicapped children. The physical educator who understands expected normal physical and motor sequences should be capable of determining where to begin an intervention program for handicapped children who demonstrate developmental delays.

Cephalocaudal

Gross motor control starts with head control and progresses down the axial skeleton to the feet. When control of the cervical region of the spine develops, head control in the prone position results. After acquiring control of the thoracic spine, the developing child can sit. During the fifth, sixth, and seventh months control of the lumbar spine should occur. Then, during the eighth to fourteenth months, control of the hips and knees is acquired.

Proximal-Distal

The principle of proximal-distal development implies that body parts closest to the midline develop first, followed by development of the shoulders, elbows, wrists, and then fingers.

General to Specific

Motor development progresses from mass undifferentiated movements, which to some degree are controlled by reflex activity, to specific voluntary motor control. The young infant responds to stimuli with a whole-body reaction. As the neuromuscular system matures, individual body parts can be controlled.

Bilateral to Unilateral to Cross-Lateral

The three stages of development that involve integration of the two sides of the body are as follows:

1. Bilateral—movement patterns in which both limbs move simultaneously
2. Unilateral—use of the limbs on one side of the body in unison, such as moving the right leg and arm simultaneously during creeping or crawling
3. Cross-lateral—use of body parts on opposite sides of the body in unison, such as swinging the right leg and left arm simultaneously when walking

Gross Motor to Fine Motor

The individual gains control over large muscles before small muscles. For example, gross-motor behavior such as striking, which involves primarily the shoulder and elbow, would develop before skills such as cutting or pasting, which require fine motor control.

Inhibition of Primitive Reflexes

Primitive reflexes appear in the process of development and facilitate early motor behaviors such as head and thorax control, rolling from front to back (and vice versa), and grasping. As the central nervous system matures, these reflexes are overridden by higher levels of the central nervous system, which control voluntary movement.

Postural Reflexes

As the primitive reflexes begin to fade, a series of automatic reactions develops that enables the child to maintain equilibrium while standing, walking, and running. Postural reflex development is believed to be closely associated with maturation of the vestibular mechanism in the inner ear. The development of postural reflexes and the vestibular system ensures the individual's ability to remain upright while executing volitional motor patterns and specific motor skills.

Continuity of Development

For the normal individual, development is a continuous process. However, the process is contingent on environmental opportunities to move about freely in a variety of conditions and the absence of pathological conditions.

Uniformity of Sequence

The sequence of development is the same in all normal children, but the rate of development varies from child to child.

Unity of Development

Development is a unified process with intellectual, physical, motor, perceptual, emotional, and social aspects intricately interrelated. If any one aspect is impaired, it may affect other aspects and interfere with the total development of the individual.

APPLICATION OF DEVELOPMENTAL THEORY

The application of the principles of development is most relevant to children at preschool ages; however, children up through the age of 12 years who demonstrate developmental delays are known to respond to application of these principles. It is widely accepted that at no time is the central nervous system more pliable than during the preschool years. Thus children who can benefit most rapidly from the application of these principles are normal preschool children, handicapped infants, and mentally retarded children who have not developed beyond preschool chronological norms.

Curriculum models have been developed from theories of growth and development. Such models are widely used in medical and therapeutic practices. It has been a traditional view that a child who expresses maldevelopment may be handicapped. Therefore a traditional procedure is to study the child in light of models of growth and development and intervene with activity at that point in the developmental process where the deficiencies occur. Indeed, knowledge of growth and development has given rise to many intervention theories by clinical practitioners, such as Kabat,[13] who formulated a system known as proprioceptive neuromuscular facilitation, Bobath,[5] and Brunstrom.[6] Theorists who tend to be more educationally oriented than medically oriented include Ayres,[3] Kephart,[15] and Getman.[9] Two theorists who have combined the medical and educational viewpoints are deQuiros and Schrager.[7]

Although there is agreement in principle among the various growth and development studies, there is considerable debate about effective systematic methods for converting these principles into practice. Since the advent of P.L. 94-142, there has been an increasing interest in application of these theories in school settings. Use of these theories may be appropriate with some children; however, their use with severely handicapped persons has been seriously challenged.[4,18,21] The empirical evidence from research raises serious questions as to the applicability of these principles to *all* children. For example, Winnick[22] studied the physical performance of orthopedically handicapped children ages 12 to 17 years. Even though these children received special education and related services under P.L. 94-142, the results of the indicated study measured regression, not development, of physical performance.

During puberty physically handicapped children have accelereated increases in body size and weight that is out of proportion to gains in strength, flexibility, endurance, and motor fitness required to control the body. As a result of these physical changes, regression of acquired development may occur. Dramatic regression was revealed in the *Armstrong v. Kline* litigation.[2] This court case revealed that adolescent handicapped students suffered such a loss of skill over a summer layoff from school that they could not recoup the loss after returning in the fall. As a result of their inability to regain their losses, they were denied educational benefits altogether.

Certain ideas, such as continuity of development, uniformity of sequence, and the concept of readiness, need to be reconsidered during the development of an IEP. Individuals who have severe disabilities that interfere with systematic development may need task-specific programming. This is not to say that these principles cannot be applied to the physical education curriculum for many handicapped children. Each principle must be selectively applied to the individual education program for each child. Only through careful monitoring of each child's progress will it become apparent whether the child is responding to application of the principle.

Careful research into the ages and types of children who can benefit from application of the principles of growth and development is still needed. The art of evaluating developmental delays and selecting appropriate intervention strategies for children with handicapping conditions is still in its infancy. We agree that the application of the principles of development is appropriate for most children; however, task analysis of functional skills is the most appropriate alternative strategy to use with school-age severely handicapped individuals. Several developmental principles and their educational implications are outlined in Tables 7-1 to 7-7. Also included are the teaching strategies for a physical educator who uses a bottom, up approach; these are contrasted with strategies that would be used in a top, down approach.

BEHAVIORAL TECHNOLOGY
Application and Use

Applying behavioral technology in the education of handicapped learners involves use of learning theory, operant conditioning, and precise objectives.[22] Behavioral technology structures the environment to produce changes in pupil behavior; this allows maximum learning to take place. The strategies and procedures have two purposes: to manage disruptive behavior and to reach the objectives specified on the IEP. The general process is the same in both instances; however, certain techniques are effective for managing disruptive behavior, whereas others are more beneficial in step-by-step learning of motor skills.

Behavior Management

The physical education teacher should establish learning environments that permit students to be productive. The environment must be arranged to facilitate skill learning and discourage disruptive behavior. Disruptive behavior by one student interferes with that student's learning as well as that of the others in the class. In such cases the teacher must design a learning environment that makes each student feel accepted when following the guidelines for acceptable behavior. Usually, if students are informed of the guidelines for behavioral management, they will accept them if they are applied fairly, equally, and consistently.

There are several strategies physical education teachers can use to manage classroom behavior; however, the most effective intervention programs are based on student performance data. A data-based system helps students control their behavior, learn new behaviors, and maintain appropriate behaviors. The data-based system involves a systematic process that (1) identifies specific behaviors, (2) analyzes the student behavior to determine any discrepancy between present behavior and desired behavior, and (3) implements interventions when necessary.

A step-by-step strategy the teacher should follow to improve behavior is listed below:

1. Identify a specific (target) behavior.
2. Select an observation system and collect baseline data on the behavior.
3. Analyze the data to determine the need for an intervention program.
4. If data indicate the need for an intervention program, select or design an intervention program that uses the most positive approach.
5. Implement the intervention program.
6. Collect data on student performance.
7. Analyze the data to determine the need to continue, modify, or terminate the intervention.
8. Take the required action.
9. When the behavior reaches the desired level and is no longer dependent on intervention, continue to collect maintenance data and return to step 4.

Identifying Specific Target Behaviors

When identifying specific behaviors, observe students as they perform. Whether the behavior involves performance on learning tasks or disruptive actions, the data collected must be precise. Precision is accomplished when the behavior is carefully defined in objective terms that can be measured. If the behavior is clearly stated, two or more observers can agree on whether the student has performed the behavior.

Collecting Baseline Data

When collecting baseline data, it is necessary first to select a measurement system and then decide who will observe and how often. Several measuring systems are available for collecting and re-

Text continued on p. 134.

TABLE 7-1
Growth and development principles

Principle	Implication	Bottom, Up Teaching Approach	Top, Down Teaching Approach
Each individual is unique.	Every child has a different motor profile.	Test for sensory input deficits and intervene to eliminate those before testing and programming for higher level abilities and skills.	Test for specific functional motor skill deficits. If some are found, probe down into specific abilities that contribute to those skills. If deficits are found, probe down into sensory input areas.
	Every child learns at his/her own rate.	Select activities that appeal to the child and use those until the deficits are eliminated.	Program activities at the highest level of dysfunction. If the child does not learn quickly, probe down into contributing components for deficits.
Children advance from one stage of development to a higher, more complex stage of development.	Activities are selected appropriate to level of development.	Select activities that are appropriate for the stage of development the child demonstrates.	Select activities specific to the skill deficits the child demonstrates. Begin an intervention program at the developmental level the child demonstrates.
	Progression to the next stage of development depends on physiological maturation and learning.	When a child appears to have mastered one stage of development, select activities appropriate for the next level of development.	When a child masters lower levels of a specific skill, select activities to promote learning of a more complex aspect of that skill.
Children learn when they are ready.	As neurological maturation takes place, we are capable of learning more. There are critical periods of learning.	Test from the bottom up and begin instruction with the lowest neurological deficit found. It is assumed the child will learn fastest if instruction is begun at the developmental stage at which the child is functioning.	Analyze a specific task from the top down until present level of educational performance is found. Level of instruction determined by empirical testing verifies that the child is ready to learn.
Development proceeds from simple to complex.	Development begins with simple movements that eventually combine with other movements to form patterns.	Eliminate reflex and sensory input delays before teaching higher level abilities and skills.	Functional skill deficits are identified. The pattern of the skill is analyzed to determine contributing components. Behavioral programs are constructed and implemented to develop pattern deficits.
	Development progresses from large to small movements (from gross to fine patterns).	Promote reflex and vestibular development to stabilize balance. Once balance becomes automatic, control of the limbs will follow.	Program to synthesize patterns that contribute to a specific skill.

TABLE 7-2
Generalization process*

Principle	Implication	Bottom, Up Teaching Approach	Top, Down Teaching Approach
Generalization procedures	Activities to promote generalization are selected in particular ways.	Activity is selected to develop sensory input systems, reflexes, and abilities that are believed to be prerequisite to many skills that could be used in a variety of environments.	Functional age-appropriate activities are selected to promote appropriate skills in a variety of natural environments.
Generalization process	There is degree to which the learning environment matches the natural environment.	At the basic levels (reflexes, sensory inputs, and abilities) the environment is controlled only to ensure that the basics are learned. No attention is paid to the type of environment the eventual skills will be used in.	Skills are practiced in environments that correspond closely to the environment in which the skill will be used (e.g., practice shooting baskets in the gym).
Retention	The more meaningful the skill, the longer it is remembered.	It is believed that once basic reflexes, sensory input systems, and abilities emerge, they remain stable (unless the child is traumatized in some way).	Activities are reviewed immediately after a lesson and then periodically to ensure retention.
Overlearning	Overlearning occurs when a skill or activity is practiced after it has been learned.	Overlearning occurs as the basic levels are interwoven into higher skill levels.	Ability levels prerequisite to skills should be substantially greater than minimum entry requirements needed to fulfill the needs of the task.

*A task is not considered learned until it can be demonstrated in a variety of environments.

TABLE 7-3
Control of sensory input

Principle	Implication	Bottom, Up Teaching Approach	Top, Down Teaching Approach
Get the attention of the learner.	Help the child attend to relevant rather than irrelevant cues.	Permit the child to participate in a free activity of his or her choice each day if the child enters the room and immediately focuses on the beginning task.	Bats, balls, and other play equipment should be kept out of sight until time of use.
	Give a signal (sometimes called a "ready signal") that indicates a task is to begin.	Structure each day's lesson the same way so the child knows that when a given activity ends, the next activity will begin.	Teach the child precise signals that indicate a task should begin.
Provide the appropriate stimulation.	Stimulate the child to focus on the desired learning task.	Make the activities enjoyable so that the child will want to continue the task.	Use precise, detailed instruction that is designed around eliciting attention through the use of the following hierarchy: 1. Visual or verbal input only 2. Combine visual and verbal input 3. Combine visual, verbal, and kinesthetic instruction

TABLE 7-4
Nature of activity and quality of experience

Principle	Implication	Bottom, Up Teaching Approach	Top, Down Teaching Approach
Learning occurs best when goals and objectives are clear.	Clear goals provide incentives for children to learn.	The desired outcome is clear to the teacher (e.g., 5 seconds of postrotatory nystagmus). The child may be advised of another goal (e.g., stay on the spinning scooter until it stops).	The goal and ongoing measurement of the attainment of the objectives that lead to the goal are shared by the teacher and the child.
The student should be actively involved in the learning process.	The greater the amount of learning time and the lesser the amount of dead time, the more learning that will occur.	The child stays active because activities that are enjoyable to the child are selected.	When and if the child learns to self-instruct and self-evaluate or do so with the help of peer tutors, the student will be active throughout the period. The well-managed class will have children work on nonspecific activities when not participating in behavioral programs.

Principle	Implication	Bottom, Up Teaching Approach	Top, Down Teaching Approach
Discourage stereotyped play activities that develop rigid behaviors.	Permitting children to participate in the same activity day after day deters learning.	The teacher must initiate new activities as soon as lack of progress is evidenced.	The ongoing collection of data makes lack of progress immediately apparent to the teacher and the child and serves notice that the activity should be changed.
Program more for success than failure.	Every satisfying experience decreases anxiety and increases confidence.	The teacher selects activities the child enjoys and gains a feeling of accomplishment from.	The increment of the step sizes in the behavioral program is constantly modified to match the ability of the learner.

TABLE 7-5
Training regimens

Principle	Implication	Bottom, Up Teaching Approach	Top, Down Teaching Approach
Rate of learning is affected by initial skill level and length of time practicing the skill.	Beginning students who are learning a new skill learn at a faster rate than intermediate and advanced learners; however, plateaus in learning do occur after initial learning.	At reflex and sensory input levels plateaus may not be seen because learning is not cognitive. At ability levels (perceptual-motor, coordination, etc.) plateaus are apparent. The teacher will have to observe progress with care and change activities if plateaus are observed.	Plateaus will be identified immediately because of the precise data being collected. Provide rest bewen training trials and terminate activity before failure sets in.
The nature of the learner, the task, and the stage of the learner in learning the task must be considered.	Some research indicates that in the initial stages of motor learning distributed practice is more effective than mass practice[19]	Use specific time frames (e.g., 5 minutes) each day for each objective.	Highly organized lessons during which accurate data on progress are gathered provide immediate feedback about the effectiveness of the practice trials. When lack of progress becomes apparent, change the activity or the learning strategy.
Stop instruction at or before the point of satiation on the task.	Short practices are better than long practices. Frequent practices are more effective than infrequent practices. Plateauing occurs when a person is satiated with learning a task.	Divide the lesson plan into several activities. Provide activities for each objective daily or several times weekly. Selecting tasks that are novel may prevent satiation. Use a variety of activities to reach the same objective.	Monitor the increment of the step size carefully because as long as the learner can be reinforced with success on challenging tasks, the child may withstand satiation. Use a variety of different types of programs for the child to move to so that satiation is countered.

Continued.

TABLE 7-5
Training regimens—cont'd

Principle	Implication	Bottom, Up Teaching Approach	Top, Down Teaching Approach
Use the method of teaching that is best for the learner (whole, part, part-whole).	When the whole method is used, the entire task is taught at one time. Usually the task is demonstrated (using visual and verbal cues), and then the child is challenged to learn the skill.	When working toward reflex normality or when stimulating sensory input systems, the entire task is presented.	Use this method when teaching complex tasks. If a child has difficulty with any part of the task, shape the response through programming.
	When the part method is used, break the task down into component parts and teach the parts using backward or forward chaining. The part-whole method involves teaching the component parts of the skill and then synthesizing the parts into the whole skill.	When teaching toward perceptual-motor abilities (e.g. size discrimination), teach the child to recognize differences between sizes. When teaching toward perceptual-motor abilities such as size discrimination, after teaching the learner to discriminate between two or three different sets of sizes, combine the sets gradually until the child can discriminate between a large set of different sizes.	Break the skill into parts and teach each specific part. Because it is difficult to establish behaviors in which one is built on the other, divide the skill into natural divisions, teach each section, and then combine them.

TABLE 7-6
Motivating children

Principle	Implication	Bottom, Up Teaching Approach	Top, Down Teaching Approach
Children will learn better if the activity is pleasurable.	As a rule, children enjoy tasks at which they can be successful and dislike tasks where the failure risk is high.	Tasks that are enjoyable to children are selected to reach the specific objective.	Learning steps are sequenced close enough to ensure success.
Provide knowledge of results on task success.	Knowledge of results provides information to the learner as to the correctness of performance. Learners tend to persist at tasks they are successful with.	The students may or may not be advised about the specific objective the teacher is trying to reach; however, the child is advised about the objective to accomplish. Example: In trying to inhibit a positive support reflex, the teacher's objective may be to have the child demonstrate ability to flex the hips, knees, and ankles when	Precise objectives should be built into the behavioral program to provide immediate feedback as to whether the task was mastered.

Principle	Implication	Bottom, Up Teaching Approach	Top, Down Teaching Approach
Apply a system of reinforcement for attainment of objectives.	Reinforcement strengthens the recurrence of behavior.	there is pressure on the bottom of the feet. The child may be told that the objective is to stop bouncing on the trampoline 3 out of 5 times on command by doing a partial squat when the feet hit the bed of the trampoline. The teacher tells the child when he or she has done a good job.	Specific behaviors in a structured hierarchy are reinforced when the behavior occurs because the learner then progresses to the next step in the hierarchy. Social conditions will be directed toward the generalizaton of social behavior that exists in natural environments.
The social context of learning should be considered.	Learning is influenced by the presence or absence of others. Each student is influenced in some way by competition/cooperation with peers and the presence or absence of spectators or the teacher.	The child is made to feel as comfortable as possible so that the activity is enjoyable. It is believed that when the child feels successful, he or she will want to engage in play/competition with peers.	

TABLE 7-7
Managing the instructional environment

Principle	Implication	Bottom, Up Teaching Approach	Top, Down Teaching Approach
Impose limits for use of equipment, facilities, and student conduct.	Children should learn to adhere to rules that are necessary in social contexts.	Students are not permitted access to equipment and areas unless they have been given permission by the teacher.	The equipment and facilities a student has access to are specified in the behavioral program.
Control the social interaction among children.	Inappropriate social behavior among children may disrupt class instruction.	The teacher must consider the performance level and emotional stability of each child when grouping children for activities.	Tasks and environments are structured to reduce adverse interaction with peers.
Do not strive for control in all situations.	Handicapped children must develop social skills that will promote social interaction in the natural environment. For this to occur, students must have an opportunity to adjust to situations independent from supervision or with minimum supervision.	Select activities that will meet the long-range goals of the students and promote social interaction. Pair children so that their interaction contributes to both students' objectives. Example: A child who needs kinesthetic stimulation might be given the task of pulling a child who needs to ride a scooter for tonic labyrinthine prone inhibition.	Permit the students to interact with others as long as progress toward short-term objectives is occurring.

cording behavior: Some of those systems are described below:

- *Permanent product recording*—a system that involves counting actual products that are produced
- *Event recording*—the number of times a specifically defined behavior occurs within a time interval (for example, counting the number of times a student steps away from a line within one class period)
- *Duration recording*—the length of time a be-

havior occurs (for example, how long a student can stay on a specific task)

- *Interval recording*—the occurrence or non-occurrence of a behavior within a specific time interval (for example, the teacher may observe that Jim was active only two of the five 1-minute observation periods)

The method selected depends on the type of behavior, the kind of data to be gathered, and the ease of implementation by the observer.

Event recording produces frequency data that

EVENT RECORDING

EXAMPLE 1: SIMPLE FREQUENCY AND PERCENT DATA

Student ____Sue____ Observer __Ms. Smith__
Behavior Observed: Objectives completed by Sue on recording sheet
Data Reported: Frequency and percentage of short-term objectives completed each day
Time of Observation: Individualized skill development and prerequisites; period of the class for 5 periods

Day	Number of Expected Objectives Achieved	Number Completed	Percentage Completed
1	4	(3)	75%
2	4	(2)	50%
3	5	(5)	100%
4	5	(4)	80%
5	5	(3)	60%

EXAMPLE 2: SIMPLE FREQUENCY

Student ____Jim____ Observer __Mr. Jones__
Behavior Observed: Talk-outs by Jim during instruction by teacher; talk-outs are verbalizations loud enough to be heard by the instructor
Data Reported: Frequency of talk-outs and rate of talk-outs per 5 minutes of instruction time
Time of Observation: Entire time teacher instructs

Day	Number of Minutes	Number of Talk-outs	Frequency
1	5		3
2	5		2
3	5		1
4	5		0
5	5		0

can be converted into percentages. Percentages and frequencies are appropriate measures for skill behaviors done in blocks of tasks. Percentages can be computed by counting the number of baskets made out of 10 shots, or the number of successful kicks out of 5 at a goal in soccer. Frequency data are simply the number of occurrences of the behavior. To compare frequencies, the observation periods should be equal in length, and the student should have the same opportunity to demonstrate the behavior during each observation period. Frequency data can be converted into rate information. Rate is simply the number of times a behavior occurs within a certain time limit, such as the number of times a student is able to set up a volleyball in 20 seconds.

Duration recordings are useful if the length of time a student engages in a behavior is of interest. For example, observers may note the amount of time a student requires to move from one ac-

tivity to the next, or how long a student is active or inactive. Duration can be recorded in actual time limits (for example, Jack was on task for 5 minutes) or in a percentage (for example, Ralph was active for 40% of the time) (see box below).

Interval recordings are particularly useful for the regular class teacher because they do not require that students be observed continuously. McLoughlin and Lewis describe advantages of this system and several of the different recording systems[17]:

This technique does not require counting or timing behaviors. Instead, the observer simply notes whether or not a behavior is present or absent during a specified time interval. For example, if a teacher is interested in observing staying on task, smiling, or swearing, the classroom day may be broken into short time periods, such as 15- or 5- or 3-minute intervals. One of several variations of interval recording can be used:

1. *Whole interval time sampling.* The observer notes whether the target behavior occurs continuously during the entire interval. That is, if 5-minute intervals are being used, the observer notes for each interval whether the behavior occurred *throughout the interval.*
2. *Partial interval time sampling.* The partial interval method requires only that the observer determines whether the behavior occurs at least once during the interval. That is, if the observation period has been broken down into 20-minute intervals, the observer notes for each interval whether the behavior has occurred at all during that time.
3. *Momentary time sampling.* In momentary time sampling, observation occurs only at the end of each time interval. That is, if the observation period is broken down into 3-minute intervals, the teacher checks the student only at the end of each interval and notes if the target behavior is occurring at that moment.

Observers must be trained to evaluate and record data accurately and consistently. The most effective data collection system requires that the students be able to evaluate themselves as to whether they did or did not demonstrate that behavior. Peer teachers and aides can also be trained to assist in and monitor the data collection. Someone other than the performer (teacher, aide, tutor) observes for only a short period each day; however, it is long enough to obtain an accurate picture of the student's behavior (Table 7-8).

DURATION RECORDING

DURATION AND PERCENT DATA

Student ____Sue____ Observer ____Jim____

Behavior Observed: Time working on self-directing task.

Data Reported: Amount of time (duration) on task; observer starts timing when child moves to learning stations.

Time of Observation: Five-minute intervals for observational periods during a class session

Day	Time	Number of Minutes	Percentage of time
1	8:00-9:05	1:00	20%
2	9:10-9:15	1:30	30%
3	9:00-9:05	1:15	25%
4	9:25-9:30	2:00	40%
5	9:20-9:25	3:00	60%

TABLE 7-8
Measures of behavior

Measure	Derivation	Example	Application
Percentage	Number of correct trials out of a block of trials	Seven basketball goals made out of a block of 10 trials $\dfrac{7}{10} \times 100 = 70\%$ accuracy	A measure of accuracy without regard for time or proficiency
Frequency	$\dfrac{\text{Count of behavior}}{\text{Observation time}}$	Pupil tutor feeds back three times in 3 minutes $= \dfrac{3}{3}$	How often a distinct behavior occurs within a period of time
Duration	Direct measures of length of time	A child is off task for 45 seconds	The total length of time a continuous behavior occurs
Intervals	Number of fixed time units in which behavior did or did not occur	Children are observed for 20 seconds; then the observer records whether behavior occurred during the interval; observers then repeat the process (usually data are expressed in terms of percentage of intervals during which behavior occurred) $\dfrac{4 \text{ intervals}}{10 \text{ intervals total}} \times 100 = 40\%$ of intervals	When behavior occurs over a time frame

Analyzing the Data

The collected data must be studied by the teacher to determine whether the behavior is effectively contributing to the learning process or deterring learning. If the behavior being observed relates to performance of a skill or learning task, the greater the number of successful occurrences the better. If the behavior being monitored is disruptive (undesirable), the fewer the number of occurrences the better (see Example 2 in the box on p. 134).

Efficient Ways of Collecting Data

It is imperative that data be collected while instruction is conducted. Three groups of persons can collect the data: physical education teachers, students who participate in activity, and peer teachers.

There are generally three types of data. One type indicates attainment of short-term objectives. Another involves observation and recording of positive social behavior that develops the individual or supports the instructional system. Disruptive behavior is the third type. Interval and time sampling techniques would be used to gather this type of information.

Data on Acquisition of Short-Term Objectives

The collection of data on the acquisition of short-term objectives should be done while the physical education class is in progress. The data sheets should be prepared before class. Checkmarks should be made during class to indicate achievement. Time usually does not permit written comments. Once a child is familiar with a score sheet, a check can be made in 2 or 3 seconds. Time intervals for recording depend on the nature of the tasks and the learner. Three suggested ways of structuring the data sheets to indicate progress are (1) to have the measurement of the task on a data sheet, (2) to convert objectives that are communicated on posters in the

---

INTERVAL RECORDING

EXAMPLE 1: WHOLE INTERVAL RECORDING

Behavior: Sam is on task
When Measured: During participation at learning station 9:00 and 9:15
Length of Interval: 5 minutes

	9:00-9:03	9:03-9:06	9:06-9:09	9:09-9:12	9:12-9:15
		X	X		
Interval	1	2	3	4	5

X = Sam was staring out the window for the entire inverval
Results: Sam stared out the window in 40% of the time intervals sampled

EXAMPLE 2: MOMENTARY TIME SAMPLING

Behavior: Sam writes on his worksheet
When Measured: Independent study times throughout the day
Length of Interval: 5 minutes

	8:00-8:00:15	8:05-8:05:15	8:10-8:10:15	8:15-8:15:15
		X		
Interval	1	2	3	4

---

physical education class to numbers on a data sheet, and (3) to have the objectives stated on a sheet that the learner carries while participating in different activities.

Measurement of the Task on the Data Sheet

Objectives should have performance measures. Many objectives build on one another to form a hierarchy. For instance, if a child was attempting to increase the distance of the long jump, the data sheet would indicate a series of measures in inches. The pupil would then indicate present status in the jumping hierarchy by placing an X over the jumping level of current instruction. If the activity was throwing a ball, distance of the throw might be marked, and a running measure might be time. If the activity was running endur-

ance, the measure might be time elapsed to run a specified distance. In this data collection system there is direct information on performance of the pupil scored on the data sheet itself. A data matrix incorporates the same principle. However, with this system several behaviors are placed in a hierarchy that forms the vertical axis of the matrix, and the performance measures of the objectives are indicated on the horizontal axis of the matrix. The student graphs or checks objectives attained with this system (Fig. 7-2) and records personal data.

Conversion of Objectives to Numbers on a Data Sheet

The objectives may be written on a sheet from which the student receives instruction. In this sys-

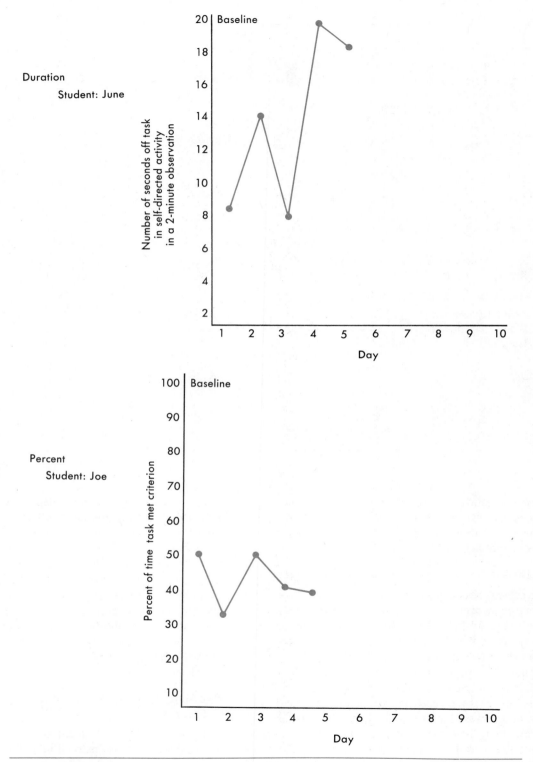

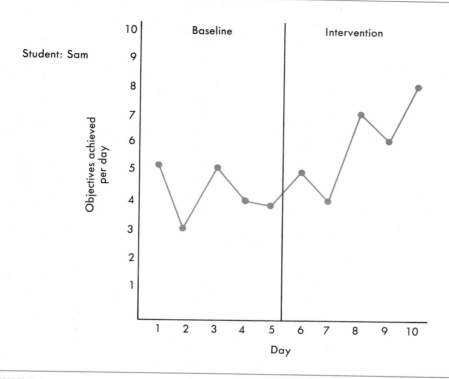

FIGURE 7-3

Graphing intervention data. Behavior observed: objectives achieved by Sam; intervention: reinforcement by peer teacher.

tem the pupil reads the objective from the sheet and checks the objective when mastered.

Data sheets can be numbers that represent tasks. A checkmark over the number on the data sheet represents acquisition of the short-term instructional objective. In this system it is necessary to have the objectives on a poster in the class setting. The pupil identifies the number of the objective in question from the poster on a specific day. The number on the data sheet is matched with the number of the objective on the poster. The objective is performed by the pupil and checked on the data sheet if mastered. The posted objectives may be written or converted to stick figures or pictures to clarify the behaviors. Use of posters requires time to teach children to match objectives on the posters with objectives on the data sheet. However, once the poster objectives are learned, the children can collect data on one another or by themselves.

Recording Data on Social Behavior

The classic manner of data collection on social behavior is for the teacher to collect information by means of interval, time sample, or event recording sheets and then graph the results. But this system may distract the teacher from instruction. The problem may be overcome if the teacher places a piece of masking tape on the student's wrist and records data on the tape with a marking pen. Appropriate and inappropriate behaviors are identified. When the pupils conduct themselves appropriately, they are given marks of one color (red). When the behaviors are inappropriate, they are awarded marks on the wrist tape of another color (green). After the class is over, the pieces of masking tape are placed on a board beside their names. The data marks may be made by a teacher or peer teachers. The marks are usually delivered immediately, do not disrupt ongoing instruction, and enable the teacher or peer teacher to deliver a consequence that relates to desired behavior. If children have severe behavioral problems, an interval or time sample or duration records are to be made.

Determining Need for an Intervention Program

The amount of productive behavior being demonstrated is the primary criterion for determining whether an intervention program is needed. To make this decision, the teacher must refer to the student's educational objectives and compare the behavior being demonstrated with those objectives. If a behavior to be learned or maintained is not being demonstrated consistently, an intervention program is needed. If disruptive behavior is occurring to the extent that meaningful learning is not occurring, an intervention program can decrease the undesirable behavior.

Selecting a Positive Intervention Program

The central purpose of the physical education program is to develop positive physical and motor behaviors that result in improved health and recreational activity. Research has demonstrated the effectiveness of several intervention techniques that can be used to promote positive behaviors. These techniques involve communication of the target task to the learner, efficiently establishing the behavior so performance can be improved, and methods to enable density of relevant programming. Following is a list of techniques that can be used to promote learning of a task. (See p. 150 for techniques to eliminate disruptive behaviors.)

Purpose	Technique
Communication of a learning task	Modeling
Establishing behavioral performance	Priming, prompting, and fading and forward and backward chaining
Density of relevant programming	Cycle constancy
Developing new behavior	Shaping

Modeling

Modeling refers to demonstration of a task by the teacher or reinforcement of another student who performs a desirable behavior in the presence of the target student. When a teacher actually performs the desirable behavior, she is teaching the target student how the task is to be performed. When another student is used as the model and performs a task correctly, the teacher praises the behavior in the presence of the target student. For example, if a teacher wants all the children to maintain a straight back while doing a sit-up, those children who keep their backs straight would be pointed out by the teacher and praised while doing their sit-ups. All other children who then perform the task correctly would also be reinforced. Modeling can lead to a fairly close approximation of the desired response. Refinement of the response could be done at another time (Fig. 7-5).

Physical Priming (Prompting)

Physical priming,[4] or prompting, involves physically holding and moving the body parts of the learner through the activity. Usually priming will enable a successful response or a close enough approximation so that shaping can be used to improve the performance level. Physical priming should be used with the idea of eliminating the primers as quickly as possible so that the learner can begin to function independently.

Prompting and Fading

Prompting and fading involve providing just enough physical assistance so that the student realizes some success at the task and then gradually withdrawing the help. The rule for prompting is to provide the minimum prompt necessary for the learner to be successful. For example, if a student tries to stand on one foot but cannot, the teacher can place his hands under the student's arms to provide support. The prompt is sequentially faded by having the teacher gradually move his hands down the student's arm to the tip of the fingers and finally letting go.

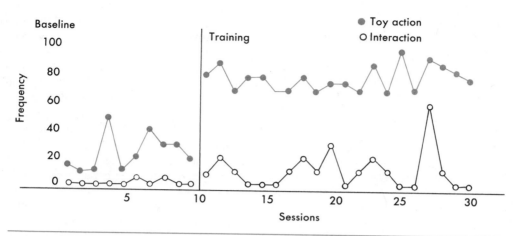

FIGURE 7-4
Graphing intervention data.

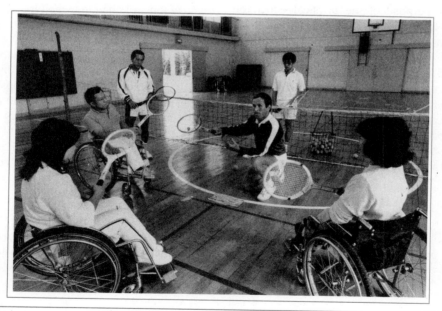

FIGURE 7-5
A coach models appropriate techniques to students learning wheelchair tennis.
(Photo by Bruce Haase; courtesy Peter Burwash International.)

Prompts are valuable if the tasks can be quickly learned. If the task is not performed in a relatively short time, the teacher probes through prerequisite components to determine which ones are missing and need to be learned before the skill can be performed.

Forward and Backward Chaining

Chaining is leading a person through a series of teachable components of a motor task. Each teachable component represents a discrete portion (link) in a task. When these portions or links are tied together, the process is known as chaining. Some skills can be broken into components and taught by the chaining process more easily than others. Self-help skills are easily broken into parts. Clearly, grasping a spoon is an essential link in the process of eating; however, it is a behavior distinctly different from scooping the food with the spoon or placing the food in one's mouth. Each of these components is a necessary link that must be tied together (chained) to accomplish the skill of self-feeding. Continuous physical skills do not break into discrete teachable components and are difficult to chain. Other physical skills, such as the lay-up shot in basketball, can be broken into discrete components that lend themselves to chaining.

When the last of the series of steps is taught first, the process is known as *backward chaining.* Teaching a basketball lay-up by means of backward chaining requires that the student (1) stand close to the basket, reach high with the arm, and shoot the basketball; (2) jump from the inside foot, reach high with the arm, and shoot the basketball; (3) run-jump from the inside foot, reach high with the arm, and shoot the basketball; and (4) dribble a ball while running, jump from the inside foot, reach high with the arm, and shoot the basketball. The value of backward chaining is that the individual is reinforced during each step by completing the task successfully.

Other skills that may be taught by backward chaining are those which are expressed in team play. Examples of the analysis of these tasks, with the terminal reinforcing behavior shown first, are listed below.

Self-help tasks such as tying a shoe and dressing are easily and effectively taught by backward chaining.

When using *forward chaining,* the first step is taught first, the second step is taught second, and so on until the entire task is learned. Most teachers use forward chaining when teaching tasks.

Cycle Constancy

Cycle constancy is the continual recurrence of a specific motor act within similar time periods. Gold[10] has indicated that cycle constancy positively affects some students' ability to learn motor tasks. The value of cycle constancy is that the learner is able to predict when stimuli will be presented and when consequences will be delivered. It is relatively easy to apply cycle constancy to

Pass-receiving in football	(1) Catch pass, (2) run and catch pass, (3) make cut, run, and catch pass, (4) release from line, run, cut, and catch pass.
Tackling in football	(1) Tackle ball carrier, (2) run pattern to intersect and tackle ball carrier, (3) release blocker, run pattern to ball carrier, and tackle ball carrier, (4) administer technique to neutralize blocker, release blocker, run pattern to ball carrier, tackle ball carrier.
Shooting a soccer goal	(1) Shoot soccer goal, (2) dribble and shoot soccer goal, (3) receive a pass dribble and shoot soccer goal.
Passing a soccer ball	(1) Pass soccer ball, (2) bring ball under control and pass soccer ball, (3) dribble, bring ball under control, and pass the soccer ball.
Leg takedown in wrestling	(1) Take opponent to the mat, (2) secure the legs and take opponent to the mat, (3) shoot move for legs, secure the legs, and take the opponent to the mat, (4) set up move, shoot the move for the legs, secure the legs, and take the opponent to the mat.
Fielding a ball and throwing a player out at first base in softball	(1) Throw to first base, (2) field the ball and throw to first base.

behavioral programming of motor tasks. To promote learning, as tasks recur, either the conditions or the criteria are altered.

Cycle constancy is most frequently used when dealing with serious emotional disturbances. Children so affected are often disruptive if their attention is not focused intently on one task. Often, when this type of child is placed in a group situation that includes some activities beyond or less than his ability level, the child becomes inattentive and begins to act out. When one child becomes disruptive in group activity, there is a tendency for others to do the same. To prevent disruptive behavior or to bring it under control, Foxx[8] proposes that a high density of relevant programming be used. This simply means that attention should be focused on activities that have meaning for the student. When these activities are coupled with predictability of the tasks and their consequences (cycle constancy), the child will focus attention on the tasks and learning will occur.

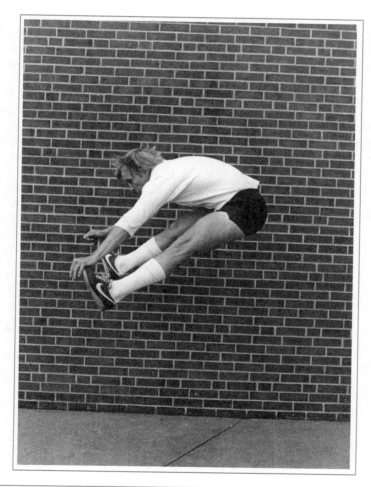

FIGURE 7-6
A student jumps and touches the toes a specific number of repetitions over a specified time frame.

Shaping

Shaping involves the reinforcing of small progressive steps that lead toward a desired behavior. Chapter 5 describes behavioral shaping programs for sensory input systems, abilities and skills; however, that same process can be applied to many other types of motor and social behaviors. The technique of shaping is used to teach new behaviors and is particularly valuable in the performance phase of acquiring a skill. When shaping a new motor response, the physical education teacher has the choice of waiting for the learner to demonstrate the next small step toward the goal or helping the learner to attain the objective through the use of a physical prompt. In either case the specifically defined task (step) must be reinforced. The procedures for shaping a behavior are as follows:

Procedure	Example
1. Define the behavior.	Balancing on one foot with eyes open for 10 seconds
2. Define a reinforcer.	Knowledge of task success
3. Determine the present level.	2 seconds on the task
4. Outline a series of small steps that lead to the desired behavior.	16 increments of ½ second each
5. Advance the learner on a predetermined criterion.	Each step three times in a row
6. Define the success level.	90%

Reinforcement

Reinforcement is a strategy that follows and strengthens a behavior. All the aforementioned procedures, except reinforcement, were discussed in Chapter 5. The discussion that follows focuses on positive reinforcers because they yield the most lasting results. Positive reinforcers include teacher or peer praise, material rewards, activities a student enjoys doing, and success on a task. Positive reinforcement is constructive because it helps individuals feel good about themselves.

Selecting reinforcers. There are intrinsic (internal) and extrinsic (external) reinforcers. Intrinsic reinforcement comes from within the learner. Often knowledge of success on a task or the satisfaction of participating is sufficient to reinforce oneself. Extrinsic reinforcement comes from outside the learner. Examples of extrinsic reinforcement are praise and other rewards from a person who acknowledges the learner's achievement. One objective of a reinforcement program is to move the learner from dependence on extrinsic reinforcers to seeking intrinsic reinforcers. Once learners no longer have to rely on teachers for feedback, they can direct their own learning. It is important that both the learner and the teachers agree on what the reinforcer will be and how the system of reinforcement will work.

Reinforcement procedures. Contingency management is a way of controlling the use of reinforcers. A *contingency* is an agreement between the student and the teacher that indicates what the student must do to earn a specific reward. A *token economy* is a form of contingency management in which tokens (external reinforcers) are earned for desirable behavior. This type of a system can be used with a single student, selected groups of students, or with classes of students. Lewis and Doorlag[16] suggest the following procedure for setting up a token economy:

1. Specify the behaviors that earn tokens.
2. Use tokens that are appropriate for the student.
3. Pose a menu (a list) of the types of available reinforcers.
4. Allow students to suggest reinforcers for the list.
5. Revise the menu regularly.
6. Use a clear record system (of distributing the tokens) that is accurate.
7. Give students frequent opportunities to cash in their earned tokens.
8. The cash-in system should take a minimal amount of time.
9. Provide clear rules to staff and peer tutors for distribution of tokens.
10. Gradually reduce the value of the tokens to increase reliance on more natural reinforcers.

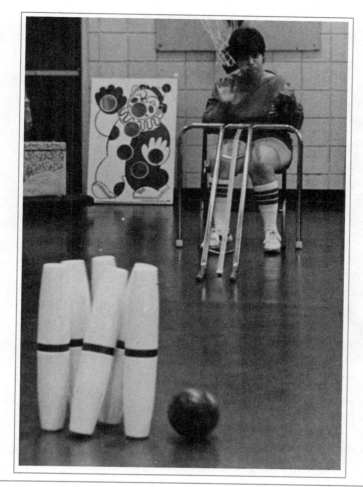

FIGURE 7-7
An unbreakable bowling set in which pins fall upon contact provides immediate reinforcement.
(Courtesy Verland Foundation, Inc.)

Table 7-9 lists several examples of different types of reinforcers appropriate for use in school settings. Social and activity reinforcers have special appeal, since they are usually available at no cost to the teacher.

Frequency of reinforcement. The frequency of distributing reinforcers should be carefully controlled so that the student continues to strive toward desirable goals. The frequency that reinforcers are given is called the *reinforcement schedule.* Schedules of reinforcement should move from continuous (a reinforcer every time the desirable behavior occurs) to a fixed interval ratio (for example, one reinforcer for every three instances of desirable behavior). The schedule should eventually be changed to a variable interval ratio (for example, one reinforcer for every three instances of desirable behavior followed by one reinforcer for every five instances of desirable behavior, or one reinforcer every minute followed by one reinforcer every 3 minutes). The variable interval ratio is the most effective because when students are unable to predict when they will be reinforced, they tend to persist at a task.

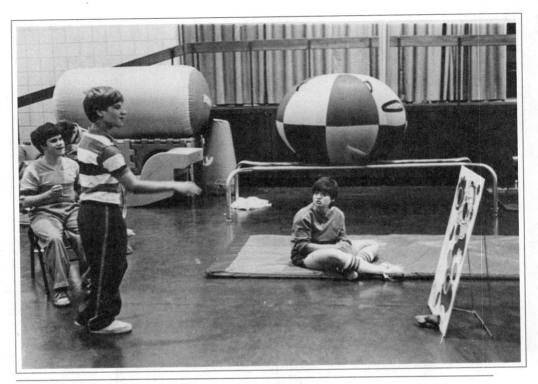

FIGURE 7-8
A child receives immediate reinforcement when the beanbag passes through the target opening.
(Courtesy Verland Foundation, Inc.)

TECHNIQUES TO ELIMINATE DISRUPTIVE BEHAVIORS

Much of the previous discussion concerns the uses of reinforcement to increase efforts toward learning tasks. Very often reinforcement procedures are used to decrease undesirable behaviors. The undesirable behaviors must be eliminated or substantially reduced so that the student can focus attention and effort on positive learning habits.

Because of self-concept problems many handicapped children disrupt classrooms and make it difficult for themselves and others to learn meaningful motor skills. When behavioral technology is applied to classroom management, it must be systematic, consistent, and concerned with both preventing disruptive behavior and promoting positive behavior. There are two levels of classroom management, one for the group and another for individuals within the group.

Controlling Group Behavior

One of the most effective techniques for controlling group behavior is preventive planning, which consists of establishing class rules and enforcing them in the least intrusive ways possible. Rules for class conduct should communicate to the students the behavior expected by the teacher. Effective class rules should be (1) few in number, (2) a statement of behavior desired from the student, (3) simple and clearly stated, and (4) guidelines that the teacher can enforce. For example, a well-stated rule is: "When lined up at the door waiting to pass to the next class, keep your hands to yourself."

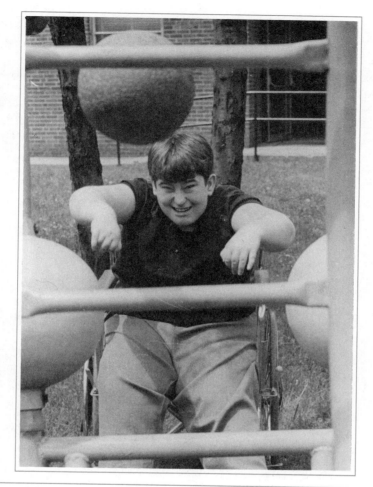

FIGURE 7-9
Intrinsic reinforcement is provided when the ball passes through the opening in the bars.

Clearly stated expectations lead to appropriate classroom behavior. They provide learners with rules of conduct and identify behavior that will be rewarded. It is suggested that a list of rules be placed where students can observe it each day. The consequences for breaking rules should also be made clear to the students. If a rule is broken, consistent consequences should follow.

Rules cannot take care of every situation; often there is disruptive behavior not covered by the rules. The difficult decision each teacher must make is whether to intervene and stop the disruptive behavior. The following suggestions can serve as guidelines for a teacher facing this decision:

♦ *Real dangers.* The teacher should intervene if children are involved in physical activity placing them in danger.
♦ *Psychological protection.* The teacher should intervene if a group gangs up on a child and uses derogatory remarks.
♦ *Protection of property.* The teacher should

TABLE 7-9
Classroom reinforcers for use in a school setting

	Social-Verbal	Manipulative	Token
Elementary Students	Hug Positive comments ("Good job" "That was a nice play") Pat on the back	Helping teacher Being team leader Time in the game center Choosing a game Extra minutes of recess X minutes of free-time activity	Paper certificate Stars Positive note sent to parents Medal
Adolescents	Gesture of approval Handshake Positive comments ("Great job" "You did it" "Great effort")	Choosing class activity	Sports equipment Posters Positive note sent to parents T-shirt

TABLE 7-10
Intermittent schedules on reinforcement

		Effects on Behavior	
Name of Schedule	Definition of Schedule	Schedule in Effect	Schedule Terminated (Extinction)
Fixed ratio (FR)	Reinforcer is given after each x responses	High response rate	Irregular burst of responding; more responses than in continuous reinforcement, less than in variable ratio
Fixed interval (FI)	Reinforcer is given for first response to occur after each x minutes	Stops working after reinforcement; works hard just prior to time for next reinforcement	Slow gradual decrease in responding
Variable ratio (VR)	Reinforcer is given after x responses on the average	Very high response rates; the higher the ratio, the higher the rate	Very resistant to extinction; maximum number of responses before extinction
Variable interval (VI)	Reinforcer is given for first response after each x minutes on the average	Steady rate of responding	Very resistant to extinction; maximum time to extinction

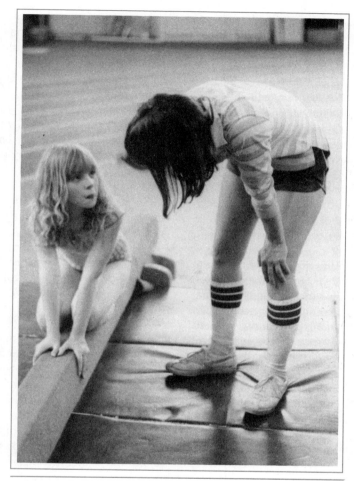

FIGURE 7-10
An instructor's close proximity may affect the behavior of the student.

intervene when it is evident that school property, equipment, or facilities are in danger of being destroyed or damaged.

♦ *Protection of the ongoing program.* Once the class is motivated in performing a particular activity, intervene if a child who is having difficulty displays disruptive behavior.

♦ *Protection against negative contagion.* The teacher should intervene if tension is mounting in an activity and a child with high social power contributes negatively to the activity.

♦ *Highlighting a value area.* The teacher may want to point to an aspect of sportsmanship or rules of the game that lie slightly below the surface of behavior.

♦ *Avoiding conflicts with the outside world.* It is expected that behavior will be controlled when the public or persons other than class members are viewing the class.

If the teacher does decide it is necessary to intervene to control disruptive behavior, several techniques are effective in controlling disturbances. Some specific techniques that have been identified from numerous authorities to manage disruptive students in a physical education setting are as follows:

♦ *Planned ignoring.* Much of children's behavior is designed to antagonize the teacher. If this behavior is not contagious, it may be wise to ignore it and not gratify the child.

♦ *Signal interference.* The teacher can use non-verbal controls such as hand clapping, eye contact, frowns, and body posture to indicate to the child disapproval and control.

♦ *Proximity control.* The teacher can stand next to a child who is having difficulty. This is to let the child know of the teacher's concern regarding the behavior.

♦ *Interest boosting.* If a child's interest is waning, involve him actively in class activities of the moment and let him demonstrate the skill that is being performed or discussed.

♦ *Reduction of tension through humor.* Humor is often able to penetrate a tense situation, with the result that everyone becomes more comfortable.

♦ *Hurdle lesson.* Sometimes child is frustrated by the immediate task she is requested to perform. Instead of asking for help, she may involve her peers in disruptive activity. In this event structure a task in which the child can be successful.

♦ *Restructure of classroom program.* If the teacher finds the class irritable, bored, or excited, a change in program might be needed.

♦ *Support from routine.* Some children need more structure than others. Without these guideposts they feel insecure. Structure programs for those who need it.

♦ *Direct appeal to value areas.* Appeal to certain values that children have internalized, such as a relationship between the teacher and the child, behavioral consequences, awareness of peer reaction, or appeal to the teacher's power of authority.

♦ *Removal of seductive objects.* It is difficult for the teacher to compete against balls, bats, objects that can be manipulated, or equipment that may be in the vicinity of in-

struction. Either the objects have to be removed, or the teacher has to accept the disorganized state of the group.

♦ *Verbal removal.* When a child's behavior has reached the point at which he will not respond to verbal controls, he may have to be asked to leave the room (to get a drink, wash up, or deliver a message—not as punishment, but to distract the child).

♦ *Physical restraint.* It may be necessary to restrain a child physically if he loses control and becomes violent.

Handling the Disruptive Student

The behavior problems of special students frequently contribute to their placement in special physical education programs. When special students return to the physical education class, teachers are often concerned that their problem behaviors will interfere with the operation of the classroom.

Behaviors that interfere with classroom instruction, impede social interaction with the teacher and peers, or endanger others are considered *classroom conduct problems.* Examples of inappropriate classroom behaviors are talking out, fighting, arguing, being out of line, swearing, and avoiding interactions with others. Breaking the rules of the game, poor sportsmanship, and immature and withdrawn behaviors also fall under this category. Behaviors that interfere with the special student's motor skill development are considered *skill problems.* Typical skill problems are poor attention and failure to attempt tasks with a best effort.

Problem behaviors are exhibited in one of three ways: (1) low rate of appropriate behaviors, (2) high rate of inappropriate behaviors, and (3) the appropriate behavior is not part of the student's repertoire. Knowing the characteristics of the behavior is important, since different management strategies are linked to each.

Low Rate of Appropriate Behaviors

Students do exhibit appropriate behaviors, but not as frequently as expected or required. A student may be able to stay on task only 50% of the time. Also, students may behave appropriately in one setting but not another. For instance, the special student may work well on individual tasks but may find it difficult to work in group games. To alleviate these problems, the teacher sets up a systematic program to generalize on task behaviors from one situation to another.

High Rate of Inappropriate Behaviors

Inappropriate behaviors that occur frequently or for long periods are troublesome to teachers. Examples are students who do not conform to class rules 30 to 40 times a week, those who talk during 50% to 60% of class instruction, those who use profanity 5 to 10 times in one class period, and those who are off task 70% to 75% of the class period. To overcome these high rates of inappropriate behavior, the physical education teacher attempts to decrease the frequency or duration of the undesired behavior by increasing appropriate behaviors that are incompatible. For instance, to decrease the incidence of hitting a peer while in class, the teacher can increase the rate of performing tasks or decrease the time between tasks.

Appropriate Behavior Not Part of Student's Repertoire

Students may not yet have learned behaviors for social interaction or classroom functioning. For instance, they may not know conduct of sportsmanship in class games. Teachers must provide instruction to help students acquire new behaviors. Behavior problems do not occur in isolation. Events or actions of others can initiate or reinforce inappropriate behaviors. To understand and manage classroom problems, examine the student in relation to the target behavior. For example, classmates who laugh at clowning or wisecracks tend to reinforce that type of disruptive behavior; as a result, the disruptive student continues to exhibit the undesirable behavior.

Students show inappropriate behavior when they have not learned correct responses or have found that acting inappropriately is more rewarding than acting appropriately. These behavior problems do respond to instruction.

Positive Methods for Decreasing Inappropriate Behavior

Positive approaches for decreasing inappropriate behavior should be tried before resorting to aversive (negative) techniques. Four techniques that can be used effectively to weaken inappropriate behavior are to provide (1) reinforcement of the incompatible behavior, (2) differential reinforcement at low rates, (3) differential reinforcement at high rates, and (4) differential reinforcement of other behaviors.

Reinforcement of Incompatible Behaviors

This method involves reinforcing appropriate behaviors that can occur only if the inappropriate behavior is not present. Examples of each follow:

Appropriate Behavior	Inappropriate Behavior
Walking	Running
Keeping hands to onself	Punching someone
Standing on a designated line for instructional purposes	Moving around the gym
Sitting	Standing

It is apparent that the appropriate behaviors are incompatiable with the inappropriate behaviors. If the teacher uses this approach, the appropriate behavior is reinforced while the inappropriate behavior is ignored.

Differential Reinforcement of Low Rates

Differential reinforcement of low rates involves reinforcing inappropriate behaviors as they are gradually decreased. For instance, a child who acts out five times in class is reinforced for acting out only four times, then three times, then two, one, and finally not at all. It is similar to a shaping procedure, but it usually deals with inappropriate behavior.

Differential Reinforcement of High Rates

This method provides reinforcers when high rates of desirable behavior are demonstrated. For instance, a disruptive child may receive reinforcement for continued activity for 10 minutes without a disruptive act, then after 12 minutes, 14 minutes, and so on until there is no disruption for the entire period. The criterion for reinforcement for demonstrating longer times of good behavior is progressively raised.

Differential Reinforcement of Other Behavior

Differential reinforcement of other behavior requires that a reinforcer be delivered after any response except the undesirable target response. The individual is reinforced for behaviors other than the target response only when he or she is not performing the target behavior. The purpose of differential reinforcement of other behaviors is to decrease the target (unreinforced) response. If the target behavior does occur within a specified time, the reinforcer is withheld. For instance, a teacher can provide a reinforcer only if the student does not strike another child with a closed fist during a 20-minute period. To further reduce

the frequency of the behavior, the time period is gradually increased.

There are two aversive procedures to decrease unwanted behaviors. One involves withholding reinforcement (extinction), and the other involves presentation of an aversive event (punishment) after the undesirable behavior.

Extinction

Extinction is the removal of reinforcers that previously followed the behavior. The behavioral technique of planned ignoring is based on the principle of extinction. When a person acts out in class and is disruptive, attention to the behavior may reinforce the behavior. When the teacher ignores the behavior, no reinforcement is provided and the disruptive behavior may diminish. Extinction procedures reduce and eliminate behavior; however, the effects of extinction procedures are

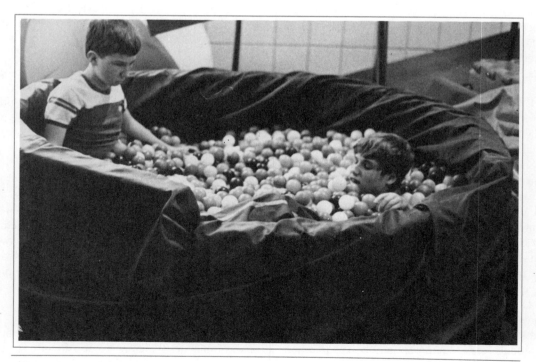

FIGURE 7-11
A person is taken out of activity to watch a peer play. This is contingent observation.
(Courtesy Verland Foundation, Inc.)

usually not immediate. An indication that the extinction procedure is working is a burst of inappropriate behavior before it extinguishes. Identification of the extinction burst is strong evidence that the behavior will extinguish. Teachers must wait out the termination of this burst.

Punishment

Punishment is an aversive event that follows an undesirable behavior, such as criticism, reprimands, and taking privileges away. Punishment should be done in the presence of a great deal of available reinforcement. The rule of thumb is at least four reinforcements to one punishment. For the punishment to be effective, it must be immediate. Furthermore, the person who does the punishing should also do the reinforcing.

There are several types of punishers. Some of the more common are response costs, contingent observation, time out, and peer isolation (Table 7-11).

Response cost. Response cost is the withdrawal of earned reinforcers or privileges follow-

ing an inappropriate behavior. A contingency management system is desirable to establish response cost weightings. To successfully implement the system, the student must already have earned reinforcers which can be withdrawn. The conditions under which the earned reinforcers are to be withdrawn must be clearly explained.

Contingent observation. In this technique an error is corrected by taking the person out of the activity so he can observe a peer performing the behavior correctly. After the observation period the person is returned to the activity. The magnitude of the punishment is determined by controlling the length of time the individual must watch. Contingent observation conducted under short duration may have little if any punishment effect. Rather, it may become a form of modeling.

Time out from reinforcement. Time out is a punishment procedure in which positive reinforcement is withdrawn for a time. The opportunity to receive reinforcement is contingent on behavior.

TABLE 7-11
Procedures and principles for weakening behavior

Learning Concepts	Educational Procedures	Effects on Behavior	Examples of Positive or Aversive Events Presented or Removed
Extinction (of behavior previously strengthened by positive reinforcement)	Behavior is not followed by positive event associated with previous occurrence	Decrease in strength of behavior	Smile, approval, affection, peer attention, bonus, special privilege
Extinction (of behavior previously strengthened by negative reinforcement)	Behavior is not followed by removal of aversion event associated with previous occurrence	Decrease in strength of behavior	Criticism, rejection, threat of loss of privileges, poor grade
Punishment: presentation of aversive events	Behavior is followed by aversive event	Decrease in strength of behavior which results in the aversive event	Criticism, poor grade, rejection by peers, threat of dismissal from club
Punishment: removal of positive events through time-out or response cost	Behavior is followed by temporary or permanent loss of positive events	Decrease in strength of behavior which results in loss of positive events	Smile, approval, affection, money, privilege, group membership

From Gardner, W.I.: Learning and behavior characteristics of exceptional children and youth, Boston, 1977, Allyn and Bacon, Inc.

Isolation from a group exemplifies time out from reinforcement. Examples in sport activity are the penalty box in hockey and being taken out of the basketball game when a player is in foul trouble. When a person is removed from reinforcing activity with a time-out procedure, it should be for a short time. An important point to remember is that there can be no time out for reinforcement if the activity from which the person is removed is not reinforcing.

Peer isolation. Peer isolation is removing an individual from a group setting. Often classrooms contain time-out areas where the student cannot see or be seen by other members of the class.

Negative Reinforcement

A negative reinforcer is an event or stimulus that, when terminated, increases the frequency of the preceding response. An example is a teacher who continually criticizes a basketball player for not having his hands up when guarding an opponent. When the player puts his hands up, the criticism stops. The event that was terminated (criticism by the teacher for not having hands up) increased the frequency of the preceding response (getting the hands up when the opponent had the ball). Another example is a student who stops talking to a friend during instruction when the teacher frowns at the person talking. Negative reinforcement increases the occurrence of a behavior by removing something that is aversive. Because it is a negative approach, it may produce avoidance, escape, or aggressive behavior on the part of the student.[20]

APPLICATION OF LEARNING PRINCIPLES TO INSTRUCTIONAL OBJECTIVES

Disruptive behavior in our public schools by non-handicapped and handicapped children is a major public concern. The application of behavior management techniques by teachers may assist in bringing structure to the environment and lead to the alleviation of disruptive student behaviors.

There is consensus that successful schools have systems of firm, consistent management. Research confirms that clearly structured, secure environments permit students to master the objectives of the program. Haring[11] indicates that "teaching . . . necessitates finding a method of instruction which allows the child to learn."

The preconditions for the application of learning principles are that there must be a precisely defined short-term instructional objective, and there must be incentives for the learner to master the objective. If either of these preconditions is not satisfied, the effect of the program is minimized.

Effective learning is the result of mutual understanding between the student and the teacher. There is a contingency relationship between what a student must do with respect to a specific consequence. Homme and co-workers[12] provide nine rules for developing contingency contracts. These principles also can be applied to the acquisition of any type of objectives by students.

1. Praise the correct objective.
2. Praise the correct objective immediately after it occurs.
3. Praise the correct objective after it occurs and not before.
4. Objectives should be in small steps so that there can be frequent praise.
5. Praise improvement.
6. Be fair in setting up consequences for achieving objectives.
7. Be honest and provide the agreed on consequences.
8. Be positive so that the child may achieve success.
9. Be systematic.

Praise the Correct Objective

To implement this principle effectively, persons involved with instruction (teachers, school administrators, parents, and related service personnel) must know precisely the objective or behavior that the learner is to carry out. That behavior must be praised only if it is achieved. The application of this principle must be consistent among all persons who work with the child.

There are two ways that this learning principle can be violated by a teacher, parent, or school administrator. First, he or she may provide praise even though the objective has not been achieved; second, he or she may neglect to provide the praise even though the objective has been achieved. In the first case the learner is being reinforced for doing less than his or her best and consequently will have a lessened desire to put forth maximum effort on subsequent trials. In the second case, if the teacher does not deliver the agreed on consequence (explicit or implicit), the student's desire to perform the instructional task again will be reduced.

Praise Immediately after Completion of the Task

Learners need to receive feedback immediately after task performance. Homme[11] indicates that reinforcing feedback should be provided 0.05 second after the task for maximum effectiveness. Immediacy of feedback on task performance is particularly important with children functioning on a lower level. If there is a delay between task performance and feedback, the child may be confused as to what the praise is for. For example, if a child walks a balance beam correctly but confirmation of task mastery is provided late (for instance as the child steps off the beam), the behavior of stepping off the beam may be strengthened to a greater degree than that of walking the beam, the desired objective. Thus the timing of the feedback (immediately after the task has been completed) is important.

Praise at the Appropriate Time

If a child is praised for performing an objective before it is completed, there is a good chance that he or she will expend less effort to meet the objective.

Objectives Should Be in Small Steps

If step size is small, there will be a greater rate of success. As has been indicated, disruptive behavior may be triggered by lack of success. The principle may therefore be applied in attempts to control disruptive behavior in the classroom. Thus if a child often exhibits many different types of disruptive behavior, objectives can be postulated to reduce the occurrence of these disruptive behaviors in small steps. For handicapped children, learning by small steps permits much needed success.

Praise Improvement

The acquisition of skill toward an objective should be praised. Providing appropriate consequences for improvement may in some instances violate the principle of praising the correct objective. However, on tasks that cannot be broken into small steps it is necessary to praise improvement. To do so, the instructor must know precisely the student's present level of educational performance. When the performance reflects an improvement on that level, the student must be reinforced with praise. Improvement means that the learner is functioning on a higher level than before. Therefore it is unwise to praise or provide positive consequences to students who perform at less than their best effort, since to do so may encourage them to contradict their potential.

Be Fair in Setting Up Consequences

When there are specific objectives to be achieved to develop skill or appropriate classroom behavior, specific consequences can be arranged to support the development of these objectives. However, if such arrangements are to be made between the learner and the teacher, there must be equity between the task and the incentives. If the learner does not have sufficient incentive to perform the tasks or to behave appropriately, he or she is unlikely to do so. This learning principle operates at very early ages.

In our clinical experience we set up a target objective for an 18-month-old boy with Down syndrome to learn to walk. The task involved walking from one chair to another, which was placed 8 feet away. If the child walked the full distance, he was allowed to play for 15 seconds with the toys that were placed on top of the chairs. When this period elapsed, he would return to the task of

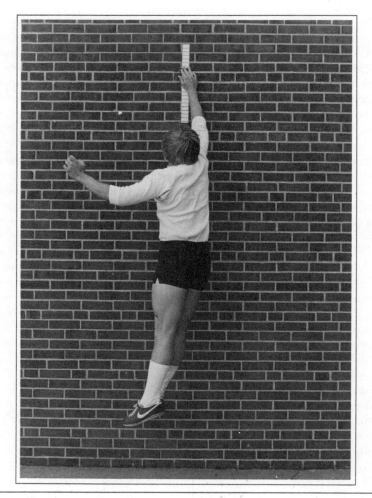

FIGURE 7-12
If the jumper hits the designated mark on the scale, his "correct behavior" should be reinforced.

walking a prescribed distance of 8 feet 1 inch, a short distance farther than the previous time. After a time the child refused to participate in the activity. The child's mother suggested that he be permitted to play with the toys for 30 seconds rather than for 15 seconds. This procedure was employed, and the child again engaged in the instructional task. It was inferred that the child would participate in tasks if the opportunity to play was commensurate with the effort put forth to master the objective. In our opinion, this is an example of equity between incentive and performance.

Be Honest

Agreements between teachers and learners must be honored by both. If there is an implicit or explicit arrangement between the teacher and the learner and the teacher does not follow through with the arrangement when the learner has upheld his or her end of the bargain, then the learning conditions will be seriously weakened. It is not uncommon for teachers to inadvertently forget the arrangements that have been made. Therefore it is important for the teacher to have records of arrangements between themselves and the learner. Forgetting the preconditions between learner and teacher may have a negative impact on the pupil's learning at a subsequent time.

If the teacher requests that a learner perform a specific task, the teacher must not provide the desirable consequences unless the learner achieves the proper objective. Honest delivery of the agreed on consequences is similar to praise for the correct behavior. However, praise for the correct behavior usually connotes a specific short-term task, whereas an agreed on consequence may involve a contractual arrangement between two parties. Principals and teachers who set policies may achieve positive results with the application of this principle.

Be Positive

The objective should be phrased positively so that the learner can achieve the stated objective, for example, "Walk to the end of the balance beam." An example of a negative statement is "Don't fall off of the balance beam." In the negative instance the child is avoiding failure, and there can be little value in mastering the desired behavior.

Be Systematic

To make the greatest positive impact on handicapped children, it is necessary to apply all the learning principles all the time. Inconsistency confuses the learner with regard to the material to be learned and the type of behavior to maintain during class. The consistent use of modern behavioral technology enhances a child's ability to learn desirable behaviors. This learning principle is the most difficult one for teachers of emotionally disturbed children to master.

SUMMARY

There is a technology based on research and demonstration that, if used in applied settings, facilitates the learning of motor skills by handicapped children. These techniques include conducting procedures that facilitate generalization of trained skills from instructional to natural environments, controlling sensory inputs, providing appropriate consequences, and controlling environmental conditions to maximize learning. Planned procedures for intervention of programs require a systematic measurement system. This measurement system may be applied to positive learning or to decreasing inappropriate behavior. Positive and unobtrusive approaches should be used first. The levels of reinforcement of learning must be determined. The implementation of contingency management systems may be necessary in some situations. Application of behavioral learning principles can enhance the learning capabilities of handicapped children.

REVIEW QUESTIONS

1. Can you explain how the top, down and bottom, up approach would apply differently to principles of growth and development?
2. What techniques can be applied to maximize student achievement in motor skill development?
3. What principles of learning can be applied to increase efficiency of training regimens that facilitate motor performance?
4. Name some techniques for providing consequences to behaviors to be learned that will facilitate motor proficiency.
5. What are some positive teacher techniques that can be used to adapt instruction to the needs of the learner?
6. What are the procedures for conducting applied behavioral programs?
7. Describe some techniques for recording data that extend present levels of performance.
8. Describe the different ways in which performance can be measured.
9. Name and describe some behavioral techniques for facilitating the development of positive behavior.
10. Indicate some principles for establishing class rules.
11. What are some techniques that can be used to manage disruptive classroom behavior?
12. Indicate some positive methods for decreasing inappropriate behavior.
13. Indicate some aversive techniques that can be used to decrease inappropriate behavior.
14. List different types of reinforcers.
15. Provide examples of the application of learning principles that can be applied to the acquisition of positive behavior.
16. What are some of the characteristics of a teacher that can maximize the development of motor and social skills for the handicapped?

STUDENT ACTIVITIES

1. Describe a case study in which tasks are taught to a handicapped child. Indicate how you could apply principles of development to instruction of the child.
2. Describe a case study in which tasks were taught to a handicapped child. Indicate how you could apply the bottom, up or top, down approach to instruction using principles of learning and development that were discussed in this chapter.
3. Select a measurement technique, collect behavioral data on a child, and graph the results.
4. Observe a teacher who is instructing a handicapped child. Record techniques used that were discussed in this chapter.
5. Make a list of class rules that might minimize disruptive behavior.
6. Set up a contingency management system for a class. Indicate procedures for the administration of the system.
7. Evaluate a person who is instructing a handicapped child with the use of instructional objectives to determine effective use of the application of learning principles.

REFERENCES

1. Affleck, H., Lowenbraun, S., and Archer, A.: Teaching the mildly handicapped in the regular classroom, ed. 2, Columbus, Ohio, 1980, Charles E. Merrill Publishing Co.
2. Armstrong v. Kline, in the United States District Court for the Eastern District of Pennsylvania Civil Action, 1979.
3. Ayres, A.J.: Sensory integration and learning disorders, Los Angeles, 1973, Western Psychological Services.
4. Bellamy, G.T., Horner, R.H., and Inman, D.P.: Habilitation of the severely and profoundly retarded, Eugene, Ore., 1977, Specialized Training Program Monograph no. 2, Center on Human Development, University of Oregon.
5. Bobath, K., and Bobath, B.: The facilitation of normal postural reactions and movements in the treatment of cerebral palsy, Physiotherapy **50:**246-262, 1964.
6. Brunstrom, S.: Motor testing procedures in hemiplegia based on recovery stages, J. Am. Phys. Ther. A., **46:**357-375, 1966.
7. deQuiros, J.B., and Schrager, O.L.: Neuropsychological fundamentals in learning disabilities, ed. 2, Novato, Calif., 1979, Academic Therapy Publishers.
8. Foxx, R.M., and Azrin, N.H.: The elimination of autistic self-stimulatory behavior by overcorrection, J. Appl. Behav. Anal. **6:**1-14, 1973.
9. Getman, G.N.: Visuomotor complex in the acquisition of learning skills, Seattle, 1965, Special Child Publishers.
10. Gold, M.: Task analysis: a statement and example using acquisition and production of a complex assembly task by the retarded blind, Institute for Child Behavior and Development, University of Illinois at Urbana-Champaign, 1975.
11. Haring, N., editor: Developing effective individualized programs for severely handicapped children and youth, Washington, D.C., 1977, United States Office of Education, Bureau of Education for the Handicapped.

12. Homme, L.: How to use contingency contracting in the classroom, Champaign, Ill., 1970, Research Press.
13. Kabat, H., and Knott, M.: Proprioceptive facilitation techniques for treatment of paralysis, Phys. Ther. Rev. **33:**53-64, 1953.
14. Kazdin, A.E.: Single-case research designs: methods for clinical and applied settings, New York, 1982, Oxford University Press.
15. Kephart, N.C.: Slow learner in the classroom, ed. 2, Columbus Ohio, 1971, Charles E. Merrill Publishing Co.
16. Lewis, R.B., and Doorlag, D.H.: Teaching special students in the mainstream, Columbus, Ohio, 1983, Charles E. Merrill Publishing Co.
17. McLoughlin, J.A., and Lewis, R.B.: Assessing special students, Columbus, Ohio, 1981, Charles E. Merrill Publishing Co.
18. Reichle, J., et al.: Curricula for the severely handicapped: components of evaluation criteria. In Wilcox, B., and York, R., editors: Quality education for the severely handicapped, Washington, D.C., 1980, U.S. Department of Education, Office of Special Education.
19. Sherrill, C.: Adapted physical education and recreation, Dubuque, Iowa, 1981, William C. Brown & Co., Publishers.
20. Sulzer-Azaroff, B., and Mayer, G.R.: Applying behavior analysis procedures with children and youth, New York, 1977, Holt, Rinehart & Winston.
21. Wilcox, B., and Bellamy, G.T.: Design of high school programs for severely handicapped students, Baltimore, 1982, Paul H. Brookes Publishing Co.
22. Winnick, J.: Project UNIQUE, Paper presented at the International Symposium Year of the Disabled Child, New Orleans, 1981.

SUGGESTED READINGS

Blankenship, C., and Lilly, M.S.: Mainstreaming students with learning and behavior problems, New York, 1981, Holt, Rinehart & Winston.

Foxx, R.M., and Azrin, N.H.: The elimination of autistic self-stimulatory behavior by overcorrection, J. Appl. Behav. Anal. **6:**1-14, 1973.

Homme, L.: How to use contingency management contracting in the classroom, Champaign, Ill., 1969, Research Press.

Kazdin, A.E.: Behavior modification in applied setting, Homewood, Ill., 1980, The Dorsey Press.

Kazdin, A.E.: Single-case research designs: methods of clinical and applied settings, New York, 1982, Oxford University Press.

Lewis, R., and Doorlag, D.H.: Teaching special students in the mainstream, Columbus, Ohio, 1983, Charles E. Merrill Publishing Co.

McLoughlin, J.A., and Lewis, R.B.: Assessing special students, Columbus, Ohio, 1981, Charles E. Merrill Publishing Co.

Seaman, J.A., and DePauw, K.P.: The new adapted physical education: a developmental approach, Palo Alto, Calif. 1982, Mayfield Publishing.

Sulzer-Azaroff, B., and Mayer G.R.: Applying behavior-analysis procedures with children and youth, New York, 1977, Holt, Rinehart & Winston.

Walker, J.E., and Shea, T.M.: Behavior modification: a practical approach for educators, ed. 3, St. Louis, 1984, The C.V. Mosby Co.

CHAPTER 8

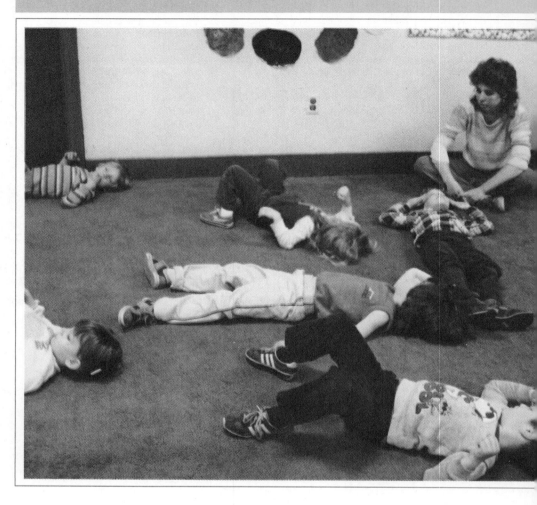

Relaxation Techniques

OBJECTIVES

♦ Know the definition of tension.

♦ Understand the seriousness of tension.

♦ Know at least five popular techniques to reduce tension that are used in modern society.

♦ Differentiate between three types of conscious control of muscular tension.

♦ List the preliminary requirements and know the principal steps to use for teaching conscious control of muscular tension.

Awareness of tension and active searching for ways to reduce tension are on the increase in the United States. There is no doubt that anxiety, increased noise levels, pace of living, crowding, and job demands produce high levels of tension. Use of prescription and illegal drugs, participation in various forms of meditation, and "hot-tubbing" are popular practices Americans employ to find relief from tension. Because tension is becoming more prevalent in our society, it is important that students be taught sound practices and techniques to reduce their tension levels. Cratty[5] has described tension as overt muscular contraction caused by an emotional state or increased muscular effort. Nervous tension results from anxiety and the hectic conditions and pace of our society.

This chapter concerns what is meant by the term *tension,* how tension affects the human body, and techniques for reducing tension. A procedure for teaching relaxation to students and evaluating its effectiveness is also presented.

CONTINUUM OF TENSION

The anxious person is one who tends to worry and has an unusual amount of undefined fear. A continual state of nervous tension may be manifested in pathological systemic conditions. Prolonged anxiety and emotional stress may also lead to psychosomatic disorders.

Selye[16] suggested the existence of a general adaptation syndrome that occurs in animals and humans when they are subjected to continual emotional stress. This syndrome is composed of three consecutive stages: (1) the alarm reaction, which represents normal body changes caused by emotion; (2) the resistance to stress, or one's adjustment to the alarm reaction, which requires considerable energy resources; and (3) the exhaustion stage, in which the store of energy is used up. The exhaustion stage may lead to the death of single cells, organs, organ systems, or the entire organism. Some authorities have suggested stress as a possible cause of hypertension, rheumatism, arthritis, ulcers, allergies, and other conditions. The overanxious person has a high level of cerebral and emotional activity, coupled with nervous muscular tension, which may eventually lead to the exhaustion stage and perhaps to psychosomatic disorders. It is commonly accepted in medicine that long-term stress may lead to one or more disease states.[16]

It is desirable for all persons to be able to consciously control their tension levels. It is particularly important for persons who have high degrees of tension attributable to some emotional or physical problem to be able to attain a relaxed state at will. Pain and nervous distress are accentuated and compounded by disorders of mind and body. Characteristically, persons with cardiovascular, respiratory, or rheumatic (as well as other) conditions need to develop the ability to reduce their tension levels.

It is important that all teachers of physical education be able to instruct their students in the skills of recognizing abnormal tensions and reducing them. It is even more important for teachers of adapted physical education, who deal with individuals with special problems, to be able to recognize overt signs of abnormal muscular tension levels and to teach ways of overcoming them.

POPULAR TENSION-REDUCING PRACTICES

Relaxation is freedom from nervous tension and anxiety. All persons seek relaxation at some time or another; however, practices leading to relief of tension differ among cultures. Many different techniques for achieving relaxation are currently in vogue in the United States. Most of these practices yield an immediate release from tension, but some result in long-range deleterious effects on the mind and body.

Pills, Powders, and Drinks

The American public annually spends millions of dollars, both legally and illegally, on drugs and alcoholic beverages to help reduce an uncomfortable sense of tension or to attain a state of euphoria. Drug abuse is an ever-pressing problem in the world today.[8] Persons seeking relief from painful anxieties and feelings of inadequacy attempt escape through drugs that alter neural activity. Common categories of agents used for relaxation and alteration of the personality are psychotomimetic drugs, narcotics, analgesics, sedatives, ataractics (tranquilizers), and depressants.

Psychotomimetic Drugs

Psychotomimetic or hallucinogenic agents such as LSD (lysergic acid diethylamide) and mescaline are often used by persons who are dissatisfied with their lives and are seeking the peace of mind and understanding that come with an expanded consciousness. Used in very small doses psychotomimetic drugs produce a toxic psychosis that may cause perceptual distortions of one or all of the senses. Users of such hallucinogens may experience a "bad trip" resulting in altered behavior, which is manifested in irrationality and uncommon fears.

Narcotics

Derivatives of opium, especially morphine, are used medically for their sedative and analgesic actions. Unfortunately, they are also sought for their euphorigenic properties (particularly in the case of heroin). Addicts of opiates and opiate-like narcotics are attempting to relieve emotional pain caused by daily anxieties and hostilities.

Marijuana, unlike the opiates, is not considered physiologically addictive. Its sole source is the plant *Cannabis sativa*. When smoked, the marijuana leaf may produce euphoria, sedation, and hallucinations. The user may display an altered consciousness, expressing feelings of lightness, gaiety, and detachment from reality.

Analgesics

Salicylates are used in a number of compounds that may be applied to the body externally or internally. Acetylsalicylic acid (aspirin) is the most common compound. Salicylates have the ability to reduce inflammation and pain. As a pain reliever, it has a definite effect on the musculoskeletal system. Although aspirin does not produce sedation or euphoria, as do the opiates, there is recent indication that it has some tranquilizing qualities.

Sedatives

Barbiturates are considered hypnotic and sedative drugs and are widely used by persons for sleep-inducing or (in smaller doses) calming effects.

The physiological effects of barbiturates are not well understood; however, there are some indications that a general depression of the central nervous system takes place. Barbiturates are highly addictive. The long-term user of barbiturates is in a constant state of severe depression, which manifests itself in numerous personality changes.

Tranquilizers

Tranquilizers, or ataractics, have become more prominent in medicine and in the patent drug industry. Used for tension and anxiety, tranquilizers affect the sympathetic nervous system by suppressing synaptic stimuli. The main use of ataractics in medicine has been in the areas of behavioral disorders and mental disease. The hyperirritable patient who becomes tranquilized is more amenable to psychotherapy. For much of the general public, tranquilizers have become a crutch frequently used for coping with daily stress.

Depressants

Ethyl alcohol has hypnotic qualities and for centuries has been used systemically as a general depressant. It is believed to block the synaptic connections of nerve impulses in the central nervous system, producing varying degrees of depression. Alcohol is an anesthetic to the higher faculties, and thus it brings about a state of temporary relaxation. Depression of the higher brain centers results in diminished control of emotional behavior and decreased movement control.

Rituals, Systems, and Methods

Most people practice various methods of achieving relaxation in daily life. Some methods may be very beneficial to health, whereas others (as mentioned before) may be deleterious to health. Some methods may be momentary, whereas others are more lasting and involve an established routine or ritual. In Western civilization many such techniques are used—for example, imagery, physical therapy, psychology and religion, and exercise.

Imagery

Imagery involves word symbolization or auditory stimulation to evoke mental pictures that are both pleasing and relaxing; for example, while in a comfortable position, a person can imagine that he or she is either floating on a cloud or becoming heavy while gradually sinking deeper and deeper. Listening to soothing music of a slow tempo may result in a state of calm; viewing a beautiful landscape painting may conjure the feelings of quiet and peace.

Physical Therapy

To achieve a relaxed state Americans use many methods that come under the classification of physical therapy. Some common methods are the use of the sauna or steam bath, hydromassage, hot water soaks, and massage.[17] For example, the Finnish sauna bath has been used for centuries as a means to decongest engorged muscles after exercise and to increase relaxation in tense musculature. The European practice of heating the body to temperatures of 185° F for 15 minutes, following this with a cool shower, and then repeating the procedure is becoming a popular technique in America. It induces a euphoric feeling of physical well-being and relaxation. Many resort hotels and spas are now offering sauna baths and hydromassage in small warm water pools, followed by an envigorating dip in a large cool water pool. Hydromassage is a popular form of relaxing the body. The water is agitated around the body by means of a machine that forces jets of water from various openings in the pool. The pressure applied to the body by the water soothe nerve endings, providing the recipient with a sense of reduced muscular tension.

Since the beginning of recorded history, some form of manual massage has been used as a means of bringing about a physiological response. Defined as the systematic manipulation of the soft tissues of the body, massage may be applied in numerous ways: through the use of mechanical vibrators, rollers, or agitated water or, most commonly, through the laying on of hands. Many experts indicate that the hands of a knowledgeable operator offer the most efficient way to apply massage. Massage can produce relaxation through physiological, mechanical, and psychological effects. The most frequently used technique is effleurage, whereby the hands glide lightly over the body in a slow rhythmical pattern, allowing passive reduction of muscular tension.

Psychology and Religion

Many persons who are seeking peace within themselves turn to religion or psychology for assistance. Millions of books are sold with themes such as achieving self-renewal, overcoming personal conflicts, and attaining peace in a tension-filled world.

Recently, some Americans have become interested in Eastern religions and philosophies, which are founded on the principles of inner contemplation and meditation. There are various forms of meditation, most of which begin with the subject assuming a comfortable posture and then focusing on some visible or imagined object. Transcendental meditation employs a *mantra,* which is a specific single sound or short phrase that is repeated many times. Focusing on an object or making a continuous sound helps the meditator avoid distracting thoughts. Scientific research has determined that meditation can significantly reduce mental anxiety and muscular tension.[11] A recent meditation approach that blends both Eastern and Western concepts is titled the *relaxation response.*[4] This method uses the three basic elements found in most meditation and conscious relaxation techniques: (1) proper posture, (2) concentration on an object or sound, and (3) assumption of a passive attitude. For the method of relaxation response the participant sits quietly in a comfortable chair with the eyes closed; progressively relaxes the muscles, starting with the feet and moving up the body; and then breathes through the nose, saying "one" mentally on each inhalation and expiration for 10 to 20 minutes.

One of the most significant biomedical advances in recent times has been the development of biofeedback methods. Through training, individuals can increase their alpha brain waves, which predominate in the mentally relaxed state.[10] By using machines that monitor the brain waves and are designed to make a sound when alpha waves are present, the subject learns to control anxiety and bring about mental and physical relaxation at will.[10]

For many persons hypnosis is a means of reducing anxieties and muscular tension psychotherapeutically. Hypnosis has ben defined as "an artificially induced passive state in which there is increased amenability and responsiveness to suggestions and commands, provided that these do not conflict seriously with the subject's own conscious or unconscious wishes."[4] During hypnosis suggestions can be made to the subject concerning such things as reducing worry, anxiety, or fear; decreasing pain; and relaxing muscles.[12,13]

Exercise

Most persons would agree that the body senses a reduction in tension after any physically fatiguing activity. Electromyographic studies show that neuromuscular tension levels decrease significantly with vigorous exercise, particularly in persons with high tension levels; however, effects are usually transitory.[6]

Some forms of exercise that result in a relaxed state are rhythmical motion, muscle stretching, and the physical exercise system of hatha-yoga, known as *asana.* Music and rhythm are used extensively to initiate coordinated movement and relaxation. Synchronization of specific movement patterns, as expressed through kinesthesia, is the basis for skilled activity. Rathbone[16] indicates that rhythmical exercise relieves the feeling of fatigue and residual tension. Activities that are based on a continuous or even sequence of movement (such as walking, dancing, swimming, and bicycle riding) result in reduced tension. Muscle stretching, which increases joint flexibility, also tends to reduce tension within the musculotendinous unit. Therefore, it is logical to presume that an articulation that is unencumbered by tight restricting tissue will also be one that is capable of relaxation. Stretching the body helps one overcome stiffness and allows the various body segments to relax. Research indicates that a steady progressive stretch tends to decrease the myotatic reflex and reduce muscle tension, whereas the ballistic or jerky stretch increases tension. Many of the asanas of hatha-yoga tend to improve joint range of motion. Each yoga posture is executed slowly and deliberately. Devotees consider that relaxation occurs as the mind and body become harmonious.

CONSCIOUS CONTROL OF MUSCULAR TENSION

The most easily learned beneficial means of reducing nervous tension is that of conscious control.[8] Physiological benefits from willed relaxation include reductions in oxygen consumption, respiratory rate, heart rate, and muscle tension.

Three excellent techniques for consciously reducing tension are progressive relaxation, autogenic training, and differential relaxation. Edmund Jacobson, a physiologist-physician, is known as the father of progressive relaxation.[9] His technique emphasizes relaxation of voluntary skeletal muscles. During progressive relaxation training an individual becomes aware of muscular tension and learns to consciously release tension in specific muscle groups. Autogenic training in relaxation was developed by H.H. Schulz, a German neurologist.[15] This technique is designed to reduce exteroceptive and proprioceptive stimulation through mental activity described as passive concentration. Using this method an individual brings to mind images that promote a relaxed state.

Jacobson's system starts with muscles of the left upper extremity and moves to the right upper extremity, followed by the left lower extremity, right lower extremity, abdominal muscles, respiratory muscles, back pectoral region, shoulder muscles, and facial muscles. Persons are encouraged to gradually stiffen each body part and then to slowly release that tension.[10]

Autogenic training begins with phrases that suggest heaviness of the whole body and the individual parts, followed by phrases that suggest warmth or regularity to the body, heart, respiratory system, and abdominal area. A third set of phrases promotes images of colors and relaxing in warm, soft, pleasant surroundings.[15]

Decreasing and increasing muscular tension levels at will require varying degrees of coordination. All skilled movement requires differential relaxation. A technique that has been found beneficial for training individuals to selectively control specific muscles is known as the muscle tension recognition and release method.[2,3] This technique starts with the subject tensing and relaxing the entire body and then learning bilateral body control (control of both upper limbs and then of both lower limbs). Following demonstration of bilateral limb control the subject advances to unilateral body control, whereby muscular tension is increased on one side of the body and completely released on the other—for example, with tensing of the right arm and leg and relaxing of the left arm and leg. From unilateral control the subject progresses to cross-lateral body control, which involves tensing of the opposite arm and leg. The last stage of differential relaxation training involves the isolation and relaxation of specific body parts at will. In general, differential relaxation training is a useful tool for developing total body control, increasing body awareness, and reducing anxiety. However, this technique should be limited to the particular developmental level of the individual. These techniques, used individually and in combination, reduce nervous tension and tactile defensive responses in children.[1]

Benefits

Learning to relax is a motor skill and must be considered an important part of the total education program or physical education program. As a skill, relaxation must be taught and practiced for competency. Too often teachers of physical education are concerned with gross movement activities alone. To lie down when tired or to practice relaxation when tense or overanxious is considered a waste of time by many teachers. This narrow point of view ignores a very important aspect of the field of physical education—that relaxation is of special importance to many atypical as well as typical students.

A number of positive benefits can be accrued by disabled children who have conscious control of their tension levels. Energy can be conserved and better control of emotions can result (fears and anxieties become less intense). Sleep comes easier, the acquisition and performance of motor skills are enhanced, pain and physical discomfort become less intense, and the ability to learn may be improved. Relaxation therefore becomes a vital tool in the total machinery of the educational process.

To the physiologist, relaxation indicates a complete absence of neuromuscular activity (zero state).[10] The relaxed body part does not resist stretch but rather reflects the lengthening of muscle fibers. An overt sign of relaxation is a limp and completely motionless body part. Through relaxation of overly tense muscles, a number of positive effects may occur in respiration, circulation, and neuromuscular coordination.

Respiration

The reduction of tension in the thorax and muscles of respiration allows for a greater capacity of inspiration and expiration. With this increased capacity, there is a more efficient exchange of oxygen and carbon dioxide within the body. For persons with breathing disorders, relaxation of the thoracic mechanism allows for a greater respiratory potential.

Circulation

Relaxation of tense skeletal muscles allows the blood to circulate unimpeded by constricted blood vessels to all the body tissues. A person with cardiovascular disease is greatly aided when the ability to reduce muscular tension at will is achieved. Blood pressure may be reduced by diminishing of outside resistance, which subsequently decreases the strain on heart and blood vessels.

Neuromuscular Coordination

In order for the body to move uninhibited, there must be a smooth synchronization of muscles. Differential relaxation or controlled tension attributable to the reciprocal action of agonist and antagonist muscles provides for coordinated movement without undue fatigue. Persons who exhibit poor coordination as a result of neuromuscular or cerebral problems must learn to relax tense muscles differentially in order for their purposeful movement to be smooth, accurate, and enduring.

TEACHING A SYSTEM OF RELAXATION

The instructor of adapted physical education can teach a variety of relaxation techniques depending on the time and conditions available. As has been described earlier in this discussion, imagery and recognition of tension provide a convenient means of learning to relax. These methods may be combined and used with success in the typical 30-minute physical education period.

Identification of abnormal tension areas in the body requires the performance of a series of muscle contractions and relaxations. In this modified system of progressive relaxation, muscle contractions should be performed gradually and slowly for 30 seconds and then the muscles should be relaxed for 30 seconds in an attempt to obtain a "negative" state. The student is reminded to tense only the muscles the instructor indicates and to keep all other body areas relaxed while tensing a single part. Special consideration is given to the areas of the body that are difficult to relax—for example, the lower back and the abdominal, shoulder, neck, and eye regions. After the guided session, the student makes a record of the areas that were difficult to relax. Eventually, with diligent practice, the student will have to tense and relax only those areas that are difficult to relax. In doing so the student can achieve at will a general decrease of muscular tonus throughout the body.

Preliminary Requirements

In order for the student to develop a keen perception of tension and learn to relax, the instructor should consider a number of environmental and learning factors that may strongly affect the ability to reduce body tension.

Room

The room in which relaxation exercises are conducted should have a comfortable temperature (between 72° and 76° F); it should be well ventilated with no chilling drafts. The light may be outside to prevent interruption of the relaxation lesson.

Dress

The student should wear comfortable, warm, loose-fitting apparel and no shoes.

Equipment

In actuality, very little equipment is needed to teach relaxation. Ideally, five small pillows or rolled-up towels and a firm mat are useful; however, relaxation can be accomplished on any comfortable surface without the use of props. All students should have a pencil and paper nearby so that they can record personal reactions after the session.

Positioning

Although a person can learn to relax while standing or sitting, the ideal position for tension recognition is that of lying on a firm mat with each body curve comfortably supported by a pillow or towel (Fig. 8-1). Contour support is afforded the curves of the cervical and lumbar vertebrae; each forearm is supported, resulting in a slight bend to each elbow; and the knees, like the elbows, are maintained in a slightly flexed position with the thighs externally rotated. With minimal support given to the body curves and limbs, free muscle contraction can take place while the individual is in a comfortable, relaxed position. However, if equipment for joint support is not available, a flat mat surface will suffice.

Sound

A number of techniques utilizing sound may be used by the teacher to aid the student in acquir-

ing the right frame of mind for relaxation. Soft music playing in the background may be beneficial. If music is not available, the monotonous pattern of a metronome clicking at 48 or fewer beats per minute may be helpful. However, the most important sound is the voice of the instructor, which should be quiet, slow, rhythmical, and distant.

Breathing

During the relaxation session the student is instructed to take slow, deep inhalations through the nose and make long, slow exhalations through the mouth. Gradually, through breathing control, the student consciously tries to let go of all the body tension. As relaxation occurs, breathing becomes slower and more shallow.

Imagery

The tension recognition technique involves two distinct phases: a contraction phase, whereby the subject contracts a particular muscle or group of muscles to sense tension; and a "let go" phase, whereby the subject seeks a complete lack of tension, or negativeness. To aid the pupil in the sec-

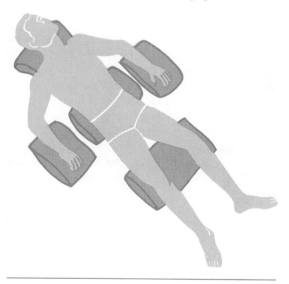

FIGURE 8-1
Basic position for tension reduction exercises (Figures 8-2 to 8-18).

ond phase the teacher encourages the use of imagery. The student is told to imagine very relaxing things. Image-inducing statements such as "your body is heavy against the floor," "your heart is beating regularly and calmly, like a clock ticking," and "listen to the sound of your breathing" may help the student relax. Children at the elementary school level have keen imaginations and respond readily to suggestions such as imagining their bodies as snowmen on a hot day or as butter in a hot pan.

Sleep

The pupil should be instructed that the main purpose of the exercise session is to develop awareness of tense body areas and the ability to relax consciously without falling asleep. However, if sleep does occur during the session, it should be considered a positive reaction.

Principles of Teaching Relaxation

There are a number of ways the instructor can proceed with relaxation guidance. The teacher can begin by having the pupils contract their facial muscles and then move downward to finish in the lower limbs or, conversely, by having them contract muscles from foot to head. If less time is available, contraction of large muscle groups with progression to the smaller muscles of the body is another alternative. Whatever the technique used, the goals are the same and the teacher will soon develop a style that seems to work best.

Because of the limited amount of time available in the physical education period, many sessions may be required before desired results are attained. A home program should be encouraged for persons who find it difficult to let go of tension.

Directions to the Student

For expediency in the physical education setting, each muscular contraction phase and each relaxation phase is conducted for approximately 30 seconds, providing a total of 1 minute for each step. During the introductory session the muscle contraction should be intense enough to cause a degree of fatigue. The tension is reduced gradually with each subsequent session, requiring a greater perceptual sensitivity. The following is a sample of a relaxation session given to a group of students in a typical school setting.

Step 1: Lie still for a minute and stare at an object on the ceiling. Do the eyes feel as though they are getting heavy? As this occurs, gradually let them close. Take five deep breaths, inhaling and exhaling slowly. Think of all the joints of the body as being very relaxed.

Step 2: Curl the toes downward and point both feet downward toward the end of the mat (Fig. 8-2). Feel the tension in the bottoms of the feet and behind the legs. Keep the mouth relaxed and continue to breathe deeply and slowly. Remember, while tensing one area of the body, all other parts should be relaxed. Now release the muscle contractions slowly, letting go to a complete relaxed state. Feel the body getting extremely heavy and sinking into the mat.

Step 3: Curl the toes and both feet upward toward the head (Fig. 8-3). Sense the tenseness on the tops of the feet and legs. Remember not to reinforce the movement by tensing other parts of the body. Breathe easily and relax. Let go of the muscle contraction, allowing the feet and ankles to go limp slowly.

Step 4: Leaving the legs in their original position, with the knees slightly bent, press the legs down (Fig. 8-4). Feel the tension in the back of the thighs and buttocks. Remember, while holding this contraction, all other parts of the body should be at ease. Relax, slowly feeling the discomfort of tension completely leave the body.

Step 5: Remain in the position as for step 4 and straighten the legs to full extension (Fig. 8-5). Feel the tightness in the tops of the thighs. Now let go. Breathing should be easy and relaxed, and a profound sense of heaviness should be present throughout the body.

Step 6: With the legs and thighs in the original resting position, draw the thighs upward to a bent-knee position, with the heels raised from the mat about 3 inches (Fig. 8-6). The tension should be felt primarily in the bend of the hip. Try to keep all other muscle groups relaxed. Return slowly to the starting position and then let go to a negative state again.

Step 7: Forcibly rotate the thighs outward (Fig. 8-7). Feel the muscle tension in the outer hip region. Do not let tension creep into other parts of the body. Now slowly relax the hip rotators. Go limp.

Step 8: Rotate the thighs inward (Fig. 8-8). Feel the muscle tension deep in the inner thighs. Relax slowly, let go of all tension, and let the thighs again rotate outward. Sense the body sinking deeper into the mat.

Step 9: Squeeze the buttocks (gluteal muscles) together tightly and tilt the hips backward (Fig. 8-9). Muscular

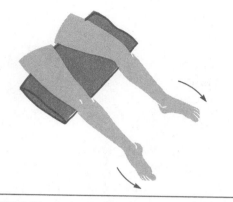

FIGURE 8-2
Step 2.

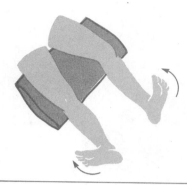

FIGURE 8-3
Step 3.

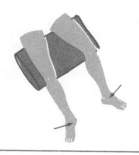

FIGURE 8-4
Step 4.

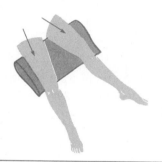

FIGURE 8-5
Step 5.

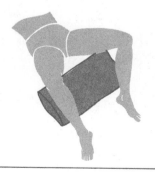

FIGURE 8-6
Step 6.

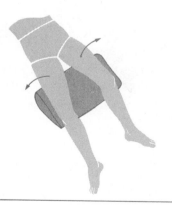

FIGURE 8-7
Step 7.

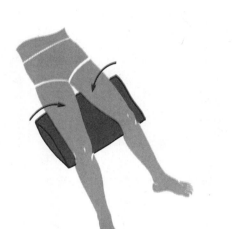

FIGURE 8-8
Step 8.

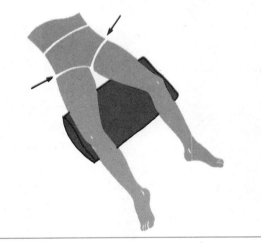

FIGURE 8-9
Step 9.

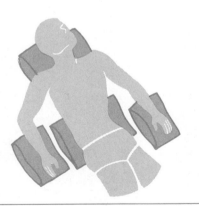

FIGURE 8-10
Step 10.

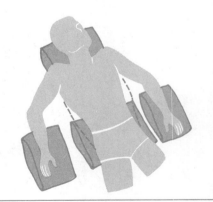

FIGURE 8-11
Step 11.

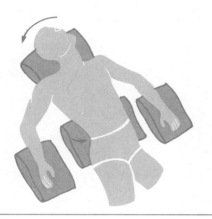

FIGURE 8-12
Step 12.

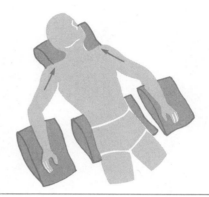

FIGURE 8-13
Step 13.

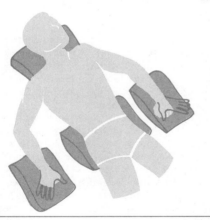

FIGURE 8-14
Step 15.

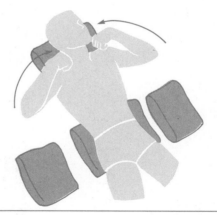

FIGURE 8-15
Step 17.

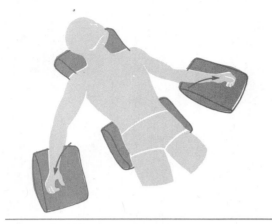

FIGURE 8-16
Step 18.

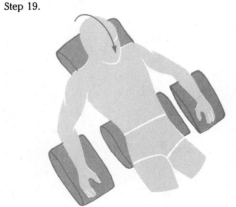

FIGURE 8-17
Step 19.

FIGURE 8-18
Step 21.

tension should only be felt in the buttocks and lower back region. Again, be aware of other tensions that may be occurring in the body. Now let go of the contraction and try to sense the joints becoming extremely loose.

Step 10: Tighten the abdominal muscles by pressing downward on the rib cage while rolling the hips backward; at the same time, flatten the lower back (Fig. 8-10). The tension is felt both in the abdominal muscles and in the lower back region. Inhale slowly and let the back settle into the mat.

Step 11: Inhale and exhale slowly and as deeply as possible three times (Fig. 8-11). A general tension should be felt throughout the rib cage. After the last forced inspiration and expiration, return to normal quiet breathing and sense the difference in tension levels.

Step 12: Accentuating the curve of the neck (cervical spine), press the head back and lift the upper back off the mat (Fig. 8-12). The tension should be felt in the back of the neck and upper back. Settle slowly back to the mat.

Step 13: Pinch the shoulders back, squeezing the two shoulder blades together. Tension is felt in the back of the shoulders. Release the contraction slowly and fall easily back to the mat. Be aware of any residual tension that might remain after returning to the mat.

Step 14: Leaving the arms in the resting position, lift and roll shoulders inward so that tension is felt in the front of the chest (Fig. 8-13). Do not allow the shoulders to drop back to the mat in the resting position. Feel the tension leave the chest.

Step 15: Spread and grip the fingers of both hands. Do this three times (Fig. 8-14). The tension is felt in the hands and forearms. As the fingers are gripped and spread, be sure not to lift the elbows from the mat. After the third series, let the hands and forearms fall limply back to their supports.

Step 16: Make a tight fist with both hands and slowly curl the wrists backward, forward, and to both sides. Tension should primarily be felt at the fist, wrist, and forearm. After these movements, allow fingers and thumbs to open gradually.

Step 17: Make a tight fist with both hands and slowly bend (flex) the arms at the elbows until the forearms rest against the upper arms, at the same time lifting the shoulders (Fig. 8-15). Tension is felt in the front part of the forearms, in the bicep regions, and in the front part of the shoulders. After the arms are slowly uncurled and returned to the resting position, relax each segment separately until they become limp, motionless, and negative.

Step 18: Make a tight fist with both hands, stiffen the arms, and press hard against the mat (Fig. 8-16). Tension should be felt in the forearms and the back of the upper arms and shoulders. Hold the pressure against the mat for 30 seconds and then release slowly.

Step 19: Shrug the right shoulder, then bend the head sideways (laterally flex neck), touching the ear to the elevated shoulder (Fig. 8-17).

Step 20: As in step 19, shrug the left shoulder; then laterally flex the neck, touching the ear to the elevated shoulder. Tension should only be felt in the upper left shoulder and the lateral muscles of the neck. Release the contraction, slowly returning the neck and shoulder to the resting position.

Step 21: Bend the head forward, touching the chin to the chest (Fig. 8-18). Tension is felt in the front of the neck. Relax and slowly return the head to the resting position. Continue to concentrate on the body as being extremely heavy and at a zero state.

Step 22: Lift the eyebrows upward and wrinkle the forehead. Feel the tension in the forehead. Let the face go blank.

Step 23: Close the eyelids tightly and wrinkle the nose. Tension is felt in the nose and eyes. Let the face relax slowly. Concentrate on the tension leaving the face.

Step 24: Open the mouth widely as if to yawn. Feel the tension in the jaw. Now let the mouth close slowly and lightly.

Step 25: Bite down hard and then show the teeth in a forced smile. Tension should be felt in the jaw and lips. Slowly allow the face to return to a blank expression. Be sure not to tense other parts of the body when contracting the facial muscles.

Step 26: Pucker the lips hard as if to whistle. Sense tension at the edge of the mouth. Let the tension melt away.

Step 27: Push the tongue hard against the roof of the mouth. Let go. Push the tongue against the roof of the mouth again as hard as possible. Relax. Push the tongue against the upper teeth. Relax. Sense the contraction of the tongue muscles. Try not to use any other body parts. Relax.

Step 28: Lie very still for a short while and try to be conscious of the body areas that were difficult to relax. Move slowly and take any position desired. Relax and rest.

Step 29: Try to hold the color of black or white in the mind's eye. Once you see one color, do not let any other color or picture slip into your mind.

Step 30: Roll to one side and sit up slowly.

Evaluation

Although the most accurate indication of abnormal tension is provided by electromyographic tests, subjective evaluation still has its place for the physical education instructor. Tension is eas-

ily observable through mannerisms such as extraneous movements or muscle twitches (eye twitches, finger movements, stiffness, changes of position, and playing with hands) and vocal sounds. The instructor should test muscle resistance by lifting the student's arms and legs after the relaxation session. Limbs that have residual tension do not feel limp or lifeless; they tend to feel stiff and unyielding. The instructor tells the student that he or she will be tested for relaxation at the end of the session. The following four factors may be made apparent by the tests: (1) whether the student assists the movement, (2) whether the student resists the movement, (3) whether the student engages in positioning body parts, or (4) whether the student ideally displays a complete lack of tension.

After the exercise session, the students are asked to answer questions about their personal reactions, writing their answers on a sheet of paper by their side. Some suggested questions include the following:

1. What was your general reaction to the session—good, bad, or indifferent?
2. Were you comfortable for the entire session? If not, what disturbed you?
3. Did you sense the tensions and relaxations at all times? If not, why not?
4. Were there areas of the body that you just could not continually relax? What were they?

Questions such as these help the student identify reactions to the relaxation session. The student may require a number of sessions before being able to identify tense body regions accurately. While learning to relax individual parts, the student will gradually be able to relax larger segments and eventually the whole body at will.

Relaxing Physically Immature Students

Conscious control of muscular tension is usually very difficult for physically immature persons. A program of relaxation training must be commensurate with the subjects' developmental and maturational levels. Before a training program can be effectively instituted, the subjects must understand what tension and relaxation are and how they contrast. The concept of relaxation can be taught by having the students pretend their arms are like rubber bands, that they are melting like snowmen on a very hot day, or that they are rag dolls that cannot stand up. Another good technique to develop the concepts of tightness and looseness is to have the participants stiffen their entire bodies for about 30 seconds and then gradually let go of the tension by pretending to be a pat of butter melting in a very hot pan. Following this activity the instructor can introduce questions such as "how does it feel to be relaxed?" or "doesn't it feel better to be relaxed than stiff and tense?" Once the subjects perceive the difference between tensing and releasing tension, the instructor can begin to develop skill programs that gradually take the students from a total body program to a segmental relaxation program.[2]

SUMMARY

Nervous tension is an overt muscular contraction caused by an emotional state. Many factors in our society contribute to abnormal muscular tension. Increased noise levels, crowding, job demands, pace of living, and anxiety are among the most prevalent of these factors. The longer nervous tension continues, the more serious and damaging the results can be. Selye[16] said that humans continually exposed to emotional stress can eventually become exhausted. Hypertension, arthritis, ulcers, and other conditions may also result from continual stress.

Americans use many different techniques to attempt to reduce tension and stress. The most popular are pills, powders, drinks, rituals, systems, and methods. Children living in our society must learn to recognize nervous tension and reduce it through conscious control. Three techniques for consciously reducing tension are progressive relaxation, autogenic training, and differential relaxation. Use of these techniques can lead to improved respiration, circulation, and neuromuscular coordination.

Instructors should teach their students how to consciously relax. All that is needed to conduct relaxation sessions is a quiet room with a comfortable temperature. The use of imagery is appealing to young children. The students are instructed to tense and then relax each muscle group in the body. The success of the relaxation period can be evaluated by manual testing of muscle resistance at the end of each session. Questioning students about their reactions to the session helps focus their attention on their level of success. Physically immature students may need additional prompts to understand the entire process.

REVIEW QUESTIONS

1. According to Selye, what are the three consecutive stages of the general adaptation syndrome?
2. What is the definition of the term *relaxation?*
3. What are three techniques used for achieving relaxation currently in use by many Americans?
4. What is the difference between narcotics and analgesics?
5. What is the difference between sedatives and tranquilizers?
6. What are three techniques for consciously reducing tension?
7. What are two benefits of conscious control of muscular tension?
8. What are the preliminary requirements for teaching conscious control of muscular tension?

STUDENT ACTIVITIES

1. Interview three friends. Ask each person what technique(s) he or she uses to relax after a tension-filled day.
2. Teach the conscious relaxation technique to one child (under 10 years of age) and one adult. Observe and record the differences in how each followed the instructions you gave them.
3. Interview three physical education teachers. Ask whether they teach conscious relaxation techniques and if so, why.
4. Examine the labels on three different brands of sleeping pills. Record the ingredients of each.
5. Read one article on the effects of narcotics or alcohol. Write a report on the negative side effects of the substance.
6. Go through a popular magazine and cut out all the advertisements for relaxants (pills, powders, or techniques). Group the advertisements according to the categories (analgesics, narcotics, sedatives, etc.) discussed in this chapter.

REFERENCES

1. Anneberg, L.: A study of the effect of different relaxation techniques on tactile deficient and tactile defensive children, Unpublished master's thesis, University of Kansas, 1977.
2. Arnheim, D.D., and Peslolisi, R.A.: Developing motor behavior in children: a balanced approach to elementary physical education, St. Louis, 1973, The C.V. Mosby Co.
3. Arnheim, D.D., and Sinclair, W.W.: The clumsy child: a program of motor therapy, ed. 2, St. Louis, 1979, The C.V. Mosby Co.
4. Benson, H.: The relaxation response, New York, 1975, Wiliam Morrow & Co., Inc.
5. Cratty, B.J.: Movement behavior and motor learning, Philadelphia, 1975, Lea & Febiger.
6. DeVries, H.A.: Physiology of exercise, ed. 3, Dubuque, Iowa, 1980, William C. Brown Co., Publishers.
7. Frederick, A.B.: Tension control, J. Health, Phys. Educ., Rec. **38**:42-44, 78-80, 1967.
8. Goth, A.: Medical pharmacology: principles and concepts, ed. 11, St. Louis, 1984, The C.V. Mosby Co.
9. Jacobson, E.O.: Modern treatment of tense patients, Springfield, Ill., 1970, Charles C Thomas, Publishers.
10. Moback, R.: the promise of biofeedback: don't hold the part yet, Psychology Today **9**:18-22, 80-81, 1975.
11. Naranjo, C., and Ornstein, R.E.: On the psychology of meditation, New York, 1973, The Viking Press.
12. Powers, M.: Advanced techniques of hypnosis, ed. 4, North Hollywood, Calif., 1956, Wilshire Book Co.
13. Powers, M.: A practical guide to self-hypnosis, North Hollywood, Calif., 1963, Wilshire Book Co.
14. Rathbone, J.L.: Relaxation, Philadelphia, 1969, Lea & Febiger.
15. Schulz, H.H., and Luthe, W.: Autogenic training, New York, 1959, George A. Straton, Inc.
16. Selye, H.: The stress of life, New York, 1976, McGraw-Hill Book Co.
17. Tappan, F.M.: Healing massage techniques, New York, 1978, Macmillan Publishing Co., Inc.

PART THREE

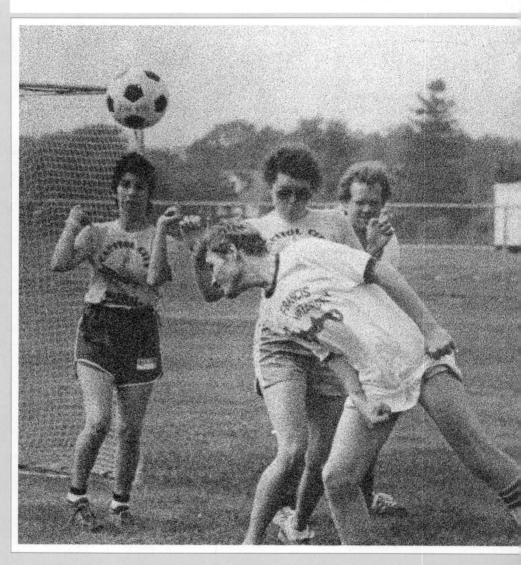

Programming for Specific Problems

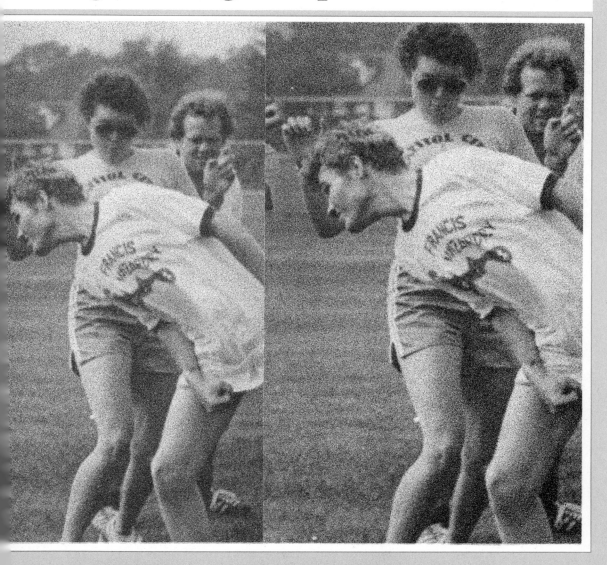

In this section specific types of disabilities are described in detail. Each condition is defined, characteristics are given, means of testing are suggested, and specific programming and teaching techniques are detailed.

CHAPTER 9

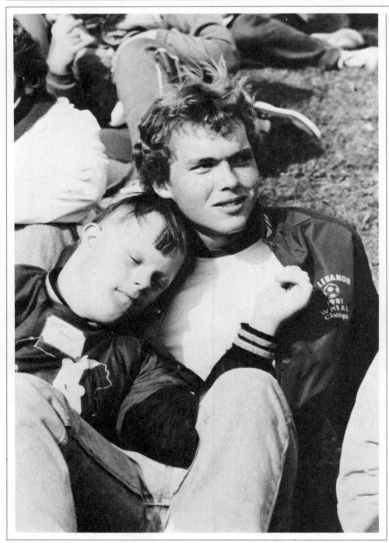

Special Olympics

Psychosocial Development

OBJECTIVES

♦ Know the kinds of social benefits that can be achieved by the handicapped through sports and games.

♦ Know the prerequisite knowledge a teacher should have to conduct an instructional process to change social behavior through sports and games.

♦ Know specific techniques to engage persons in social interaction.

♦ Know how to write social goals that involve sports and games.

♦ Know how to generalize social behavior from sports and games to other environments.

Many educators view schools as the vehicle for transmitting social and cultural values to children. This may be done through an instructional process similar to that for teaching motor skills to handicapped children. It involves (1) identifying the social abilities to be transmitted to handicapped children, (2) identifying a sequence of microsocieties capable of transmitting the social abilities, (3) identifying necessary prerequisites of social participation in sports, games, and play, (4) using procedures to assess the present level of performance on ability traits and behavior in the sequence of games and play activity, (5) determining social goals, and (6) intervening with specific techniques and strategies to achieve the social goals.

FACTORS THAT CONTRIBUTE TO PSYCHOSOCIAL DELAYS
Social Maldevelopment

The environmental conditions enjoyed by the handicapped often are not conducive to positive social development. Some factors that can deter social development are overprotection by parents and teachers, exclusion from play and other social activity, and rejection by peers and authority figures. Teachers should have adequate information about what to expect from the handicapped. The lack of appropriate information may limit intervention strategies by the teacher to lessen fears and prejudice among those with whom handicapped persons interact socially. The lack of acceptance has a negative effect on self-concept and physical performance.[4] Participation may be inhibited, and the talents and needs of the handicapped may be overlooked.

Social Problems

The handicapped generally experience more problems in individual and social development and adjustment than do their nonhandicapped peers.[10] Many do not look or act like other students. Some of the ways in which they differ socially from others are as follows:
1. They may lack ability to relate to others and respond appropriately.

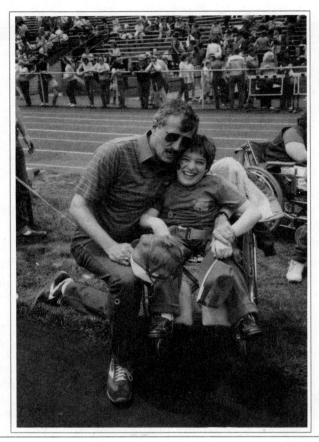

FIGURE 9-1
Acceptance of the handicapped may increase their desire to participate in physical activity.
(Courtesy Western Pennsylvania Special Olympics.)

2. They may fail to conform to the expectations of the school and society.
3. They may have particular difficulty in social interactions with peers and teachers.
4. They may encounter continued failure throughout the school years.
5. They may feel inferior, resulting in withdrawal from physical activity.

Labeling

Handicapped children must be labeled as such to receive an individual physical education program. More often than not, the labeling process influ-

ences teacher attitudes.[1] In many instances labeling interferes with objective observation. It is not uncommon for teachers to lower their expectations for persons if they are labeled handicapped. Teachers and peers of the handicapped are often misled by the label, and it delays initial social acceptance.[14] Therefore the teacher must plan specific interventions to counter the labeling effect the handicapped child carries.

Teacher Problems

Physical educators should structure situations that guide the handicapped through social development. This is often difficult because differences in behavior and appearance expressed by the handicapped may create apprehension on the part of both the teacher and peers initially. The teacher must be careful not to display negative attitudes about certain children; in the case of mainstreaming, it may reduce the chance of successful integration.[4] Teachers need to acquire the specific skill of socially integrating children. If their training is lacking, it is difficult for physical education teachers to provide an appropriate learning situation.[9]

SOCIAL BENEFITS OF SPORTS AND GAMES

The development of social capability of handicapped children is an important objective of the physical education program. Social skills improve the chances of social acceptance by others. Seaman and DePauw[12] and Oliver[11] indicate that physical education is an efficient medium through which these children can realize social and emotional growth. Some social benefits that might be outcomes of a physical education program follow:

- It enables a display of socially acceptable characterisics.[5]
- It enables a variety of social experiences and interactions.[11]
- It enables the handicapped and their peers to learn of their capabilities.[7]
- It enables them to be contributors to team and group efforts.[2]
- It enables them to become intelligent spectators in the sport activities in which they participate.

SEGREGATED AND INTEGRATED CLASSES

Regular physical education programs are often restricted to nonhandicapped persons, and thus the two groups are not able to share experiences. Handicapped children should take their physical education in the regular class if possible. If they are removed from regular class, their IEP should provide them with the skills they lack. Eventually they can participate successfully in the regular class setting.

The attitudes of the regular students are often discriminatory.[13] But these attitudes can be improved if the teacher employs appropriate strategies. Before the handicapped are placed in the regular class, provide the regular students with information about the handicapping condition. The regular physical education teacher or the adapted physical education teacher of the handicapped-only class can be responsible, or both may work together.[5]

SOCIAL INTEGRATION OF THE HANDICAPPED PERSON

The Amateur Sports Act of 1978 (P.L. 95-606) encourages the integration of handicapped and nonhandicapped persons in sport competition. The United States Olympic Committee provides assistance to amateur athletic programs for inclusion of the handicapped in competition with the nonhandicapped. This theme is also expressed in the Rehabilitation Act of 1973 (P.L. 93-112) and P.L. 94-142. In some cases integration requires creative strategies. Handicapped children may be delayed in social development as well as motor development. Poor social skills are a factor in their rejection. Many handicapped children are not as capable as regular class children in initiating and sustaining appropriate social relationships; some children lack language skills. The handicapped may fail to develop social skills because they have fewer friends and are rated significantly lower in sociometric status than their peers. Or it may be that special students have difficulty using social cues; some misperceive their social standing and feel that they are better accepted by peers than they actually are.[4] Friendless students have little opportunity to develop social skills, and those with poor skills are unlikely to form friendships.

At the secondary level these problems might increase. In adolescence social interaction with peers becomes extremely important. Handicapped students who have spent the majority of their educational career segregated from age peers can find the transition to a mainstream environment arduous. They may not only fail to share a common experiential background with regular class students, but also might not yet have acquired important social skills. These problems, combined with the barriers to acceptance, magnify the difficulty in promoting social acceptance.

Research indicates that regular students and teachers do not consistently accept the special student.[4] Teachers and peers are more likely to ignore social interactions initiated by the handicapped. Teachers are more critical of their behavior, provide less praise, and consider them less desirable as students.

INSTRUCTIONAL PROCESS FOR SOCIALIZATION

Socialization is the process of learning how to behave appropriately in social settings, that is, how to interact with others.[12] Social skill instruction follows the same procedures as those for teaching motor skills. In the process the learner interacts with a social environment (the game or play activity), adapts to the characteristics of the environment, and thus changes actions so that he is better able to engage in the social process. Fostering, nurturing, guiding, influencing, and controlling social behavior are possible in a designed environment with practical objectives structured by the physical educator. If the teacher is successful, handicapped children move to higher levels of social skills. The prerequisites for such a process are as follows:

1. Skill, physical, and cognitive prerequisites to participate in an activity
2. A taxonomy of social objectives/behavior
3. A sequence of environments where more elaborate social skills, which are task analyzed, are required
4. A procedure for assessing the present level of performance

5. Intervention strategies by the teacher
6. Skills to accommodate social and skill deficiencies
7. Management procedures to structure the social environments

Skill Prerequisites

Handicapped children can apply their skills in social play and recreational sport activity. In the event that the skill level of a person is very low compared with those of the group, there may be diminished opportunity for social facilitation. Therefore the skill levels must be assessed for each individual in comparison with persons that individual might participate with.

Physical Prerequisites

In addition to knowledge of rules and strategies of games and play, there are usually prerequisite skills. In the event that students have not acquired sufficient skill to participate in the sport or game, task analyses of the skills should be conducted and instruction should begin at the present level of performance of the individual (see Chapter 7). To review, the process of task analysis involves the following steps:

1. Specification of terminal objectives in behavioral terms
2. Division of the terminal objective into a series of less and less complex responses
3. Sequencing the series of less complex responses
4. Verification of the student's ability to perform each response in the series
5. Teaching the student to perform each response in serial order
6. Recording performance during each training phase so that adjustments can be made during the teaching process

Cognitive Prerequisites for Playing Games

Rules and strategies incorporated in games require cognitive comprehension. Many nonhandicapped children learn rules and strategies incidently, but handicapped students may not. Some of the basic cognitive abilities that a student must possess to play games effectively follow:

1. Respond to one's name.
2. Follow simple directions: line up, stop, throw the ball, etc.
3. Line up or remain in assigned areas of the classroom.
4. Respond to start and stop cues.
5. Be aware of the behavior of others in relation to one's own behavior.
6. Respond to modeling.
7. Respond to signs that cue behavior.
8. Understand the boundaries for games.
9. Understand winning and losing.
10. Understand signs that communicate movement (forward/backward, fast/slow, run, jump, throw, catch, etc.).

Social Taxonomy

The adaptive social behavior of a person has the power to make the individual handicapped or not handicapped. Before a person is classified as mentally retarded, there must be impairment in adapted social behavior. This is also true for emotional disturbances and other handicapping conditions. Thus, if the components of adapted behavior can be defined and behavior ascribed to each of these components, it may be possible to design intervention programs to develop behavior that can be generalized to social abilities. Games are usually microsocieties in which rules of interaction and behavior are required for successful participation. A list of social abilities that impair adapted behavior and make individuals with sub-average intelligence mentally retarded has been developed from the American Association on Mental Deficiency classification of mental retardation.[3]

There are two ways of developing social behavior. One is to treat the specific, operationally defined behavior (task-specific approach). The other is to develop social behavior that relates to a common ability and generalize the ability to other environments. For instance, if a person can be taught to cooperate in a game of basketball by passing to the most appropriate person, the cooperation developed in the microsociety of basketball might transfer to other situations if it is planned. Suggested lists of ability traits follow. Most games that involve social interaction generate behavior that can be classified in one of these categories of social ability.

Internal Traits

These six social abilities are internal traits that are not necessarily expressed around other persons. They are assessed and can be developed individually as persons perform sport tasks.

1. *Delay of gratification:* the ability to control emotional responses so one's social status in the group is not jeopardized or the goals of the group are not deterred (exercising self-control, not losing one's temper or acting out). Common violations: (a) loses temper at a referee's decision, (b) does not attend to tasks, (c) does not participate with vigor in competition because of fatigue.
2. *Responsibility:* carrying out the role that has been assigned by an authority figure as a member of the society. Examples: (a) does not play assigned positions in a sport or game, (b) does not carry out assigned functions associated with participation in the game, (c) may withdraw from difficult assigned duties when the activity is underway.
3. *Reliability:* the consistency with which one carries out assigned responsibilities. This relates to the qualitative aspects of performance. Example: consistency in the successful execution of tasks for which one is responsible, such as (a) high batting and fielding averages in baseball, (b) high shooting percentages in basketball, (c) high percentages of successful execution of assignments in football.
4. *Pride in accomplishment:* internal satisfaction of having completed a task to the maximum of one's capability. This requires assessment of one's capability and the efforts that one must put forth to achieve a desired

outcome. Accomplishment is a function of effort. Examples: (a) meeting a standard in the physical education class as a result of hard practice, (b) winning a medal in the Special Olympics as a result of participation in a training program for the event.

5. *Control of personal feelings for the good of the group:* reaching the goals of the group are primary. Persons cooperating together can achieve goals that the individual cannot. Therefore it may be necessary for persons to give up their own personal feelings to enhance the goals of the group. Example: cooperating with another person within the game, such as (a) passing to a teammate who has a better shot, even though the player wants to shoot, (b) playing a position that will make the team stronger but is not that person's choice.

6. *Long-range goals:* delay of immediate needs and desires to reach a future goal. Examples: (a) working at physical fitness programs to improve sport skills, (b) practicing hard in Special Olympic training regimens.

External Traits

Each of these traits has a developmental structure that can be identified while students participate in games. If there is a behavioral violation of the traits, an intervention program can be implemented (see Chapter 7).

1. *Response to authority:* abiding by the decisions of those in authority by virtue of office (official in a game, coach, physical education teacher, squad leader, peer teacher). Examples: (a) abiding by the decision of an official in a game, (b) following directions of the teacher in the organization of games, (c) appropriate responses to squad leaders and peer teachers.

2. *Cooperation:* the ability to work with other members of a group to achieve a common goal. Examples: (a) taking turns while participating in an activity, (b) participating in a dance activity, (c) participating as a team member, (d) fitting well into the group structure.

3. *Competition:* the willingness to enter into a game in which there can be only one winner, regardless of whether the competitors' abilities are equitable. Examples: (a) maximizing efforts when games are close, (b) maximizing effort when behind, (c) maximizing efforts when the other person is the better player, (d) maximizing efforts when the individual is inferior.

4. *Leadership:* recognition of group goals and determination of the way to achieve the goal; motivation of the group to undertake a plan of action to achieve the goal. Examples: (a) providing a role model for others, (b) providing a plan of action for others, (c) assuming roles such as captain or exercise leader for the group.

5. *Asocial behavior:* not knowing the expected normative behavior of the group. Examples: (a) demonstration of any inappropriate behavior that can be corrected, (b) nonparticipation in or withdrawal from activity.

6. *Antisocial behavior:* planned action to undermine the rules and strategies for achieving the social structure or the achievement of group goals. Examples: (a) disobeying rules of conduct of a game in a premeditated fashion, (b) breaking training rules set up by a coach.

Social Sequence

There appears to be a developmental sequence of social behavior. The lowest form of development occurs when the person engages in social behavior through the initiative of another. The higher forms of social behavior require adaptation to environments with complex rules, skills, and judgment. These behaviors are required for participation in highly organized sport activity. However, each sport activity, game, or play situation might be placed on a social continuum that requires more or less complex social behavior. The following is a hypothetical sequence of social behavior for which there are many subdivisions. Stages of social development with substages are described.

Adult-Initiated Activity

In this case the social activity is initiated by someone other than the individual. Social behavior depends on the teacher or a group leader. The more severely handicapped persons often function at this level of social development. To advance from this stage of development, persons must have interests and skills to interact with the social environment.

Self-Initiated Activity

At this level of social development the person voluntarily chooses activity that is within her range of interest and capability. There are at least four distinct substages at the self-initiated level:

1. *Observer.* The individual is involved with activity but only as a spectator. The person does not interact with the environment but can learn about social behavior through observation.
2. *Nonpurposeful activity.* The individual becomes active in the exploration of self and the environment, but it is nonpurposeful. The activity usually involves objects or body parts.
3. *Purposeful solitary activity.* The activity has a definite purpose (bouncing a ball, kicking a ball, building blocks). There is usually an observable outcome of the activity.
4. *Elaborate solitary activity.* The self-initiated activity involves a wide range of activities and materials. It expands the existing repertoire of skills to prepare for later social interaction.

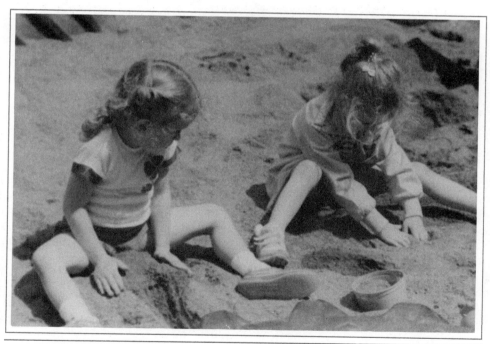

FIGURE 9-2
Children participate in socially acceptable parallel play. One child models for the other.

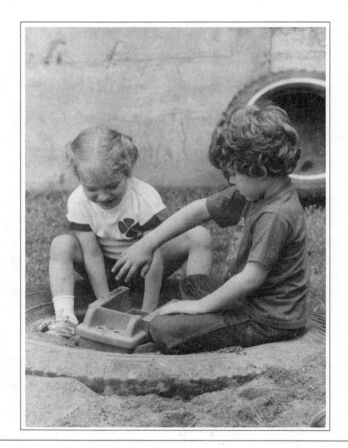

FIGURE 9-3
Two children play cooperatively with one another. Such cooperation may generalize to other areas of social life.

Parallel Activity

This category involves play with objects. The activity takes place at the ability level of the individual in observable proximity to other persons. There is a tendency for persons to get closer together as they mature socially, which permits reciprocal modeling of one another's behavior. A considerable amount of learning can occur under these circumstances. Movement education is based on parallel activity.

Social Interaction

At this stage of social development persons interact with one another. Its purpose is the achievement of mutual satisfaction. There are usually few, if any, rules to the interaction. The social situation is discontinued when either party is no longer interested in the activity. The social interaction level is usually spontaneous rather than planned activity.

Organized Social Games and Sports

Organized social games and sports can be arranged on a continuum from low to high organization. The characteristics that make games more or less socially complex are as follows:

- *The level of skill:* the less skill, the simpler the game.

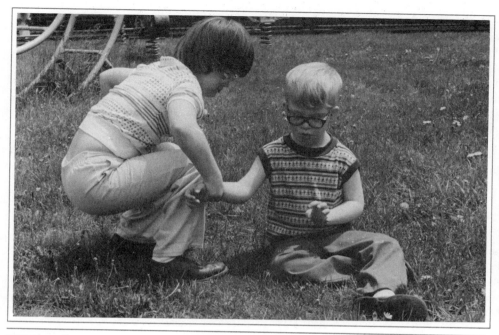

FIGURE 9-4
Children at the social interaction level of play.

♦ *The number of social interactions with others:* the more interactions, the more socially complex the game. Examples: Hot Potato, rolling the ball to another person (simple); quarterback in football (complex) (1) snap from center, (2) handoff or fake to backs, (3) follow blockers who protect on a pass, (4) hand off to backs, (5) throw passes to receivers, (6) execute plays called by the coach, etc.

♦ *The number of rules to the game:* there are few in Hot Potato, but an extensive rulebook for football.

♦ *The complexity of strategies:* there are few strategies for Hot Potato and complex strategies for football.

♦ *The interdependency of persons in the group:* there are few interdependencies in Hot Potato but many in football; the center's snap to the quarterback must be proper, the quarterback's fake to a back and handoff to

the ball carrier must be proper, the blockers must carry out assignments for the back, and the back must run the appropriate route of the designed blocking scheme.

♦ *The consequence of winning or losing:* there is no winning in Hot Potato, but there can be great social consequence for losing an important interscholastic game.

♦ *The structure of training regimens:* the more structure, the more complex the microsociety.

A hierarchy of social games can be developed so that persons can participate in games that meet their social needs. Under these conditions games and sports are not merely recreational but also have a valuable social purpose. Playing games can also be used to teach strategies and rules and to apply acquired sport skills from instruction. However, these are objectives separate and distinct from social considerations.

Social adjustment requires adaptation to the

rules of the game or the microsociety. A socially immature person has difficulty comprehending rules. Later, rules are regarded as absolute. Although the rules of a game may remain absolute, the values expressed through the social ability structure becomes more relative as the person gains social experience. There is a concomitant self-accepted moral principle.

Constructing a Game to Develop Social Skills

There are many games designed for elementary children, but the rules and strategies are often not well defined. Games of higher organization in interscholastic athletic competition are well structured and defined. Games of lower organization can be designed so that the structure permits analysis of social behavior. A procedure and format for construction of games for diagnostic-prescriptive programming are presented below:

Name the Game

Each game should be labeled or named. This communicates to the students the rules, strategies, and formations of games that have already been learned.

Objectives of the Game

Most games have objectives for the students and their teams. For instance, in basketball the players on offense must score a basket and those on defense prevent opponents from scoring. The objective of bowling is to attain more points than the opposition. The objective of the low organization game Hot Potato is to get rid of the ball so you are not the last person to touch it before the whistle is blown. Groups of persons or individuals try to achieve the target objectives of the microsociety.

Rules of the Game

Each game must have rules, just as does society at large. Breaking rules may be willful or accidental. Therefore the physical education teacher, to minimize accidents and rule breaking, must make the rules precise, enforce them during play, and watch for deficient social ability reflected in rule violation.

Strategies

Many games have rules that require cooperative strategies among members of the team. The implementation of these strategies in some cases requires complex social behavior of students playing the game, which can be judged against the social abilities.

Description of the Game

The description should include the formation required to play the game, how the game is started, what the opposing players do, how the game is terminated, how the game is scored, and the consequence for losing. Descriptions for Hot Potato follow:
1. Formation: circle formation, persons close enough so the ball can be handed to one another, one person in the center of the circle.
2. Start: ball is passed around the circle at the command of the person in the middle.
3. Participation: the ball is moved from one person to another as quickly as possible.
4. Termination: person in the middle says "stop."
5. Consequence: person holding the ball on command "Stop" goes to the middle.

Procedures for Teaching the Game

The persons who teach the game must know the exact procedures so they can conduct the game. The specific procedures enable peer tutors to conduct the games. If peer and cross-age tutors can learn to conduct the games, then several different games may be played at the same time. This allows more students to participate at their social ability level. The procedures are step-by-step analysis of what the leader must do to teach the game. The teaching procedures for Hot Potato follow:
1. Instruct the children to form a circle by joining hands.
2. Identify one person for the middle to start the game.
3. Instruct the person holding the ball to pass it to the right and keep the ball moving.
4. Instruct the person in the middle to close her eyes.
5. Tell the person in the middle to say "Stop" within the next 10 seconds.
6. Tell the person who last held the ball to move to the center.
7. Keep track of the persons who have been in the center.
8. The person who has been in the center the fewest times wins.

Diagram of Starting Position

A diagram of the starting position is prerequisite information to initiate the game. The components of the diagram should include the different players, the formation, and permanent equipment.

Diagram of the Game While in Progress

There should be a diagram of the game while it is in progress. It is desirable to indicate movement of the players and equipment in relation to the formation of the game.

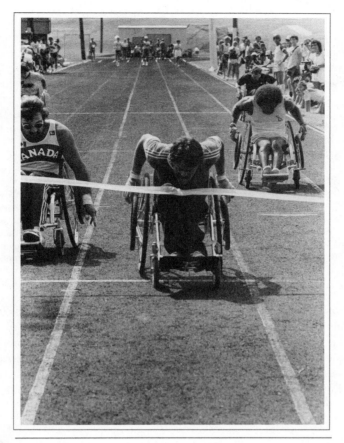

FIGURE 9-5
An organized competitive event for wheelchair athletes.
(Courtesy United Cerebral Palsy Associations, Inc.)

Variation of Rules to Make the Game More Complex

The rules of a game can be varied to increase demands for higher skills or require more sophisticated social behavior. Below are variations of hot potato that may make the game more or less complex.

Use two balls	Improved perceptual skills are required because the visual mechanism must focus on two objects.
Clap hands before passing	There are three components to the task instead of two (that is, receive-clap-pass versus receive and pass).
Smaller circle	The amount of movement necessary to pass the ball is reduced.

Cognitive Analysis

The cognitive information that an individual must master to play the game effectively should be analyzed. Cognitive analysis has been discussed previously. The specific cognitive component that is most difficult in Hot Potato is remembering the score and using this knowledge as an incentive to participate.

Relationship of Game Behavior with Social Abilities

The game should be analyzed to determine potential social traits that can be violated. These may be predicted by study of the desired behaviors of the rules and the strategies of the game. These two features of play tend to govern social interaction. An analysis of social abilities for playing Hot Potato follows. The positive and negative behaviors are linked with specific social abilities.

Ability	Positive Behavior	Negative Behavior
Cooperation	Passes ball to next person	Holds or throws the ball
Competition	Moves ball as fast as possible	Does not try to pass ball fast
Responsibility	Maintains proper position in formation throughout the game	Moves from the formation
Delay gratification	Attends to the game	Inattentive to the conduct of the game

Prerequisite Skills

The prerequisite skills for game participation should be noted. This includes all of the skills that enable successful participation in the activity. For Hot Potato the prerequisite motor skills are receiving and passing (hand to hand). Any skill can be analyzed into skill components.

Prerequisite Abilities

In the event a person cannot successfully perform the skills required for participation in the game, a prerequisite analysis is desirable. The analysis should be made in perceptual-physical-psychomotor area. A prerequisite analysis for Hot Potato appears below. The ability trait is described in relation to the activity involved in the game.

Ability	Activity
Visual tracking	Following the ball with the eyes around the circle
Hand-eye coordinaton	Receiving and passing the ball
Speed of limb	Moving the ball fast so the person will not be "it"
Manual dexterity	Manipulation of the ball (physical)

Interrelationship Skills and Abilities and Social Behavior

Skills and abilities are prerequisites for acceptable social behavior in group play. To determine the present level of performance of a child in a social game, it is desirable to know the game

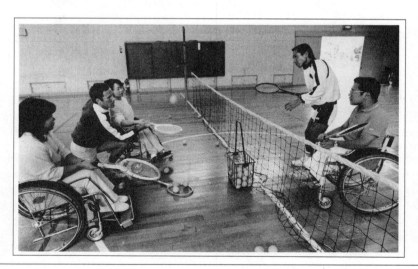

FIGURE 9-6
When the handicapped learn the skills of tennis, several cognitive skills will be needed to play wheelchair tennis.
(Photo by Bruce Haase; courtesy Peter Burwash International.)

thoroughly and then analyze the game in relation to skills and abilities for engagement in social behavior in the sport or game. The game should be designed with enough specificity that peer or cross-age tutors can conduct it. The physical education teacher should be trained with the skills to analyze the behavior of the children as the game unfolds and make prescriptive judgments of social needs for the children.

PSYCHOSOCIAL ASSESSMENT

There are two approaches to psychosocial assessment. One involves the use of standardized norm-referenced testing. The other uses content-referenced testing, in which the assessment of social behavior is made from existing and ongoing physical education curricula from sports and games. The standardized tests involve general social behaviors independent of a specific social context. The content-referenced testing is game specific.

Norm-Referenced Social Assessment

Selected norm-referenced social assessment instruments are the Detroit, Brigance, Vineland Social Maturity Scale, the American Association on Mental Deficiency (AAMD) Adaptive Behavior Scales, and the Gesell Developmental Schedules. Most of these tests have subtests that represent domains of social behavior. Some of the domains on these tests are personal independence, socialization, self-direction, language development, number and time concepts, self-help, communication, and locomotion. The norm-referenced tests are descriptive of the individual in general areas. However, for the most part they work with specific behavioral characteristics rather than social abilities that generalize across persons, environments, and activities. Examples of standardized games from which social assessments can be made appear on pp. 192-196.

Content-Referenced Social Assessment

Content-referenced social assessment requires the acquisition of information about what an in-

dividual can and cannot do within the context of social sport and play activity of the specific physical education curriculum of a given school district. The information received from such an assessment may be used to make relevant instructional decisions to enhance social behavior. The prerequisites for such an assessment of individual social abilities within the context of sport and games are as follows:

1. Operationally defined social abilities to be developed
2. A sequence of games/play activities that progress from lower to higher demands for social skills of participants
3. Entry procedures to determine present level of sport/play abiity of the learner and the specific deficient social behavior within a specific social context

Analyzing Games for Social Demands

It is difficult to structure spontaneous play; the sports and games social curriculum is a sequence of simple to complex activity. Some of the characteristics that make a sport or game more or less complex are skills required by the learner, rule complexity, strategy level, social responsibility for a function, and number of structured interactions. These characteristics are translated into more difficult social abilities that students must display to successfully participate in the games. The considerations for ordering games from less to greater complexity are as follows:

1. Ascribe a degree of difficulty for each social ability for each game on an arbitrary scale of 0 to 4.
2. Tabulate the total raw score for each game.
3. Order the games in sequence.

The box on p. 197 shows a battery of 40 social games that have been arranged according to an arbitrarily assigned difficulty score. Keep in mind that when a game is expressed by a single score, there is no indication as to which specific social abilities contribute to the difficulty of the game. An ability analysis of 18 games of cooperation, responsibility, response to authority, and competition appears in Table 9-1. A comprehensive

Text continued on p. 198.

HOT POTATO (SEATED)

Game classification: individual competition; sub.
Materials needed for the game: 1. __8" ball__ 2. _____ 3. _____ 4. _____ 5. _____

OBJECTIVE OF THE GAME

To hit the ball before the signal for termination of the game.

DESCRIPTION OF THE GAME

Circle formation, one child in the center with eyes closed. Ball is passed around the circle. Person in middle says "go" and then calls out "stop"; the person caught with ball in his hands or whoever touches it last must go to the center of the circle. Game is started over again.

RULES OF THE GAME

1. Must remain in the circle.
2. Must move the ball when the signal to begin game is given.
3. Ball must stay on the floor.

PROCEDURES FOR TEACHING THE GAME

1. Instruct them to form a circle by joining hands by the time the instructor counts to 10.
2. Identify one person to be in the middle.
3. Instruct the person holding the ball to pass it to his right (point).
4. Instruct person in center to close his eyes, start and stop the game.
5. Give the group a "do it" signal. Keep score as game proceeds.

VARIATION OF RULES TO MAKE THE GAME MORE OR LESS COMPLEX

1. Use two balls.
2. Before passing the ball, clap hands.
3. Count before passing the ball.
4. Form a smaller circle.

SOCIAL STRATEGIES ASSOCIATED WITH THE GAME

There are few social strategies.

Traits	Positive Description	Description of Social Deficiency
Cooperation	Hits balls that are in his area	Refuses to participate
Competition	Tries to move the ball as fast as possible	Does not fully attend to the game at all times; moves ball slowly
Responsibility	Maintains proper position throughout game	Moves out of position when game is under-way

DUCK, DUCK, GOOSE

Game classification: individual competition

Materials needed for the game: 1. ___none___ 2. _____ 3. _____ 4. _____ 5. _____

OBJECTIVES OF THE GAME

1. The runner avoids the tag of the person who is "it."
2. The person who is "it," the goose, must chase and tag the runner.

DESCRIPTION OF THE GAME

Group sits in circle with one person standing (goose). Goose walks around circle tapping sitters on the head and saying "duck." When goose gets to the person who is to chase, the command "goose" is given. The person tagged by the goose must chase her around the circle. If the chaser cannot tag the goose before she gets to the chaser's place, then he becomes the goose.

RULES OF THE GAME

1. Everyone sits in circle except one person, who is the goose. She must tap others on head and say "duck."
2. When she comes to the person who is to be "it," the runner taps him on the head and says "goose."
3. Person must chase tagger around circle; if chaser catches the goose, she's still "it."

PROCEDURES FOR TEACHING THE GAME

1. Hold someone else's hands.
2. Make a circle.
3. Back up as far as possible while still holding hands.
4. Sit on the floor.
5. Designate a "goose."
6. Say "Do what I do" (walk around circle and say "duck, duck").
7. Instruct those sitting that they are to run around the circle once and tag the goose before she sits on the spot where the chaser started.
8. Instruct the goose to walk around the circle and say "duck, duck."
9. If the child walks more than once around the circle, identify a chaser.

VARIATION OF RULES TO MAKE THE GAME MORE OR LESS COMPLEX

1. Run around circle twice.
2. Hop around circle.
3. Sitters raise arm when goose comes by and lower arm when chaser comes by.

SOCIAL STRATEGIES ASSOCIATED WITH THE GAME

There are no social strategies for this game.

Traits	Positive Description	Description of Social Deficiency
Cooperation	Cooperates in the formation of the game	Does not hold hands during organization of the game
Competition	Competes against the other person	Runs for the sake of running; does not try if behind
Sportsmanship	Tags persons of equal competition	Tags someone when the outcome is not in doubt
Responsibility	Maintains appropriate position throughout the game	Moves out of position in the circle

JUMP THE BROOK

Game classification: individual competition
Materials needed for the game: 1. __ropes (2)__   2. _____   3. _____   4. _____   5. _____

OBJECTIVES OF THE GAME

1. Jump as far as one can.
2. Jump farther than everyone else.

DESCRIPTION OF THE GAME

Two ropes are laid parallel to each other. The players take turns jumping over the ropes. After all have gone through the first time, the ropes are moved farther apart and jumping is repeated. Jump until there is failure to make it over both ropes. This procedure goes on until one person is left. He is the winner.

RULES OF THE GAME

1. Two ropes are placed parallel to one another, 1 foot apart.
2. All players line up behind the ropes.
3. The players attempt to jump over the two ropes.
4. Take off before the first rope and land after the second rope.
5. Widen the distance between the ropes 2 inches after each person in the group has jumped.
6. Jump until there is a miss. The last player who has made all attempts is the winner.

PROCEDURES FOR TEACHING THE GAME

1. Set the ropes parallel, 1 foot apart.
2. Line the pupils behind ropes.
3. Teach the rules of the game as it develops.

VARIATION OF RULES TO MAKE THE GAME MORE OR LESS COMPLEX

1. Shorten the running space.
2. Move the rope 6 inches each time.
3. Perform blindfolded.

SOCIAL STRATEGIES ASSOCIATED WITH THE GAME

There are no tactical social strategies associated with this game.

Traits	Positive Description	Description of Social Deficiency
Delay of gratification	Is under emotional control at all times	Does not want to participate
Sportsmanship	Engages in fair endeavor with others	Poor evaluation of self mastering the task; will not leave game on a miss
Pride in individual accomplishment	Puts forth effort	Does not value successful performance, misses early in the game without effort
Individual responsibility	Is considerate in giving other performers room to jump	Fails to stay behind the restraining line or wait turn in line to jump
Response to authority figures	Abides by the referee's decision on make or miss	Refuses to go out of game when the teacher indicates failure
Competition	Participates with intensity on each jump that challenges	Will not try when task is difficult

CIRCLE STRIDE BALL

Game classification: competition between players
Materials needed for the game 1. __volleyball__ 2. _____ 3. _____ 4. _____ 5. _____

OBJECTIVES OF THE GAME

1. The player in the center of the circle rolls the ball through the legs of players in the circle.
2. The players in the center of the circle prevent the ball from being rolled through their legs.

DESCRIPTION OF THE GAME

There is a circle of players; "it" is in the center. The circle players take a stride-stand position with the feet touching those of the person beside them. The center player attempts to roll the ball through the legs of the players in the circle.

RULES OF THE GAME

1. Players in the circle can use only their hands to stop the ball.
2. Players in the circle cannot move their feet.
3. The player in the center of the circle must roll the ball underhand.
4. The player in the center of the circle must stay in the center.
5. If the ball goes through the legs of a player in the circle, places are traded with the player in the center.
6. Player returns ball to "it" when ball is stopped.

PROCEDURES FOR TEACHING THE GAME

1. Instruct the players to join hands and form a circle.
2. Designate one person as the center person.
3. Instruct the players in the circle to spread their legs so feet touch one another.
4. Instruct the center player to roll the ball through the legs of the circle players.
5. Clarify the rules as the game progresses.

VARIATION OF RULES TO MAKE THE GAME MORE OR LESS COMPLEX

1. Change the size of the balls.
2. Change the number of persons who are in the circle.

SOCIAL STRATEGIES ASSOCIATED WITH THE GAME

This is an individual game in which there is little interdependency among players.

Traits	Positive Description	Description of Social Deficiency
Competition	Plays intensely at all times to win	Is sporadic in attempts to score
Sportsmanship	Gracious winner and loser	Ungracious winner and loser

BOWLING

Game classification: cooperation; team responsibilities
Materials needed for the game: 1. ___6 pins___ 2. ___bowling ball___ 3. _____
4. _____ 5. _____

OBJECTIVE OF THE GAME

1. To knock down more pins than the other team within a specified time.

DESCRIPTION OF THE GAME

There are three players on each team: one bowler, one ball retriever, and one pin setter–scorer. The bowler rolls the ball down and knocks as many pins over as possible, being sure not to cross the line. Retriever throws back ball as quickly as possible. Pins are reset, and score is kept by the pin setter. The bowler knocks as many pins over as possible in 15 seconds. At end of 15 seconds, players change places. This procedure is repeated until each person has bowled.

RULES OF THE GAME

1. Three players on a team: bowler, retriever, pin setter.
2. Ball must be rolled.
3. Count pins knocked over in a 15-second time frame.
4. Bowler may not cross the restraining line.

PROCEDURES FOR TEACHING THE GAME

1. Divide or instruct three persons to stand behind the bowling pins.
2. Ask no. 1's to raise their hands, then stand behind the bowling line.
3. Ask no. 2's to raise their hands, then be a pin setter and count the total number of pins knocked down.
4. Ask no. 3's to raise their hands, then tell them to retrieve the ball after it hits the pins.
5. Instruct them to knock down as many pins as possible in 15 seconds.

VARIATION OF RULES TO MAKE THE GAME MORE OR LESS COMPLEX

1. Bowl ball a different distance.
2. Increase or decrease time allowance.
3. Use smaller or larger ball.
4. Knock down more pins.

SOCIAL STRATEGIES ASSOCIATED WITH THE GAME

The strategies depend on the techniques an individual possesses in carrying out functions.

Traits	Positive Description	Description of Social Deficiency
Cooperation	Develops a system to interrelate functions	Tends to perform independently of other teammates
Competition	Tries on all tasks all of the time	Does not get involved in the contest; performs poorly when behind
Objectivity in meeting team goals	Performs the function assigned to best ability	Overtly shows impaired performance in unappealing task
Sportsmanship	Is willing to abide by rules of fair competition	Gains undue advantage, violates restraining line
Reliability	Always performs the functions assigned	Sporadic in performing the assigned roles in the game
Responsibility	Understands the function that is to be performed and does it	Does not fulfill the roles assigned in the game

DIFFICULTY RATING OF SOCIAL GAMES

1. Movement Imitation	3.2
2. Simon Says	3.8
3. Hot Potato	3.8
4. Duck, Duck, Goose	3.8
5. Drop the Handkerchief	3.8
6. One, Two, Three	4.3
7. Musical Chairs	4.5
8. Movement Imitation II	4.6
9. Squirrels and Trees	4.9
10. Cat and Mouse	5.0
11. Hoop Tag	5.2
12. Jump the Brook	5.3
13. Steal the Bacon	5.5
14. Jump the Bean Bag	5.6
15. Streets and Alleys	5.9
16. Run and Catch	6.0
17. Crows and Cranes	6.1
18. Running Bases	6.2
19. Sick Cat	6.6
20. Circle Stride Ball	6.8
21. Fish Net	7.6
22. Scooter Relay	7.7
23. Round the World	8.0
24. Four Square	8.0
25. Club Guard	8.5
26. Tag End Person	8.5
27. Tug of War	8.9
28. Wheelbarrow Relay	9.0
29. Whiffle Baseball	10.1
30. Bowling	10.3
31. Air Ball	11.0
32. Kickball Soccer	11.9
33. Scooter Basketball	12.4
34. Scooter soccer	12.7
35. Kickball	12.8
36. Badminton	12.9
37. Dodge Ball	12.9
38. Keep Away	13.1
39. Newcombe Volleyball	13.2
40. Basketball	14.4

TABLE 9-1
Social games developmental scale

Game	Total Score	Competition	Responsibility	Response to Authority	Cooperation
Hot Potato	2.7	0.0	1.5	0.5	1.0
Duck, Duck, Goose	2.0	0.0	0.5	0.5	1.0
Green Light	2.5	0.0	0.5	1.0	0.7
Squirrel Trees	3.9	0.7	1.2	0.5	1.5
Hoop Tag	4.5	0.5	0.5	1.0	2.5
Steal the Bacon	4.8	0.3	0.5	1.0	3.0
Crows and Cranes	5.0	0.5	1.0	1.0	2.5
Scooter Relay	5.2	0.5	1.5	0.7	2.5
Streets and Alleys	6.3	2.0	2.0	1.0	1.3
Over and Under	7.5	1.5	2.0	1.5	2.5
Dodge Ball	7.5	1.0	1.3	1.7	3.5
Four Square	8.0	0.0	3.5	1.0	3.5
Tag End Person	9.3	2.5	2.5	1.3	3.0
Bowling	10.0	3.0	3.5	0.8	2.7
Newcombe Volleyball	12.5	3.5	3.0	2.5	3.5
Kickball	14.3	3.3	4.0	3.0	4.0
Scooter Soccer	15.5	4.0	4.5	3.0	4.0
Scooter Basketball	15.5	4.0	4.5	3.0	4.0

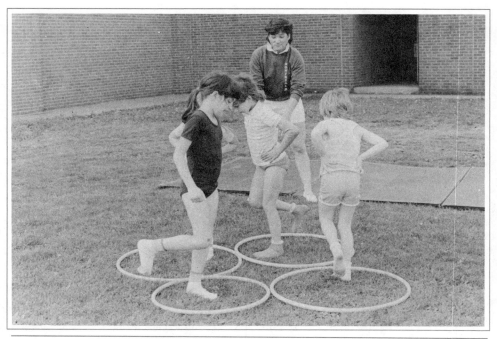

FIGURE 9-7
An organized game of hopping overtake can be placed on a continuum of games that require greater or less social development of the participants.

analysis of games would require an analysis of all abilities. With the profile of weighted traits for each game, activities can be selected according to specific social abilities needed by specific individuals. The problem of entry becomes one of determining which games are beneficial for the social development of each child.

The sequence of social activity of games and sports enables rough judgments to be made on the nature of activity in which individuals may and may not be successful. Determining the social needs through games and sports requires two types of information. One is the complexity of games that are commensurate with the social abilities of the individual. The other is the specific social ability traits that may be deficient in a person for a specific activity.

Analysis Through Observation of Play

The placement of a person in the sequence of games is conducted by having children partici-

pate in the games and observing social deficiencies as they play. If the individual has little or no social deficiency in a specific game, it can be assumed that less difficult games may also be played with success. Of course, this is not always true, since the skills and specific social abilities for each game vary. Therefore a specific match between characteristics of the game and the child may be present in a more complex game and not in a less complex one. However, knowing which abilities are needed to participate in a game is valuable for selecting games on a social continuum.

The identification of social deficits observed as specific behaviors that link with ability traits requires documentation of specific behaviors as the game is being played. An inference must also be made as to the link of the behavior with the social ability trait. For instance, in the game of Hot Potato, if a child breaks formation and withdraws from the game momentarily, the teacher may infer, based on previous observation, that the child is defying authority of the teacher or is attending to more interesting stimuli in the environment and cannot delay the gratification until termination of the game. These are judgments that need to be made by the teacher. The professional judgment that links behavior with social abilities is important for generalization of the social ability rather than just for treating a social behavior. Therefore social assessment involves finding out which games can be played by the children and the specific nature of the deficit (if one exists).

It is important to standardize the administrational procedures for the games when entering persons in the sequence. This enables better control of the variables of the social situation. Those who conduct the games must practice implementation for consistency. A procedure for teaching the game is to present the game rules succinctly as possible and engage the children in activity. They should see a model of the game when it is underway. Then prompt the behavior of the individuals into the activity and fade instructor assistance. Under these conditions every person has an opportunity to be successful. If children cannot perform the skills and social requirements of the games after the prompt and fade procedure, there is most likely a deficiency in social, skill, or prerequisite abilities.

Persons who provide instructional services to develop social abilities should have an extensive activity curriculum. Following are procedures for the selection and design of the social activities:

1. Identify the activities from the literature or make them up.
2. Pilot the activities in small groups.
3. Write the specifications for administration.
4. Play the game with other populations.
5. Finalize the administration procedures.
6. Conduct an analysis of the game and enter it into the sequence of social games.

DEVELOPMENT OF INCENTIVES FOR SOCIAL PARTICIPATION IN GAMES

There may be a developmental hierarchy of incentives for participation in social activity.

Kohlberg[8] suggests the following sequence of psychosocial development. The range of social responsibility is from participation based on avoidance of punishment to maintaining the self-respect on a voluntary basis.

1. Obey rules to avoid punishment. — If there is no punishment, the rules will not be obeyed.
2. Conform to obtain rewards. — If there are no rewards, there may be inappropriate social behavior.
3. Conform to obtain approval from others. — If there is little recognition from the group, there is little incentive to maximize participation.
4. Conform to avoid censure by authority figures. — If there is no authority censure, there is insufficient incentive to participate.
5. Conform to maintain respect of social community. — If the social community cannot express respect, there is insufficient incentive to participate.
6. Conform to maintain self-respect and integrity. — If there is little desire to be a person of integrity, there is less incentive to participate.

WRITING SOCIAL GOALS

The standard procedure for developing social behavior is through application of behavioral principles to a behavior that is to be changed. This is usually directed toward disruptive or self-abusive behaviors, which are negative and should be brought under control. The development of positive social goals suggests a different approach. A goal that involves social development possesses the following characteristics:

♦ It should contain a social ability that can be generalized from the microsociety of sport and games to a macrosociety.
♦ It should be observable in the sports and games in physical education classes and in generalized environments.
♦ It should be measurable to determine the effectiveness of the proposed strategies for intervention.
♦ It must have the capability of being developed through classroom intervention.
♦ It must represent a social ability concept as well as a specific behavior in the class.

For example, in Hot Potato the child will demonstrate the responsibility (1) of staying in circle formation (2) for three (3) 1-minute games. All the criteria for writing a social goal are met in this statement. No specific applied behavioral intervention would be planned. If one technique fails, another is attempted.

SELECTION OF THE APPROPRIATE SOCIAL ACTIVITY

The activities involved in sports and games should be commensurate with the abilities of each handicapped person. Components in the implementation of social activity that should be synthesized are (1) the assessed need of the learner, (2) the specific activity that will meet the need, (3) the deficient behavior that reflects a social disability, (4) the nature of the social group who will assist with transmission of the appropriate social behavior, and (5) teacher techniques for intervention. Following is a hypothetical application of the procedures in a game of Hot Potato when a person will not exchange the ball with the person who is to receive it:

1. Assessed needs	The child cannot participate in the game of Hot Potato.
2. Specific activity of need	Pass the ball to the next person upon receiving it; do not hold it
3. Deficient ability	There is a lack of cooperation.
4. Nature of social group	All other persons have capability to pass the ball. They become the model for the target student.
5. Teacher techniques	Model, prompt, and reinforce appropriate behavior.

TECHNIQUES TO PROMOTE SOCIALIZATION
Peer Tutoring

The general process of socialization is one of children modeling an activity for their peers. Under such conditions, those who have appropriate social behavior can transmit it to those who possess inappropriate behavior. The persons who receive the most social benefit are those who learn

from the group with appropriate social behavior. There is impressive evidence favoring the value of peer instruction.[15] To accommodate the needs of any children, it is desirable for peer tutors and cross-age peers to learn to administer social activity. Ideas for training peer tutors to administer the games are included in the following list:

1. Learn the rules, formation, and procedures of the game.
2. Define the teacher responsibilities in the game, such as getting the equipment, setting up the equipment, and keeping score.
3. Assign the responsibilities to specific peer teachers.
4. Train them to secure the equipment.
5. Train them to set up the instructional environment.
6. Teach them to score the game.
7. Teach them to conduct the game.
8. Teach them how to evaluate their performance in the conduction of the game.

The specifications and the structure of the games enable a peer tutor system to operate within the social activity.

Staff Skills

A team of persons may be involved with the conduction of social programming. Staff efforts should complement one another. The staff should know the games thoroughly and be consistent in the application of language cues and reinforcers of the correct social behavior. A list of guidelines for conduction of social instruction follows:

1. All staff should know thoroughly the social games.
2. All staff should be consistent in instruction.
3. Effective reinforcers should be applied expressively and immediately.
4. Language cues should be consistent, short, and relevant.
5. Extra visual and language cues should be provided if necessary.

Social Communication Skills

Handicapped persons must possess social prerequisites before they can enter into meaningful

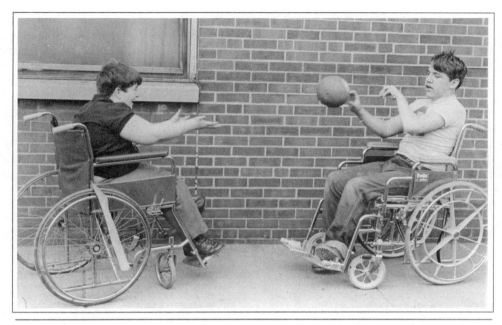

FIGURE 9-8
A goal can be written to express the social concept of cooperation in activity.

social interaction. Some of the prerequisites are as follows:

♦ *Verbalization.* This is the best means of communicating with another person. Signing is a substitute for the deaf who cannot speak.

♦ *Visual onlooking.* This is the ability to interpret the modeling process of another person.

♦ *Imitation.* This is the ability to reproduce behavior of another through the modeling process.

♦ *Smiling.* This communicates the approval of one person of the actions of another.

♦ *Token giving.* Giving something to another person establishes a commonality between them.

♦ *Affection.* Smiles, hugs, and kisses reinforce the behavior of another.

The social interaction process involves ways of receiving information from another person and also ways of feeding back to the other person approval for their behavior. Visual onlooking enables the assessment of social information from others. The other prerequisites of social interac-

tion are means of initiating social activity or giving feedback on the appropriateness of another's social behavior.

♦ *Sharing materials (toys).* This involves materials of mutual interest to two persons when they share them and engage in social interaction.

♦ *Appropriate physical contact.* A handshake or another sign of approval of a behavior can be used.

♦ *Complimentary comments.* Say something nice about another person. This may be something that the person wears or has, but the most appropriate compliment involves something the person can do.

♦ *Peer reinforcement.* Reinforcing a peer for an appropriate behavior will strengthen that behavior. A compliment is not directed at strengthening any particular behavior.

Structuring Social Interactions

Social interactions between handicapped and nonhandicapped persons have a greater chance of success if instructors provide guidelines. When initial social contact is purposeful and well structured, positive social development is likely to occur. Techniques for structuring these interactions appear in following sections.

Cooperative Learning

In cooperative learning students work together on teams and carry out their responsibilities. These teams are small groups of students with a wide range of abilities. Cooperative learning provides practice in learning motor skills and social interactions to promote social acceptance. The instructor establishes and guides the cooperation. Gottlieb and Leyser[3] suggest the following steps:

1. Teacher specifies instructional objectives on the learning task.
2. Teacher selects the group size most appropriate for the game.
3. Students are assigned to the teams or groups.
4. Roles are structured among the groups.
5. Requirements are made for each child.
6. The appropriate equipment is provided for each group.

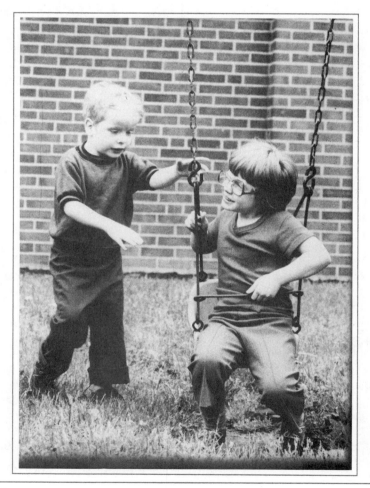

FIGURE 9-9
Children provide social reinforcement for one another.

7. The task and cooperative goal structure are explained.
8. Peers are trained if necessary.

As an example, consider bowling as the instructional task for the group.

Instructional objective	Group knocks a bowlng pin down 15 times in a specified time.
Group size	Three persons in each group.
Group assignment	Heterogeneous.
Structured roles	Bowler rolls ball from 10 feet to knock down the pin.
	Pin setter sets the pin up each time it is knocked down.
	Retriever rolls the ball back to the bowler.
	Counter counts the number of pins knocked down.
	Timer determines how long it took the group to knock down the pins 15 times.
	Manager keeps the group informed as to whose turn it is to bowl. (Each person bowls until 5 pins are knocked down.)
Requirements	Each person performs to the above specifications.
Equipment	Ball and bowling pin.
Explanation	Describe the game and the responsibility of each person.

Group Rewards

In a group reward system games are won not only by team score but also for appropriate social behavior. There are two winners—a social winner and a game winner. Class members pool their positive and negative points. This approach increases the number of positive social interactions during the play of the activity and helps improve the attitudes of all students.[4]

Cognitive Training

Another approach to the development of social skills is the use of cognitive behavior modification to develop skills that can be used in a variety of settings. Students are involved as active participants in sports and games. They are aware of the behaviors targeted for change and receive training in how behaviors change.[6] Cognitive training programs may teach self-evaluation and self-instruc-tion strategies. In self-evaluation, students may record their own inappropriate behaviors and reinforce themselves for acceptable performance. This type of program requires that teachers reward students for accurate evaluation of their own behaviors.

Cognitive training is an efficient approach with handicapped children of higher intellectually functioning. Teachers can train students to become responsible for their own behavior in the instructional program, and the teacher then assumes a monitoring role. Typical cognitive training includes:

- ◆ Problem definition
- ◆ Goal statement
- ◆ Impulse delay (stop and think before you act)
- ◆ Consideration of consequences (think of the different consequences that may follow each solution)
- ◆ Implementation
- ◆ Recycling (use self-evaluation and error-correcting options)[7]

TECHNIQUES TO CHANGE SOCIAL MISBEHAVIOR

There are several techniques that can be used by instructors to change social behavior of handicapped children.[16] Each technique has different applications. A description of some of these techniques follows:

Proximity Control

This involves placing persons who are isolated from group activity closer to the activity. This may facilitate opportunity for peer modeling and social interaction. The strategy can be used when attempting to move a person from self-initiated activity to parallel or social interaction levels.

Peer-Mediated Reinforcement

Peers are trained to reinforce specific social behaviors of a pupil. This procedure has powerful generalization effects.

Peer-Mediated Reinforcement and Self-Recording

In this procedure peers reinforce the behavior, but the pupil makes records of the successful event. The pupil is actively involved in assessing his own behavior.

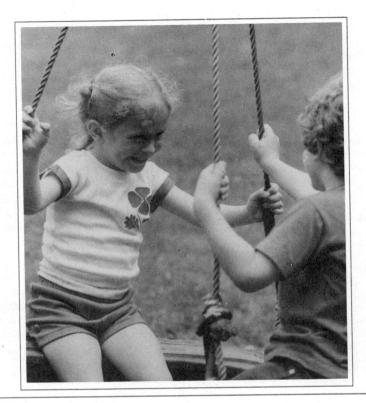

FIGURE 9-10
Peers smile to communicate approval and affection for one another.

Mutual Peer Reinforcement

Peers are trained to mutually reinforce one another.

Model-Prompt-Reinforce

The instructor models the appropriate behavior, physically prompts the pupil in the behavior, and then quickly reinforces the behavior. It is important that latency (time between model and prompt), prompt and reinforcement be minimal.

Stimulus Pairing

This is a positive event paired with an opportunity to play or participate in an activity. Example: Isolated child offered candy to playmates just before play period. There was over a 400% increase in the amount of play time of the isolate child with the peers.

Film-Mediated Models

Observational learning includes both incidental and controlled interaction among children. Social patterns undergo modifications as a direct result of observing another's behavior and its consequences. In this case films depict appropriate peer interaction.

Direct Shaping of Behavior

This technique involves establishing or identifying a social behavior and then making it more or less frequent with a program of small steps.

Direct Shaping of Prerequisite Behavior

There are occasions when the desired social behavior cannot be emitted. Under these conditions it is necessary to shape the prerequisite behaviors, such as onlooking.

Increase Number of Objects/Materials for Interaction

The range of options for social activity may be limited. Therefore an increase in the number of objects and materials may provide the novelty for interaction. This technique can be used to move the person to the self-initiated social activity level.

Limit Number of Options for Play

There are times when the materials of the environment should be limited. If a person is repetitiously engaged with activity with a single object and purpose, this imposed limit may increase the range of skills and interests. The preferred objects can be removed to facilitate interaction with other materials. Specific strategies need to be paired with specific purpose.

Activities of Similar Stimulus Characteristics

If a person has favored materials or activities, those of similar stimulus characteristics may be well accepted by the pupils. Example: If a person or group has a favorite game, alter the game so that the objectives, skills, and social interactions are different.

Materials that Require Two Persons to Participate

Certain activity requires the participation of two persons. Engagement in this activity facilitates social interaction. Examples: Teeter-totter, throwing and catching a ball, tandem bicycle riding.

Mix High and Low Socially Developed Persons

Persons who are to develop social behavior through modeling need to participate with those who can provide the models. This technique is effective for social development in games.

Confederate Peer Initiates Activity

A peer is trained and integrated into a group to initiate activity.

Two Peers Trained by One Adult

The instructor structures the social interaction between two peers who are participating in an activity. The interaction capability of each peer must be determined. The specific social behaviors of each peer must be defined before this procedure is attempted.

Reciprocally Reinforcing Activity to Prompt Taking Turns

The behavior of one child sets the stage for reinforcing a partner. Examples: Teeter-totter, play catch with a ball, and table games. A natural cue prompts a child to take turns and initiate interaction.

GENERALIZATION

Issues related to successful implementation of social programming are the generalization and maintenance of behavior outside of the play, sport, and game environments of instruction. The generalization of social behavior is a product of complex interactions between a number of factors, such as the following:

1. *The level of the behavioral handicap.* Data indicate that the more severe the handicap, the more difficult the generalization process.

2. *Reduction of the discrepancy between the training and the generalization setting.* This refers to similarity of the stimulus characteristics of the environment, the similarity in response and reinforcement properties of the tasks of the training, and natural environments.

There are techniques for generalizing social behavior within and external to the instructional setting. The mission of generalization of social behavior within the instructional setting is to enable the behaviors to be demonstrated independent of the training staff. For low functioning persons it is often necessary to have staff and trained peers involved in the process of social development. Techniques for generalization involve fading (gradually eliminating) peers and trainers from the social activity. Some specific techniques for generalization of social behavior in the instructional setting are to (1) fade the number of trainers in a social game, (2) fade the number of higher functioning peers, (3) fade the amount of time a trainer spends in activity, and (4) increase the number of peers and decrease the number of staff involved in the game. Once the social behavior in play and game activity are established in the instructional setting, attempts should be made to generalize the behaviors across other persons and environments. Some considerations for generalization of social behavior and abilities outside of the instructional setting are:

1. Practice the skills in different environments (intramurals, other facilities).
2. Practice the skills in the home with parents, siblings, and relatives.
3. Practice the skills in the neighborhood and community environments.

ORGANIZATION OF SOCIAL GROUPS

Social development requires participation in microsocieties—play settings or sports activity. To maximize opportunity for social development, activities should be carried out in a variety of settings, such as the instructional school program, the intramural program, and extramural participation. The intramural program is an outgrowth of the physical education instructional program that takes place within one school and involves voluntary participation. Extramurals are an extension of activity beyond one school. Special Olympics is an example. Community activity involves participation with YMCAs, YWCAs, church groups, and community recreation programs. In these circumstances socialization is not under control of personnel associated with the physical education instructional program. In addition to generalizing the social opportunities beyond the school instructional program, another problem is equalizing competition in sports activity by functional skill level. Each child should be able to compete regardless of the level of skill. To make provision for competition, attempts should be made to equalize age and performance level, with encouragement of each individual to improve within the divisional rankings. Special Olympics is a good example of such a structure. There are five divisions based on skill level for each age for both boys and girls. Such an arrangement enables participation by those who have severe handicaps. The purpose of such organization is inclusion in sports to facilitate social opportunities.

SUMMARY

Handicapped individuals sometimes demonstrate delayed psychosocial development. Factors that contribute to this delay include differences in appearance and behavior, overprotective environments, lack of opportunity to interact with others in play, and rejection by others.

Psychosocial development can be promoted through participation in games and sports. To enable such growth it is necessary to determine which psychosocial skills are lacking, set clear-cut goals, and design instructional environments that favor development. Both internal and external social traits as well as each individual's placement on a social continuum must be determined. Once functioning levels are determined, clearly stated social goals are developed. Appropriate games and activities are selected and sequenced to promote specific goals. Peer tutoring, total staff involvement, prerequisite communication skills, cooperative learning, group rewards, and cognitive training facilitate psychosocial growth and development.

The use of specific techniques to change social misbehavior and knowledge of techniques to generalize social behavior contribute to the durability of appropriate behaviors and continued psychosocial development.

REVIEW QUESTIONS

1. What are some social benefits that can be derived from sports and games?
2. Describe an instructional process for developing social skills of children.
3. What is one way to improve the attitude of regular students toward handicapped students who will be joining an integrated class?
4. List some specific social traits that may be generalized from the microsocieties of games to other aspects of social life.
5. What are the six stages of social development?
6. Construct a standardized social game from which social development can be measured.
7. What are some different methods of assessing social behavior?
8. Write a social goal.
9. What are the necessary steps to follow when constructing a game to develop social skills?
10. Suggest a procedure to structure cooperative learning.
11. What are some techniques that can be used to change social behavior?
12. How can social behavior be generalized from games and sports to other social environments?
13. What should be included in a social goal?

STUDENT ACTIVITIES

1. Interview a teacher of an integrated class. Find out what social problems (if any) handicapped students just joining the class demonstrate. Ask

how the teacher prepares the class members when a handicapped student will be joining the class. Find out what the teacher does when social problems between handicapped and non-handicapped occur.

2. Observe a handicapped student at play with other children. Note whether the handicapped child demonstrates any delays in external social interaction traits. Note the student's reaction when responding to authority, cooperating and competing with others, and when given an opportunity to lead the group.

3. Observe three groups of children of different ages at play. Identify which stage of social development each group demonstrates (adult-initiated activity, self-initiated activity, parallel activity, or social interaction).

4. Analyze two games. Determine what social strategies, physical skills, and cognitive skills are required for each game.

5. Write three social goals that include the five characteristics given in this chapter.

6. Observe a handicapped individual at play. Identify which social communication skills the person demonstrates.

7. Simulate a game situation that includes students and teacher. Have one individual "act out" specific types of asocial behavior. Have the teacher use at least four different techniques to change the social misbehavior. After the game is over, have the class members name the techniques used and discuss the effectiveness of each.

REFERENCES

1. Donaldson, J., and Martinson, M.C.: Modifying attitudes toward physically disabled persons, Except. Child. **43**:337-341, 1977.
2. Fait, H., and Dunn, J.: Special physical education, Philadelphia, 1984, Saunders College Publishing.
3. Gottlieb, J., and Leyser, Y.: Facilitating the social mainstreaming of retarded children, Except. Educ. Q. **1**(4):57-70, 1981.
4. Grossman, H.: Manual on terminology and classification in mental retardation. Washington, D.C., 1977, American Association on Mental Deficiency.
5. Henker, B., Whalen, C.K., and Hinshaw, S.P.: The attributional contexts of cognitive intervention strategies, Except. Educ. Q. **1**(1):17-30, 1980.
6. Heron, T.E., and Harris, K.C.: The educational consultant: helping professionals, parents, and mainstreamed students, Boston, 1982, Allyn & Bacon.
7. Kneedler, R.D.: The use of cognitive training to change social behavior, Except. Educ. Q. **1**(1):65-73, 1980.
8. Kohlberg, L.: The cognitive-development approach to moral education. In Values, concepts, and techniques, Washington, D.C., 1971, National Education Association.
9. Lewis, R.B., and Doorlag, D.H.: Teaching special students in the mainstream, Columbus, Ohio, 1983, Charles E. Merrill Publishing Co.
10. Meisgeier, C.: A social/behavioral program for the adolescent student with serious learning problems, Focus Except. Child. **13**(9):1-13, 1981.
11. Oliver, J.: Physical activity and the psychological development of the handicapped. In Kane, J.E., editor: Psychological aspects of physical education and sport, Boston, 1972, Routledge and Kegan.
12. Seaman, J.A., and DePauw, K.: The new adapted physical education, Palo Alto, Calif., 1982, Mayfield Publishing Co.
13. Sherrill, C.: Adapted physical education and recreation, ed. 2, Dubuque, Iowa, 1985, William C. Brown & Co., Publisher.
14. Simpson, R.L.: Modifying the attributes of regular class students toward the handicapped, Focus Except. Child. **13**(3):1-11, 1980.
15. Strain, P.S.: Peer-mediated treatment of exceptional children's social withdrawal, Except. Educ. Q. **1**(4):93-105, 1981.
16. Wheman, P.: Helping the mentally retarded acquire play skills, Springfield, Ill., 1977, Charles C Thomas, Publishers.

SUGGESTED READINGS

Bryant, L.E., and Budd, K.S.: Teaching behaviorally handicapped preschool children to share, J. Appl. Behav. Anal. **17**:45-56, 1984.

Cooke, T.P., and Apolloni, T.: Developing positive social-emotional behaviors: a study of training and generalization effects, J. Appl. Behav. Anal. **9**:65-78, 1976.

Egel, A.L., Richman, G.S., and Koegel, R.L.: Normal peer models and autistic children's learning, J. Appl. Behav. Anal. **14**:3-12, 1981.

Lancioni, G.E.: Normal children as tutors to teach social responses to withdrawn mentally retarded schoolmates: training maintenance and generalization, J. Appl. Behav. Anal. **15**:17-40, 1982.

Morris, R.H., and Dolker, M.: Developing cooperative play in socially withdrawn retarded children, Ment. Retard. **12**:24-27, 1974.

Peck, C.A., et al.: Teaching retarded preschoolers to imitate the free play behavior of nonretarded classmates: trained and generalized effects, J. Spec. Educ. **12**:195-207, 1978.

Stainback, S.B., Stainback, W.C., and Hatcher, C.W.: Non-handicapped peer involvement in the education of severely handicapped students, J. Assoc. Severely Handicapped Persons **8**:39-45, 1983.

CHAPTER 10

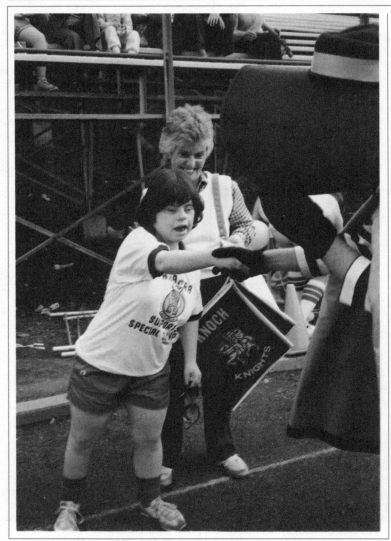

Special Olympics

Mental Handicaps

OBJECTIVES

♦ Understand the definition of mental retardation.

♦ Understand the variability among individuals who are mentally handicapped.

♦ Recognize the need for differential programming for mentally handicapped individuals.

♦ Select appropriate activities depending on the age and level of functioning of each retarded person.

It is now recognized that mental retardation is not a fixed, unalterable condition that condemns an individual to a static, deprived lifetime of failure to achieve. Rather, today we understand that cognitive, psychomotor, and affective behaviors are dynamic processes that, if properly stimulated, can be developed further than ever before imagined. Early concepts of mental retardation viewed the condition as an inherited disorder that was essentially incurable. This notion resulted in hopelessness on the part of professionals and social and physical separation of persons who were mentally retarded. After years of research and innovative programming, it is now recognized that intelligence and other functions are dependent on the readiness and experience of the child, the degree and quality of environmental stimulation, and many other variables.

In the late 1960s and early 1970s institutions that served retarded persons began designing and implementing educational programs intended to develop independent living skills of retarded persons to enable them to function in community settings. As institutionalized retarded individuals rose to the challenge of these educational pro-grams, a movement began to promote their placement in communities. Thousands of persons were removed from the institutions and allowed to take their rightful place as contributing members of communities.

As institutions began to develop viable educational programs, public schools took up their responsibility toward young mentally handicapped children living in the communities. Professionals trained in appropriate teaching techniques were hired by the school systems to provide educational opportunities for retarded children. As a result of efforts by both institutions for retarded persons and public school systems, all except the most severely involved mentally handicapped individuals are living, going to school, and working in the community. Thus, mentally retarded persons today have more opportunities than ever before for optimal social interaction.

DEFINITION AND DESCRIPTION

In 1973 the American Association on Mental Deficiency (AAMD) redefined mental retardation as follows: "Mental retardation refers to subaverage general intellectual functioning existing concurrently with deficits in adaptive behavior, and manifested during the developmental period." This same definition was incorporated into P.L. 94-142, in 1975.

Terms used in the definition have important implications for all educators working with the mentally retarded because they project the dynamic nature of the condition. Specifically, the following concepts should be noted:

- *Mental retardation:* This term implies a slowness in development rather than the static descriptors used historically, such as amentia, feeblemindedness, mental deficiency, mental subnormality, idiocy, imbecility, and moronity.

- *Subaverage:* The mental retardate's functioning is lower than normative expectancies for the society. That is, performance is more than one standard deviation below the mean of a given age group on a standardized IQ measure.

- *General intellectual functioning:* Determination of intellectual functioning requires an assessment of overall cognitive performance on one or more of the various objective tests developed for that purpose.

- *Deficits in adaptive behavior:* Adaptive behavior is the ability to cope with the natural and social demands of the environment. A deficit exists when a person lacks average ability to adjust responses to environmental demands. Inability to effectively modify behavior may result from any or all of the following: (1) a delay in acquiring early perceptual-motor skills that are prerequisite to commanding physical and intellectual tasks; (2) a lack of knowledge because of limited experience; and (3) a lack of understanding of social behaviors needed to maintain oneself in the community, in gainful employment, and during exchange with other members of the community.

- *Manifested during the developmental period:* That behavior is an orderly predictable sequence is acknowledged in this phrase. It is generally agreed that the developmental period refers to the first 18 years of life. Sometimes slow development is evident during infancy. Delayed sitting, crawling, and walking are often the first clues that a child may be mentally retarded. The slowness in acquiring knowledge becomes most apparent when a child reaches school age and his or her performance is compared with that of others in a structured group setting.

Inherent in the 1973 definition is that mental retardation is simply a slowness to demonstrate performance levels expected from the majority of persons of a given age. Gone are the implications that the mental retardate is "stuck" at a certain age level, that social interaction is undesirable, and that development of cognitive, psychomotor, and affective abilities is not possible. Rather, we are provided with an image of a condition that slows the development of an individual along a continuum. Given this definition, the educator's role becomes one of utilizing appropriate techniques to ensure the greatest possible progress for the mentally retarded student.

The levels of IQ and expected adaptive behavior are as follows[4]:

- *Level I:* Includes mildly retarded individuals with IQ ranges from 52 to approximately 68 or 70. These individuals show few, if any, early motor delays and often are not identified until they enter school. They can learn academic skills up to the equivalent of a sixth grader and often achieve social and vocational skills equivalent to the average adult in society.

- *Level II:* Includes moderately retarded individuals with an IQ range from 36 to 51. This population can learn to walk and communicate, although prevalence of speech impediments is high. These individuals usually acquire minimal academic skills (approximately second grade level) and are capable of developing a semi-skilled vocation and semi-independent living skills.

- *Level III:* Is made up of severely retarded persons with IQs ranging from 20 to 35. As children these individuals demonstrate markedly delayed motor development and often must learn signing to augment their limited speaking ability. Severely retarded persons can learn rudimentary tasks but need constant supervision at work and in their learning environment. They constitute approximately 3.5% of the retarded population.

♦ *Level IV:* Represents the lowest functioning (profoundly) retarded persons. Extensive neurological damage often limits motor control and cognitive development is often present in this population. Their IQs are below 19. They may respond to some basic training and therapeutic intervention, but seldom achieve the ability to care for themselves even with concerted training.

Despite the wide acceptance of the adaptive behavior classifications delinineated above, the educator should be cautioned against using these guidelines as definitive limitations. As was indicated earlier in this chapter, deficits in adaptive behavior may result from maturational delays, limited learning experience, or lack of social skill. In the 1980s, thanks to Child Find and similar nationwide programs, high-risk children who demonstrate developmental delays early in life are being identified and provided with intervention programs to stimulate their growth and development. The physical educator is able to contribute to these youngseters' development by promoting sensorimotor function during the preschool years. The earlier the potentially retarded person is identified through motor evaluation techniques and appropriate intervention is implemented, the greater the motor development progress. Benefits in learning ability can also be expected to accrue.

INCIDENCE

Estimates of the number of retarded individuals in the population range between 2.5% and 3.0%. Of this number approximately 89% are classified as mildly retarded, 6% as moderately retarded, and 5% as severely or profoundly retarded.[9]

TESTING TO DETERMINE FUNCTIONING LEVELS

Development of the IEP requires that present functioning levels be determined. Several formal tests that can be used with mentally handicapped students are listed in Table 6-1 of this text. Other acceptable ways to evaluate the functioning levels of this population are task analysis and observation of the students as they perform a hierarchical sequence of activities. These techniques have been described in Chapter 7.

One of the most difficult problems of testing mentally handicapped individuals is deciding whether poor comprehension or poor motor development is the reason for their inability to perform a specific task. Because it is difficult to determine whether a mentally handicapped student understands directions given during test situations, the following suggestions may help the evaluator elicit the best performance possible:

1. If after the student has been told what to do the response is incorrect, demonstrate the position or movement.
2. If demonstration does not elicit the correct performance, manually place the student in or through the desired position or pattern.
3. Use positive reinforcement (praise, tokens, free play) to encourage the student.

When severely or profoundly handicapped students are tested, it may be necessary to use an anatomical task analysis (see Chapter 6) to determine their level of capability.

TEACHING STRATEGIES

Physical education programs should be based on the nature and needs of the learner. As mentioned previously there is great variability among the mentally retarded population. This is attributable to inherent differences between mild and more severe retardation, causes, and the many

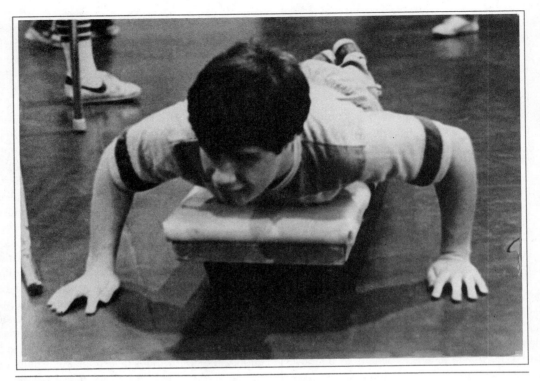

FIGURE 10-1
Select activities that are both safe and beneficial for the learner. A scooter board is a safe vehicle that is beneficial for development of movement and coordination of the arms.
(Courtesy Verland Foundation, Inc.)

other disorders that accompany mental retardation.

Disorders associated with mental retardation may be sensory impairments such as blindness, being hard-of-hearing, or deafness; emotional disturbances; and neurological disorders such as cerebral palsy, muscular dystrophy, and problems in perception. It becomes apparent that physical education programs for mentally retarded persons must meet a multitude of needs at all age levels and all levels of intellectual and physical development.

The mentally retarded are a very heterogeneous group. Many techniques of instruction are necessary to elicit a desired response. Therefore, it is difficult to make generalizations that may be helpful in the instruction of physical education activi-

ties for mentally retarded persons. However, as a guide, some teaching hints follows:

1. Consider individual differences when selecting the activities. There are many games that allow for differences in abilities among class members.
2. Select activities according to the needs of the mentally retarded.
3. Select activities to meet the students' interest levels. However, precaution should be taken against participation in one particular activity to the exclusion of others. Be aware of the retarded student's tendency to favor the single activity with which he or she is most familiar.
4. Do not underestimate the ability of mentally retarded students to perform skilled

movements. There is a tendency to set goals too low for these children.

5. Select sensory-perceptual-motor activities to promote specific and general development of the young retarded child and develop recreational skills of older students to make it possible for these individuals to integrate socially with peers and members of their families now and in later life.

6. Select activities primarily on the basis of the development of motor skills. Do not let mental and chronological ages bias your selection of activities.

7. Structure the environment in which the activity takes place so that it challenges the students yet frees them from the fear of physical hurt and gives them some degree of success.

8. Analyze tasks involved in activities to be sure you are clear about all the components of the skill you are about to teach.

9. Remember that mentally retarded children with lower functioning must be taught to play. This means that physical education programs are responsible for creating the play environment, developing basic motor skills that are the tools of play, identifying at what play level (self-directed, onlooker, solitary, paralleled, associative, or cooperative) the child is functioning, and promoting development from that point.

10. Create a safe play environment, but do not necessarily provide security to the extent that the children are unduly dependent on you for physical safety.

11. Use manual guidance as a method of instruction. The proprioceptors are great teachers of movement. Manual guidance is more important for the younger and more severely mentally retarded children. The less ability the child has to communicate verbally, the more manual guidance should be considered as a tool for instruction.

12. Work for progression in skill development. For preschool retardates use sensorimotor activities that contribute to skills found on motor development scales; for mentally retarded children functioning above the preschool level, use task analysis and progression methods commonly employed for typical children.

13. Work for active participation on the part of all mentally retarded children. Active involvement contributes more to neurological development than does passive movement.

14. Modify the activity so that each child can participate up to his or her ability level.

15. Convey to mentally retarded persons that they are persons of worth, reinforcing their strengths and minimizing their weaknesses.

16. Be patient with smaller and slower gains in more severely retarded persons. Often gains that seem small when compared with those of typical children are tremendous for the more severely mentally retarded.

17. Use strong visual and auditory stimuli for the more severely retarded children, as these often bring the best results.

18. Use demonstration as an effective instructional tool.

19. Have many activities available, because attention span is short.

20. Keep verbal directions to a minimum. They are often ineffective when teaching more severely retarded children.

21. Provide a broad spectrum of activities that have recreational and social significance for later life.

Adaptations for Mildly Retarded Students

The largest number of retarded students in the school system demonstrate mild degrees of retardation. In some cases the physical educator will have a difficult time picking out the mildly retarded children by just observing their movement patterns. In other cases the differences between the mildly retarded child and students with normal intelligence becomes more apparent.

In 1970 Rarick, Widdop, and Broadhead[8] re-

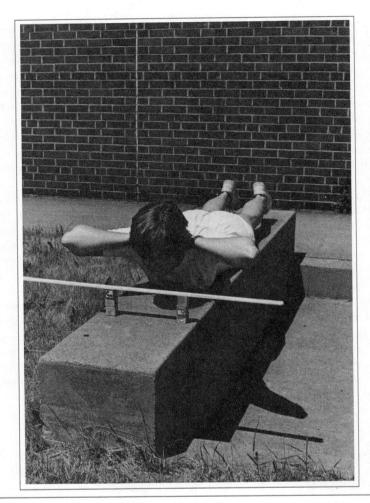

FIGURE 10-2
The objective of raising the chin above the marker is adapted to the ability level of the learner.

ported that the performance of mildly retarded boys, although lower than that of boys with normal intelligence, was within one standard deviation from the mean in the majority of cases. However, 95% of the mildly retarded girls averaged almost two standard deviations below the mean of their counterparts with normal intelligence.

A more recent study by Dobbins, Carron, and Rarick[3] found that after corrections were made for body size there were no differences between ed-

ucable mentally retarded boys and intellectually normal boys between the ages of 6 and 9.9 years on the measures of speed, knee flexion and extension strength, and abdominal strength. They did find significant differences between the groups in body fat, grip strength, and performance of tire run, scramble, standing long jump, vertical jump, and softball throw. The authors pointed out that the fact that the educable mentally retarded boys were, on the average, one standard deviation above the mean of the normal boys on three measures of body fat could in itself account for the observed performance differences.

The most apparent difficulty the mildly retarded student demonstrates is comprehension of complex playing rules and strategies. Often the mildly retarded student who is placed in the mainstream is accused inappropriately of trying to cheat, when in reality, he or she honestly does not understand what the rule or proper move is. Such accusations by peers or teachers often lead to momentary or prolonged rejection of the retarded child. Rejection leads to feelings of low self-esteem, which contribute directly to withdrawal or retaliation on the part of the retarded student. Acting out then becomes an everyday occurrence, and before long they are perceived by peers or teachers as troublemakers. The vicious cycle can be avoided if the teacher anticipates comprehension difficulties and acts to counter them before they occur. Some suggestions for dealing with lack of understanding of rules or playing strategies are as follows:

1. Place the student in a less demanding position.
2. Overteach and constantly reinforce cognitive aspects of each game.
3. Help the other students in the class develop an understanding and sensitivity toward the retarded student's learning difficulties.

If, as the Dobbins, Carron, and Rarick study[3] suggests, the mildly retarded child has a propensity toward excessive body fat, this problem will be detected when the American Alliance for Health, Physical Education, Recreation, and Dance (AAHPERD) Health Related Fitness Test or a similar assessment is given early in the school year to all students. Every child identified as having excessive body fat should be provided with appropriate aerobic activities and, possibly, nutritional counseling to reduce body fat stores. The authors' observation points out the need for routine health-related testing of all students in all schools, at every level. The sooner children learn the importance of controlling body fat levels through diet control and exercise, the better the

chance that these good habits will carry over to adulthood.

Should other types of testing (motor skills, balance, coordination) be deemed necessary by the physical educator, developmental delays may be found in mildly retarded students. The reader may refer to Table 6-1 for appropriate tests to use with this population. Appropriate intervention strategies such as direct teaching of the specific basic motor components found to be deficient in a variety of abilities and skills will benefit these students greatly.

To enhance the probability that retarded children will interact with their families and peers in healthful leisure time pursuits, care must be taken to teach the retarded student to play games and sports that are typically pursued in community settings. The child who finds success and enjoyment in vigorous activity at a young age will continue participation as an adult.

Adaptations for Moderately Retarded Students

Probably the most heterogeneous group within the retarded population is the group classified as moderately retarded. Several different causative factors including environment, chromosome abnormalities, infections, metabolism and nutrition, brain disease, and gestational disorders contribute to the intellectual limitations of moderately retarded individuals.[4] The largest single category within this population is Down syndrome. The condition results from a chromosome abnormality and is most prevalent in children born to women younger than 16 years or older than 40 years. The physical characteristics of persons with Down syndrome include small head and ears, flat nose, small mouth with protruding tongue, fine hair, small and square hands with a crease across the palm, and short and stocky body. Congenital heart defects and poor orthoptic vision are common among Down syndrome individuals.

Moderately retarded students' performance ranges from very poor motor skill and physical fitness levels to quite acceptable performance

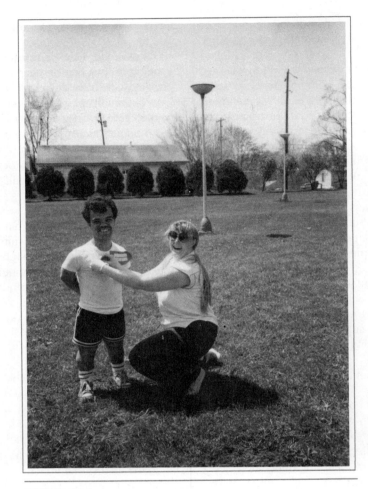

FIGURE 10-3
Volunteers assist with the conduction of Special Olympics.
(Courtesy Western Pennsylvania Special Olympics.)

ability. Traditional studies done by Hayden,[5] Cratty,[2] and Rarick[7] showed the motor development of moderately retarded child to lag 2 to 4 years behind that of children with normal intelligence. However, the performance level of the moderately retarded may indeed reflect the type of motor development programs afforded them.

At least one study has shown that moderately retarded children are capable of academic achievement at a level nearly equal to that of mildly retarded children.[1] Appropriate motivation, high teacher expectations, and carefully designed learning sequences appear to be the keys to promoting learning among the moderately retarded population.

It is true that these youngsters often demonstrate delayed motor development milestones early in life and learn at about one-half the rate of normal children. However, the early childhood intervention programs that are gaining in popularity in the 1980s may help to offset the marked motor delays moderately retarded children demonstrate when they reach school age.

The physical educator is cautioned against

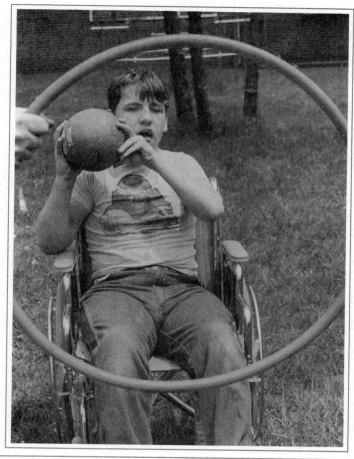

FIGURE 10-4
Time may not be sufficient to enable some children to attain motor skills for self-sufficiency. They need modified tasks that maximize performance toward the goal. This child participates in a modified basketball shooting program.

generalizing about the motor functioning level and learning capability of the moderately retarded student. As in all cases of students with handicapping conditions, the moderately retarded child should be thoroughly tested for motor skill functioning level and physical fitness before decisions are made as to what type of physical education program is needed. If testing shows a moderately retarded student to be deficient in areas of motor behavior performance, a thorough task analysis should be completed before the student's program is determined.

Adaptations for Severely Retarded Students

Severely mentally impaired children with limited motor skills are now in our public schools. Many of these children cannot walk or engage in self-help skills; development of motor skills is one of their most critical needs. Increased opportunities for physical educators to participate in the motor development of severely handicapped children constitute a great challenge.

When designing the physical education program, the physical educator should work closely with both the physical and occupational therapists, who very often test severely retarded students to determine range of motion and level of reflex development. Consultation with the therapists and creative modification of traditional physical education activities will benefit severely mentally retarded students. Some common activities used by physical and occupational therapists with this population follow*:

1. To relieve hip and knee flexors remove the nonambulatory severely mentally retarded student from a sitting position and allow him or her to stretch out on a mat.

2. To improve range of motion encourage the individual to reach for an object held just a few degrees beyond the range of capability. To hold interest, permit the person to reach the object occasionally.

3. Place the student face down on the mat and place a pillow or bolster under the upper chest. Encourage the student to look up (lift head) from this position as often as possible.

4. Place the severely mentally retarded student face down on a long scooter. Pull the scooter and encourage the individual to try using hands and feet to propel himself or herself.

5. Place the student in a supine position on an air mat or trampoline. Gently bounce the surface around the student.

6. Praise every attempt the severely mentally retarded student makes to initiate movement.

7. Hook a lightweight Theraband strip or an elastic loop around each of the student's limbs (one at a time) and encourage him or her to pull against the loop.

THE PHYSICAL EDUCATION PROGRAM

If at all possible, mentally handicapped children should be integrated with their peers in regular

*An excellent resource to use when working with this population is *Gross Motor Management of Severely Multiply Impaired Students* by Fraser, Galka, and Hensinger (see Suggested Readings at the end of this chapter).

physical education classes. If they cannot participate successfully in regular classes, they should be given special developmental physical education commensurate with their capacity and needs. It is recognized that the regular physical education class may not provide adequate placement for all mentally retarded children. These children are below the social and physical norms to the extent that they are not motivated to participate with members of the regular class. Consequently, they often are found on the periphery of activity and do not involve themselves in the games and activities of the physical education class. An effort must be made to integrate mentally retarded persons into regular class activities; however, if this is not possible, special physical education programs should be adapted to the particular needs of the children.

It is also suggested that any mentally retarded children who can be successfully integrated socially in the unrestricted physical education program, but who have physical or motor deficiencies, receive supplementary physical education to remedy or ameliorate the particular diagnosed motor deficiency. Erroneous assumptions are often made relative to the physical abilities of a person labeled mentally retarded. In many instances mentally retarded children from special classes are proficient athletes in interscholastic athletics.

OPPORTUNITIES BEYOND FORMAL EDUCATION

Opportunities to learn motor skills and participate in recreation using those skills should be available to all persons beyond the normal years of public-sponsored education. After leaving school, individuals must be able to find recreation using the skills and activities taught during the formal years of schooling. Opportunities for such recreation should be available to mentally retarded persons of all ages. Physical education for the mentally retarded is a relatively recent development. Those who have been deprived of opportunities to participate and to learn motor skills should be provided with opportunities to learn

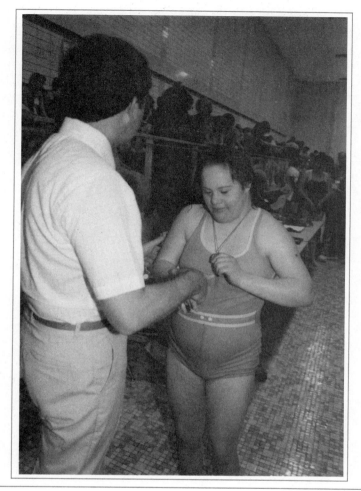

FIGURE 10-5
Special Olympics results in positive interpersonal relationships between volunteers and mentally retarded athletes.
(Courtesy Western Pennsylvania Special Olympics.)

these skills and ways of using leisure time for physical activity. The desired aspects of physical fitness for the particular age and characteristics of a retarded person should be a part of the extended physical education program.

Recreation

Recreational opportunities for mentally retarded children should be provided after the school day terminates, during school vacations, and after formal educational training. There should be adequate provision in the recreation program for vigorous activity such as sports, dancing, active games, swimming, and hiking. Intramural and community sports leagues should be provided to reinforce skills developed in the instructional program. In addition, winter snow games should be made available. Camping and outdoor education programs are other ways of affording expression of skills and interests.

In conjunction with the recreation program, special events scheduled throughout the school

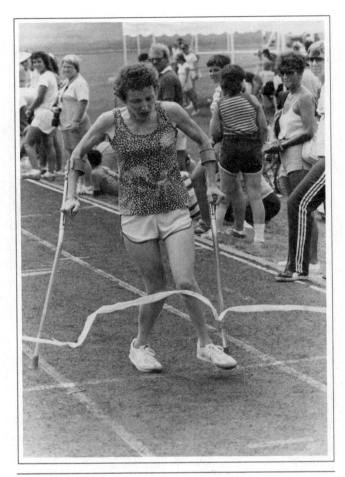

FIGURE 10-6
A handicapped runner completes her event.
(Courtesy United Cerebral Palsy Associations, Inc.)

year serve to stimulate interests, motivate the children, and inform the community about the progress of the physical education program and about the abilities of mentally retarded children. Examples of such events are demonstrations for PTA meetings, track and field meets, swimming meets, play days, sports days, pass-punt-kick contests, hikes, and bicycle races.

Programs

Severely retarded children often require individual attention. Volunteers trained in specific duties can be of assistance to the instructional program as well as to after school and vacation recreation programs. Parents of retarded children, members of high school and college service clubs, and scouting groups are becoming increasingly active as volunteers. Instructors can seek out these people and ask them to become involved with the programs for the mentally retarded. A 1- or 2-hour training session can be planned to teach these volunteers what needs to be done, how to do it, what to expect from retarded individuals, and how to deal with behavior problems.

THE HOME PROGRAM

The amount of time that the physical educator will be involved personally with the mentally retarded children is relatively small. If maximum benefits are to be derived from programs, it is necessary to have a follow-up of activities taught in the form of a home program. Therefore, an educational program for parents describing the children's program and its purpose should be provided for implementation in the home. Parents should receive direction and assistance in methods for involving their children in physical activity taking place in the neighborhood and the home. The "Let's-Play-to-Grow" materials published by the Joseph P. Kennedy, Jr., Foundation are an excellent source of information for parents of handicapped children.[6]

SPECIAL OLYMPICS

Probably no single program has done as much to foster the participation of retarded individuals in physical activities as has the Special Olympics program. This program, which is now international in scope, was begun in 1968 by the Joseph P. Kennedy, Jr., Foundation.* The program includes training in physical fitness and sports and provides competition for mentally retarded children and adults at the local, district, state, national, and international levels.

Fourteen official sports are offered—alpine and Nordic skiing, basketball, bowling, diving, Frisbee throwing, floor hockey, gymnastics, ice skating, poly hockey, soccer, swimming, track and field events, volleyball, and wheelchair events.

*Information about Special Olympics can be obtained by writing to Special Olympics, Inc., Joseph P. Kennedy, Jr., Foundation, 1701 K. Street, N.W., Suite 205, Washington, DC 20006.

Competition is conducted according to the following age groupings: 8 to 9 years, 10 to 11 years, 12 to 13 years, 14 to 15 years, 16 to 17 years, 18 to 19 years, 20 to 29 years, and 30 years and older. To qualify for competition, students' records of performance levels during practice must be submitted (in most cases) on an entry form. Assignment to a division by the meet director is based on these scores. Girls and boys compete separately, and every participant is recognized in some way.

SUMMARY

Mental retardation is subaverage general intellectual functioning accompanied by deficits in adaptive behavior that become manifest during the developmental period. The prevalence of mental retardation in the population is approximately 3%. Four levels are recognized—mildly retarded, moderately retarded, severely retarded, and profoundly retarded. Persons of all levels, with the possible exception of the last, can be expected to learn and develop to some extent.

Physical educators can expect to be called on to serve mildly, moderately, and severely retarded students in the public school system. Carefully selected teaching strategies and program adaptations will yield very positive motor development results. Retarded students should be tested to determine their specific motor strengths and weaknesses, as is true for most performance abilities. Physical education programs should be designed around these test results. Outside recreation, home programs, and participation in Special Olympics should be encouraged.

REVIEW QUESTIONS

1. What is the history of the social perception of mentally retarded persons as contributing members of the community?
2. What are the essential concepts for determination of who is mentally retarded?
3. What are the intellectual and adaptive response levels of the mentally retarded?
4. What are five specific teaching strategies that can be used with mentally retarded persons?
5. How are adaptations for physical activity different for mildly, moderately, and severely mentally retarded persons?
6. What is the need or lack of need for supplementary programs outside of school and beyond formal education for the mentally retarded?
7. What are the activities and participation age ranges of the Special Olympics program?

STUDENT ACTIVITIES

1. Interview parents of mildly and severely mentally retarded adults. Determine differences on the following:
   a. When did mental retardation first become apparent?
   b. What problems did each person in the family have with adapting to the neighborhood?
   c. What was the nature of the schooling at each level?
   d. What services are being provided at present?
   e. What are the prospects for future or continued self-sufficiency in the community?
2. Learn more about agencies and organizations in your community that provide services for the mentally retarded. In most areas there are agencies of both state and local governments that service mentally retarded adults. Most communities have associations for retarded citizens. Many mentally retarded persons are multihandicapped and have access to services for the physically handicapped, deaf, blind, and emotionally disturbed.
   a. What services do these agencies provide?
   b. How does one go about receiving these services?
3. Locate one of the journals that deals with mental retardation. (Some of these journals are *Exceptional Children; Retardation; Education and Training of the Mentally Retarded;* and *American Journal of Mental Deficiency.*) Look through recent issues for articles that present teaching techniques that might be applied to conducting physical education programs for the mentally retarded.
4. Visit classes in which mentally retarded children are mainstreamed. Compare the progress of these children with that of children in special, handicapped only, adapted physical education classes. Compare the following factors for each class:
   a. The nature of the activity.
   b. The interaction with peers and with the teacher.
   c. The degree to which there is active participation.
   d. What steps could be taken to improve instructional efficiency.
5. Visit classes of mildly, moderately, and severely handicapped children. Describe the physical, intellectual, and behavioral characteristics of each group.
6. Talk with a physical education teacher who has worked with mentally retarded children and ask which teaching strategies have proven successful with specific types of learners on specific tasks.
7. Observe a Special Olympics meet. Describe how the meet was conducted to accommodate the different abilities of the participants so all could engage in meaningful competition.

REFERENCES

1. Birnbrauer, J., and Lawler, J.: Token reinforcement for learning, Ment. Retard. **2:**275-279, 1964.
2. Cratty, B.J.: Motor activity and the education of retardates, ed. 2., Philadelphia, 1974, Lea & Febiger.
3. Dobbins, D.A., Carron, R., and Rarick, G.L.: The motor performance of educable mentally retarded and intellectually normal boys after covariate control for differences in body size, Res. Exerc. Sport **52:**1-8, 1981.
4. Grossman, H.J.: Manual on terminology and classification in mental retardation, ed. 3, Baltimore, 1977, Garamond and Pridemarks Press.
5. Hayden, F.: The nature of physical performance in the trainable retardate, Paper presented at the Joseph P. Kennedy, Jr., Foundation Third International Scientific Symposium on Mental Retardation, Boston, 1966.
6. Joseph P. Kennedy, Jr., Foundation: Let's-play-to-grow, Washington, D.C., 1978, Joseph P. Kennedy, Jr., Foundation.
7. Rarick, G.L.: The factor structure of the motor domain of trainable mentally retarded children and adolescents, Unpublished study, University of California at Berkeley, 1977.
8. Rarick, G.L., Widdop, J., and Broadhead, G.D.: The physical fitness and motor performance of educable mentally retarded children, Except. Child. **36:**509-519, 1970.
9. Sherrill, C.: Adapted physical education and recreation, ed. 3, Dubuque, Iowa, 1985, Wm. C. Brown Co., Publishers.

SUGGESTED READINGS

Abeson, A., Bolick, H., and Hass, J.: A primer on due process: education decisions for the handicapped, Except. Child. **42:**68-74, 1975.
American Alliance for Health, Physical Education, and Recreation: Special Olympics instructional manual—from beginners to champions, Washington, D.C., 1972, American Alliance for Health, Physical Education, and Recreation.
Carrier, N., Malpass, N., and Orton, K.: Responses to learning tasks of bright, normal, and retarded children, Technical Bulletin, Project 578, OE-35073, Washington, D.C., 1961, U.S. Office of Education Cooperative Research Program.
Corman, L., and Gottlieb, J.: Mainstreaming mentally retarded children: a review of research. In Elli, N.R., editor: International review of research in mental retardation, New York, 1978, Academic Press, pp. 251-257.
Fraser, B., Galka, G., and Hensinger, R.: Gross motor management of severely multiply impaired students, Baltimore, 1980, University Park Press.
French, R., and Jansma, P.: Special physical education, Columbus, Ohio, 1982, Charles E. Merrill Pub. Co.
Moran, J., and Kalakian L.: Movement experiences for the mentally retarded or emotionally disturbed child, ed. 2, Minneapolis, Minn., 1977, Burgess Pub. Co.
Robinson, N., and Robinson, H.: The mentally retarded child, ed. 2, New York, 1976, McGraw-Hill Book Co.
Seaman, J.A., and Depauw, K.: The new adapted physical education: a developmental approach, Palo Alto, Calif., 1982, Mayfield Pub. Co.
Sherrill, C.: Posture training as a means of normalization, Ment. Retard. **18:**235-238, 1980.
Sontag, E., Certo, N., and Button, J.: On a distinction between the education of the severely and profoundly handicapped, Except. Child. **45:**604-616, 1979.
Staugaitis, S.: New directions for effective weight control with mentally retarded people, Ment. Retard. **16:**157-162, 1978.
Wehman, P.: Helping the mentally retarded acquire play skills, Springfield, Ill., 1977, Charles C Thomas, Publisher.

CHAPTER 11

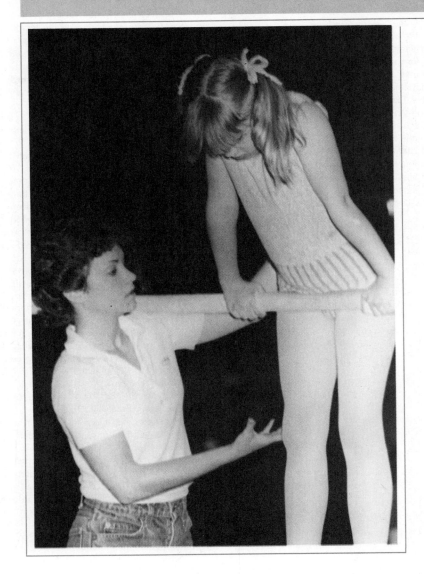

Specific Learning Disabilities

OBJECTIVES

♦ Know how the term *specific learning disability* is defined in P.L. 94-142.

♦ Understand the contemporary controversy about the importance of motor development to the functioning of individuals with specific learning disabilities.

♦ Understand the variety of motor development delays demonstrated by individuals classified as having specific learning disabilities.

♦ Know at least five teaching strategies to use when working with specific learning disabled students.

Probably no handicapping condition has proven to be more controversial nor has undergone more name changes than what we now call *specific learning disability*. Confusion about the condition is reflected in the number of terms associated with disability. Over the past 30 years individuals with these disabilities have been classified as perceptually handicapped, brain injured, brain damaged, minimal brain dysfunctionate, dyslexic, and/or developmentally aphasic. In every case each term has been selected in an attempt to convey the fact that persons with a specific learning disability have normal intelligence but fail to demonstrate the same academic competencies as do the majority of individuals whose IQs fall within the normal range.

Estimates of the prevalence of the condition range from 3% to 20% of the population, depending on the number of characteristics included in the definition.[6,21] Regardless of which characteristics are included, it is widely accepted that 70% to 90% of the children identified as having a specific learning disability are male. We do not know why this is the case.

What is known is that children who were once believed to be daydreamers, inattentive, mischievous, or just plain "dumb" in school do indeed have an organic basis for their behaviors.[15] However, the true reasons for their learning problems are far from proven. The best we can do at this point is to describe the condition and postulate reasons why persons with specific learning disabilities do not learn cognitive information as adeptly and easily as do others.

DEFINITION

Specific learning disability is defined as a "disorder in one or more of the basic psychological processes involving understanding or in using language, spoken or written, which may manifest itself in an imperfect ability to listen, think, speak, write, spell, or do mathetmatical calculations."[22] According to this definition, the term does not include learning problems that are primarily the result of visual, hearing, or motor handicaps; mental retardation; or environmental, cultural, or economic disadvantage.

225

Unfortunately, some educators have interpreted the qualifications surrounding this definition to mean that individuals with a specific learning disability do not demonstrate any visual, hearing, or motor handicaps. In truth, the individual who has a specific learning disability may indeed demonstrate any one or all of these conditions. The difficulty rests with sorting out whether the visual, hearing, or motor handicaps are causing the learning difficulty or whether the problem is one of processing information that has arrived at the brain relatively intact.

It is easier to determine the presence of visual and hearing factors than it is to distinguish motor involvement. As visual specialists become more adept at evaluating orthoptic visual problems that interfere with an individual's ability to fixate on the printed word and smoothly track a series of written words, individuals with visual problems can be distinguished from those with specific learning disabilities.[3] As hearing specialists learn to use sophisticated equipment that actually determines where, neurologically, the auditory signal is being thwarted, the truly hearing impaired can also be identified. Distinguishing motor impairment from imperfect ability to listen, think, speak, write, spell, and understand mathematical concepts will not be accomplished as easily because of the complexity of neural interactions between sensory and motor components that may indeed contribute directly or indirectly to cognitive functioning and the difficulty in measuring basic sensory and motor components.

COGNITIVE-MOTOR RELATIONSHIPS

No attempt will be made in this text to resolve the controversy concerning whether specific learning disabilities have a direct relationship with sensory-perceptual-motor functioning; however, it is important that the physical educator be aware of the historical perspectives surrounding the controversy. Initially, the reason many special educators took such a firm stand against the position that motor impairments may affect cognitive processing dates back to the 1960s. During that de-

cade the perceptual-motor theories of Kephart[13] and Frostig[8] were emerging. These two pioneers proposed that the basic "stuff" from which cognitive information was constructed included perceptual and motor components. Special educators with little or no background in motor development seized on these theories as the possible answer to resolving the academic learning problems manifested by learning disabled populations. In an attempt to "cure" the learning disabled individuals, Kephart's and Frostig's programs of activities were tried on groups of learning disabled students. Almost without exception, the wholesale application of these theories proved disappointing. In most cases the learning disabled student improved in motor function but demonstrated no immediate change in reading or mathematical ability. As a result, many special educators abandoned the notion that there could be a causative relationship between motor and cognitive functioning.

However, researchers with extensive knowledge about neurological functioning have not been so quick to rule out the possibility of a very real and powerful relationship between the basic sensory and motor components and cognitive functioning. Prominent advocates of a definitive relationship between the domains are Ayres[1,2] and deQuiros and Schrager.[7] Ayres, a well-known researcher in the area of sensory integration therapy, has for many years advocated that "learning and behavior are the visible aspects of sensory integration"[2] and that sensory integration results from sensory stimulation and motor activity. Schrager and deQuiros continue to propose that primary learning disabilities have their bases in vestibular dysfunctions, perceptual modalities, and cerebral dysfunctions. They advocate the use of sensory-perceptual-motor activities to assuage vestibular and perceptual problems. A third researcher, Buckley,[5] proposes that the hyperkinetic child will sometimes demonstrate clumsiness and problems with writing, reading, spelling, and mathematical concepts. However, the "pure" learning disability type will exhibit writing, reading, and spelling disabilities but rarely demonstrate poor motor coordination. Children who are both hyperkinetic and learning disabled will usually exhibit poor motor coordination and writing, reading, and spelling disabilities.

Obviously, the controversy will not be easily settled. Carefully designed research studies that delineate specific types of motor components and their possible effect on cognitive functions will need to be completed and replicated. Longitudinal studies that follow individuals who have been exposed to contemporary sensory-perceptual-motor intervention programs will need to be carried out. Dialogue among educators, neurologists, visual and hearing specialists, and researchers will need to be initiated and fostered. The questions to be answered must be approached with open minds, honest and critical analysis, and persistence.

PSYCHOMOTOR, COGNITIVE, AND BEHAVIORAL CHARACTERISTICS

The psychomotor, cognitive, and behavioral characteristics of children with specific learning disabilities are not clear-cut. This is because the label covers a variety of conditions that interfere with these individuals' learning ability.

Hallahan and Cruikshank[9] cited seven social-psychological-behavioral characteristics that are prevalent among children with specific learning disabilities: hyperactivity, attention problems (short attention span, distractibility, perseveration), impulsivity, poor self-concept, low socioeconomic status, social imperception, and delay in social play development.

Hyperactivity and *short attention span* are usually grouped together. These two behaviors are characterized by constant fidgeting and moving around with a tendency to mentally jump from one subject to another. Many children with these problems are referred to physicians, who often prescribe medication to slow the children down. A survey done in Baltimore County from 1971 to 1981 found that the practice of medicating hyperactive students increased twofold to threefold during the decade.[17] Methylphenidate (Ritalin)

hydrochloride, dextroamphetamine sulfate (Dexedrine), and pemoline (Cylert) are the three most common drugs prescribed for the control of hyperactivity.[14]

Distractibility is the tendency to be distracted by stimuli such as sounds, colors, and movement. *Perseveration* is the opposite of distractibility. Children who perseverate tend to continue to repeat an action even though the task has, according to instructions, reached completion.

Impulsivity is characterized by jumping to a conclusion or apparently acting without careful thought as to how a task should be completed.

Poor self-concept means that a person perceives herself or himself as a failure. Their attitude of "I can't do it" often leads to withdrawal or aggressive behavior—avoidance tactics that often keep the child from participating with peers.

Low socioeconomic status means the child's family has a below-average income. This characteristic has not been validated by other studies. Pyfer and Alley found that among the 263 children they tested, all socioeconomic levels were represented fairly equally.[18]

Social imperception refers to the inability to recognize the meaning of body language and vocal tones of others. The child who cannot perceive such differences does not discriminate between friendly and unfriendly or open and threatening situations.

Delay in social play development refers to the failure to have moved through the stages of play. Too often the child with a specific learning disability continues to play alone or parallels others' play rather than interact with peers.

Other authors[6,20,21] agree that the specific learning disabled student may demonstrate cognitive processing problems, perceptual difficulties, hyperactivity, and clumsy motor performance. Any one or all of these factors may affect the design and success of the physical education program. Children with cognitive processing problems may not understand or remember instructions. Perceptual difficulties lead to spatial awareness or body image problems. Hyperactivity interferes with a student's ability to attend to instructions about, or

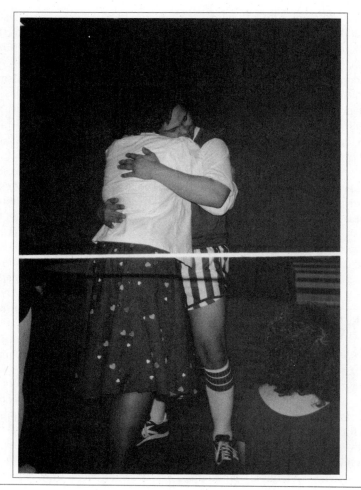

FIGURE 11-1
All children need positive reinforcement. This child is reinforced after a good throw.
(Courtesy Western Pennsylvania Special Olympics.)

persistence at, a task. Clumsy motor performance directly influences a student's ability to master basic movement tasks and to combine those tasks into complicated patterns necessary to succeed in sports or leisure time activities. Researchers who have tested children with specific learning disabilities agree that their motor problems include equilibrium problems, difficulty with controlled visual-motor movements, fine motor coordination delays, and delayed bilateral coordination.[4,11,12]

Other studies show that it is difficult to group all specific learning disabled children together when trying to determine precisely what movement difficulties they will demonstrate. In an attempt to determine whether there is a clear-cut motor profile demonstrated by this population, Pyfer and Alley[18] administered a wide variety of tests to 263 children with specific learning disabilities. Pyfer[15] later repeated the study with an additional 126 children. The results of these two studies revealed three very distinct groups of learning disabled children. Approximately 12% demonstrated no motor delays, 75% scored average on some tests but below average on other tests, and the remaining 13% were severely delayed in all areas tested. When all of the subjects were analyzed together to determine what type of motor performance characterizes specific learning disabled children, it was found that these students have developmental delays, they tend to be in the perceptual-motor (body image, visual-motor control, spatial awareness), balance, and fine motor areas of performance. Although these findings agree with those of the studies cited earlier in this chapter, it must be pointed out that no one performance profile characterizes all specific learning disabled children. These children constitute a heterogeneous group and as such need to be treated as individuals. Haubenstricker[9] proposes that before appropriate prescriptive activities are selected, efforts must be made to determine particular movement characteristics of the students with specific learning disabilities. He proposes that the earlier the problem is identified and the longer the remediation is carried out, the better the chances for eliminating the problems.

TESTING TO DETERMINE MOTOR FUNCTIONING LEVELS

Appropriate tests to use with this population include the Purdue Perceptual Motor Survey, the Frostig Developmental Test of Visual Perception, and the Bruininks-Oseretsky Test of Motor Proficiency. If time or expense only permits one test to be administered, the Bruininks-Oseretsky Test (entire battery) will probably provide the greatest number of clues as to the motor functioning level of the child with a specific learning disability.

INTERVENTION PROGRAMS

Two types of intervention commonly used with specific learning disabled students are perceptual-motor programs and sensory integration programs. Some research studies support the value of these programs and others give reasons to question their value. Until more evidence is available it is reasonable to conclude that each of these programs has some value for some specific learning disability children.

Perceptual-Motor Program

A perceptual-motor program is usually made up of activities believed to promote development of balance, body image, spatial awareness, laterality, directionality, cross-lateral integration, and so on. Sometimes intact perceptual-motor programs such as those developed by Kephart[13] or Frostig and Maslow[8] are used. Other times physical educators select perceptual-motor activities from a variety of sources. Activities used include balance beam tasks, making forms and shapes with the body, hand-eye coordination tasks, and moving through obstacle courses. Very often these activities are taught via an indirect approach such as movement education. Such activities can benefit the specific learning disabled child if the child has been assessed as deficient in any one or more of these areas and if there are no underlying deficiencies (such as vestibular, kinesthetic, visual, or reflex delays). However, if underlying deficiencies are found, the physical education program should include activities to promote development of the deficient systems.

Sensory Integration Program

A sensory integration program is made up of activities believed to promote processing of sensory stimuli. The activities used are based on Ayres' theory of sensory integration.[2] This theory, which has been evolving over the past 20 years, proposes that sensory input systems such as the kinesthetic, vestibular, and tactile systems must be fully developed and integrated before an individual can build cognitive structures needed to accurately interpret the environment. Selection of appropriate intervention activities is determined from results of the Southern California Tests of Sensory Integration (see Chapter 6). Usually only occupational or physical therapists are trained and certified to administer and interpret these tests. Activities included in a sensory integration

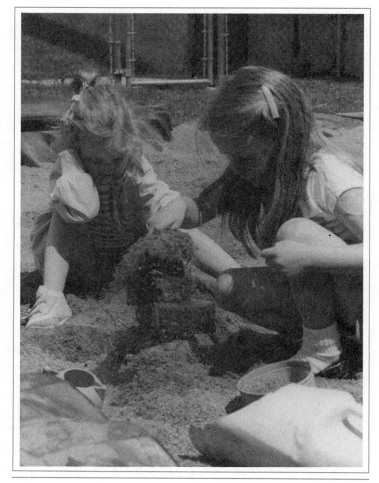

FIGURE 11-2
Activities in which children play together are beneficial.

program include rolling, spinning, turning, balancing on unstable bases, rubbing the body with different textures, and many activities with scooter boards.[2]

The primary criticism of use of the sensory integration tests and program concerns the tendency of some therapists to decide that every specific learning disabled child they test has developmental delays and needs a sensory integration program. Therapists well schooled in the use of the theory and tests are less adamant about every child needing the program. If a sensoy integration program is being used in a school, the physical educator should discuss with the therapist how best to coordinate the adapted physical education program with the therapies being used.

TEACHING STRATEGIES

Regardless of what type of program a physical educator favors, tests should be administered to determine the motor functioning level of the child with a specific learning disability. After areas of

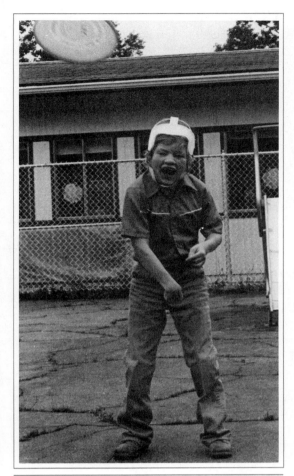

FIGURE 11-3
Always reinforce legitimate efforts made by the children.

text in Chapter 6. General points to keep in mind when working with these students follow:

♦ To reduce interference from hyperactive (hyperkinetic) tendencies, select a larger number of different activities and spend less time on each than you would with other children the same age.

♦ Use a positive behavior modification program to get the students to finish tasks (for instance, use tokens or let them select their favorite activity once each day if they stay on task).

♦ Incorporate 3 to 5 minutes of conscious relaxation instruction/practice into each class period (preferably at the end of the lesson).

♦ Use a very structured, one-on-one teaching/ learning arrangement whenever possible. Do not permit these students to participate in group activities that are beyond their capabilities. Such practices only reinforce the feeling that the children are different from their normal peers.

♦ Design your programs to promote sensory input functioning before concentrating on perceptual-motor integration or motor output behaviors. The greatest amount of carryover will occur if you "fill in the blanks" of missing sensory and perceptual components before teaching motor output behaviors.

♦ Give brief instructions and ask the children to repeat those instructions before starting an activity. By doing this you prevent problems that arise from the limited memory some of the children demonstrate.

♦ To enhance the children's self-concept, use very small learning steps and praise every legitimate effort the students make.

deficiencies have been identified, activities can be selected to promote development in problem areas. If appropriate activities are selected and carefully taught, the prognosis for the motor development of these students is quite good. At least one study reported that once perceptual and motor deficiencies of specific learning disabled children were resolved through a well-designed motor development program, the children developed motor ability along age-expected levels.[16]

Specific activities to use with students with specific learning disabilities can be found in this

SUMMARY

Specific learning disability is a condition that is manifested through disabilities in listening, thinking, writing, speaking, spelling, mathematical calculations. The majority of children with this disability also demonstrate sensory-perceptual-motor problems. There is widespread disagreement about the relationship between the cognitive and psychomotor problems demonstrated by children with specific learning disabilities. The controversy does not dismiss the reality of poor perceptual and motor coordination displayed by many of these children. Before an appropriate physical education program can be developed for the person with a specific learning disability, testing must be done to determine type and extent of the perceptual and motor disabilities. Activities should be selected on the basis of test results and carefully sequenced to produce optimum results.

REVIEW QUESTIONS

1. What is the relationship between perceptual-motor abilities and cognitive functioning?
2. What are some psychomotor, cognitive and behavioral characteristics of children with specific learning disability?
3. What are some specific components of the perceptual-motor structure and test items?
4. What are the ways in which learning disabled children may differ as the result of perceptual-motor testing?
5. What are some teaching strategies that can make learning more effective for children with specific learning disability?

STUDENT ACTIVITIES

1. Select one of the journals that focus on learning disabilities or physical education and recreation journals that which may discuss learning disabled persons. Some are *Journal of Health, Physical Education, and Recreation, Journal of Learning Disabilities, Learning Disability Quarterly,* and *Academic Therapy.* Look through articles that discuss the relationship between perceptual-motor activity and learning disability. Discuss the implications of the findings.
2. Talk with physical education teachers who have worked with learning disabled children. Discuss the strategies they used to enable participation at the children's ability levels in the physical education class.
3. Observe a class with learning disabled persons. List some of the characteristics of these children as they participate in physical activity. Describe the social and physical-motor characteristics. Describe differences among the learning disabled persons.
4. Observe the conduction of a perceptual-motor program. Describe the types of activities in which the class participated.
5. Visit with a person who has learning disabilities. Discuss the physical-motor and social problems this person had in school, community, physical education, and sports programs. List the specific accommodations and strategies employed to accommodate the specific needs by teachers and those who conducted the programs.

REFERENCES

1. Ayres, A.J.: Sensory integration and learning disorders, Los Angeles, 1972, Western Psychological Services.
2. Ayres, A.J.: Sensory integration and the child, Los Angeles, 1980, Western Psychological Services.
3. Broxterman, J., and Stebbins, A.J.: The significance of visual training in the treatment of reading disabilities, Am. Correct. Ther. J. **35**(5):122-125, 1981.
4. Bruininks, V.L., and Bruininks, R.L.: Motor proficiency and learning disabled and nondisabled students, Percept. Mot. Skills **44**:131-137, 1977.
5. Buckley, R.E.: The biobasis for distraction and dyslexia, Acad. Ther. **16**:289-301, 1981.
6. Cratty, B.J.: Adapted physical education for handicapped children and youth, Denver, 1980, Love Publishing Co.
7. deQuiros, J.B., and Schrager, O.L.: Neuropsychological fundamentals in learning disabilities, Novato, Calif., 1979, Academic Therapy Publications.
8. Frostig, M., and Maslow, P.: Movement education: theory and practice, Chicago, 1970, Follett Publishing Co.
9. Hallahan, D., and Cruickshank, W.: Psychoeducational foundations of learning disabilities, Englewood Cliffs, N.J., 1973, Prentice-Hall Inc.
10. Haubenstricker, J.L.: Motor development of children with learning disabilities, J. Phys. Educ. Rec. Dance **53**(5):41-43, 1983.
11. Haubenstricker, J., et al.: The efficiency of the Bruininks-Oseretsky Test of Motor Proficiency in discriminating between normal children and those with gross motor dysfunction, Paper presented to the Motor Development Academy at the annual convention of the American Alliance for Health, Physical Education, Recreation, and Dance, Boston, 1981.
12. Kendrick, K., and Hanten, W.: Differentiation of learning disabled children from normal chldren using four coordination tasks, Phys. Ther. **60**(6):787, 788, 1980.
13. Kephart, N.: The slow learner in the classroom, Columbus, Ohio, 1971, Charles E. Merrill Publishing Co.
14. Learning disabilities: integrating the handicapped student in physical education, Columbus, 1983, Department of Education, Ohio State University.
15. Leary, P.M., and Batho, K.: The role of the EEG in the investigation of the child with learning disability, S. Afr. Med. J. June 1981, pp. 867-868.
16. McLaughlin, E.: Followup study on children remediated for perceptual-motor dysfunction at the University of Kansas Perceptual-Motor Clinic, Microfische, Eugene, 1980, University of Oregon.
17. Pyfer, J.L. : Sensory-perceptual-motor characteristics of learning disabled children: a validation study, Unpublished paper, Texas Woman's University, Denton, 1983.
18. Pyfer, J.L., and Alley, G.: Sensory-perceptual-motor dysfunction of learning disabled children, Paper presented at the First World Congress of the Council for Exceptional Children, Stirling, Scotland, 1978.
19. Safer, D., and Krager, J.: Trends in medication of hyperactive school children, Clin. Pediatr., vol. 22, no. 7, July 1983.
20. Seaman, J.A., and DePauw, K.P.: The new adapted physical education: a developmental approach, Palo Alto, Calif., 1982, Mayfield Publishing Co.
21. Sherrill, C.: Adapted physical education and recreation, ed. 3, Dubuque, Iowa, 1985, Wm. C. Brown Co., Publishers.
22. U.S. Department of Health, Education, and Welfare, Fed. Reg., vol. 4, Aug. 23, 1977.

SUGGESTED READINGS

Arnheim, D., and Sinclair, W.: The clumsy child, ed. 2, St. Louis, 1979, The C.V. Mosby Co.

Barsch, R.: Achieving perceptual motor efficiency: a space-oriented approach to learning, vol. 1, Seattle, 1967, Special Child Publications.

Cratty, B.: Adapted physical education for handicapped children and youth, Denver, 1980, Love Publishing Co.

Cruickshank, W.: Psychology of exceptional children and youth, Englewood Cliffs, N.J., 1980, Prentice-Hall Inc.

French, R., and Jansma, P.: Special physical education, Columbus, Ohio, 1982, Charles E. Merrill Publishing Co.

Gallahue, D., Werner, P., and Luedke, G.: A conceptual approach to moving and learning. New York, 1975, John Wiley & Sons Inc.

Geddes, D.: Future directions: physical activity for ld children, Acad. Ther. **16**:5-9, 1980.

Myers, P., and Hammill, D.: Methods for learning disorders, ed. 2, New York, 1976, John Wiley & Sons Inc.

Mykelbust, H., editor: Progress in learning disabilities, New York, 1975, Grune & Stratton Inc.

Rapport, L., et al.: Children's descriptions of their developmental dysfunctions, Am. J. Dis. Child. **137**:369-374, 1983.

Wallace, G., and McLoughlin, J.: Learning disabilities: concepts and characteristics, ed. 2, Columbus, Ohio, 1979, Charles E. Merrill Publishing Co.

CHAPTER 12

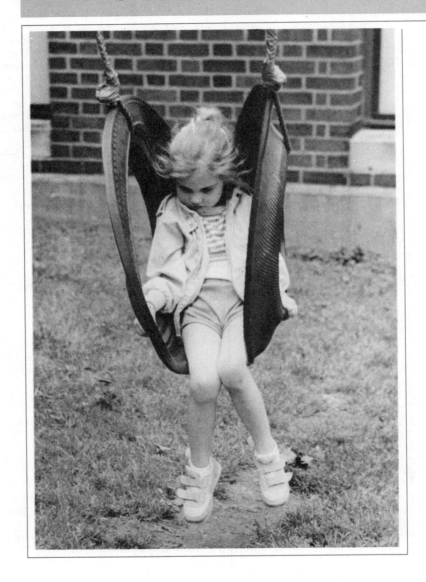

Emotional Disturbances and Behavior Disorders

OBJECTIVES

♦ Demonstrate knowledge of the scope and types of emotional disturbance.

♦ Demonstrate knowledge of the characteristics of emotionally disturbed persons.

♦ Understand the techniques used for conducting programs of physical education for the emotionally disturbed.

♦ Demonstrate knowledge of the relationship among the teacher, services, and programming for the emotionally disturbed.

There are several terms in the literature that have parallel meaning to the term *emotionally disturbed*. Some of these terms are *emotionally disordered, behaviorally disordered, behaviorally disabled, emotionally handicapped, psychologically disordered,* and *mentally ill.* For the purposes of this discussion, the term *emotionally disturbed* incorporates all of these terms.

According to P.L. 94-142, Section 121a.5(b)(8), serious emotional disturbance is defined as follows[15]:

(i) The term means a condition exhibiting one or more of the following characteristics over a long period of time and to a marked degree, which adversely affects educational performance.
   (A) Inability to learn which cannot be explained by intellectual, sensory, or health factors.
   (B) An inability to build or maintain satisfactory interpersonal relationships with peers and teachers.
   (C) Inappropriate types of behavior or feelings under normal circumstances.
   (D) A general pervasive mood of unhappiness or depression; or
   (E) A tendency to develop physical symptoms or fears associated with personal or school problems.

(ii) The definition includes children who are schizophrenic or autistic. The terms does not include children who are socially maladjusted, unless it is determined that they are seriously emotionally disturbed.

CONTINUUM

Emotional functioning may be viewed as a continuum of demonstrated behavior from normal to abnormal and socially unacceptable. Usually, the greater the deviance from the norm, the greater the need for resources to maintain or provide remedial services. French and Jansma[5] describe a continuum of emotional disturbance based on the percentage of inappropriate behavior. Most persons can be placed on this continuum; however, persons do fluctuate on the scale. According to the French and Jansma continuum, persons who demonstrate inappropriate behavior within the 0% to 50% range are considered normal; when inappropriate behavior falls between the 50% to 80% range, a person is perceived as neurotic; inappropriate behavior in excess of 80%

would be labeled as psychotic (out of touch with reality).

The severity of the emotional disturbance is another important variable that reflects placement on a continuum. When acts that result from an emotional disturbance present a danger to self and to others, such behavior is said to reflect deep-seated emotional problems.

Kalakian and Eichstaedt[7] make a distinction between having an emotional disturbance and being emotionally disturbed. Having an emo-

tional disturbance in response to frustration is expected and normal. The state of being emotionally disturbed is characterized by behavior that is disordered to a marked degree and that occurs over a protracted period of time.

INCIDENCE

There is disagreement among authorities as to the incidence of emotional disturbance. Morse[11] has indicated that the incidence ranges from 0.1% to

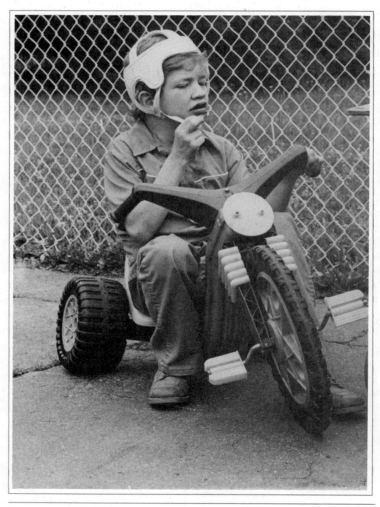

FIGURE 12-1
Organic brain involvement may cause emotional disturbance.
(Courtesy Children's Rehabilitation Center, Butler, Pa.)

30%. However, a conservative estimate of school-age populations of seriously emotionally disturbed children is 2%. It is also estimated that 3% of these students are labeled juvenile delinquents.[4] Other estimates indicate that 10% to 15% of school-age children need some form of psychiatric help to function optimally.[14] When short-term and long-term disturbances of varying extremes are counted, the incidence of emotional disturbance would perhaps be between 7% and 15%. These figures would include delinquents who often present characteristics of the emotionally disturbed in classrooms, such as defiance, impertinence, uncooperativeness, irresponsibility, antisocial behavior, hyperactivity, and restlessness. In addition, they may display characteristics of shyness, hypersensitivity, and high levels of anxiety. A common ratio given in the literature of the incidence of emotional disturbance in boys and girls is 4:1.

CAUSES

When working with emotionally disturbed children, teachers sometimes find it helpful to know the causes of the emotional disturbances. This may help them to form prognoses and to be aware of circumstances that may aggravate existing conditions.

There is disagreement among authorities as to the cause of behavioral disorders in young people. However, hereditary, organic, and functional causes are reported to exist. Meyen[9] has recognized the importance of both predisposing factors (a condition that may cause disturbance) and precipitating factors (a specific condition, a stressful moment) as they relate to the cause of emotional disturbance. An *organic* cause might be brain involvement resulting from disease, trauma, injury, infection, neurological degeneration, poor nutrition, chemical imbalances, or glandular dysfunctions. *Environmental* or *functional* causes are behavioral disorders caused by real or imagined pressures from peers, parents, teachers, or other authority figures or child abuse, poverty, discrimination, peer pressure, breakdown in the family unit, or perception of self as

being of limited value. Many clinicians place emphasis on locating a hypothesized environmental source of the disturbance. It is suggested that additional emotional blocks to learning of environmental nature might be parental ambitiousness, awareness of the impending birth of a sibling, or inability to adapt to a change in surroundings.

There are differing points of view regarding the predominant cause of the more severe emotional disturbances of childhood. Many authorities trace the cause of emotional disturbance to environmental circumstances that occur early in life. Faulty parental relationships, in particular, are believed by some authorities to account for the cause of a great portion of emotional disturbance in children. Some authorities estimate that 75% of the children who are disruptive in school come from broken homes.[8]

USE OF TEST INFORMATION TO LABEL

Psychological tests are required to establish the presence of emotional disturbance. However, the psychological data and the label associated with the data do not provide specific information to assist the physical education teacher in planning instruction. Without a behavioral assessment and programming relevant to skills that are a part of the physical education program, the label is of limited value. Once a pupil is placed in a class as emotionally disturbed, a correlation should be made among behavioral activity, diagnostic data concerning functional activity, and instructional strategies.

CHARACTERISTICS OF THE EMOTIONALLY DISTURBED

The physical education teacher may identify emotionally disturbed children as they participate in activity through observation of adverse performance or abnormal behavior. Identifying emotional disturbance during the initial stages is difficult because behavior is similar to that of normal persons. However, timeliness in identification of emotional disturbance is essential for effective treatment. A list of characteristics that can be observed by physical education teachers and that can be used to assist with early identification of emotional disturbance follows. A child is considered emotionally disturbed if he or she exhibits one or more of the following characteristics over a long period of time to a marked degree:

♦ An inability to learn that cannot be explained by intellectual, sensory, or health factors. Emotional factors play a part in the learning of the child. Inability to learn is a readily observable characteristic among all emotionally disturbed children. A child's inability to learn at the expected rate might indicate some handicapping conditions, one of which may be emotional disturbance.

♦ An inability to build and maintain satisfactory interpersonal relationships with peers and teachers. The result of an emotional disturbance may thus be some type of antisocial or asocial behavior, which has an adverse effect on the child's interaction with others at school. Unsatisfactory personal relationships of children with one another and the teacher are easily observed.

♦ Inappropriate types of behavior or feelings under normal circumstances. Such characteristics indicate that an individual reacts to the environment differently than do others. Emotionally disturbed children may act aggressively or totally withdraw from activity.

♦ A general and pervasive mood of unhappiness or depression. Such persons display characteristics of unhappiness.

♦ A tendency to develop physical symptoms or fears associated with personal and school problems. This may be due to long-term anxiety, excessive or unrealistic fears, or anxieties stemming from perceived stress.

Emotionally disturbed children constitute a heterogeneous group. This becomes apparent when a person compares the behavior of an emotionally disturbed child who is hyperactive with the behavior of an emotionally disturbed child who is withdrawn. There are many behavioral characteristics that are prevalent among the emotionally disturbed; however, all emotionally disturbed children do not possess all these characteristics.

Characteristics that may interfere with the learning of motor skills and the management of physical education classes are the following:

1. Learning
   a. Poor work habits in practicing and developing motor skills and aspects of physical fitness
   b. Lack of motivation in achieving goals not of an immediate nature
   c. Disruptive class behavior on the part of students who are hyperactive
   d. Lack of involvement on the part of students who are withdrawn
   e. Inability to follow directions or seek help despite demands for constant attention
   f. Short attention span
   g. Poor coordination
   h. Development of physical symptoms (stomachache, headache, etc.) when confronted with physical activities with which the person is not secure
   i. Overactivity
   l. Restlessness
   k. Distractibility
2. Interpersonal relationships
   a. Lack of conscience
   b. Loss of emotional control
   c. Formation of superficial relationships
   d. Shyness
   e. Sensitivity
   f. Detachment
   g. Unsocialized aggressiveness
   h. Hostility
   i. Quarrelsomeness
   j. Destructiveness
   k. Temper tantrums
   l. Hostile disobedience
   m. Physical and verbal aggressiveness
   n. Holding group values of delinquency
3. Inappropriate behavior under normal conditions
   a. Unhappiness or depression
   b. Inconsistencies in responses

   c. Rigid expectations of everyday life
   d. Carelessness, irresponsibility, and apathy
   e. Immaturity
   f. Timidity
   g. Feelings of rejection
4. Physical and motor characteristics
   a. Poor physical condition caused by withdrawal from activity
   b. Retardation of motor skill development caused by withdrawal from activity

Identification

The early identification of children who are emotionally disturbed is extremely important. It is recognized that the earlier educators and mental health specialists can attack this problem, the greater the prospect for ameliorating or remedying it. In many instances the treatment and education of emotionally disturbed persons involve the unlearning of behavioral patterns. If identification is made early, less unlearning is necessary.

It is important that teachers know their role in screening. The purpose of screening is to determine which children are not functioning properly, not to determine what caused the difficulty. The purposes of identifying children with emotional disturbances are as follows:

♦ To identify children with emotional problems that impair their learning.
♦ To identify children with emotional problems that disrupt classroom management and prevent others from learning.
♦ To permit intervention to control the disturbance with remedial services (special or adjunctive physical education services).
♦ To place children in the educational environment in which they can best develop their potential.

It is not easy to determine which children have problems that require special educational services. Usually, a problem in physical education classes is manifested by disruption of the student's work, of the desirable cooperation of the group, or of the individual's ability to function ad-

equately. Buhler, Smitter, and Richardson[2] describe the following sequence of behavioral patterns that lead to a severe disturbance, which may assist educators in identifying the severity of a disturbance:

1. Trivial everyday disturbances such as giggling or the lack of concentration that teachers cannot study in detail; action can be met with counteraction to eliminate this form of disturbance
2. Repetitious behavior that must be interpreted as a sign of deeper underlying tension
3. Repetitious behavior accompanied by a serious single disturbance, a tantrum, or breaking into tears
4. A succession of different disturbances on different days such as talking when roll is taken, poking the person standing nearby, and staring into space; indicates deep-seated tension and requires the experience of a psychologist or a psychiatrist

The other characteristics previously listed will also provide assistance in identifying emotionally disturbed children. More often than not, the teacher makes the initial identification of the disturbance and then refers the case to the school psychologist. There is a great need to develop sensitivity to the characteristics of emotionally disturbed children in teacher training programs so that these children may be better served in a public school setting.

Emotionally disturbed children possess a multitude of traits. Consequently, the label *emotionally disturbed* tells little about a particular person.

It has been traditional to classify emotionally disturbed children with a label describing their behavior. Suggested categories that may be of significance to the physical educator of emotionally disturbed children are the following:

♦ *Dimension of personality afflicted:* Personality characteristics associated with emotional disturbance may be immaturity of physical, emotional, social, or psychological traits. Each trait has implications for physical education programming. Social immaturity lim-

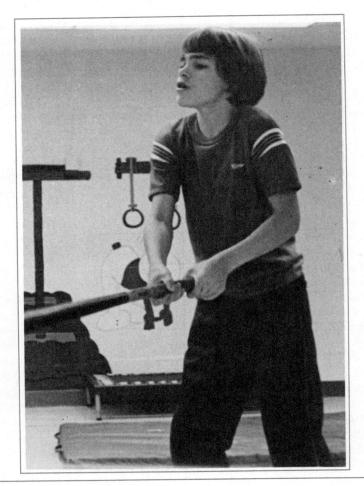

FIGURE 12-2
Teachers of the emotionally disturbed should be responsible for directing play.
(Courtesy Slippery Rock University Laboratory School for Exceptional Children.)

its the child's participation in a hierarchy of social games requiring team play and adherence to discipline with regard to obeying rules. The psychological problems are often perceptual in nature, making it difficult to match perception with motor skills that are associated with many sports activities. In many instances the child's emotional instability may affect his or her physical development.

♦ *Overt behavior patterns:* Emotionally disturbed children tend to be on a continuum

from hyperactivity to withdrawal. Children at each end of this continuum pose different types of problems to the physical educator with regard to program implementation for optimal development.

♦ *Degree of emotional disturbance:* Neurosis is a less severe form of emotional disturbance than psychosis. The psychotic child loses touch with reality and poses a more difficult problem for the physical educator than does the neurotic child.

♦ *Associated deficiencies:* In some instances

emotional disturbance is accompanied by other disorders such as mental retardation, sensory deterioration, perceptual problems, epilepsy, and obesity.

Definitions and classifications by the American Psychiatric Association[1] have identified three types of mental illness: *neuroses,* or mild aversions, phobias, and compulsions found in a large percentage of children and adults; *psychoses,* or losing touch with reality; and *personality disorders,* which reflect obvious social maladaptive behaviors in educational settings.

Although emotional disorders are well classified, it is suggested that maladaptive emotional behavior be viewed on a continuum with strategies and specific techniques applied to each child. The *Diagnostic and Statistical Manual of Mental Disorders*[1] stresses consideration of the individual first ("an individual with schizophrenia" instead of "a schizophrenic"). Thus the groups of disorders discussed in the following sections should be viewed as symptoms of poor mental health rather than a classification system for labeling.

Neuroses

Persons with neuroses exhibit personality problems but are usually able to function independently and retain contact with reality. Neuroses usually do not cause serious personality disorganization and do not cause persons to function abnormally. The neurotic person tends to ignore reality, whereas the psychotic person denies it. A wide range of behavioral deviations have been classified by the American Psychiatric Association[1] under the category of neuroses. Only the most prevalent types will be discussed.

Phobias

Phobias are abnormal fears of specific objects, people, or situations and may severely interfere with the child's education. Such phobias may include fear of taking a shower, fear of heights, fear of sport activity involving contact, or inversion of the posturing mechanism in an activity such as gymnastics. Some children have fears such that

they refuse to go to school.[3] School personnel, parents, and physical education teachers should be aware of conditions that may contribute to phobias.

Obsessions and Compulsions

Obsessive-compulsive reactions are usually characterized by persistent, unwanted repetitive impulses that the individual is unable to control. The reactions may interfere with behavior during instruction. Children who are inattentive, yet not disruptive, to the activity in the physical education classes may have such problems. Repetitious behaviors are also considered a form of compulsion.

Hysteria

Hysteria is an involuntary loss of motor or sensory function or alteration in state of consciousness. Some of the symptoms include sleepwalking and emotional outbursts that are extremely out of character for the individual. Other common neurotic behaviors are reactions marked by anxiety that is out of proportion to obvious causes and depressive reactions that result from real or imagined loss of personal relationships or possessions.

Neurotic symptoms may appear in one setting but not in others, and neurotic types may appear in combination or separate. Therefore, the physical education teacher is in a position to observe the onset of neurosis, recommend psychological intervention, and assist with proposed treatments.

Psychoses

Psychosis constitutes a more serious form of emotional disturbance than neurosis. Persons suffering from psychotic disorders lose touch with reality and demonstrate abnormal and antisocial behavior. They are so impaired that the daily routines and ordinary demands of life are no longer attended to. Some of the characteristics of psychotic persons are inappropriate interpersonal relationships, withdrawal, deficits in perception, and limited language and memory. Intense psychiatric attention and possibly confinement are often indicated. Support services are usually needed for normal life.

Although there are various types of psychosis including maladaptive character disorders and emotional affective disorders, schizophrenia is the most common functional disorder. It is estimated that 1% of the persons in the world suffer from schizophrenia at one time or another. One-half of all patients with mental disorders are schizophrenic.[14] These persons can benefit from specially designed instruction to develop their physical and social skills.

Personality Disorders

Personality disorders are long-term maladaptive behavioral patterns that are culturally and socially unacceptable. These behavior patterns are usually learned and are so ingrained that they are normal for that person. They include alcoholism, drug dependence, and unacceptable sexual behavior and usually lead to social and economic inadequacies.

Schizophrenia

Schizophrenia involves abnormal behavior patterns with personality disorganization. There is usually less than adequate contact with reality.

There are at least nine types of schizophrenia. However, at a minimum, there are four identifiable symptoms common to all types. These four symptoms are known as "splits," and they include the following diverse behaviors: (1) split of affect—lack of integration between thoughts and feelings; (2) split of association—thoughts isolated from logical associations or reasoning; (3) split of attention—inability to focus on one topic, and (4) split sense of reality—retreating from the real world to a make-believe world.[13] Characteristics associated with schizophrenia follow:

- *Physical and motor ability:* Characteristics include poor physical fitness, poor posture, inaccurate movements, and poor motor coordination.
- *Social behavior:* Typical social behavior patterns include depression, withdrawal, difficult social interactions, and moodiness.

- *Speech:* Speech patterns include echolalia and incoherent speech.
- *Interpretation of reality:* Characteristics include bizarre thoughts, hallucinations (perceiving something that does not exist), delusion (interpreting events in an unrealistic way), persistent erroneous beliefs, and stupor (mental inability to interpret the environment).

Schizophrenic disorders have been classified by special characteristics that are observable to the physical educator. There are four common forms of schizophrenia: catatonic schizophrenia, paranoid schizophrenia, hebephrenic schizophrenia, and undifferentiated schizophrenia.

Catatonic schizophrenia. The catatonic schizophrenic person withdraws from or inappropriately relates to reality. In the catatonic state the person withdraws and may be inattentive and in a stupor. This person will not recognize or relate to others and is very difficult to stimulate. The individual will often sit in a rigid posture in one place or position for hours.

Paranoid schizophrenia. The characteristics of the paranoid person are fear of others, distrust of others, and hostility toward others. The paranoid person believes that others present a clear danger to his or her well-being. The theme of persecution dominates the characterization of the paranoid schizophrenic.

Hebephrenic schizophrenia. Hebephrenia involves a defense mechanism that results in regression to childish behaviors such as inappropriate laughter, giggling, and bizarre language. This may be due to inability to cope with behavior that is socially acceptable for the individual's specific age. The regression is believed to be an attempt to return to a time in life when stress and responsibility were less threatening.

Undifferentiated schizophrenia. The category of undifferentiated schizophrenia is associated with behavior that cannot be classified in the other three categories. These persons may exhibit characteristics common to two or all of the three previously mentioned types of schizophrenia. The diagnosis of acute undifferentiated schizophrenia

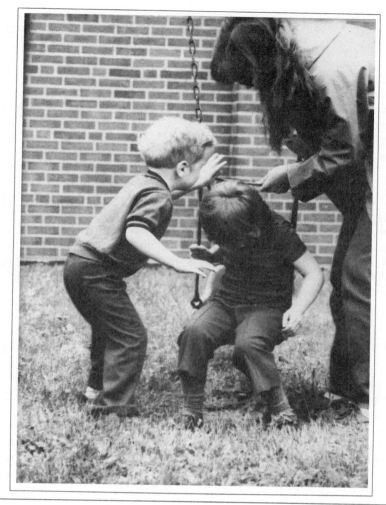

FIGURE 12-3
Inaccurate movements and poor motor coordination may be associated with emotional disturbance.
(Courtesy Slippery Rock University Laboratory School for Exceptional Children.)

is made when the symptoms appear and disappear suddenly in a brief period of time.

Conduction of programs with schizophrenic persons is difficult. Each person to be instructed must have an individual assessment of learning characteristics and needs. The application of sound behavioral principles after consultation with persons responsible for psychiatric care is recommended.

THE TEACHER

The teacher of an emotionally disturbed child bears great responsibility. The teacher organizes physical activities, directs play, and, what is more critical, provides patterns of behavior for the child to emulate. It is from the teacher that immature children learn how the environment works and how persons cope.

The teacher of an emotionally disturbed child

must be stable, flexible, and understanding toward atypical behavior and must be able to perceive what the child is experiencing. Such a teacher provides a medium through which the child may better understand his or her own behavior and modify it. This is no easy task. Being in contact with anxiety-provoking persons often stretches the teacher's emotional capacities. Some of the child's behaviors that the teacher often must tolerate are implied rejection, conflicting demands ranging from demands that immediate needs be met to severe withdrawal, aggressive tactics, and immature behaviors. Regular classroom teachers may be unaccustomed to these behaviors. However, to succeed in working with these children, teachers must understand and accept their atypical behavior patterns. It may be necessary for teachers to receive special guidance and support to prevent reaching a emotional breaking point.

COORDINATION OF SERVICES

Several different persons including psychological support service personnel usually provide services to emotionally disturbed children. The physical education teacher often has a better opportunity to contribute to the solution of these children's problems because of the universal appeal of play to school-age children. Appropriate use of the appeal of activity can result in a successful program that the child finds interesting. However, it must be noted that the physical education teacher or program content may have either positive or negative influences on emotionally disturbed children. Thus it is suggested that all changes in behavior, for better or worse, be closely observed. Consultation with other personnel involved with the child, including those in psychological services, should be on a regular basis.

BENEFITS OF SPORT ACTIVITY

Sport and physical activities are important for emotionally disturbed persons because there is potential for the development and restoration of physical and emotional characteristics. Sport and physical activities provide a wide variety of opportunities to meet the interest of these children. Some of the benefits of programs of sports and physical activities for the emotionally disturbed are as follows:

- The program may provide incentive for acceptable modes of conduct during sport activity.
- Aggressive tendencies may be expressed in socially acceptable ways because of controlled rules.
- Games and activities may provide oportunities for the development of social characteristics such as cooperation and competition.

Sports, games, and physical activity benefit the emotionally disturbed at least as much as they benefit nonhandicapped children.

THE PHYSICAL EDUCATION PROGRAM
Objectives

The objectives of a physical education program for emotionally disturbed children are the same as those for typical children. The program for emotionally disturbed children should stress the development of motor skills and physical fitness, social competence, and personal adequacy. The objectives should be to develop personal and social competencies that will make the children aware of their own resources and potential for self-development. Physical activities fostering desirable relationships between self and both peers and persons in authority should be provided. Physical activities should also provide constructive and positive new experiences that enhance the concept of self and provide a feeling of worth.

The approach to the education of emotionally disturbed individuals is a central problem needing resolution. The difference between medical and educational models for emotionally disturbed children is adequately described by Hobbs,[6] who indicates that education places the emphasis on health rather than on illness, on teaching rather than on treatment, on learning rather than on fundamental personality reorganization, on the present and future rather than on the past, and on the operation of the total social system of which the child is a part rather than on the intrapsychic processes exclusively. The primary purpose of the physical educator is to deal with the process of education, not with therapeutic treatment, when implementing programs.

Principles of Teaching

To conduct a developmental curriculum in physical education for emotionally disturbed children, it is necessary to understand their learning characteristics in the development of motor skills and to apply principles taking these characteristics into consideration. The principles of good teaching of emotionally disturbed children in physical education are as follows:

1. Provide the appropriate stimulation. Many emotionally disturbed children need a strong prompt to focus their attention on the activity at hand. Use tactile stimulation in teaching if the child does not attend to the task. However, avoid overstimulation of the hyperactive emotionally disturbed child.
2. Use activity and a variety of games that will accommodate the students' different physical, social, and emotional developmental levels. The short attention span of these children makes it necessary to have several games on hand so that their interest can be recaptured when an initial activity is no longer productive. Novelty in activities is a great aid in holding attention.
3. Remove distracting objects. The attention span can be increased if seductive objects are removed from the environment because the possibilities of involvement in other activity are reduced. Bats, balls, and other play equipment should be kept out of sight until the time of use, if possible.
4. Provide manual guidance when teaching basic skills to some emotionally disturbed children. This is not necessarily a good procedure for all disturbed children. A rapport must first be built between the child and the instructor before use of manual guidance or the kinesthetic method of teaching motor skills becomes effective. This method is particularly effective with *autistic* children. Manual guidance is less effective with hyperactive children than with those who are withdrawn.
5. Impose limits with regard to conduct and use of equipment and facilities. Undue expectations with regard to developmental level of emotions should not be made. However, each child should adhere to behavioral limits within his or her capabilities. Responsible behavior in the use of equipment and fa-

cilities involved in play activity affords opportunities for the development of positive attitudes.
6. Work with motor skills and games that allow some degree of success. Every satisfying experience makes for decreased anxiety and increased confidence.
7. Know when to encourage a child to approach, explore, and try a new activity or experience. A new experience is often met with resistance. In such instances it is wise to build guarantees of success into the new experience. Subsequent involvement becomes much easier for the emotionally disturbed child. The child who witnesses peers participating successfully in activities sometimes receives impetus to participate with them.
8. Discourage stereotyped play activities that develop rigid behavioral patterns. Emotionally disturbed children often tend to respond to the same objects or activities day after day. After a skill or activity has been well mastered, it may deter initiation of other activities.
9. Do not necessarily strive for control in all situations. One major goal of education for persons who are emotionally disturbed is to affect adequate social adjustment. This does not imply strict obedience to authority but the ability of the individual to adjust to situations independently of supervision. Control should be of such a nature that the preconceived goals of the IEP are being achieved.
10. Discourage inappropriate interaction among the children. Such interaction may result in conflicts that disrupt the whole class. It may be necessary to separate children who interact in a disruptive manner.
11. Provide activities within individual ability and levels of development. The instructor should know the developmental level of the child's social, emotional, and motor patterns; should be aware of how the child responds to various stimuli and activities; and should plan the program around the child's abilities and disabilities.
12. Identify specific disruptive behaviors that can be brought under control. If disruptive behaviors can be identified and defined, intervention strategies from applied behavioral analysis can be used to control the disruptions (see Chapter 6 for the application of these principles).
13. Expect aggressive behavior during specific periods of time. Depending on specific conditions, aggressive and disruptive behaviors may fluctuate. It is important that trends of the strength and frequency of the aggressive or disruptive behavior be monitored and linked with specific behavioral techniques and strategies.
14. Do not stress elimination of neurotic behavior but build positive behavior.[15] It may be difficult to build positive behavior and extinguish neurotic behavior

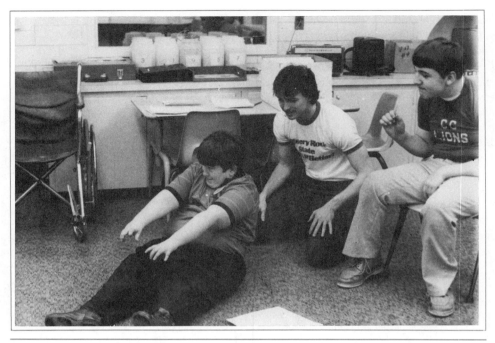

FIGURE 12-4
Performance signals should be no stronger than are needed to elicit the response.
(Courtesy Slippery Rock University Laboratory School for Exceptional Children.)

at the same time. Careful strategies must be developed to ensure that attempts are not made to bring too much behavior under control at one time. Eventually, neurotic behavior can be reduced within the context of a carefully thought out plan and strategies.

15. Use activities that provide immediate consequences of the child's performance. The child should receive some feedback as to the limit of capability and the degree of success that was achieved on the task.

It is recognized that the emotionally disturbed population is an extremely heterogeneous group that possesses varying traits. Therefore, the principles mentioned above are obviously not applicable to all emotionally disturbed children. They are to serve only as a guide to the implementation of programs of physical education for the emotionally disturbed.

Teaching Strategies

Physical activity in the form of play and dance has traditionally been used by mental health spe-

cialists both as a tool in diagnosis and as therapy for emotionally disturbed persons. The qualitative aspects of play and the development of motor skills in disturbed persons have not always received a great deal of attention in the past. However, educators of emotionally disturbed children now recognize that play is not an intermittent freedom from the discipline of academic tasks but is of educational value.

There is a qualitative aspect to the nature of physical activity in play that can contribute to the well-being of disturbed children. Constructive play of a higher order implies the socialization of children. Usually, emotionally disturbed children must be taught how to play and enjoy physical activity. Once constructive play is learned, it provides a medium through which the children may experiment with self-control and with the control of the environment. Play also offers opportunity for social learning and tension release. Because emotionally disturbed children strain the educational program, they are often left out of the extra-curricular and intramural activities of a regular school. This is in reverse order of their basic needs for experience in community living.

To enable successful classroom participation of the emotionally disturbed, a primary consideration is that of managing behavior during instruction. To manage behavior efficiently, it is often necessary to highly structure environments. Such structure, in and of itself, may control hyperactive and aggressive behaviors. When emotionally disturbed children are "on task," disruptive behavior is incompatible with the activity. However, when emotionally disturbed children are not performing tasks, there is opportunity for behavior that may disrupt instruction.

The management of a classroom can be improved if there are designated spots on the floor or specific locations where the children are to be when they are not performing a learning task. Such an arrangement enables greater behavior control during the slack times when the occurrence of disruptive behavior is probable. Pupils may be placed so that they are spread over an area or are close together.

Signals that indicate the beginning and end of activity and movement of the children from one part of the play area to another part increase the structure of the play environment. The characteristics of signals for providing structure to the instructional environment are as follows:

1. The command signals should be short and concise.
2. The signals should be no stronger than needed to elicit the response.
3. Signals may be needed to secure attention (such commands as "listen" and "look" may be needed to secure the attention of the more severely emotionally disturbed persons).
4. Feedback signals about task mastery are needed to provide information to the learner; through the use of these signals, the teacher should indicate to the student the level of success he or she is experiencing.

Analytical techniques for applying tentative principles of behavior to improve behavior are well understood and widely practiced. The application of applied behavioral analysis requires objective definition of the behavior to be changed, an intervention procedure, and a design or schedule to follow during the intervention. Treatment decisions are based on observable behavior that is to be changed, not on medical data.

Developing Socialization Skills

There are specific techniques and procedures that physical education teachers can use to develop socialization skills of the emotionally disturbed. Severely emotionally disturbed persons may have impaired ability to relate to persons and may choose, instead, to relate to inanimate objects. To facilitate interpersonal relationships during play, another person can be paired with the inanimate object that is the focus of the emotionally disturbed pupil's attention. In some cases there may be positive transfer from the inanimate object to the person paired with the object. Such a transfer could constitute the beginning of an interpersonal contact for the emotionally disturbed person.

It should also be noted that team membership in sports may place social controls on behavior to such an extent that unsocialized behavior is curbed. However, the composition of the membership of the team is important. When emotionally disturbed children are grouped together, it is extremely difficult to predict group behavior. In fact, it is not uncommon to see that emotionally disturbed children who have been grouped together contribute to one another's problems as they infect one another with inappropriate behavior.[7]

If emotionally disturbed children are placed in groups of persons with emotional maturity, group behavior becomes more predictable, especially if the nonhandicapped students are sensitive regarding accommodation of the emotionally disturbed students in the play environment. Also, good role models by the nonhandicapped students may be of value for social development of the emotionally disturbed children. Thus social development through games for disturbed children can best be accomplished in play with their normal peers where planned strategies between the teacher and normal peers occurs. It is important to foster sport skill development and basic levels of social skills because they are prerequisites for play in organized sport activity.

Development of Self-concept

Emotionally disturbed persons often possess poor self-concepts. This may be due to previous failure on physical education tasks, which creates anxiety. Levels of anxiety and failure can be lessened through individualization of instruction and provision of activity in small steps that slightly extend (shape) present levels of performance (see Chapter 6). Through this procedure, failure can be controlled and learning measured. Such successful experiences may alleviate anxiety and improve the self-concept.

AUTISM
Definition

Autism is a severely incapacitating lifelong disability that usually appears during the first 3 years of life.[12] It is characterized by severe problems in communication and inability to relate to others in a normal manner.

Little is known about the possible causes or conditions preceding autism. This disorder can be suspected a few months after birth. However, in most cases, autistic behavior is diagnosed when the child is between the ages of 2 and 5 years.[14] It is a condition in which a person is dominated by subjective, self-centered trends of thought and behavior. Two different autistic syndromes have been identified. Early autism appears during the first year of life. These children walk before they develop useful language, and they may not demonstrate meaningful communicative skills.

Psychomotor, Cognitive, and Behavioral Characteristics

There is considerable information concerning the abilities of autistic children. However, the data from the literature conflict with respect to general aptitude on specific motor traits. There is agreement that autistic children usually possess limited motor abilities as compared with other children of the same chronological age. There is some evidence, although scanty, that autistic children possess greater variance in profiles of abilities than do normal children. In many instances, they possess uneven profiles of abilities and tend to convert their assets into obvious talents, whereas other aspects of their behavior may become poorly developed.

Other disabilities in the motor area include postural insecurity, distorted body image, irregularities in passing major developmental milestones, and lack of gross and fine motor coordination essential to performance of activities of daily living. There are indications that through proper application of learning principles and developmental curricula, autistic children can learn gross motor activity. Miller and Miller[10] indicate that autistic children are capable of learning manual skills and generalizing concepts at significant levels of proficiency.

Perceptual-motor Ability

There is information that autistic children possess distinct limitations in matching perceptual inputs with motor outputs. Some of the limitations are as follows:

1. Inability to clap hands to music, reflecting auditory-motor disability
2. Inability to manipulate objects, the result of visual-motor disability
3. Inability to translate imitation of movement into similar motor patterns, a further example of visual-motor disability
4. Inability to perform self-help skills, the result of impairment in gross and fine motor skills

The autistic child, as a rule, possesses a set of limited motor characteristics. The physical educator thus has a challenge in the development of a most worthy aspect of the functions of everyday living. The application of physical training programs to autistic children possesses great possibilities for exploration.

Attention Span

Autistic children have difficulty focusing attention on learning tasks. Some of the characteristics that interfere with attending to tasks are poor or deviant eye contact, lack of a startle reaction, overattention to objects, abnormal response to sound, a mix of sensitivity and insensitivity, and perseveration.

Language

Many autistic children cannot understand spoken words. Some remain mute. Other characteristics that relate to language development are echolalia (repetition of words and phrases), inappropriate use of personal pronouns, arrhythmical speech, and speech lacking in emotion and affect.

Socialization and Play

The autistic child often is out of touch with reality and therefore finds it difficult to socialize with other children. Stereotyped activity of the autistic child prevents the optimal development of skills. This limitation of skills also inhibits social interaction. Team or group interaction depends on the severity of the disability and acquisition of skills. Competitive situations are often frightening and demoralizing to the child and tend to increase withdrawal.

Instructional activities that enable the autistic child to play effectively are essential. A clear, systematic instructional system is needed in which programs for socialization and motor skills can be developed with full knowledge of missing prerequisite behaviors.

Some characteristics of the autistic child that reduce social opportunities are as follows:

♦ *Social withdrawal and unresponsiveness:* Social withdrawal and unresponsiveness often make autistic children inaccessible to their peers, their parents, and other adults.
♦ *Behavioral inflexibility:* Autistic children appear to function best in highly structured environments in which predictable routines are established. Changes in routine or in the environment tend to upset many autistic children.

♦ *Stereotyped behavior:* Many autistic children engage in stereotyped behaviors in which a specific act is repeated many times. These behaviors often are bizarre and further reduce the social acceptance of the children by others.
♦ *Self-mutilating behavior:* Self-mutilating behaviors involve acts that injure the children. Some examples of such activity are head banging and biting and hitting oneself. All these behaviors make it more difficult for the children to engage in social activity.

In normal play, rules that most children pick up easily cause autistic children great difficulty. Many autistic children have difficulty in adopting social play behaviors appropriate to the situation, which often results in withdrawal. Thus there is a need for a systematic planning of social interaction.

Inasmuch as play is a medium in which the inabilities of autistic children can be identified, it may be a medium through which positive social behavior can be fostered. There are sequences of play and prescriptive techniques to promote social behavior in microsocial environments. These techniques are worthy of trial with autistic children (see Chapter 6).

Concerted efforts should be made to move autistic children from adult-initiated and side-by-side play to cooperative play with others. This is a formidable challenge. The play of autistic children weakens without novelty in the environment. Novelty can be introduced in several ways to foster the play behavior:

1. Skills within the ability levels of the children can be developed so that the children may invent novel ways of manipulating the environment.
2. New playthings may be added to the environment.
3. The children can be introduced to different social settings.
4. Different environmental events may be structured.

Novelty can be added in other ways. To foster play development, it is important to pair the play materials with the skill levels of the children. Otherwise, it may be very difficult to motivate the children to experiment with the play materials so that skill and social development may occur. For instance, children can use a playground ball in many novel ways and thus accommodate low levels of skill. However, a baseball requires a baseball glove or bat for participation. Both pieces of equipment need to be manipulated in task-specific ways that require skill and limit novelty.

Teaching Strategies

Individual activity requires fewer social skills than do activities involving team sports. Therefore, the social level of the child needs to be matched with the nature of the activity. Autistic children with limited social abilities might best participate in individual activities such as gymnastics, track, and swimming. When they acquire social skills, they may be able to participate in games such as basketball and softball. The skill and social levels of the child, to a great extent, determine the appropriateness of the physical activity.

There are several strategies that may be used to conduct instruction with autistic children. One is a nondirective approach, in which the teacher takes the cue from the learner and pursues the interest of the child. Another is the application of techniques of direct instruction in which specific objectives are to be achieved by the learner.

The literature indicates that if accepted principles of learning are applied to the instruction of children with autism and if target objectives are within their capabilities, progress in learning tasks is feasible. The effective use of shaping procedures in the teaching of motor skills to autistic children has already been mentioned (see Chapter 6). Shaping requires movement of the learner through sequential activities. The children progress at their own rates through the sequence. Another technique is modeling the behavior to visually communicate to the children tasks that they are to perform. The use of aversive stimuli—that is, an avoidance type of learning—may be successful but should be a last resort. Therefore, with the proper application of learning principles to programming, productive positive learning results can be achieved with autistic children.

There are indications that tasks which are rather comlex and require complicated processing of information by the learner often are too difficult for the autistic child. Activities that require quick decisions and changing situations are usually too advanced for the autistic child. Therefore, when tasks are selected for the child, they should be analyzed according to their complexity in relationship to the child's ability.

Several instructional techniques can be used with autistic children; however, directions should be presented clearly, concisely, and simply with a multisensory approach. Activities should be presented in such a way that there is not a reversal or mirror image effect—that is, the instructor should plan to present visual information so that children view the behavior from the rear of the instructor.

Many autistic children respond to activity that provides strong sensory signals. Dance and music provide strong auditory signals that are accompanied by kinesthetic and vestibular sensation. This meets the sensory needs of many autistic children. Balance beam activity challenges the balancing mechanism and also provides vestibular and kinesthetic information to the autistic children.

SUMMARY

Emotionally disturbed children may exhibit unsatisfactory relationships with teachers and peers, inappropriate types of behavior, or a pervasive mood of depression or may even develop physical symptoms or fears associated with school problems. These characteristics result in inability to learn.

Emotional disturbance may be viewed on a continuum of demonstrated behavior from normal to abnormal and socially unacceptable, where the pupil is a danger to himself or herself and others. Neurosis is a less severe form of emotional disturbance in which an individual can usually function independently, while psychosis constitutes a more serious form in which the person loses touch with reality. Schizophrenia is the most common type of psychosis.

The program objectives for emotionally disturbed children are similar to those for nonhandicapped children. They can benefit equally with nonhandicapped peers in sports activities and physical activities designed to meet their interests and needs.

The central problem that needs to be addressed by physical educators working with emotionally disturbed persons is management of abnormal behavior in the classroom. There are several techniques and procedures that can be used to manage fear, withdrawal, aggressiveness, and hyperactivity. Among these are accepted principles of classroom management, desensitization to alleviate fears, and shaping with 90%:10% success/failure ratio, which may build self-concept and counter withdrawal from activity caused by previous failure.

REVIEW QUESTIONS

1. What are some causes of emotional disturbance?
2. Describe some different types of neuroses.
3. Describe some characteristics of schizophrenics.
4. What are the different types of schizophrenia?
5. What are the personal-social and physical-motor characteristics of the emotionally disturbed?
6. What are some behavioral patterns of children that may indicate the severity of emotional disturbance?
7. When is it important to identify persons who are emotionally disturbed?
8. What are some characteristics of a physical education teacher of the emotionally disturbed?
9. What are some benefits of sport for the emotionally disturbed?
10. What are the objectives of a physical education program for disturbed persons?
11. What are some teaching principles for instructing the emotionally disturbed?
12. Describe psychomotor, cognitive, and behavioral characteristics of autistic persons.
13. What are some teaching strategies that could be used with autistic students?

STUDENT ACTIVITIES

1. Observe a physical education teacher who conducts programs for the emotionally disturbed. Describe the following:
   a. The nature of the class (special or integrated class).
   b. The manner of instruction (individual, small groups, or as a total class).
   c. The ways in which the physical and motor needs are met.
   d. Strategies the teacher employed during instruction.
   e. Disruptive pupil behaviors.

2. There are several organizations designed to serve emotionally disturbed or autistic persons. Identify the local chapters of such groups in your area. Contact a local or national office of such an organization. Inquire about the services that they render for specific clientele.
3. Read two articles that discuss techniques for working with students with behavioral disorders. The *Journal of Applied Behavioral Analysis* and *Behavioral Disorders and Behavior Therapy* are journals in which such articles often appear. Describe how these techniques may be applied to a physical education program with children who have emotional disturbance or autism.
4. Interview a teacher who works with children with behavior disorders and ask for recommendations of appropriate techniques and learning strategies based on experience. Write a summary of the interview and discuss any of the points with which you disagree.
5. Talk with teachers or other professionals from different schools about ways to improve social acceptance of emotionally disturbed children in special and integrated classes. Indicate their suggestions and methods they have tried in the past that have worked. Indicate the activities they provide for parents, classroom teachers, students, and others.
6. Contact a local school district and determine the types of physical education programs for behaviorally disordered persons. Compare your findings with those of another person who has studied another district.
7. Interview an adult person with mental health problems. Try to determine the following:
   a. The nature of the person's physical education program.
   b. Whether the person was taught in an integrated setting.
   c. The person's perception of how teachers and peers view him or her.

REFERENCES

1. American Psychiatric Association: Diagnostic and statistical manual of mental disorders, ed. 3, Washington, D.C., 1980.
2. Buhler, C., Smitter, F., and Richardson, S.: What is a problem? In Long, H.J., editor: Conflict in the classroom, Belmont, Calif., 1965, Wadsworth Publishing Co. Inc.
3. Cratty, B.J.: Adapted physical education for handicapped children and youth, Denver, 1980, Love Publishing Co.
4. Craven, R.S., and Ferdinand, T.M.: Juvenile delinquency, ed. 3, New York, 1975, Harper & Row, Publishers Inc.
5. French, R.W., and Jansma, P.: Special physical education, Columbus, Ohio, 1982, Charles E. Merrill Publishing Co.
6. Hobbs, N. How the Re-ED plan developed. In Long, H.J., editor: Conflict in the classroom, Belmont, Calif., 1965, Wadsworth Publishing Co. Inc.
7. Kalakian, L.H., and Eichstaedt, C.B.: Developmental/adapted physical education, Minneapolis, 1982, Burgess Publishing Co.
8. Klein, C.: A summary of remarks at the House-Senate Education Committee hearing, Senator Reibman, Chairperson, Senate Bill 1214, Harrisburg, Pa., 1978.
9. Meyen, E.L.: Exceptional children and youth, Denver, 1978, Love Publishing Co.
10. Miller, S., and Miller, E.E.: Cognitive-developmental training with elevated boards and sign language, Journal of Autism and Childhood Schizophrenia 3(1):65-85, 1973.
11. Morse, W.C.: The helping teacher/crisis teacher concept, Focus on Exceptional Children 8:1-11, 1976.
12. National Society for Autistic Children: Fact sheet: autism, Washington, D.C., 1980, National Society for Autistic Children.
13. Seaman, J.A., and DePauw, K.P.: The new adapted physical education, Palo Alto, Calif., 1982, Mayfield Publishing Co.
14. Sherrill, C.: Adapted physical education and recreation, ed. 3, Dubuque, Iowa, 1985, Wm. C. Brown Co., Publishers.
15. U.S. Department of Health, Education, and Welfare: Regulations for the Education for All Handicapped Children Act of 1975, Fed. Reg., Vol. 4, Aug. 23, 1977.

SUGGESTED READINGS

American Alliance for Health, Physical Education, and Recreation: Physical education, recreation, and related programs for autistic and emotionally disturbed, Washington, D.C., 1976, American Alliance for Health, Physical Education, and Recreation.

Baker, A.: Congitive functioning of psychotic children: a reappraisal, Except. Child. 45:344-348, 1979.

Clarizio, H.F., and McCoy, G.F.: Behavior disorders in children, ed. 2, New York, 1976, Crowell.

Ferdinande, R., and Coligan, R.: Psychiatric hospitalization: mainstream reentry planning for adolescent patients, Except. Child. 46:544-548, 1980.

French, R., and Jansma, P.: Special physical education, Columbus, Ohio, 1982, Charles E. Merrill Publishing Co.

Gallagher, P.: Teaching students with behavior disorders, Denver, 1979, Love Publishing Co.

Haring, N.G., and Schiefelbusch, R.L., editors: Methods in special education, ed. 2, New York, 1975, McGraw-Hill Book Co.

Hewett, F.: The emotionally disturbed child in the classroom, ed. 2, Boston, 1980, Allyn & Bacon Inc.

Kauffman, J.M.: Characteristics of children's behavior disorders, Columbus, Ohio, 1977, Charles E. Merrill Publishing Co.

Kugelmass, N.I.: The autistic child, Springfield, Ill., 1974, Charles C Thomas, Publisher.

Moran, J.M., and Kalakian, L.H.: Movement experiences for the mentally retarded or emotionally disturbed child, ed. 2, Minneapolis, 1977, Burgess Publishing Co.

Mosher, R.: Perceptual-motor training and the autistic child, J. Leisurability 2:29-35, 1975.

Shea, T.: Teaching children and youth with behavior disorders, St. Louis, 1978, The C.V. Mosby Co.

Sherrill, C.: Adapted physical education and recreation, ed. 3, Dubuque, Iowa, 1985, Wm. C. Brown Co., Publishers.

Swanson, H.L., and Reinert, H.: Teaching strategies for children in conflict, St. Louis, 1979, The C.V. Mosby Co.

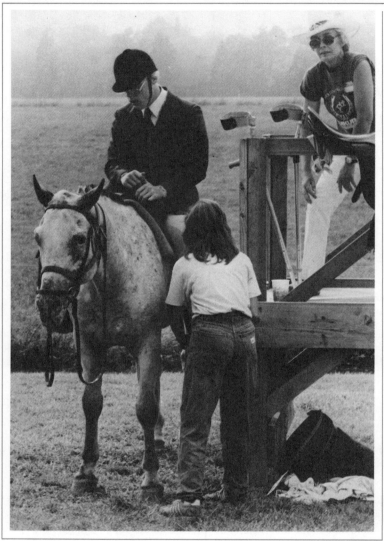

CHAPTER 13

United Cerebral Palsy Associations, Inc.

Orthopedically Handicapping Conditions

OBJECTIVES

♦ Understand a variety of physically handicapping conditions.

♦ Know which physical activities are contraindicated for specific types of orthopedically handicapping conditions.

♦ Select appropriate developmental activities associated with specific types of orthopedic handicaps.

♦ Understand variations of physical characteristics among persons with orthopedic handicaps.

♦ Know how to adapt activity to maximize participation in sports and games.

There are many different types of orthopedically handicapping conditions. Afflictions can occur at more than 500 anatomical sites. Each person who has an orthopedically handicapping condition has different physical and motor capabilities.

Each handicapped person must be treated in such a manner that his or her unique educational needs are met. In this chapter we suggest a procedure to accomplish this task. The goals of this procedure are to (1) identify the specific clinical condition of the child, (2) determine which activities are contraindicated based on medical recommendations, (3) determine the functional motor skills needed, (4) determine the activities that will assist the development of the desired motor skills, and (5) determine aids and devices that will enable the child to secure an education in the most normal environment.

There are two broad aspects of the physical education program. In one portion of the program the student engages in activity to develop skills and abilities. In the other portion the student expresses the skills attained through instructions in the playing of games. A student may develop individual skills during play, but because of the lack of control of specific conditions, skill acquisition may be due to chance. The primary values of playing a game are to learn rules and strategies and to benefit from the social interaction with teammates.

Accommodations must be made for physically handicapped persons so they may participate in games and sports. It is desirable to include a program of modified games and sports for these students for many reasons:

1. Handicapped students need activities that have carryover value. They may continue exercise programs in the future, but they also need training in sports and games that have recreational potential which will be useful to them in later life.

2. Modified sports have therapeutic value if they are carefully structured for the students.

3. Modified sports and games should help physically handicapped persons learn to handle their bodies under a variety of circumstances.

4. There are recreational values in games and sports activities for students who are facing the dual problem of getting a good education and overcoming a handicap.

5. A certain amount of emotional release takes place during play, and this is important to students who are physically handicapped.

6. The modified sports program, regardless of the frequency with which it is provided, tends to relieve the boredom of a regular exercise program. No matter how carefully a special exercise program is planned, it is difficult to maintain a high level of interest if the students participate in this kind of activity on a daily basis.

Included in this chapter are definitions and descriptions of specific types of orthopedically handicapping conditions, types of medical treatment used for each condition, and suggestions for therapeutic and adapted activities that will benefit persons with specific conditions.

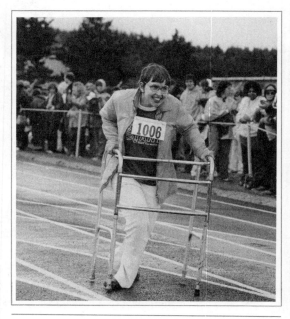

FIGURE 13-1
A walker enables a physically handicapped person to compete in a race.
(Courtesy H. Armstrong Roberts.)

DEFINITION AND SCOPE

There are several specific physically handicapping conditions that are the result of orthopedic conditions. By federal definition the term *orthopedic impairment* means "a severe orthopedic impairment which adversely affects a child's educational performance."[8] The term includes impairments such as clubfoot, absence of appendages, poliomyelitis, bone tuberculosis, and impairments from other causes (for example, cerebral palsy, amputations, and fractures, burns, or injuries that cause contractures). Muscular dystrophy, arthritis, Legg-Perthes disease, Osgood-Schlatter conditions, spina bifida, brittle bone disease, curved joints, multiple sclerosis, osteomyelitis, rickets, and spinal cord injuries are also discussed.

Orthopedic handicaps may occur at more than 50 anatomical sites. Orthopedic problems affect the use of the body as a result of deficiencies to the spine, muscles, bones, and/or joints. The three main sources of neuromuscular impairments are neurological impairments, musculoskeletal conditions, and trauma. Persons with musculoskeletal conditions are so diverse in character that individual programming is required. However, some of the conditions focus on a specific part of the anatomy, and have similar characteristics, which permits broad recommendations to be made for pairing appropriate types of activity with conditions.

CONTINUUM OF PHYSICAL DISABILITY

The effects of physical disability on the performance of physical education tasks are considerable. Many persons with physical handicaps have impaired performance on physical tasks; however, many may excel at such tasks. Of course, those who are totally paralyzed cannot perform physical tasks at all. Thus persons with physical handicaps have diverse abilities to perform motor tasks.

INCIDENCE

For many years federal agencies have estimated that approximately 0.5% of school-age children (5 children in 1000) are physically handicapped.[2] About half of the physically handicapped children have cerebral palsy or other crippling conditions. The other half have chronic health problems or other diseases. An increase in physical handicaps during the recent decades has been reported by some health agencies.[12] This may be because many severely and profoundly handicapped individuals in the past would not have survived or would not have been kept alive.[10]

CAUSES

There are two principal causes of orthopedic handicaps—congenital defects, in which children are born with an orthopedic handicap, and trauma, which damages muscles, ligaments, tendons or the nervous system and results in physical impairment.

TESTING FOR IDENTIFICATION

There are two sources to determine orthopedic handicaps by testing—the physician and the physical educator. The physician may use numerous tests to determine the specific neurological, physiological, and anatomical aspects of the orthopedic condition. Medical techniques such as electroencephalography, electromyography, x-ray examination, and reflex testing as well as other procedures can be used.

The physical educator, on the other hand, assesses the child's performance on the specific motor tasks of the physical education curriculum. A mild orthopedic handicap may be the reason for poor performance. Some physical handicaps are obvious because the children cannot participate in physical tasks that are part of an unrestricted program.

CEREBRAL PALSY

Cerebral palsy is a condition rather than a disease. The term *cerebral palsy* is used to denote conditions that stem from brain injury, including a number of types of neuromuscular disabilities characterized by disturbances of voluntary motor function.

Statistical estimates indicate that approximately 1 in 14,000 births in the United States results in severe brain injury. Conditions that give rise to these disorders may be operative during the prenatal, natal, or postnatal period. Authorities believe that approximately 30% of the cases are due to prenatal causes, 60% to natal causes, and the remaining 10% to postnatal causes. Prenatal causes include maternal infection such as rubella, syphilis, and toxoplasmosis; metabolic malfunction; toxemia; diabetes; placental abnormalities such as fetal anoxia; and excessive radiation.

Motor Characteristics

The degree of motor impairment of children with cerebral palsy may range from serious physical disability to little physical disability.

Since the extent of the brain damage that results in neuromotor dysfunction varies greatly, diagnosis is related to the amount of dysfunction and associated motor involvement. Severe brain injury may be evident shortly after birth. However, cases of children with cerebral palsy who have slight brain damage and little motor impairment may be difficult to diagnose. In the milder cases developmental lag in the motor and intellectual tasks required to meet environmental demands may not be detected until the children are 3 or 4 years old. As a rule, the clinical signs and symptoms of cerebral palsy reach maximum severity when the children reach the age of 2 to 4 years.

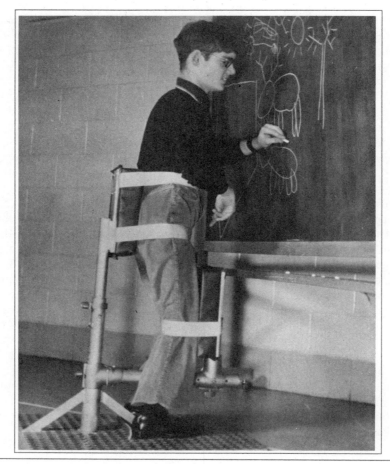

FIGURE 13-2
Some cerebral palsied children have perceptual-motor problems because of developmental delays in hand-eye coordination.
(Courtesy Achievement Products Incorporated.)

Nonmotor Characteristics

Cerebral palsy can include mental retardation, convulsive disorders, impulsive disorders such as hyperkinetic behavior, and learning disabilities such as minimal cerebral dysfunction and visual, auditory, and perceptual problems. Some of the secondary impairments that may accompany motor involvement are mental retardation, hearing and vision loss, emotional disturbance, loss of perceptual ability, and inability to make psychological adjustments.

Various authors agree that more than 50% of children with cerebral palsy have oculomotor defects. In other words, children with brain injury often have difficulty in coordinating their eye movements. The implications of this condition for physical activities that involve a great deal of oculomotor tracking of projectiles point to a need for programs that train for ocular control.

Emotional disturbances constitute another concomitant to cerebral palsy. Children with cerebral palsy are often afflicted with significant impairment that may deprive them of opportunities for ordinary social experience and thus restrict normal social maturation. An interrelated maldevelopment in the physical and social spheres may be retarded emotional development. The basic needs of the child with cerebral palsy—recognition, esteem, and independence—all require fulfillment and are an integral part of the experiences of childhood.

Classification

Hard Signs of Neuromotor Disorders

The different clinical types of cerebral dysfunction involve various obvious motor patterns, commonly known as hard signs. There are six clinical classifications—spasticity, athetosis, rigidity, ataxia, tremor, and atonia. Of persons with cerebral palsy, 50% are clinically classified as spastic, 25% as athetoid, and 13% as rigid; the remaining 12% are divided among ataxic, atonic, tremulous, and mixed and undiagnosed cerebral palsy conditions.

Spasticity. Muscular spasticity is the most prevalent type of hard sign among persons with cerebral palsy. One characteristic of spasticity is that muscle contractures that restrict muscular movement give the appearance of stiffness to affected limbs. This makes muscle movement jerky and uncertain. Spastic children have exaggerated stretch reflexes that cause them to respond to rapid passive stimulation with vigorous muscle contractions. Tendon reflexes are also hyperactive in the involved part. When the spastic condition involves the lower extremities, the legs may be rotated inward and flexed at the hips, knees may be flexed, and a contracted gastrocnemius muscle holds the heel off the ground. Lower leg deficiency contributes to a scissors gait that is common among persons with this type of cerebral palsy. When the upper extremities are involved, the characteristic forms of physical deviation in persons with spastic cerebral palsy include flexion at the elbows, forearm pronation, and wrist and finger flexion. Spasticity is most common in the antigravity muscles of the body. Contractures are more common in children with spastic cerebral palsy than in children with any of the other types of cerebral palsy. In the event contractures are not remedied or programmed for, permanent contractures may result. Consequently, good posture is extremely difficult to maintain. Because of poor balance among reciprocal muscle groups, innervation of muscles for functional motor patterns is often difficult. Mental impairment is associated with spasticity more than with any other clinical type of cerebral palsy, so the incidence of mental retardation among this group is high.

Athetosis. Athetosis is the second most prevalent clinical type of severe cerebral palsy. The distinguishing characteristic of the athetoid individual is recognizable incoordinate movements of voluntary muscles. These movements take the form of wormlike motions that involve the trunk, arms, legs, or tongue or muscle twitches of the face. The unrhythmical, uncontrollable, involuntary movements seem to increase with voluntary motion and emotional or environmental stimuli. Because of the athetoid individual's inability to control muscles and the presence of primitive reflexes, posture is unpredictable and poses a problem. Impairment in the muscular control of hands, speech, and swallowing often accompanies athetosis.

Rigidity. A central feature of the rigid type of cerebral palsy is the functional incoordination of reciprocal muscle groups. There is great resistance to slow motion, and the stretch reflex is impaired. Mental retardation often accompanies this clinical type of cerebral palsy.

Ataxia. A primary characteristic of the ataxic type of cerebral palsy is a disturbance of equilibrium, which impairs the ability to maintain balance. This impairment in balance becomes evident in the walking gait. The gait of the person with ataxic cerebral palsy is unstable, which causes weaving about during locomotion. Standing is often a problem. Kinesthetic awareness seems to be lacking in the ataxic individual. Also, muscle tone and the ability to locate objects in three-dimensional space are poor in persons with ataxic cerebral palsy.

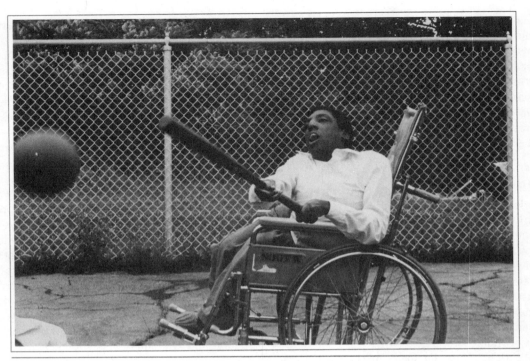

FIGURE 13-3
Handicapped persons with cerebral palsy can participate in adapted sports and games.
(Courtesy Children's Rehabilitation Center, Butler, Pa.)

Tremor. Tremor is evidenced by a rhythmic movement that is usually caused by alternating contractions between flexor and extensor muscles. Tremors appear as uncontrollable pendular movements.

Atonia (flaccidity). Atonia is characterized by a lack of muscle tone. The muscles of the atonic person are often so weak that the activities of daily living are severely hampered.

Alternate Systems

Another means of classifying persons with cerebral palsy concerns the limbs that are affected. The classifications are as follows:

- *Paraplegia:* Legs only
- *Diplegia:* Legs mainly, arms slightly
- *Quadriplegia:* All four extremities
- *Hemiplegia:* One half of the body or the limbs on one side of the body

- *Triplegia:* Both legs and one arm, or both arms and one leg
- *Monoplegia:* One extremity

A third way in which individuals with cerebral palsy are classified is based on the anatomical part that contributes to the palsy. There are three primary classifications:

- *Pyramidal cerebral palsy,* usually characterized by spasticity
- *Extrapyramidal* or *basonuclear cerebral palsy,* characterized by athetosis, tremors, and rigidity
- *Cerebellar cerebral palsy,* characterized by ataxia

Medical Treatment

The four procedures prevalent in medical treatment of orthopedically handicapped persons are bracing, drug therapy, operation, and rehabilitation. Braces are important as an aid in teaching joint function as well as in assisting in the locomotion of patients who are severely handicapped. Another use for bracing is the prevention of deforming contractures. Drug administration usually serves two functions—aiding in relaxation of muscle groups when neuromuscular exercise therapy is attempted, and controlling epileptic seizures through the use of anticonvulsant drugs.

There are various opinions as to the value of orthopedic surgery for persons with cerebral palsy. Certain types of operative procedures have met with considerable success, especially with particular types of cerebral palsy. The physical growth of children affects the efficiency of muscle and tendon surgery; however, operation, for the most part, is not curative but rather assists the functional activities of daily living. Tenotomy (tendon cutting) of the hip adductor and hamstring muscles seems to be the most valuable surgical procedure for adults.

Therapeutic Treatment

There is no treatment for the repair of a damaged brain. However, the portion of the nervous system that remains intact can be made functional through a well-managed training program. Intervention by the physical educator and other personnel is needed to build functional developmental motor patterns with the operative parts of the body. Each child should be evaluated closely and programs that foster those functional abilities should be formulated. Developmental programs should be constructed to correct deficiencies that respond to treatment. The specific child should be considered when determining the exercise regimen. Because of their numerous involuntary muscular activities athetoid children are much more active than spastic, ataxic, and rigid children, who are inhibited regarding physical activity.

There is growing evidence that some of the perceptual characteristics can be improved through training. Perceptual training techniques are developed primarily through visuomotor and sensorimotor training programs. The aspects of such a program include reducing primitive reflex involvement, developing locomotor patterns, balancing, performing actively to rhythm, developing ocular control, and using devices that detect form perception. All of these perceptual activities are inherent in most physical education programs. However, the quality of physical education programs could be improved by implementation of programs of activities that might enhance these particular perceptual characteristics.

The IEP is designed to meet the unique needs of each child. Therefore, special physical education and related services include many types of physical activity. Some of the therapeutic activities and techniques include the following:

1. Muscle stretching to relieve muscle contractures, prevent deformities, and permit fuller range of purposeful motion
2. Gravity exercises that involve lifting the weight of the body or body part against gravity
3. Muscle awareness exercises to control specific muscles or muscle groups
4. Neuromuscular reeducation exercises that are performed through the muscles' current range to stimulate the proprioceptors and return the muscles to greater functional use
5. Reciprocal exercises to stimulate and strengthen the action of the protagonist
6. Tonic exercises to prevent atrophy or to maintain organic efficiency
7. Relaxation training to assist in the remediation of muscle contractures, rigidity, and spasms
8. Postural alignments to maintain proper alignment of musculature
9. Gait training to teach or reteach walking patterns
10. Body mechanics and lifting techniques to obtain maximum use of the large muscle groups of the body
11. Proprioceptive facilitation exercises to bring about maximal excitation of motor units of a muscle with each voluntary effort to overcome motor functioning paralysis

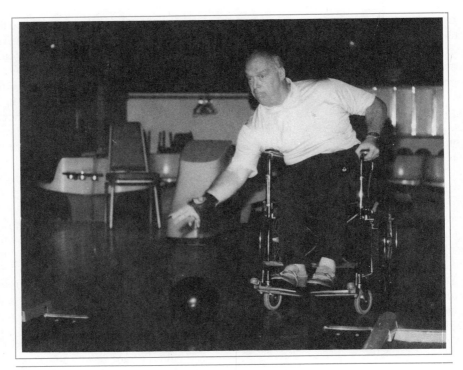

FIGURE 13-4
Physically handicapped persons can participate in organized bowling.
(Courtesy Daryl Pfister, American Wheelchair Bowling Association.)

12. Ramp climbing to improve ambulation and balance
13. Progressive, resistive exercise to develop muscle strength

There is impressive evidence that motor skills, muscular endurance, and strength can be developed in children with cerebral palsy through progressive exercise. Failure to conduct such exercises may leave the children short of their potential development. The opportunities for adapted physical education to maximize the physical development of these children are great. Furthermore, children with cerebral palsy frequently do not develop adequate basic motor skills because of their limited play experiences.

Adapted Physical Education Program

When a child with cerebral palsy participates in group activity, it may be necessary to adapt the activity to the child's abilities or modify the rules of environment. An example of rule adaptation for the handicapped child in soccer would be narrowing the goal area that must be defended. Another strategy of activity adaptation might be to require the child with cerebral palsy to play in a position that requires a slower pace or demands less activity than does some other position in the game. An example of this might be the position of goalkeeper in a soccer game, which is usually less active than the other positions on the team. Positions in many sports vary in the degree of mobility required to play them.

In addition to use of rule modification and adaptation of activity, the capabilities of each individual must be considered. Children with spasticity, athetosis, and ataxia differ greatly in function. For instance, the spastic child finds it easier to engage in activities in which motion is continuous. However, in the case of the athetoid child, relaxation between movements is extremely important to prevent involuntary muscular contractions that may thwart the development of skills.

Ataxic children have different motor problems—they are usually severely handicapped in all activities that require balance. The motor characteristics of the basic types of cerebral palsy, as well as of each individual child, are important variables in the selection of activities. Rest periods should be frequent for children with cerebral palsy. The length and frequency of the rest periods should vary with the nature of the activity and the severity of the handicap. The development of a sequence of activities varying in degree of difficulty is important. This sequencing provides an opportunity to place each child in an activity that is commensurate with his or her ability and proposes a subsequent goal to work toward.

Physical activities described under the definition of physical education in P.L. 94-142 are appropriate for children with cerebral palsy. At the early elementary level, appropriate activities might include fundamental motor patterns such as walking, running, jumping, skipping, and hopping and fundamental motor skills such as throwing, kicking, and catching. The junior high school level curriculum should be in keeping with the activities of the development of physical fitness levels, body mechanics, and games that lead to highly organized sports activities. In the high school program, it is important that students with cerebral palsy maintain adequate levels of physical fitness as well as learn carryover rhythms, and sports such as bowling, archery, badminton, swimming, shuffleboard, and golf. These activities provide interaction and worthy fulfillment of leisure time in postschool years.

For optimal development of sport skills, opportunities should be extended to the individual with cerebral palsy beyond the period of formal education. Acquisition of skills usually takes longer for such children than for nonhandicapped children. Recreational services should then be provided commensurate with their abilities. To date, greater emphasis has been placed on recreational

services for young children with cerebral palsy rather than for the adult handicapped population.

MUSCULAR DYSTROPHY

Muscular dystrophy is a disease of the muscular system characterized by weakness and atrophy of the muscles of the body. Although the exact incidence of muscular dystrophy is unknown, estimates place the number of persons with the disorder in excess of 200,000 in the United States. It is estimated that more than half those cases known fall within the age range of 3 to 13 years.

The etiology of muscular dystrophy is not known. Speculation regarding the exact cause includes faulty metabolism (related to inability to utilize vitamin E), endocrine disorders, and deficiencies in the peripheral nerves. There is some indication that an inherited abnormality causes the body's chemistry to be unable to carry on proper muscle metabolism.

Physical Description

The physical characteristics of persons with muscular dystrophy are relevant to the degenerative stage as well as type of muscular dystrophy. In the late stages of the disease connective tissue replaces most of the muscle tissue. In some cases deposits of fat give the appearance of well-developed muscles. Despite the muscle atrophy, there is no apparent central nervous system impairment.

The age of onset of muscular dystrophy is of importance to the total development of the children. Persons who contract the disease after having had an opportunity to secure an education, or part of an education, and develop social and psychological strengths are better able to cope with their environments than are those who are afflicted with the disease prior to the acquisition of basic skills.

Although the characteristics of patients with muscular dystrophy vary according to the stage that the disease has reached, some general characteristics are as follows:

1. There is a tendency to tire quickly.

2. There may be a tendency to lose fine manual dexterity.
3. Intelligence is normal, but there is a lack of motivation to learn because of isolation from social contacts and limited educational opportunities.
4. Progressive weakness tends to produce adverse postural changes.
5. Emotional disturbance may be prevalent because of the progressive nature of the illness and the resulting restrictions placed on opportunities for socialization.

Classification

There are numerous classifications of muscular dystrophy based on the muscle groups affected and the age of onset. However, four main clinical types of muscular dystrophy have been identified: the psuedohypertrophic (Duchenne) type, the facioscapulohumeral type, the juvenile type, and the mixed type.

Pseudohypertrophic Type

The pseudohypertrophic type is the most prevalent type of muscular dystrophy and is usually recognized when the child is between the ages of 4 and 7 years. It occurs primarily in males. Symptoms that give an indication of the disease are the following:

1. Decreased physical activity as compared with activity of children of commensurate age
2. Delay in the age at which the child walks
3. Poor motor development in walking and stair climbing
4. Little muscular endurance
5. A waddling gait with the legs carried far apart
6. Walking on tiptoe
7. Moving to all fours and then "climbing up the legs" when changing from a prone to a standing position
8. Weakness in anterior abdominal muscles
9. Weakness in neck muscles, which makes it difficult to sit erect

10. Pseudohypertrophy of muscles, particularly in the calves of the leg, which are enlarged and firm on palpation
11. Pronounced lordosis and gradual weakness of lower extremities

As the disease progresses, imbalance of muscle strength in various parts of the body occurs. Deformities develop in flexion at the hips and knees. The spine, pelvis, and shoulder girdle also eventually become atrophied. Contractures and

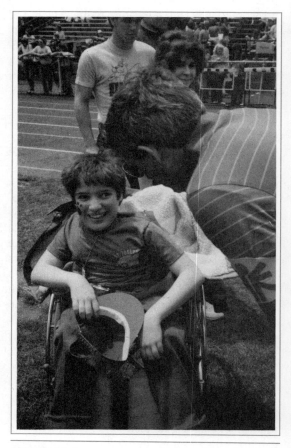

FIGURE 13-5

Children with progressive muscular weakness have an opportunity to participate in Special Olympics competition.
(Courtesy Western Pennsylvania Special Olympics.)

involvement of the heart may develop with the progressive degeneration of the disease. In general, the later the age at which the disease is observed, the slower the disease progresses. Consequently, persons who are affected later in life may perform functional activities longer.

Facioscapulohumeral Type

The facioscapulohumeral type of muscular dystrophy is the second most common type. The onset of symptoms or signs of the facioscapulohumeral type is usually recognized when the person is between the ages of 3 and 20 years, with the most common age of onset between 3 and 15 years. Both genders are equally subject to the condition.

This form of muscular dystrophy affects the shoulder and upper arm, and the person may have trouble in raising the arms above the head. There is also a weakness in the facial muscles and the child may lack the ability to shut the eyes, close the eyes completely when sleeping, whistle, or drink through a straw. A child with this type of disease often appears to have a masklike face that lacks expression. Later, involvement of the muscles that move the humerus and scapula will be noticed. Weakness usually appears later in the abdominal, pelvic, and hip musculature. The progressive weakness and muscle deterioration often lead to scoliosis and lordosis. This type of muscular dystrophy is often milder than the pseudohypertrophic type, and some persons with it have been able to live productive lives. Facioscapulohumeral muscular dystrophy usually progresses slowly, and psuedohypertrophy of the muscles is very rare.

Juvenile Type

The juvenile type of muscular dystrophy begins in late childhood, adolescence, or early adulthood. Muscle atrophy is more general, with the muscles of the shoulder girdle being affected first. The progression is usually slower than the types mentioned previously, and persons afflicted with this type live longer.

Mixed Type

The mixed version of muscular dystrophy may occur between the ages of 30 and 50 years. Effects are most likely to appear in the area of the scapula and pelvis. Persons with this type may take on many of the characteristics of the pseudohypertrophic type.

Prognosis

Muscular dystrophy is probably the most serious disabling condition that can occur in childhood. Although not fatal in itself, the disease contributes to premature death in most known cases because of its progressive nature.

Medical Treatment

Nothing currently known will arrest muscular dystrophy once it begins. The negativism prevalent in some cases as a result of the inability of children with muscular dystrophy to serve a social purpose has been a serious deterrent to expansion of educational plans for these patients. However, it is worth noting that scientific research may be close to solving unanswered questions regarding the disease, and eventually the progressive deterioration of muscles may be halted.

Contraindications

Progressive weakness and muscle deterioration make the child with muscular dystrophy particularly susceptible to respiratory infections. Therefore, the physical educator and therapist should be particularly alert not to expose these children to damp environments or to situations that are conducive to respiratory infections.

Therapeutic Treatment

Inactivity seems to contribute to the progressive weakening of the muscles of persons with muscular dystrophy. Exercise of muscles involved in the activities of daily living to increase strength may permit greater functional use of the body. Furthermore, exercise may assist in reducing excessive weight, which is a burden to those who have muscular dystrophy. The diet should be closely monitored. Control of excess weight is essential to the success of the rehabilitation program of persons with progressive muscular dystrophy. For individuals whose strength is marginal, any extra weight throws an added burden on ambulation and on activities for daily living.

A great deal can be done to prevent deformities and loss of muscle strength from inactivity. If a specific program is outlined during each stage of the disease, it is possible that the child may extend the ability to care for most daily needs for many additional years. In addition to the administration of specific developmental exercises for the involved muscles, exercises should include development of walking patterns, posture control, muscle coordination, and stretching of contractures involved in disuse atrophy. However, it should be noted that all exercises should be selected after study of contraindications specified by a physician. Rusk[5] has stressed that variations in prognosis determine the ambulatory activities and restrictions that should help educators and therapists in program planning. It may be desirable to blueprint the activities around the remaining strengths so that enjoyment and success can be achieved.

Adapted Sports Program

One must recognize that all the types of muscular dystrophy cannot be considered the same; therefore, the physical and social benefits that children can derive from physical education and recreation programs are different. Children who have milder forms of muscular dystrophy, which progress slowly, can derive many benefits from well-constructed adapted physical education and therapeutic programs and should be allowed to play as long as they can.

ARTHRITIS

The term *arthritis* is derived from two Greek roots—*arthro-*, meaning joint, and *-itis*, meaning inflammation. It has been estimated that more than 12 million persons in the United States are afflicted with some form of arthritis disease. Since arthritis inflicts a low mortality and high morbidity, the potential for increasing numbers of those afflicted and disabled is great.

It is assumed that a great many factors may predispose one to arthritis. Major contributors could be infection, hereditary factors, environmental stress, dietary deficiencies, trauma, and organic or emotional disturbances.

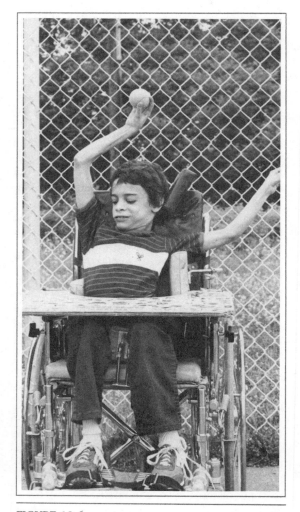

FIGURE 13-6
Persons can participate in adapted sports even if they are in wheelchairs.
(Courtesy Children's Rehabilitation Center, Butler, Pa.)

Classification

The American Rheumatism Association indicated that the three most prevalent forms of arthritis are arthritis from infection, arthritis from rheumatic fever, and rheumatoid arthritis. Arthritis after trauma and degenerative joint disease of the elderly also have a high incidence among the general population.

Infectious Arthritis

Arthritis from infection is usually caused by staphylococci and streptococci. The disease appears as an acute inflammatory condition with joints becoming swollen, hot, red, and painful. Associated muscle tendons may also become inflamed, resulting in contractures, inactivity, and, subsequently, muscle atrophy. Uncontrolled infection eventually results in bone deterioration.

Arthritis from Rheumatic Fever

Arthritis caused by rheumatic fever involves many joints but does not involve the chronic effect of degeneration of articular tissue. The highest incidence of rheumatic fever occurs in children. After a general systemic reaction of sore throat and fever, a transitory polyarthritis travels from one joint to another. Carditis may later be manifested by the appearance of murmurs, tachycardia, and chest pain.

Rheumatoid Arthritis

Rheumatoid arthritis represents the nation's number one crippling disease, afflicting more than 3 million persons. It is a systemic disease of unknown cause. Seventy-five percent of the cases occur between the ages of 25 and 50 years and in a ratio of $3:1$, women to men. A type of rheumatoid arthritis called Still's disease, or juvenile arthritis, attacks children before the age of 7 years.

Physical Characteristics

In most cases arthritis is progressive, gradually resulting in general fatigue, weight loss, and muscular stiffness. Joint impairment is symmetrical, and characteristically, the small joints of the hand and feet are affected in the earliest stages. Tenderness and pain may occur in tendons and muscular tissue near inflamed joints. As the inflammation in the joints becomes progressively chronic, degenerative and proliferative changes occur to the synovial tendons, ligaments, and articular cartilages. If the inflammation is not arrested in its early stages, joints become ankylosed and muscles atrophy and contract, eventually causing a twisted and deformed limb.

Prognosis

The majority of persons afflicted with rheumatoid arthritis recover almost totally with only minor residual effects. However, it has been estimated that about 10% to 15% of persons become crippled to the point of invalid status. For the most part, the course of the disease is unpredictable, with spontaneous remissions and exacerbations.

Medical Treatment

Medical treatment of patients with rheumatoid arthritis involves proper diet, rest, drug therapy, and exercise. Because of its debilitating effect, prolonged bed rest is discouraged, although daily rest sessions are required to avoid undue fatigue. A number of drugs may be given to the patient, depending on individual needs; for example, salicylates such as aspirin relieve pain, gold compounds may be used for arresting the acute inflammatory stage, and adrenocortical steroids may be employed for the control of the degenerative process.

There are drugless techniques of controlling arthritis pain, such as biofeedback, self-hypnosis, behavior modification, and transcutaneous nerve stimulation. Such techniques are often used as an adjunct to other more traditional types of treatment.

Therapeutic Treatment

Physical therapy is primarily concerned with preventing contracture deformities and muscle atrophy by the use of heat, massage, and graded exercise. The exercises required by arthritic patients fall into three major categories: exercises that prevent deformity, exercises that prevent muscle atrophy, and exercises that maintain joint range and basic function. The physical educator can use gradual or static stretching, isometric muscle contraction, and graded isotonic exercises to advantage.

Preventing deformity is a major concern of the arthritic patient. In the acute stage, when muscle contractures are prevalent, splinting is a common practice. The patient is encouraged to engage in muscle tensing exercises numerous times during the day while lying in bed and splinted. Such a program tends to prevent general weakness and maintains a balance of strength.

Preventing muscle weakness from inactivity is very important if the arthritic patient is to maintain joint function. Muscle-setting exercises, isometrics, and isotonic exercises must be employed throughout the patient's convalescence. Particular emphasis is paid to the gluteus and knee extensor muscles, which are extensively used in ambulation.

Maintenance of normal joint range of movement is of prime importance for establishing a functional joint. Stretching is first employed passively.

An individual with arthritis may need rest periods during the day. These should be combined with a well-planned exercise program. Activity should never increase pain or so tire an individual that normal recovery is not obtained by the next day.

Because of the nature of arthritis, an activity program must be based on the particular requirements of the individual. If the disease has been arrested from the acute stage, a variety of sports and game activities may be initiated; however, abnormal physical stress or injury must be avoided at all costs. Swimming is an excellent activity for the arthritic person; however, the water must not be chilling. Additional sports might include archery, golf, badminton, tennis, or weight training. Exercises that improve joint range of movement should be conducted daily. Posture training and good body alignment must be stressed in all aspects of the arthritic's daily living.

HIP DISORDERS

Developmental hip dislocation, commonly called congenital hip dislocation, refers to a partially or completely displaced femoral head in relation to the acetabulum (Fig. 13-7). It is estimated that it occurs six times more often in females than in males; it may be bilateral or unilateral, occurring most often in the left hip.

The cause of congenital hip dislocation is unknown, with various reasons proposed. Heredity seems to be a primary causative factor in faulty hip development and subsequent dysplasia. Actually, only about 2% of developmental hip dislocations are congenital.

Physical Description

Generally, the acetabulum is shallower on the affected side than on the nonaffected side, and the femoral head is displaced upward and backward in relation to the ilium. Ligaments and muscles become deranged, resulting in a shortening of the rectus femoris, hamstring, and adductor thigh muscles and affecting the small intrinsic muscles of the hip. Prolonged malpositioning of the femoral head produces a chronic weakness of the gluteus medius and minimus muscles. A primary factor in stabilizing one hip in the upright posture is the iliopsoas muscle. In developmental hip dis-

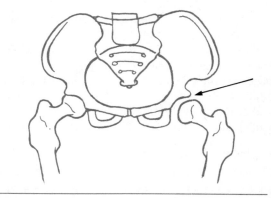

FIGURE 13-7
Developmental hip dislocation.

location, the iliopsoas muscle serves to displace the femoral head upward; this will eventually cause the lumbar vertebrae to become lordotic and scoliotic.

Detection of the hip dislocation may not occur until the child begins to bear weight or walk. Early recognition of this condition may be accomplished by observing asymmetrical fat folds on the infant's legs and restricted hip adduction on the affected side. The Trendelenburg test will reveal that the child is unable to maintain the pelvis level while standing on the affected leg. In such cases, weak abductor muscles of the affected leg allow the pelvis to tilt downward on the nonaffected side. The child walks with a decided limp in unilateral cases and with a waddle in bilateral cases. No discomfort or pain is normally experienced by the child, but fatigue tolerance to physical activity is very low. Pain and discomfort become more apparent as the individual becomes older and as postural deformities become more structural.

Medical Treatment

Medical treatment of the developmental hip dislocation depends on the age of the child and the extent of displacement. Young babies with a mild involvement may have the condition remedied through gradual adduction of the femur by a pillow splint, whereas more complicated cases may require traction, casting, or operation to restore proper hip continuity. The thigh is slowly returned to a normal position.

Therapeutic Treatment

Active exercise is suggested along with passive stretching to contracted tissue. Primary concern is paid to reconditioning the movement of hip extension and abduction. When adequate muscle strength has been gained in the hip region, a program of ambulation is conducted, with particular attention paid to walking without a lateral pelvic tilt.

A child in the adapted physical education or therapeutic recreation program with a history of developmental hip dislocation will, in most instances, require specific postural training, conditioning of the hip region, continual gait training, and general body mechanics training. Swimming is an excellent activity for general conditioning of the hip, and it is highly recommended.

Contraindications

Activities should not be engaged in to the point of discomfort or fatigue.

COXA PLANA (LEGG-PERTHES DISEASE)

Coxa plana is the result of osteochrondritis dissecans, or abnormal softening, of the femoral head. It is a condition identified early in the twentieth century independently by Legg of Boston, Calvé of France, and Perthes of Germany. Its gross signs reflect a fattening of the head of the femur, and it is found predominantly in boys between the ages of 3 and 12 years. It has been variously termed osteochondritis deformans juvenilis, pseudocoxalgia, and Legg-Calvé-Perthes disease. (See Fig. 13-8.)

The exact cause of coxa plana is not known; trauma, infection, and endocrine imbalance have been suggested as possible causes.

Medical Description and Prognosis

Coxa plana is characterized by degeneration of the capital epiphysis of the femoral head. Os-

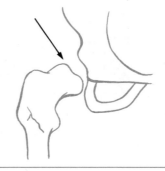

FIGURE 13-8
Coxa plana.

teoporosis, or bone rarefaction, results in a flattened and deformed femoral head. Later developments may also include widening of the femoral head and thickening of the femoral neck. The last stage of coxa plana may be reflected by a self-limiting course in which there is a regeneration and an almost complete return of the normal epiphysis within 3 to 4 years. However, recovery is not always complete and there is often some residual deformity present. The younger child with coxa plana has the best prognosis for complete recovery.

Physical Description

The first outward sign of this condition is often a limp favoring the affected leg, with pain referred to the knee region. Further investigation by the physician may show pain upon passive movement and restricted motion upon internal rotation and abduction. X-ray examination will provide the

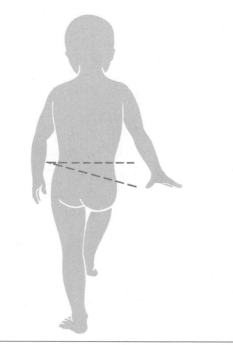

FIGURE 13-9
Trendelenburg test.

definitive signs of degeneration. The physical educator or therapist may be the first person to observe the gross signs of coxa plana and bring it to the attention of parents or physician.

Whatever the mechanism of injury, the individual with coxa plana experiences progressive fatigue and pain upon weight bearing, progressive stiffness, and a limited range of movement. A limp is apparent, which reflects weakness in the hip abductor muscles and pain referred to the region of the knee. With displacement of the epiphyseal plate, the affected limb tends to rotate externally and to abduct when flexed.

Medical Treatment

Treatment of coxa plana primarily entails the removal of stress placed on the femoral head by weight bearing. Bed rest is often employed in the acute stages, with ambulation and non–weight-bearing devices used for the remaining period of incapacitation. The sling and crutch method for non–weight bearing is widely used for this condition.

Contraindications

Weight-bearing exercise is contraindicated until the physician discounts the possibility of a pathological joint condition.

Therapeutic Treatment

The individual with an epiphyseal affection of the hip presents a problem of muscular and skeletal stability and joint range of movement. Stability of the hip region requires skeletal continuity and a balance of muscle strength, primarily in the muscles of hip extension and abduction. Prolonged limited motion and non–weight bearing may result in contractures of tissues surrounding the hip joint and an inability to walk or run with ease. Abnormal weakness of the hip extensors and abductors causes the individual to display the Trendelenburg sign. (See Fig. 13-9.)

A program of exercise must be carried out to prevent muscle atrophy and general deconditioning. When movement is prohibited, muscle-tensing exercises for muscles of the hip region are conducted, together with isotonic exercises for the upper extremities, trunk, ankles, and feet.

When the hip becomes free of symptoms, a progressive, isotonic, non–weight-bearing program is first initiated for the hip region. Active movement emphasizing hip extension and abduction is recommended. Swimming is an excellent adjunct to the regular exercise program.

The program of exercise should never exceed the point of pain or fatigue until full recovery is accomplished. A general physical fitness program emphasizing weight control and body mechanics will aid the student in preparing for a return to a full program of physical education and recreation activities.

Adapted Activity

Principles described in the opening section of this chapter may be applied to persons with coxa plana to include them in games and sports. To the greatest extent possible, children with coxa plana should be taught activities that parallel those of normal school children.

COXA VARA AND COXA VALGA

In adults the normal angle of inclination of the femoral head, or neck of the femur, is about 128 degrees. An abnormal increase in this angle is

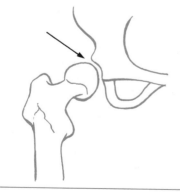

FIGURE 13-10
Coxa vara.

called coxa valga and a decrease is called coxa vara. (See Fig. 13-10.)

The acquired type of coxa vara is, by far, the most prevalent and occurs most often in adolescent boys between 10 and 16 years of age. It is commonly termed adolescent coxa vara.

The pathological mechanics of coxa vara and coxa valga result from the combined stresses of an abnormal increase or decrease in weight bearing. A variation of more than 10 to 15 degrees can produce significant shortening or lengthening of an extremity.

Coxa valga and coxa vara can be caused by many etiological factors—for example, hip injury, paralysis, non–weight bearing, or congenital malformation. Coxa vara and coxa valga are described according to where the structural changes have occurred in the femur—that is, neck (cervical), head (epiphyseal), or combined head and neck (cervicoepiphyseal).

Adolescent coxa vara is found in boys who have displacement of the upper femoral epiphysis. Boys who are most prone to adolescent coxa vara have been found to be obese and sexually immature or tall and lanky, having experienced a rapid growing phase. Trauma such as hip fracture or dislocation may result in acute coxa vara. More often, through constant stress, a gradual displacement may take place.

Classification

Coxa vara and coxa valga are disturbances in the proximal cartilage or epiphyseal plate of the femur that result in alteration in the angle of the shaft as it relates to the neck of the femur. Two types of conditions have been recognized—the congenital type and the acquired type. The congenital type may be associated with developmental hip dislocation.

Medical Treatment

Management in the early stages of coxa vara involves use of crutches and the prevention of weight bearing to allow revascularization of the epiphyseal plate. Where deformity, displacement, and limb shortening are apparent, corrective surgery may be elected by the physician.

OSGOOD-SCHLATTER CONDITION

Many terms have been applied to the Osgood-Schlatter condition; the most prevalent are apophysitis, osteochondritis, and epiphysitis of the tibial tubercle. It is not considered a disease entity but the result of a separation of the tibial tubercle at the epiphyseal junction.

The cause of this condition is unknown, but direct injury and long-term irritation are thought to be the main inciting factors. Direct trauma (as in a blow), osteochondritis, or an excessive strain of the patellar tendon as it attaches to the tibial tubercle may result in evulsion at the epiphyseal cartilage junction.

Osgood-Schlatter condition usually occurs in active adolescent boys and girls between the ages of 10 and 15 years who are in a rapid growth period.

Physical Description

Disruption of the blood supply to the epiphysis results in enlargement of the tibial tubercle, joint tenderness, and pain upon contraction of the quadriceps muscle. The physical educator may be the one to detect this condition from the complaints of the student, who should be immediately referred to a physician.

Prognosis

If the Osgood-Schlatter condition is not properly cared for, deformity and a defective extensor mechanism may result; however, it may not necessarily be associated with pain or discomfort. In most cases, Osgood-Schlatter condition is acute, is self-limiting, and does not exceed a few months' duration. However, even after arrest of symptoms, Osgood-Schlatter condition tends to recur after irritation.

Contraindications

Local inflammation is accentuated by leg activity and ameliorated by rest. The individual may be unable to kneel or engage in flexion and extension movements without pain. The knee joint must be kept completely immobilized when the inflammatory state persists. Forced inactivity, provided by a plaster cast, may be the only answer to keeping the overactive adolescent from using the affected leg.

Therapeutic Treatment

Early detection may reveal a slight condition in which the individual can continue a normal activity routine, excluding overexposure to strenuous running, jumping, and falling on the affected leg. All physical education activities must be modified to avoid quadriceps muscle strain while preparing for general physical fitness.

While the limb is immobilized in a cast, the individual is greatly restricted; weight bearing may be held to a minimum, with signs of pain at the affected part closely watched by the physician. Although Osgood-Schlatter condition is self-limiting and temporary, exercise is an important factor in full recovery. Physical education activities should emphasize the capabilities of the upper body and nonaffected leg to prevent their deconditioning.

After arrest of the condition and removal of the cast (or relief from immobilization), the patient is given a graduated reconditioning program. The major objectives at this time are reeducation in proper walking patterns and restoration of normal strength and flexibility of the knee joint. Strenuous knee movement is avoided for at least 5 weeks and the demanding requirements of regular physical education classes may be postponed for extended periods, depending on the physician's recommendations. Although during the period of rehabilitation emphasis is placed on the affected leg, a program must also be provided for the entire body.

The criteria for the individual to return to a regular physical education program would be as follows:

1. Normal range of movement of the knee
2. Quadriceps muscle strength equal to that of the unaffected leg

3. Evidence that the Osgood-Schlatter condition has become asymptomatic
4. Ability to move freely without favoring the affected part

Following recovery, the student should avoid all activities that would tend to contuse, or in any way irritate again, the tibial tuberosity.

Modified Sports Program and Adapted Activity

Principles described in the opening section of this chapter may be applied to persons with Osgood-Schlatter condition to include them in games and sports. To the greatest extent possible, children with Osgood-Schlatter condition should be taught activities that parallel those of normal school children.

CLUBFOOT

One of the most common deformities of the lower extremity is clubfoot. This deformity is characterized by plantar flexion or dorsiflexion and inversion or eversion of the foot. The clubfoot defor-

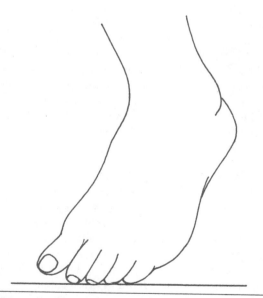

FIGURE 13-11
Clubfoot.

mity, if not corrected, would force the individual to walk on the side of the foot or on the ankle rather than on the sole of the foot. (See Fig. 13-11.)

This defect can be acquired or congenital. The acquired type of clubfoot can develop from a spastic paralysis, as in cerebral palsy or other neuromuscular diseases, which may eventuate in bone and soft tissue changes. Congenital clubfoot is by far the most prevalent type. Talipes equinovarus has the highest incidence, amounting to 70% among the congenital forms of clubfoot.

Prognosis

If talipes equinovarus is not corrected early in life, the individual develops an awkward gait and walks on the outside of the foot and ankle.

Medical Treatment

If the deformity is recognized soon after birth, a plaster cast is employed to retain the foot in an overcorrected position. Special clubfoot shoes with a rigid steel pole may be employed for the prewalker to help maintain the proper position of the foot. Various corrective shoes may be worn and splints applied to continue the development of proper foot alignment until amelioration is achieved.

Modification of Activities

The pupil's limitations and capabilities will depend on the extent of residual derangement and deformity. A handicapped child with a severe malformation may be restricted from standing for long periods or may be unable to walk without fatigue. Activities requiring running and jumping must be modified. Team and individual sports activities are beneficial for the pupil with clubfoot, but they have to be adapted to prevent the deleterious effects of extensive running, jumping, and kicking.

Therapeutic Treatment

Exercise cannot be considered a means for correcting a clubfoot. However, a graded program should be given to the pupil that will maintain or improve muscle tone, ambulation, body mechanics, posture, and physical and motor fitness.

SPINA BIFIDA

Spina bifida is the most common congenital defect occurring to the spine. Spina bifida implies congenital malformation of the posterior aspects of the spinal column, in which some portion of the vertebral arch fails to form over the spinal cord. (See Fig. 13-12).

Spinal bifida occulta is the unfused condition of vertebral arches without any cystic distension of the meninges.

The incidence of spina bifida is estimated at 0.02%, making it one of the most common birth defects causing physical disability.

Characteristics

In any type of spina bifida, spinal cord defects may produce varying degrees of neurological impairment ranging from mild muscle imbalance and sensory loss in the lower limbs to complete paraplegia. In almost half the children with spina bifida, a hydrocephalic condition also exists. In these cases shunting is mandated to prevent irreversible brain damage. However, neurological disturbances may be completely absent in cases

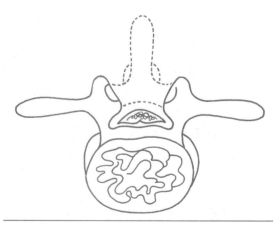

FIGURE 13-12
Spina bifida occulta.

of spina bifida occulta or may not become symptomatic until later in life.

Children who are paraplegic from spina bifida are often able to move about with the aid of braces and crutches. There may or may not be changes in the overlying skin, neurological signs, or pathological changes in the spinal cord.

Therapeutic Treatment

No particular program of physical education or therapy can be directly assigned to the student with spina bifida. Some students have no physical reaction and discover the condition only by chance through x-ray examination for another problem. On the other hand, a person may have extensive neuromuscular involvement requiring constant medical care. A program of physical education or therapeutic exercise based on the individual needs of the person should be planned.

Medical Treatment

Activities that could distress placement of any shunts or put pressure on sensitive areas of the spine must be avoided. Of considerable concern is the prevention of contractures and associated foot deformities (for example, equinovarus) through daily passive flexibility exercises.

Adapted Activity

Adapted physical education programming is often not required for pupils with spina bifida occulta or meningocele acquired at infancy. However, children with myelomeningocele need programs that are modified to their needs and that stress intensive development.

Social Problems

Many social problems result from spina bifida. In addition to the physical handicap, there are often problems associated with control of bowels and bladder, which draw further attention to the children as they function in a social environment. In many cases this has a negative social impact on the children. Often, children with spina bifida need catheterization. If someone must do it for them, the attention of others is drawn to these circumstances. However, in many cases the children may be able to catheterize themselves. The physical handicaps and the associated physiological problems stress social situations where groups must adapt to the needs of spina bifida children. Social circumstances can be made more favorable if these children are integrated into regular classes in the early grades, and social integration strategies are employed (see Chapter 9).

OSTEOGENESIS IMPERFECTA (BRITTLE BONE DISEASE)

Osteogenesis imperfecta is a condition marked by both weak bones and elasticity of the joints, ligaments, and skin. It is apparently inherited, although at times it seems to be caused by spontaneous changes in the genes (mutation).

Classification

There are two main types of osteogenesis imperfecta. One is evident at birth (congenital) and the other occurs after birth. Children with the congenital type are born with short, deformed limbs, numerous broken bones and a soft skull, which if they live, tends to grow in a triangular shape, broad at the forehead and narrow at the chin. Many babies with this condition die at birth, however.

Physical Characteristics

The bones of children with this defect are in many ways like those of the developing fetus, and the immaturity is caused by reduction in bone salts (calcium and phosphorus) rather than any defect in the calcification mechanism. The underlying layer of the eyeball (choroid) shows through as a blue discoloration.

As growth occurs in individuals with either type of the disease, the limbs tend to become bowed. The bones are not dense, and the spine is rounded backward and often evidences scoliosis. The teeth are in poor condition, easily broken, discolored, and prone to cavities. The joints are excessively mobile, and the positions that the children may take show great flexibility.

Medical Treatment

No known chemical or nutrient has been shown to correct osteogenesis imperfecta, and the most

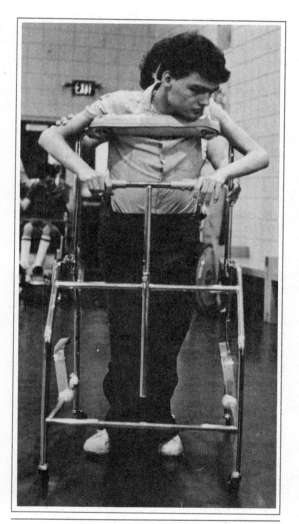

FIGURE 13-13
Children with spina bifida often lack independent mobility and require physical and social assistance from others. *(Courtesy Verland Foundation, Inc.)*

satisfactory treatment is the surgical insertion of a steel rod between the ends of the long bones. This treatment, plus bracing, permits some youths to walk.

Aids

Many persons with brittle bone disease need a wheelchair at least part of the time, and those with severe cases require a wheelchair exclusively.

Contraindications

Some authorities have suggested that physical activities are to be ruled out for this population, while others suggest that persons who have undergone surgical insertion of the steel rod may participate in specialized programs of aquatics and activities taking place in special facilities. The condition of children who have undergone operation tends to stabilize as the children grow older; they incur fewer fractures, and they may attend a regular school.

Mild activity, or even attempts to stand or walk, can cause fractures throughout the bony framework. Many children with osteogenesis imperfecta are unable to walk. Pillows are kept around both sides of the bed as well as at the head and feet. Heavy books and toys are not allowed.

Adapted Activity

Adapted physical education teachers should be sensitive to the presence of older children with this condition in their classes and to the presence of other children whose bones may be highly susceptible to injury, trauma, or breakage because of this and related conditions. The child who approaches normalcy in other areas continues to require a highly adapted physical education program that is limited to range of motion exercises. Although the diagnosis of osteogenesis imperfecta is assigned only to severe cases, many children seem to have a propensity for broken bones. Physical educators should take softness of bones into consideration when developing the physical education prescriptions for children.

ARTHROGRYPOSIS (CURVED JOINTS)

Arthrogryposis is a condition of flexure or contracture of joints (joints of the lower limbs more often than joints of the upper limbs). When several limbs are in contracture, the condition is referred to as multiple congenital contracture. Sherrill[6] reports that each year approximately 500 children are born in the United States with arthrogryposis. The cause is unknown, and the contractures may be observed relatively early in fetal life because of either a primary muscle disease or a spinal cord disease of cells controlling muscle contraction.

Physical Conditions

The limbs may be fixed in any position. However, the usual forms are with the shoulders turned in, elbows straightened and extended, forearms turned with the palm outward (pronated), and wrists flexed and deviated upward with the fingers curled into the palms. The hips may be bent in a flexed position and turned outward (externally rotated), and the feet are usually turned inward and downward. The spine often evidences scoliosis, and the limbs are small in circumference, and the joints appear large and have lost their range of motion.

Several physical conditions are associated with arthrogryposis, including congenital heart disease, urinary tract abnormalities, respiratory problems, abdominal hernias, and facial abnormalities. Children with arthrogryposis may walk independently but with an abnormal gait, or they may depend on a wheelchair.

Prognosis

The literature states that articular surfaces do deteriorate with age. Therefore, developmental exercises may assist in amelioration of deficient motor ability.

Medical Treatment

Surgery is often used to correct hip conditions as well as knee and foot deformities and is sometimes used to permit limited flexion of the elbow joint as well as greater wrist mobility.

Physical Education Program

The awkwardness of joint positions and mechanics causes no pain, and therefore children with arthrogryposis are free to engage in most types of activity.[6]

MULTIPLE SCLEROSIS

Multiple sclerosis is a chronic and degenerative neurological disease primarily affecting older adolescents and adults. It is a slowly progressive disease of the central nervous system leading to the disintegration of the myelin coverings of nerve fibers, which results in hardening or scarring of the tissue that replaces the disintegrated protective myelin sheath.[3] The cause of multiple sclerosis and other related diseases, such as amyotrophic lateral sclerosis (Lou Gehrig disease), is not known.

Physical Symptoms

The symptoms of multiple sclerosis include sensory problems, tremors, muscle weakness, spasticity, speech difficulties, dizziness, mild emotional disturbances, partial paralysis, and motor difficulties.

Prognosis

Multiple sclerosis generally appears when the person is between the ages of 20 and 40 years and results in incapacitation and eventual death.

Therapeutic Treatment

There is no treatment that can repair the damage to the nervous system caused by degeneration. However, each person should be evaluated individually and therapeutic programs of resistive exercise administered to maintain maximal functioning. The goal of these programs is to maintain functional skills, strength of muscles, and range of motion. Inactivity may contribute to the progressive weakening of the muscles needed for daily activity. Braces may be introduced at the later stages of the disorder to assist with locomotion.

OSTEOMYELITIS

Osteomyelitis is an inflammation of a bone and its medullary (marrow) cavity. This condition is occasionally referred to as *myelitis*. It is caused by *Staphylococcus, Streptococcus,* or *Pneumococcus* organisms.

Classification

In its early stages osteomyelitis is described as acute. If the infection persists or recurs periodically, it is called chronic. Since chronic osteomyelitis may linger on for years, the physical educator should confer with the physician about the nature of an adapted program.

Physical Description

The bones most often affected are the tibia, femur, and humerus. Pain and tenderness are present, and heat is felt through the overlying skin. Soft tissues feel hard, and neighboring joints may be distended with clear fluid.[6] There are limited effects on range of joint movement. The child may limp because of the acute pain.

Contraindications

Exercise is always contraindicated when infection is active in the body.

Medical Treatment

If medical treatment is delayed, abscesses work outward, causing a sinus (hole) in the skin over the affected bone from which pus is discharged. This sinus is covered with a dressing that must be changed several times daily. The medical treatment is rest and intensive antibiotic therapy. Through surgery, the infected bone may be scraped to evacuate the pus.

Adapted Sports Activity

Rehabilitation activity can restore motor functions so that normal activity can be resumed. However, under certain conditions the child with osteomyelitis can participate in most developmental and recreational activities that allow the affected limb to be mobilized.[5]

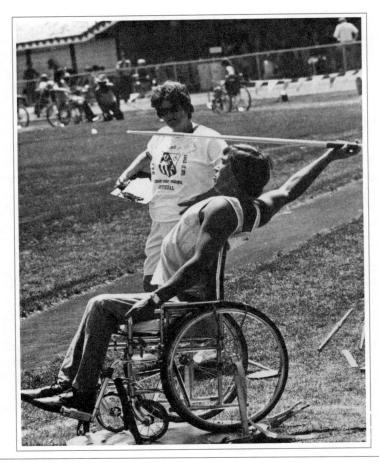

FIGURE 13-14
Adapted sports and activities in track and field can accommodate persons with physical handicaps.
(Photo by Curt Beamer; courtesy Paralyzed Veterans of America: Sports 'n Spokes Magazine.)

POLIOMYELITIS

Poliomyelitis is a disease that causes damage to the central nervous system. An inflammation affects the motor cells in the spinal cord, which in turn affects the muscles. Polio is caused by a filterable virus that attacks the anterior horn of the spinal cord.

Classification

There are three prevalent classifications of poliomyelitis—abortive, nonparalytic, and paralytic.

The symptoms of abortive poliomyelitis are headache, fever, and nausea.

Nonparalytic poliomyelitis involves the central nervous system but does not damage the motor cells permanently. In addition to the symptoms of abortive poliomyelitis, the victim might experience general and specific pain and acute contractions of one or more muscle groups located in the upper and lower extremities, neck, and back.

Paralytic poliomyelitis includes three afflictions: spinal poliomyelitis, which involves upper limbs, lower limbs, respiratory muscles, and trunk muscles; bulbar poliomyelitis, which affects the muscles of the respiratory center; and, spinal-bulbar poliomyelitis, which involves a combination of voluntary and involuntary muscles (the most serious of the three paralytic forms).

Prognosis

Sherrill[6] reports that approximately 6% of the persons who contract polio die, 14% have severe paralysis, 30% suffer mild aftereffects, and 50% recover completely.

Medical Treatment

Tendon transplants and arthrodesis are commonly performed during the chronic stage.

Therapeutic Treatment

Exercise programs should focus on motor tasks that develop strength, endurance, flexibility, and coordination.

Adapted Sports Activities

Orthopedic deformities do not totally restrict movement. Children learn quickly to compensate for the inconvenience of an impaired foot or arm. At the elementary school level, many children with polio can achieve considerable athletic success. However, as they progress through school life, accumulated developmental lags as a rule influence skill development enough so that successful participation in competitive sports cannot be achieved. Wheelchair sports are popular for polio victims who cannot walk.

RICKETS

Rickets is characterized by an abnormal bowing of the longer bones of the body. The condition may be caused by nutritional problems, inborn metabolic anomalies, or congenital kidney impairment. By far, the latter two causes of rickets are the most prevalent in the United States.

Medical Treatment

The medical treatment for rickets involves a diet containing supplementary vitamin D.

Contraindications

Strenuous weight-bearing activity may be contraindicated in some instances.

Therapeutic Treatment

Children with bowed limbs can be aided by developmental exercises rather than strenuous weight-bearing activity.

DWARFISM

Dwarfism is retarded physical growth that is more than three standard deviations from the mean for the age. The two main causes of growth retardation in children are heredity and endocrine disturbances. Steindler[7] reports more than 100 syndromes characterized by either abnormal shortness or dwarfism, many of which are congenital.

Physical Activity

Dwarfs can participate in physical activities to the same extent as normal persons with only occasional problems because of disproportionately short limbs. Size is the only restriction.

SPINAL CORD INJURIES

Spinal cord injuries usually result in paralysis or partial paralysis of the arms, trunk, legs, or any particular combination thereof depending on the locus of the damage. The spinal cord is housed in the spinal or vertebral column. Nerves from the spinal cord pass down into the segments of the spinal column. Injury to the spinal cord affects innervation of muscle. The higher up the vertebral column the level of injury, the greater the restriction of body movement. Persons with spinal cord injuries are usually referred to as *paraplegics* or *quadriplegics*. A paraplegic is one who has the legs paralyzed. The quadriplegic has both the arms and legs affected.

Classification

Spinal cord injuries are classified according to the region of the vertebrae affected. The regions

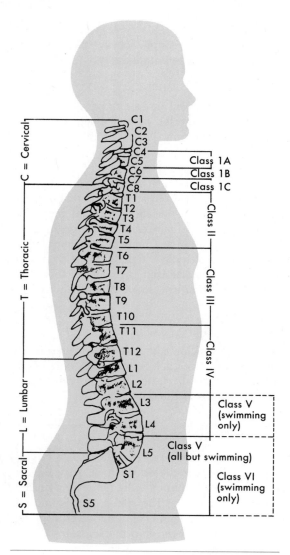

FIGURE 13-15
Classification for wheelchair sports.
(Redrawn from Sherrill, C.: Adapted physical education and recreation, ed. 3, Dubuque, Iowa; Copyright 1985, William C. Brown Publishers.)

affected are cervical, thoracic, lumbar, and sacral regions. A description of the movement capability at each level of the lesion appears below.

- ♦ *Fourth cervical level:* Use of only the neck muscles and the diaphragm.

- ♦ *Fifth cervical level:* Use of deltoid muscles of the shoulder and biceps muscles of the arm. Can perform activities with the arm. It is difficult to engage in manipulative tasks.
- ♦ *Sixth cervical level:* Gains the use of the wrist extensors. Can push a wheelchair.
- ♦ *Seventh cervical level:* Gains extension of the elbow and flexion and extension of the fingers.
- ♦ *Upper thoracic level:* Gains total movement capability in the arms but none in the legs.
- ♦ *Lower thoracic level:* Gains control of the abdominal muscles that right the trunk as well as the muscles that control the upper back.
- ♦ *Lumbar levels:* Gains control of the hip joint. May have fairly good walking ability.
- ♦ *Sacral levels:* Gains control of the bowels and bladder.

Physical Characteristics

The physical characteristics of a specific person with a spinal cord injury are related to the level of the lesion. However, collectively, the physical characteristics are as follows:

1. Inappropriate control of the bladder and digestive organs
2. Contractures (abnormal shortening of muscles)
3. Heterotopic bone formation, or laying down of new bone in soft tissue around joints (during this process the area may become inflamed and swollen)
4. Urinary infections
5. Difficulty in defecation
6. Decubitus ulcers on the back and buttocks (caused by pressure of the body weight on specific areas)
7. Spasms of the muscles
8. Spasticity of muscles that prevent effective movement
9. Overweight because of low energy expenditures

Therapeutic Treatment

Therapeutic treatment should be based on a well-rounded program of exercises for all the usable body parts, including activities to develop strength, flexibility, muscular endurance, cardiovascular endurance, and coordination. Cardiovascular development may be attained through arm pedaling of a bicycle ergometer, pushing of a wheelchair over considerable distances, and agility maneuvers with the wheelchair. Paraplegics can perform a considerable number of physical activities.

Adapted Sports Activity

Paraplegics can perform most physical education activities from a wheelchair. For younger children, fundamental motor skills such as throwing, hitting, and catching are appropriate. Once these skills are mastered, games that incorporate these skills may be played. Modifications of games that have been previously described are appropriate for children in wheelchairs. Children in wheelchairs can participate in parachute games and target games without accommodation. They can maintain fitness of the upper body through the same type of regimens as do the nonhandicapped. Strengthening of the arms and shoulder girdle is important for propulsion of the wheelchair and for changing body positions when moving in and out of the wheelchair. Swimming is a particularly good activity for the development of total physical fitness.

Several organizations promote competition for persons in wheelchairs. These events include archery, bowling, basketball, table tennis, racing in wheelchairs, and track events. A classification system based on the levels of injury has been developed for equitable competition. The classification system is indicated in Fig. 13-15.

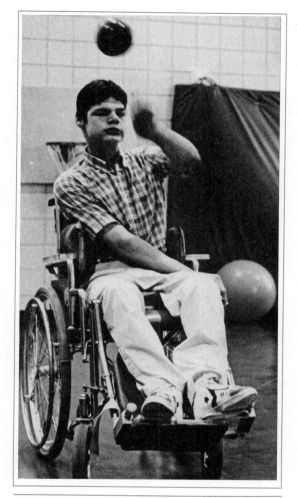

FIGURE 13-16
Knowledge of measured performance of throwing a ball from a wheelchair enables placement in groups for equitable competition.
(Courtesy Verland Foundation, Inc.)

SPONDYLOLYSIS AND SPONDYLOLISTHESIS

Spondylolysis and spondylolisthesis result from a congenital malformation of one or both of the neural arches of the fifth lumbar vertebra or, less frequently, the fourth lumbar vertebra. Spondylolisthesis is distinguished from spondylolysis by anterior displacement of the fifth lumbar vertebra on the sacrum. Spondylolysis may be accompanied by pain in the lower back.

Forward displacement may occur as a result of sudden trauma to the lumbar region. The vertebrae are moved anteriorly because there is an absence of bony continuity of the neural arch and the main support is derived from its ligamentous arrangement. In such cases, individuals often appear to have a severe lordosis.

Characteristics

Many individuals have spondylolysis, or even spondylolisthesis, without symptoms of any kind, but a mild twist or blow may set off a whole series of low back complaints and localized discomfort of pain radiating down one or both sides.

Medical Treatment

The pathological condition may eventually become so extensive that surgical intervention will be required.

Therapeutic Treatment

Proper therapy may involve a graduated exercise program that may help prevent further aggravation and, in some cases, remove many symptoms characteristic of the condition. A program should be initiated similar to that of ameliorating the postural malalignment of lordosis (with primary concentration on the strengthening of abdominal muscles, the lengthening of low back muscles, and the segmental realignment of legs, pelvis, and spine).

Contraindications

Games and sports that overextend, fatigue, or severely twist and bend the low back should be avoided. In most cases the physician will advise against contact sports and heavy weight lifting.

AMPUTATIONS

Amputation is the loss of part or all of a limb (Fig. 13-17). Amputation may be performed to arrest a malignant condition caused by trauma, tumors, infection, vascular impairment, diabetes, or arteriosclerosis. There are more than 300,000 amputees in the United States.

Classification

Amputations can be classified into two categories—acquired amputation and congenital amputation. The amputation is acquired if one has a limb removed by operation and congenital if the child is born without a limb.

Congenital amputations are classified according to the site and level of limb absence. When an amputation is performed through a joint, it is referred to as a disarticulation.

Medical Treatment

Medical treatment involves the design of a prosthetic appliance. The purpose of the prosthetic device is to enable the individual to function as normally as possible. The application of a prosthetic device may be preceded by surgery to produce a stump. After the operation the stump is dressed and bandaged to aid shrinkage of the

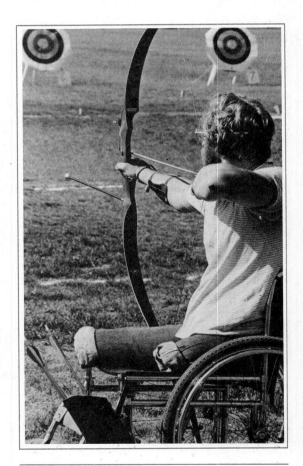

FIGURE 13-17
A person with amputated legs participates in archery.
(Photo by Curt Beamer; courtesy Paralyzed Veterans of America: Sports 'n Spokes Magazine.)

stump. Following the fitting of the prosthesis, the stump must be continually cared for. It should be checked periodically and cleaned to prevent infection, abrasion, and skin disorder.

The attachment of a false limb early in a child's development will encourage the incorporation of the appendage into natural body activity more than if the prosthesis is introduced later in life.

Prosthesis Training

Amputees must develop skill to use prostheses; effective use demands much effort. Training should be directed toward daily living skills such as eating, drinking, and dressing and recreational skills that can be taught in physical education. Prostheses often result in problems of ambulation. These problems vary with the specific level of amputation.

Gait Training

Most gait deviations result from problems with the alignment of the prosthesis. Deviations may include rotations of the foot at heel strike, unequal timing, side walking base, abducted gait, excessive heel ride, instability of the knee, excessive knee flexion, hyperextension of the knees, excessive pronation of the foot, foot slap, and rotation of the foot with continuing whip.[1]

Persons with amputations below the knee can learn ambulation skills well with a prosthesis and training. Persons with amputation above the knee but below the hip may have difficulty in developing efficient walking gaits. Amputations at this level require alteration of the gait pattern. Steps are usually shortened to circumvent lack of knee function.

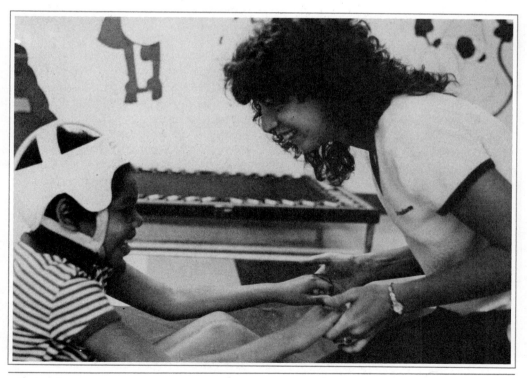

FIGURE 13-18
A child receives a physical prompt in the performance of a sit-up.
(Courtesy Children's Rehabilitation Center, Butler, Pa.)

Aids

Aids may be designed to assist prostheses of the legs or the arms. Assistive devices may be used to aid locomotion when the legs are debilitated. Some assistive devices are canes and crutches. A major problem for students who use canes and crutches is the need to learn balance to free one hand for participation in activity. Use of the Lofstrand crutches, which are anchored to the forearms, enables balance to be maintained by one crutch. This frees one arm and enables participation in throwing and striking activities.

Although it is difficult to substitute for the human hand and fingers, it is possible to achieve dexterity with the use of a utility arm and split hook. These aids enable the use of racquets for paddle games if both arms are amputated. Persons who have lost a single arm can play most basic skill games and participate in more advanced sports activity without modifications. Special devices can be built by an orthotist to fit into the arm prosthesis to hold sports equipment such as gloves.

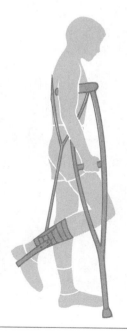

FIGURE 13-19
Sling and crutch for hip conditions.

Therapeutic Treatment

Amputees are often exposed to beneficial exercise through the use of the prosthesis. Exercises should be initiated to strengthen muscles after a stump heals. Training also enhances ambulation, inhibits atrophy and contractures, improves or maintains mechanical alignment of body parts, and develops general physical fitness.

Adapted Sports Activity

Authorities agree that children with properly fitted prostheses should engage in regular physical education activities. Amputees have considerable potential for participation in adapted sports and games. There are opportunities for persons with prostheses to participate in official sports competition. Persons with above-knee amputations can walk well and engage in swimming, skiing, and other activities with the proper aids. Arm amputees who have use of their feet can participate in activities that require foot action such as soccer and running events as well as other activities that involve exclusively the feet.

There are several adaptations of physical activity that can be made for children with impaired ambulation. For these children the major disadvantages are speed of locomotion and fatigue to sustained activity. Some accommodations that can be made are shortening the distance the player must travel and decreasing the speed needed to move from one place to another.

BRACES AND WHEELCHAIRS

Many physically handicapped children who participate in physical education programs use a wheelchair for locomotion or wear braces, and some children require both devices. The physical educator should have a working knowledge of the care and maintenence of lower extremity braces and wheelchairs. One of the teacher's responsibilities is daily observation of the student's use and care of ambulation equipment. In conjunction with related services, the child's classroom teacher, family, and physical educator should develop a program to maximize the use of ambulation devices in the physical education setting and beyond the school boundaries. In addition, any problems that arise with the ambulation devices should be communicated to the special or regular class teacher or the parents.

Leg Braces

Leg braces are metal or plastic support frames that are strapped to the body above and below specific joints to assist with ambulation. The main purposes of lower extremity braces are to support the weight for ambulation, to control involuntary movements, and to prevent or correct deformities.

In general, there are three classifications of lower leg braces—short leg braces, long leg braces, and hip braces.

Short Leg Brace

A short leg brace is appropriate when the disabling condition occurs at the ankle joint. Although there are several different types of short leg braces, the simplest form consists of a single metal upright bar attached to the shoe with a cuff around the calf of the leg. When more stability is needed, double upright bars are used. The design of this type of brace should facilitate the control of four movements of the ankle joint. Leather straps attached to the metal uprights and strapped around the ankle assist with control of the ankle joint. (See Fig. 13-20.)

Long Leg Brace

The long leg (knee-ankle-foot) brace assists with control of the ankle and knee joint. The fundamental purpose of the long leg brace is to prevent hyperextension of the knee caused by weak extensor muscles. The brace must be in different positions when the student is sitting as compared to standing. To accommodate the different positions of the knee, various types of locks are placed at the knee joints, the most common of which is a sliding metal lock that is easily locked and unlocked by hand. The knee joint of the long leg brace is locked when the individual is sitting in a chair. Locking devices may also be used to control the ankle when this type of brace is used. (See Fig. 13-21.)

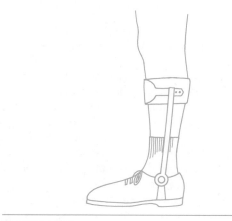

FIGURE 13-20
A short leg brace.

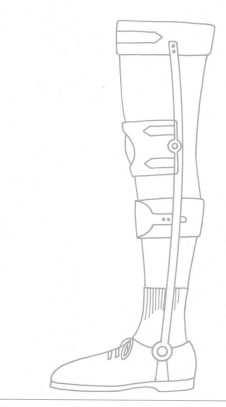

FIGURE 13-21
A long leg brace.

Long Leg Brace with Pelvic Band

The long leg brace may extend from below the ankle to above the hip. Such a brace is called a hip-knee-ankle-foot long leg brace. The purpose of such a brace is to control movements of the hip joint as well as the knee and the ankle. To assist with the control of the hip joint, a pelvic band is attached to the top of the upright bar.

The physical education teacher should have a working knowledge of the functions of leg braces. Some of the characteristics that can be observed are as follows: (1) brace joints work easily, (2) brace and anatomical joints coincide, (3) upright conforms to the leg, (4) brace is of correct length, and (5) upright coincides with the midline of the leg. A more detailed view of characteristics of leg braces is on p. 285.

Wheelchairs

The purpose of wheelchairs is to provide a means of locomotion for persons who lack strength, endurance, or flexibility of muscles prerequisite for ambulation. Persons who can walk but cannot rise from a seated position to a standing position or those who need to transport objects but cannot do so may also need a wheelchair.

There are several types of wheelchairs. However, the most common are made of metal and have four wheels. The two back wheels are large, and the two front wheels are small and mounted on casters that pivot freely. Two or more separate rims that can be grasped to propel the chair are mounted to the back wheels.

Wheelchair design is a continuous process, the goal of which is to make the wheelchair more functional. Many special features can be added to make a wheelchair more functional or comfortable, including armrests, footrests, legrests, and headrests, all of which can be removed. Leg spreaders have also been incorporated into some wheelchairs to prevent the scissoring of legs. Many wheelchairs can be folded for easy storage. There are now motorized wheelchairs to accommodate persons who have severe afflictions of the upper extremities. Some other features of wheelchairs are unique folding mechanisms that allow

it to double as a stroller or car seat, adjustable Velcro fasteners, pads, and attachable trays. The boxed material on pp. 287-289 contains a checklist that will enable physical education teachers to assess wheelchairs and braces as they relate to optimal functioning and comfort of the individual.[9]

Adapted Sports Activity

Physically handicapped persons should develop skills that can be expressed in recreational activity in the community. One of the desired outcomes of the acquisition of sport skills is participation in competitive sports. Therefore, the instruction in the physical education program should match opportunities for sport participation in the community. The generalization of the sport skills acquired by the physically handicapped in the instructional phase of the physical education program requires close study of several

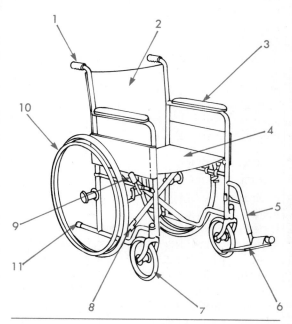

FIGURE 13-22

Parts of a wheelchair. *1*, Handgrips/push handles; *2*, back upholstery; *3*, armrests; *4*, seat upholstery; *5*, front rigging; *6*, footplate; *7*, casters; *8*, crossbraces; *9*, wheel locks; *10*, wheel and handrim; *11*, tipping lever.

CHECKLIST FOR BRACES AND WHEELCHAIRS

SHORT LEG (ANKLE-FOOT) BRACE

A. With the brace off the student
   1. Do joints work easily?
   2. Can shoes be easily removed?
   3. Is the workmanship good?
      a. No rough edges
      b. Straps secure
      c. Leather work stitched properly
B. Student standing with brace on
   1. Are the sole and heel flat on the floor?
   2. Are the ankle joints aligned so that they coincide with the anatomical joints?
   3. Is there ample clearance between the leg and the brace (one finger width)?
   4. Does the T strap exert enough force for correction without causing deformity?
   5. Do the uprights conform to the contour of the leg?
   6. Do the uprights coincide with the midline of the leg when viewed from the side?
   7. Is the brace long enough?
      a. It should be below the bend of the knee so the student can bend the knee comfortably to 120°.
      b. It should not be lower than the bulky part of the calf muscle.
C. Student walking with brace on
   1. Is there clearance between the uprights and the leg?
   2. Are there any gait deviations?
   3. Is the brace quiet?

LONG LEG (KNEE-ANKLE-FOOT) BRACE

A. With the brace off the student
   1. Do joints work easily?
   2. Can shoes be easily removed?
   3. Is the workmanship good?
      a. No rough edges
      b. Straps secure
      c. Leather work stitched properly
B. Student standing with brace on
   1. Are the knee joints aligned at the approximate anatomical joints?

   a. There should be no pressure from the thigh band when knee is bent (if so joints are too high).
   b. There should be no pressure from calf band when knee is bent (if so joints are too low).
   c. There should be no pressure on calf (if so joints are too far forward).
   d. There should be no pressure on shin or knee cap (if so joints are too far backward).
   2. Are locks secure and easy to work?
   3. Is the brace long enough?
      a. Medial upright should be up into groin region but should not cause pain.
      b. Lateral upright should be 1 inch longer.
   4. Are the thigh bands and calf bands about equal distance from the knee?

LONG LEG BRACE WITH PELVIC BAND (HIP-KNEE-ANKLE-FOOT ORTHOSIS)

A. With the brace off the student
   1. Do joints work easily?
   2. Can shoes be easily removed?
   3. Is the workmanship good?
      a. No rough edges
      b. Straps secure
      c. Leather work stitched properly?
B. Student with brace on
   1. Is the pelvic band located below the waist?
   2. Is the student comfortable sitting and standing?
   3. Are the hip joints in the right place and do the locks work easily?

OTHER POINTS TO CHECK

A. Do the shoes fit and are they in good repair?
B. Do reddened areas go away after the brace has been off 20 minutes?
C. Is the student comfortable?
D. Is the brace helping the student?

From Venn, J., Morganstern, C., and Dykes, M.K.: Teach. Except. Child., Winter 1979, pp. 51-56. Copyright 1979 by The Council for Exceptional Children. Reprinted with permission.

Continued.

CHECKLIST FOR BRACES AND WHEELCHAIRS—cont'd

PLASTIC BRACES

A. Does the brace conform to and contact the extremity?
B. Is the student wearing a sock between foot and brace?
C. Does the brace pull away from the leg excessively when the student walks?
D. Do reddened areas go away after the brace has been off 20 minutes?

LOWER EXTREMITY PROSTHETICS

A. Is the student wearing prosthesis (frequency)?
B. Does the student use assistive devices with prosthesis (crutches, canes, one cane, other)? If so, what does he or she use and how often?
C. Is the prosthesis on correctly?
   1. Is the toe turned out about the same as the other foot?
   2. When the student sits is the knee in alignment?
D. Does the leg appear the same length as the normal leg?
   1. Does the student stand straight when bearing weight on the prothesis?
   2. Are the shoulders even when leg is bearing weight (one shoulder does not drop)?
   3. When the student walks does the knee stay straight without turning out or in?

GAIT DEVIATIONS

A. Does the student stand straight when bearing weight on the prosthesis?
B. Does the artificial leg swing forward without turning in or out?
C. Does the student swing the artificial leg through without rising up on the foot of the normal leg?
D. When the student walks does the leg swing straight forward? (It should not swing out in an arc.)
E. When the student stands are the feet a normal distance apart? (The stance should not be too wide.)
F. Does the knee bend and straighten like a normal leg?

CONDITION OF THE PROSTHESIS

A. Do the suspension joints appear to be in good condition (leather, joint, band)?
B. Does the leg stay in place when the student is standing and sitting?
C. Does the knee bend appropriately?
D. Are the joints quiet when moved?
E. Do the foot and ankle appear to be in one piece?
F. Is the shoe in good condition (heel, sole)?

WHEELCHAIR

A. Arms
   1. Are the armrests and side panels secure and free of sharp edges and cracks?
   2. Do the arm locks function properly?
B. Back
   1. Is the upholstery free of rips and tears?
   2. Is the back taut from top to bottom?
   3. Is the safety belt attached tightly and not frayed?
C. Seat and frame
   1. Is the upholstery free of rips and tears?
   2. Does the chair fold easily without sticking?
   3. When the chair is folded fully are the front post slides straight and round?
D. Wheel locks
   1. Do the wheel locks securely engage the tire surfaces and prevent the wheel from turning?
E. Large wheels
   1. Are the wheels free from wobble or side-play when spun?
   2. Are the spokes equally tight and without any missing spikes?
   3. Are the tires free from excessive wear and gaps at the joined section?
F. Casters
   1. Is the stem firmly attached to the fork?
   2. Are the forks straight on sides and stem so that the caster swivels easily?
   3. Is the caster assembly free of excessive play both upward and downward as well as backward and forward?
   4. Are the wheels free of excessive play and wobble?
   5. Are the tires in good condition?

CHECKLIST FOR BRACES AND WHEELCHAIRS—cont'd

G. Footrest/legrest
  1. Does the lock mechanism fit securely?
  2. Are the heel loops secure and correctly installed?
  3. Do the foot plates fold easily and hold in any position?
  4. Are the legrest panels free of cracks and sharp edges?

WITH STUDENT SITTING IN WHEELCHAIR

A. Seat width
  1. When your palms are placed between the patient's hip and the side of the chair (skirtguard), do the hands contact the hip and the skirtguard at the same time without pressure?
  2. Or, is the clearance between the patient's widest point of either hips or thigh and the skirtguard approximately 1 inch on either side?
B. Seat depth
  1. Can you place your hand, with fingers extended, between the front edge of the seat upholstery and to the rear of the knee with a clearance of three or four fingers?
  2. Or, is the seat upholstery approximately 2 to 3 inches less than the student's thigh measurement?

C. Seat height and footrest
  1. Is the lowest part of the stepplates no closer than 2 inches from the floor?
  2. Or, is the student's thigh elevated slightly above the front edge of the seat upholstery?
D. Arm height
  1. Does the arm height not force the shoulders up or allow them to drop significantly when the student is in a normal sitting position?
  2. Is the elbow positioned slightly forward of the trunk midline when the student is in a normal sitting position?
E. Back height
  1. Can you insert four or five fingers between the patient's armpit area and the top of the back upholstery touching both at the same time?
  2. Is the top of the back upholstery approximately 4 inches below the armpit for the student who needs only minimum trunk support?

WITH STUDENT PUSHING OR RIDING IN WHEELCHAIR

A. Is the wheelchair free from squeaks or rattles?
B. Does the chair roll easily without pulling to either side?
C. Are the large wheels and casters free of play and wobble?

---

variables. Some considerations might be the nature of the specific disability, the equipment required for participation (wheelchairs and ancillary equipment), and ways of structuring competition to maximize fulfillment for the individual.

Opportunities for Participation

Physically handicapped persons need opportunities to express attained sport skills in competition. Many public schools have limited numbers of physically handicapped persons of similar ages and ability. This makes organized competition difficult. Therefore, cooperative efforts need to be made among schools to provide opportunities for competition among the athletes. Special Olympics, in some states, provides this opportunity. Wheelchair sports events are staged for competition. Several colleges and universities have intercollegiate wheelchair sports programs. The University of Illinois has developed one of the best intercollegiate wheelchair sports programs. Several other universities also have well-developed intercollegiate athletic programs.

There are two national organizations for wheel-

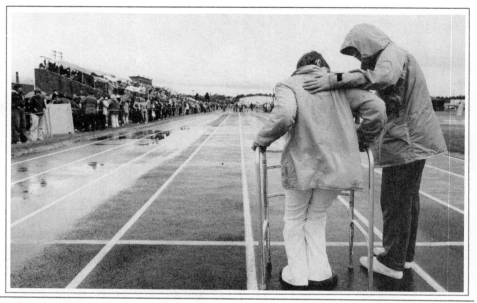

FIGURE 13-23
The physically handicapped can learn to use walkers over considerable distances and thereby engage in competition.
(Courtesy H. Armstrong Roberts.)

chair sports—the National Wheelchair Athletic Association and the National Wheelchair Basketball Association (see Appendix). The mission of both of these organizations is to promote competition in which persons confined to wheelchairs may participate. These organizations provide a forum and incentive to maximize proficiency in sports for competition. Higher forms of competition may be expressed at the International Sports Organization for the Disabled. Thus opportunities exist for many physically disabled individuals to participate in competitive sports at their ability level with incentive to increase skills to a world class level.

Nature and Scope of Program

Wheelchair sports are designed to accommodate persons with significant, permanent physical disability of the lower extremities that prevents full participation with able-bodied peers. Persons who may be included in this group are those with cerebral palsy, muscular dystrophy, or spinal

cord injuries. Many of these persons may not use wheelchairs but qualify for competition because of inability to engage in full participation with able-bodied peers.

The sports activity program involves sports that do not require use of the legs and can be performed from the wheelchair. Some of the sports activities of the National Wheelchair Athletic Association are target archery, table tennis, swimming, weight lifting, and selected field events. Other activities for which adaptation can be made are fencing, bowling, badminton, volleyball, floor hockey, and miniature golf.

Differences in Abilities

Official wheelchair sports competition is based on a medical classification system. The purpose of the classification system is to allow for fair competition. Tests are administered to determine the level of muscular function. Such tests do not take into account the proficiency of the athletes in competition. Clearly, children in wheelchairs

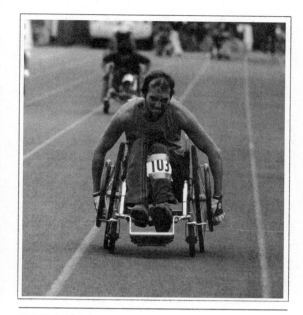

FIGURE 13-24
Gloves are desirable equipment for competition in
wheelchair racing events.
(Courtesy H. Armstrong Roberts.)

do not have equal abilities. Therefore, to provide
equitable competition in school-based wheelchair activities it may be necessary to test skill
performances and group the participants according to ability in the individual sports.

Amputees are considered to possess a lesser
handicap when compared with other athletes
confined to wheelchairs. In some instances they
play sports such as volleyball standing up.[11] In
efforts to equate competition they are classified
according to the number of amputations and the
location and the length of the stumps. Amputations may occur on one or both sides of the body,
above or below the knees.

Another group of persons in wheelchairs have
severe impairment of the upper appendages. They
may have spasticity or contractures. It is not uncommon for these children to adopt unique
throwing patterns to maximize performance.
Their physical structure rules out the teaching of
mechanically sound sport skill patterns. Specific
techniques must be determined for each child.

Adaptation of Equipment

The physical limitations of orthopedically handicapped children are related to opportunity for
participation in games. It may be necessary to
adapt equipment to include children in sports activity. For instance, there are several commer-
cially available pieces of equipment that enable
handicapped persons to participate in bowling.
Some of the adaptations are a bowling bowl with
handles, a ramp that allows the handicapped
person to push the bowling ball as in shuffleboard, and a ramp that enables gravity to act on
the ball in place of the force provided by movement. Each of these adaptations in equipment
accommodates for a specific physical problem
related to bowling. The adapted equipment for
bowling is paired with the nature of the physical
problem.

Equipment	Accommodation of Disability
Handles	Needs assistance with the grip but has the use of the arm and wrist
Fork	Has the use of the arm but has limited ability to control the wrist and an underhand throwing pattern
Ramp	Has limited use of the arm, wrist, and fingers as they apply to an underhand movement pattern

Assessment of Skills Needed for Participation

Many children with severe physical handicaps
can engage in games and sports with few adaptations. Most can enjoy swimming activities. However, persons restricted to wheelchairs should be
appraised to determine their functional movement capability. Motor programs should then be
developed to meet their unique needs. The assessment should provide information about the
potential for movement of each action of the
body. This would involve knowledge of strength,
power, flexibility, and endurance of specific muscle groups. In addition, there should be information about which movement actions can be coordinated to attain specific motor outcomes. For
instance, several throwing patterns that children
with severe impairments use when participating

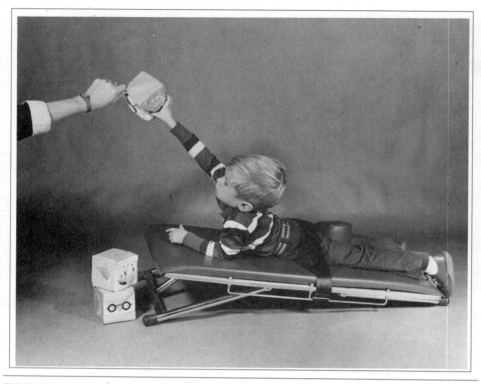

FIGURE 13-25

A bolster chair assists with the alignment of the legs and facilitates more efficient ambulation. *(Courtesy Achievement Products Incorporated.)*

in the Special Olympics can help circumvent movements problems of the arms and hands. The desired throwing pattern is one of extension of the arm and elbow and flexion of the wrist. If either of these actions is impaired, alternate throwing patterns need to be found. Some throwing patterns developed to circumvent extreme disability of arm, elbow, and wrist are underhand movement, horizontal abduction of the arm/shoulder, flexion of the arm and elbow (over the shoulder), horizontal abduction of the arm (side arm), and overhand movement with most of the force from a rocking motion of the trunk. To maximize the potential of each of these types of throwing patterns, it is necessary to conduct training programs that will consider each child's assets and develop them fully. However, another option is to provide therapeutic exercise for each of the desired actions and then teach it as a functional, normalized movement pattern.

The ability prerequisites of strength, flexibility, endurance, power, and coordination can be applied to many wheelchair activities. Some of these activities involve (1) transfer skills from and to the wheelchair, (2) performance on mats, (3) performance on gymnastics apparatus, (4) ability to maneuver vehicles, (5) motor capabilities in a swimming pool, (6) walking with aids, and (7) the ability to push and pull objects. The ability prerequisites for each fundamental movement pattern should be studied to identify specific problems so that appropriate intervention can be undertaken. Below are examples of each of the categories of activities or abilities.

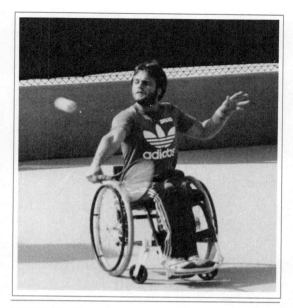

FIGURE 13-26
Tennis is a popular wheelchair activity.
(Photo by Wendy Parks; courtesy National Foundation of Wheelchair Tennis.)

1. Transfer skills
    a. Standing from a wheelchair
    b. Moving from a wheelchair to another chair
    c. Moving from a wheelchair to mats
    d. Moving from a wheelchair to different pieces of equipment
2. Performance on mats
    a. Forward and backward rolls
    b. Partner activity
    c. Climbing on low obstacles and elevated mats
3. Performance on gymnastics apparatus
    a. Rings
    b. High bar
    c. Parallel bars
4. Ability to maneuver vehicles
    a. Floor scooters
    b. Hand-propelled carts
    c. Tricycles
    d. Upright scooters with three wheels
5. Swimming pool activity
    a. Getting into and out of the pool
    b. Use of the railing for resting
    c. Swimming
6. Walking with aids
    a. Different types of canes
    b. Crutches
    c. Walkers
7. Ability to push and pull objects
    a. Throw a ball or push a ball
    b. Propel scooters with the hands
    c. Push a cage ball

Each of the above-mentioned behaviors should be analyzed to see if the student's strength, flexibility, endurance, power, and coordination are sufficient for acquisition and proficiency of these functional activities.

ADAPTING ACTIVITY FOR THE ORTHOPEDICALLY HANDICAPPED LEARNER

Many games and sports in which students regularly participate in physical education classes can, with minor modification, be made safe and interesting for orthopedically handicapped persons. In general, the rules, techniques, and equipment of a game or activity should be changed as little as possible when they are modified for handicapped students. Some of the ways that regular physical education and sports activities can be modified are the following:

1. The size of the playing area can be made smaller, with proportionate reduction of the amount of activity
2. Larger balls or larger pieces of equipment can be introduced to make the game easier or to slow down the tempo so physical accommodations can be made
3. Smaller, lighter balls or striking implements (plastic or Styrofoam balls and plastic bats) or objects that are easier to handle (a beanbag or Nerf ball) can be substituted
4. More players can be added to a team, which reduces the amount of activity and the responsibility of individuals

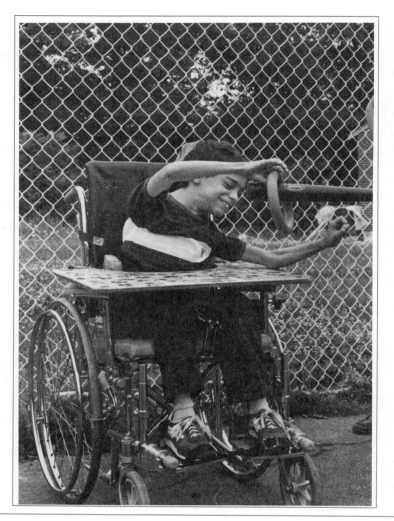

FIGURE 13-27
The distance the bat is from the performer controls the space the ring must travel for a successful trial.
(Courtesy Children's Rehabilitation Center, Butler, Pa.)

5. Minor rule changes can be made in the contest or game while as many of the basic rules as possible are retained
6. The amount of time allowed for play can be reduced via shorter quarters, or the total time for a game can be reduced to allow for the onset of fatigue
7. The number of points required to win a contest can be reduced
8. Free substitutions can be made, which allows the students alternately to participate and then rest while the contest continues

These modifications can be made in a game or contest whether the student participates in a handicapped-only class or regular physical education classes. If the handicapped child participates in a handicapped-only class, it is possible to provide activities similar to those of regular

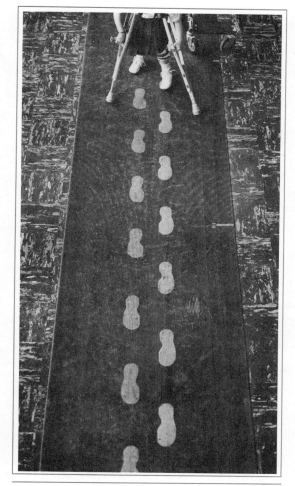

FIGURE 13-28
Footprints help a child to develop a rhythmical walking pattern.
(Courtesy H. Armstrong Roberts.)

ties can be designed to accommodate physical limitations (Table 13-1). Students with temporary injuries may become more skillful in various activities so that when they return to an unrestricted class they may participate in the whole game or sport with a reasonable degree of success.

Procedure for Adapting Sports and Games

Teachers who attempt to include handicapped children in games and sports in the regular physical education class must be able to apply principles of adapting the sports and games to each child. It is beyond the scope of this book to compile adaptations of games for a wide range of handicapping conditions for specific activities. Below is a suggested procedure for adapting a sport or game for a handicapped child:

1. Select and analyze the sport or game to be played
2. Identify the problems the individual child will have in participating in the sport or game
3. Make the adaptations to the sport or game
4. Select principles of adaptation that may apply to the specific situation

Adaptations for Children with Limited Movement

There are several options to accommodate individual problems for children with limited movement. First, games may be selected that circumvent the inability to move. This enables handicapped children to participate in a normal environment with their peers. However, it is obvious that such activity will comprise but a small part of the games and sports of the total physical education program. Second, in team sports it is not uncommon for specific positions of a sport to require different degrees of movement; thus children who have limited movement capability should assume positions that require less movement. Third, the rules of the game can be modified, enabling equitable competition between handicapped and the nonhandicapped persons. Fourth, aids can be introduced that accommodate inability so that adjustments can be made to the game. Any one or

physical education classes by practicing many of the culturally accepted sport skills in drill types of activities. An example would be playing such basketball games as "twenty-one" and "around the world" or taking free throws as lead-up activities to the sport. Pitching, batting, throwing, catching, and games such as "over the line" can be played as lead-up activities for softball. Serving, stroking, volleying, and the like can be practiced as lead-up activities for tennis. Such activi-

TABLE 13-1
Principles for adapting physical activity

Activity	Modification	Consequence
Reduce Size of Playing Area		
Soccer	Reduce size of field	Less distance to cover; ball moves from one end of field to other faster
Soccer	Reduce size of goal commensurate with student's movement ability	Less distance to cover
Badminton	Reduce size of court	Less distance to cover; accommodation can be made to equate movement capability of handicapped student with that of nonhandicapped student
Softball	Shorten distance between bases when handicapped person bats	Handicapped student has equitable amount of time to reach base
Introduce Larger Pieces of Equipment		
Softball	Use balloon or beach ball	Speed of the object and tempo of game are reduced
Softball	Use larger ball	Chance of success is enhanced and tempo of game is reduced
Soccer	Use larger ball	Area where ball can be propelled successfully is increased
Volleyball	Use beach ball	Area of contact is increased, enhancing success and requiring less finger strength to control ball
Introduce Lighter Equipment		
Softball	Use lighter bat	Bat can be moved more quickly so there is greater opportunity to strike ball
Soccer	Use lighter ball	Speed is reduced and successful contact is more likely
Bowling	Use lighter ball	Weaker persons have greater control of ball
Archery	Use lighter bow	Weaker person can draw bow
Tennis	Use aluminum racquet	Weaker person can control racquet
Modify Size of Team		
Volleyball	Add more players	Less area for each person to cover
Soccer	Add more players	Distance each person must cover in team play is reduced
Softball	Add more players	Less area for each person to cover
Handball/tennis	Play triples	Less area for each person to cover
Make Minor Rule Changes		
Wrestling	Use physical contact on takedown for blind persons	Blind person will always be in physical contact with opponent, enable him or her to know where opponent is at all times
Volleyball	Allow person with affliction in arms/hands to carry on a volleyball hit	Opportunity for success is greater
Soccer	Reduce size of goal	Opportunity for success is greater
Gymnastics	Strap legs of paraplegic together	Strap controls legs when body moves

TABLE 13-1
Principles for adapting physical activity—cont'd

Activity	Modification	Consequence
Reduce Playing Time		
Basketball/soccer	Substitute every 3 or 4 minutes	Accommodation is made for fatigue
Swimming	Swim beside pool edge and rest at prescribed distances of travel or time intervals	Accommodation is made for fatigue
Reduce Number of Points Required to Win Contest		
Handball/paddleball/tennis	Lessen number to fatigue level of individual	Physical endurance will not be factor in the outcome of game
Basketball	Play until specified number of points are made	

a combination of these principles of adaptation may be employed to enable handicapped children to participate in regular classes.

Computer-Controlled Movement of Paralyzed Muscles

In the past it was thought that paralyzed muscles could not contract to produce purposeful movement. The development of electrical stimulation procedures to muscles and computer technology have opened a new era for the prospect of functional movement for persons who are paralyzed.[4]

The application of robotic technology to prosthesis is not new; however, the application of computer technology to electrical stimulation of paralyzed muscles is currently being developed. The Research Institute for Biomedical Engineering at Wright State University is in the process of designing microprocessors to control the stimulation of paralyzed muscles. The research at the institute has followed a logical evolution to develop techniques that will make paralyzed muscle functional, thereby allowing paralyzed persons to achieve proficiency on motor skills needed for self-sufficient living. The steps that led to computer-controlled functional walking of paralyzed persons required the synthesis of several techniques. The basis of computer-controlled ambu-lation is artificial stimulation of muscle. Once this technique was established to contract muscle, the problem was one of controlling the stimulation so that functional movement of paralyzed muscles would occur. The application of computer technology to control muscle function has led to the possibility of useful movements to enhance self-sufficient living. Microprocessors are now being used to control stimulation of the muscles that are used for walking. Computers to control functional movement of paralyzed muscles are currently in the early stages of development.*

SUMMARY

There are many different types of orthopedically handicapping conditions. Afflictions can occur at more than 500 anatomical sites. Each orthopedically handicapped student has different physical and motor capabilities and is to be provided with special accommodations that enable participation in modified games and sports activity.

There are certain fundamental considerations that teachers must make to meet the unique phys-

---

*Further information on current research may be acquired from the Research Laboratory of Dr. J.F. Petrofsky at Wright State University in Dayton, Ohio.

ical education needs of the child. When developing programs for orthopedically handicapped persons, the teacher must avoid contraindicated activity, as identified by medical personnel.

Furthermore, physical educators must address two types of program considerations to meet the physical education needs of the orthopedically handicapped. One is to develop therapeutic programs that enhance sport skills, prerequisite motor patterns, and physical and motor fitness. The other is to structure the environment so that orthopedically handicapped children can derive physical benefits through expression of their skills in adapted sport activity (this may be facilitated by the use of aids for specific types of activities and handicaps).

The physical educator should be ready to accommodate the individual program needs of orthopedically handicapped persons by adapting activity and environments in integrated classes, handicapped-only classes, and special settings.

REVIEW QUESTIONS

1. What are some principles for adapting physical activity for the orthopedically handicapped?
2. Apply these principles for adapting physical activity for a specific handicap in a specific activity.
3. What are some motor and nonmotor characteristics of the cerebral palsied?
4. What are the clinical classifications of cerebral palsy?
5. List some types of physical activity that can be provided to remedy physical deficiencies of the orthopedically handicapped.
6. What are the physical characteristics of persons with muscular dystrophy?
7. Describe different types of muscular dystrophy.
8. What are the physical characteristics of arthritis, the prognosis for the disorder, and medical and therapeutic treatment?
9. What are the physical characteristics of developmental hip dislocations? Describe medical and therapeutic treatments.
10. What are some orthopedic conditions of the lower extremity? Describe the physical characteristics, medical prognosis, contraindications,

therapeutic treatments, and the application of principles for adapting physical activity.
11. Describe two spinal column malformations. Indicate the physical characteristics, medical prognosis, contraindications for physical activity, therapeutic exercises, and principles for adapting to physical activity.
12. Arthrogryposis, multiple sclerosis, osteomyelitis, poliomyelitis, and rickets may result in orthopedic handicaps. Describe the physical characteristics of each condition, medical prognosis, and therapeutic treatments that can be provided for each disorder.

STUDENT ACTIVITIES

1. Arrange a visit with a physical education teacher who has physically handicapped children in a class. Inquire about the types of activities the teacher provides and about whether the class is a special adapted class or an integrated regular class. What is the relationship with the physical therapist and other medical services?
2. Select one or two major journals in the field of physical or special education. Some of these journals are *Journal of Health, Physical Education, and Recreation; Teaching Exceptional Children;* and *Education and Training of the Mentally Retarded.* Look through the issues from the past few years for articles that present useful suggestions for adapting instruction for physically handicapped students. Make a file of these suggestions.
3. There are several organizations designed to serve parents of orthopedically handicapped persons. Some of these are Easter Seals, Association for Muscular Dystrophy, and United Cerebral Palsy Associations, Inc. Contact a local or national office to learn the purpose of these groups. Do they provide information about these orthopedically handicapped groups or serve as advocates for parents? What should physical education teachers know about these organizations?
4. Talk to an adult who is physically disabled. Ask about the ways in which the physical disability affects recreational activity and activity in the domestic and community environments. If the person was physically disabled as a child, ask about school experiences. Were adapted physical education services available? What were the effects of the services or lack of services on adult life?

5. Do a task analysis of a hypothetical orthopedically handicapping condition. Identify the muscles that must be strengthened and stretched and the prerequisite motor behaviors that need to be developed and integrated into a functional skill.
6. Visit a school, shopping center, or municipal building. Are there architectural barriers that would deny access to some handicapped individuals? Watch for stairs, curbs, and steep inclines. What types of activities might enable orthopedically handicapped persons gain access to these facilities through therapeutic programming?

REFERENCES

1. Daniels, L., and Worthingham, C.: Muscle testing, ed. 4, Philadelphia, 1980, W.B. Saunders Co.
2. Hallahan, D.P., and Kaufman, J.M.: Exceptional children, Englewood Cliffs, N.J., 1982, Prentice-Hall, Inc.
3. Meyen, E.L.: Exceptional children and youth, Denver, 1978, Love Publishing Co.
4. Petrofsky, J.S., and Phillips, C.A.: Computer controlled walking in the paralyzed individual, IEEE NAECON Rec. **2:**1162-1165, 1983.
5. Rusk, H.A., and Taylor, E.J.: Rehabilitation medicine, ed. 4, St. Louis, 1977, The C.V. Mosby Co.
6. Sherrill, C.: Adapted physical education and recreation, Dubuque, Iowa, 1981, William C. Brown Publishers.
7. Steindler, A.: Kinesiology of the human body, Springfield, Ill., 1955, Charles C Thomas, Publishers.
8. U.S. Department of Health, Education and Welfare. Fed. Reg., vol. 4, Aug. 23, 1977.
9. Venn, J., Morganstern, L., and Dykes, M.K.: Checklist for evaluating the fit and function of orthoses, prostheses, and wheelchairs in the classroom, Teach. Except. Child., pp. 51-56, Winter 1979.
10. Verhaaren, P., and Connor, F.: Physical disabilities. In Kaufman, J.M., and Hallahan, D.P., editors: Handbook of special education, Englewood Cliffs, N.J., 1981, Prentice-Hall, Inc.
11. Vodola, T.: Motor disabilities or limitations, Oakmont, N.J., 1976, Project Active.
12. Wilson, M.I.: Children with crippling and health disabilities. In Dunn, L.M., editor: Exceptional children in the schools, ed. 1, New York, 1973, Holt, Rinehart, & Winston.

SUGGESTED READINGS

Cratty, B.J.: Adapted physical education for handicapped children and youth, Denver, 1980, Love Publishing Co.
Licht, S., editor: Therapeutic exercise, ed. 2, New Haven, 1965, Elizabeth Licht, Publisher.

CHAPTER 14

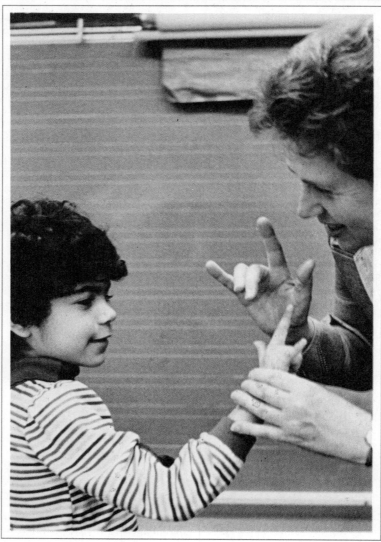

Photo by Erika Stone, Peter Arnold, Inc.

Hearing Impairments

OBJECTIVES

♦ Know the physical, psychological, and social characteristics of persons with hearing impairments.

♦ Know how to determine hearing loss through informal assessment.

♦ Know instructional techniques and methods for communicating with the hearing-impaired individual.

♦ Know how to apply principles for adapting instruction and activity for the hearing-impaired student.

Hearing is one of the strongest lines of communication between persons and the world in which they live. Children who have permanent hearing impairment are afflicted with handicaps that often have an impact on their total development, adjustment, and personality. The purpose of this chapter is to provide a background into the nature of hearing impairments and the needs of persons who are deaf and hard-of-hearing and to discuss the role of physical education in meeting these needs as part of the total educational process. Formal and informal tests, classifications of hearing loss, characteristics of hearing-impaired individuals, and teaching techniques and principles are discussed.

DEFINITION

According to P.L. 94-142,

"Deaf" means a hearing impairment which is so severe that the child is impaired in processing linguistic information through hearing, with or without amplification, which adversely affects educational performance (Section a.5.b.3) . . . . "Hard of hearing" means a hearing impairment whether permanent or fluctuating, which adversely affects a child's educational performance but which is not included under deaf in this section (Section 121a.5.b.3).[17]

This definition is useful to physical educators because it requires focus on the child as he or she participates in tasks in physical education. If there is performance deficiency, the question can be asked, "Is the deficiency the result of hearing loss?" If the answer is "Yes" special accommodation for the child should be made.

CONTINUUM OF DISTURBANCE

The continuum of degree of hearing loss and ability to understand speech ranges from that of little significance to that of extreme handicap, whereby an individual cannot understand amplified speech. Table 14-1 indicates the relationship between decibel loss, degree of handicap, and the ability to understand speech.

Children classified as having a marked handicap may be educationally deaf in academic subjects. Intensity (decibel) is one measurable attribute of sound. Others are frequency, which refers to perception of high and low pitch, and spec-

Table 14-1
Continuum of hearing impairment

Degree of Handicap	Range of Decibel Loss	Ability to Understand Speech
Not significant	0-25	No significant ability with faint speech
Slight handicap	25-40	Difficulty only with faint speech
Mild handicap	40-55	Frequent difficulty with normal speech
Marked handicap	55-70	Frequent difficulty with loud speech
Severe handicap	70-90	Can only understand shouted or amplified speech
Extreme handicap	> 90	Usually cannot understand even amplified speech

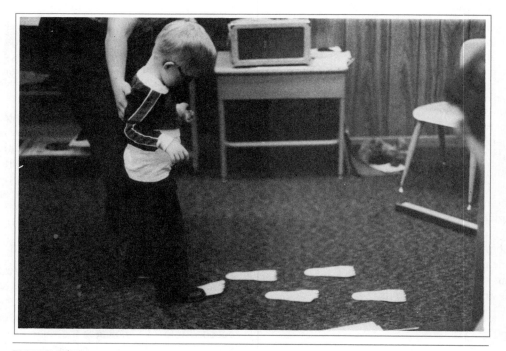

FIGURE 14-1
Footprints for the training of a walking gait provide visual and tactile information. Hearing-impaired children need visual and tactile cues for instructional purposes.

trum or timbre, which encompasses different tonal qualities ranging from a tone of single frequency to complex tones such as speech.

INCIDENCE

The prevalence of persons in the population who are hard-of-hearing is 3.2%, and those who are deaf represent 0.87% of the population.[16] In the cases of hard-of-hearing, adaptive procedures must be considered in the educational setting. However, only a few cases of hearing loss require completely altered educational methods.

CAUSES

There are two general categories of hearing loss—congenital defects, whereby children are born deaf or with a hearing loss, and deafness or hearing loss acquired after birth. Some individuals with congenital hearing defects have hereditary causes. Many can be traced to some form of disease. Rubella (German measles) in the mother is the most frequent disease that causes hearing loss as a prenatal infection. Syphillis is also a prenatal cause of hearing loss.

There are several causes of acquired deafness, including the following:

1. The presence of foreign objects in the external ear (paper, pins, crayons, etc.)
2. Tumors of the external auditory canal
3. Excessive buildup of ear wax
4. Perforation of the eardrum from a blow to the head or excessive pressure in the middle ear
5. Infections that spread to the middle ear from the eustachian tube (otitis media)
6. Allergies that make the eustachian tube swell
7. Viral infections such as mumps and measles
8. Bacterial infections such as meningitis and encephalitis

There is a relationship between the cause of hearing impairment and the degree of hearing loss. The most devastating losses occur because of meningitis, maternal rubella, and hereditary factors.[4]

TESTING FOR IDENTIFICATION

There are two purposes in the assessment of hearing loss—to determine how well the person's hearing serves the process of communication and to determine what can be done in terms of auditory rehabilitation. The educator is mainly concerned with hearing tests for the purposes of communication. It is desirable to have children diagnosed at the earliest possible age so that correctable defects may be treated adequately. If this is done, the impairment will not interfere greatly with the child's development. Knobloch and Pasamanick[9] have suggested the following list of signs of hearing loss:

1. Hearing and comprehension of speech
   a. General indifference to sound
   b. Lack of response to the spoken word
   c. Response to noises as opposed to words
2. Vocalization and sound production
   a. Monotonal quality
   b. Indistinct speech
   c. Lessened laughter
   d. Meager experimental sound play
   e. Vocal play for vibratory sensation
   f. Head banging, foot stamping for vibratory sensation
   g. Yelling, screeching to express pleasure or need
3. Visual attention
   a. Augmental visual vigilence and attentiveness
   b. Alertness to gesture and movement
   c. Marked imitativeness in play
   d. Vehement gestures
4. Social rapport and adaptation
   a. Subnormal rapport in vocal games
   b. Intensified preoccupation with things rather than persons
   c. Puzzling and unhappy episodes in social situations

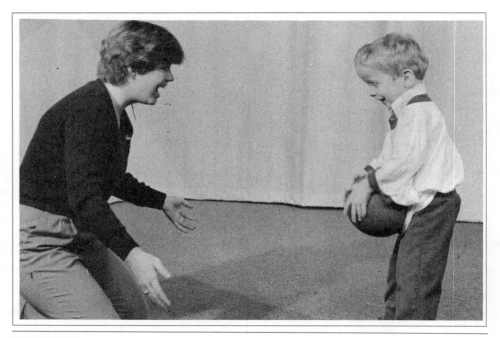

FIGURE 14-2
Visual attention to the instructor is necessary if hearing-impaired children are to receive quality instruction.

d. Suspiciousness and alertness, alternating with cooperation
e. Marked reaction to praise and affection
5. Emotional behavior
   a. Tantrums to call attention to self or need
   b. Tensions, tantrums, resistance, due to lack of comprehension
   c. Frequent obstinance, irritability at not making self understood

French and Jansma[3] cite additional behavioral characteristics that might indicate referral to an audiologist for a hearing test. They are poor speech, leaning toward the source of sound, request for repeated statements, recurring earaches, fluid draining from the ear, inattention, and poor balance.

Informal Methods

The electric audiometer is the most refined instrument for the detection of hearing loss. However, informal methods may still be of use for the rough appraisal of a child's hearing. Some of the tests are as follows:

♦ *Watch tick test:* A watch is brought progressively closer to the child's ear until he or she acknowledges the sound of the watch.
♦ *Coin click test:* A coin is brought in contact with a hard surface that is placed progressively closer to the child's ear to detect hearing loss of high-frequency sounds.
♦ *Conversational test:* The child is placed 20 feet from the teacher and is spoken to in a regular conversational tone. In the event the child cannot hear the teacher, the teacher moves closer and closer. If the child has difficulty hearing at 10 or 20 feet, he or she should be referred for a more thorough examination.
♦ *Whisper test:* The whisper test is administered in a manner similar to the conversational test except that the teacher uses a whisper.

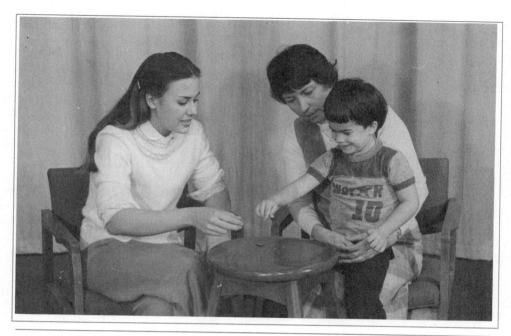

FIGURE 14-3
The coin click test may evaluate informally the ability of a child.

CLASSIFICATION

The acquisition of speech and language skills is basic to the subsequent development of the individual. Therefore, the time of onset of deafness is a critical factor in determining the effects that it may have on the learning situation. Meyen[11] indicates that if hearing loss occurs before or at birth, there is no chance for language to be heard normally or for incidental learning to occur. A child who is afflicted with a hearing loss early in development progresses more slowly than does one who is afflicted with a loss later in the developmental process.

Persons whose sense of hearing is nonfunctional for the ordinary purposes of life may be grouped in two distinct classes according to time of onset. They are the congenitally deaf and the adventitiously deaf. Congenitally deaf persons are born deaf. Adventitiously deaf persons are born with normal hearing but incur the hearing loss after birth.

Proper diagnosis of hearing defects may provide assistance for development of physical education programs. Each type of deafness, accompanied with the uniqueness of each deaf child, requires individualized treatment by teachers. Categories of deafness that should be considered in the educational planning for the student are the following:

- *Psychogenic deafness:* A condition in which the receptive organs function adequately and there is no damage to the nervous system, but, for emotional reasons, the person does not respond to sound.
- *Central deafness:* A condition in which the receiving mechanism of hearing is functioning properly, but an abnormality in the central nervous system prevents the person from hearing. This disorder is often referred to as auditory or sensory aphasia, or word deafness.
- *Perceptive or sensorineural deafness:* A condition caused by a defect of the inner ear or

of the auditory nerve in transmitting the impulse to the brain.

♦ *Conductive deafness:* A condition in which the intensity of sound is reduced before reaching the inner ear, where the auditory nerve begins. Since hearing loss is a multidimensional problem, it is important that the educator form no generalized concept regarding the deaf or hard-of-hearing child without considering such relevant factors as degree of hearing loss, age of onset, and type of hearing loss.

Conductive hearing losses are usually the result of dysfunction of the outer or middle ear. Vibrations of sound waves are prevented from reaching the inner ear. The most prevalent cause of conductive hearing loss is infection of the middle ear, which is called *otitis media.* Another infection that may cause conductive hearing loss is *mastoiditis.* Mastoiditis occurs when there is chronic inflammation of the middle ear and spreads into the air cells of the mastoid process within the temporal bone. Other causes of conductive hearing loss are cerebral tumors or abscesses, arterial sclerosis, cerebral hemorrhage, and multiple sclerosis.

Sensorineural hearing loss is a dysfunction of the inner ear in which the main problem is discrimination among speech sounds. Sound can be heard, but persons often cannot derive meaning from high-frequency sounds. Hearing aids are of limited value to remedy this type of hearing loss.

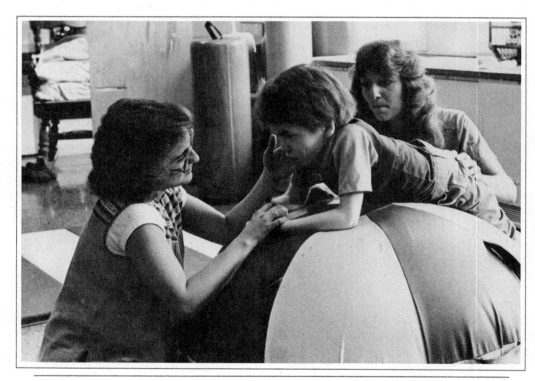

FIGURE 14-4
A cage ball stimulates the vestibular systems, and visual information from the instructor's lips replaces auditory feedback.
(Courtesy Children's Rehabilitation Center, Butler, Pa.)

Personality disorders generally associated with neuroses may contribute to the form of deafness known as psychogenic deafness.

PSYCHOLOGICAL AND BEHAVIORAL CHARACTERISTICS

Hearing loss can have profound consequences on a person's behavior. Hearing loss affects language and speech development, intellectual ability, and social adjustment. The areas most affected by hearing impairment are those of comprehension and production of the *English* language. Jensema, Karchmer, and Trybus[6] have indicated that of the hearing-impaired persons they studied, 15.4% were very intelligible, 29.4% were intelligible, 21.9% were barely intelligible, 20.5% were not intelligible, and 12.8% would not speak. Three reasons that may account for language deficit are that hearing-impaired persons do not receive adequate auditory feedback when they make sounds, that they receive inadequate verbal reinforcement from adults, and that they are unable to hear adequately an adult language model.

The intellectual ability of hearing-impaired children has been the subject of controversy over the years. The once popular view that hearing-impaired are somewhat deficient intellectually has been challenged. Several intelligence tests rely heavily on verbal skills. Many professionals hold the view that IQ tests do not assess the hearing-impaired child's true capability. The results of nonverbal tests favor the view that hearing-impaired children are not intellectually retarded.

Social personality development in the normal population is dependent on communication. Social interaction is the communication between two or more people, and language is the most important means of communication. Therefore, the personality and social characteristics of hearing-impaired persons often differ from those of people who have normal hearing ability. Hoeman and Briga[5] indicate that hearing-impaired persons develop behavioral problems based on how well others in the environment accept the disability.

Hearing-impaired children frequently grow up in isolation from others. The physical education program has the potential through games and sport to provide opportunity for much-needed social interaction.

Developmental Factors

Hearing loss that afflicts youngsters in the early phases of development impairs the total developmental process. One of the effects of deafness is to limit the children's play experience with other children. Play in the preschool years is important for learning of social skills and for development of motor skills. In play situations deaf children are often uncertain as to the part they should play in the game, and therefore they often withdraw from participation. Thus the role of play, which is important to the social, psychological, and motor aspects of development in typical children, is usually limited for deaf children.

The social benefits of play experienced by typical children are not experienced to the same degree by deaf children. Consequently, social development occurs more slowly in deaf children. It is in social maturation that the handicap of deafness is most apparent. This retardation is probably partially caused by language inadequacy that results from the hearing loss.

Because of their impaired ability to function socially with their peers and because of their restricted developmental experiences, deaf children are likely to be subjected to more strain than are hearing children. Therefore, young deaf children may be less emotionally mature than hearing children of the same age.

IMPORTANCE OF CASE HISTORY

Case histories often provide valuable information about children with limited hearing. The following information may be of relevance to the educational process:

1. Type, degree, cause, and age of onset involved in hearing impairment
2. Psychological impact of the onset of hearing loss on the student and the family

3. Major modes of communication and problems arising from the student's communication limitations
4. Effects of the disability in the social, educational, recreational, and domestic spheres
5. Behavior, attitudes, achievements, and aspiration of the student
6. History of diagnostic experiences and rehabilitative measures, including special education
7. Attitudes, motivations, and problems concerning education
8. Presence of other disabilities (visual defects and organic brain damage)
9. Health and medical problems

These data, if obtainable, should provide comprehensive information and may assist the future educational and rehabilitative program.

COMMUNICATION AIDS

The two prevalent methods of educating deaf persons are known as *oralism* and *manualism*. The oral method involves the media of lip reading and facial gestures for communication, with no associated use of hand signs. The manual method makes use of hand signals (signing) to express thoughts. Some educators of deaf or hard-of-hearing persons have stressed the importance of total communication. Thus the child is taught to use all these avenues of communication: lip reading, facial and body gestures, and hand signs (with verbalization, when possible).

Children with a hearing loss should be taught to make as much use of their residual hearing as possible. This method of teaching is called, *auditory training,* and it consists of improving listening skill by systematically developing the children's discrimination of gross sounds and rhythm patterns of speech. In addition to auditory training, which is designed to enhance the communication process, lip reading and speech training are also used. As a rule, special skills training takes up little program time. However, some authorities believe that this form of compensatory education is the most important part of the plan to prepare hard-of-hearing children for life in a hearing world and that some time should be devoted to such programs. Effective and efficient communication with hearing-impaired persons is a great challenge to teachers. Physical education teachers may improve their instructional ability by learning to communicate in a variety of ways to accommodate a wide range of pupils. Communication through hand signals may assist in communication with hearing-impaired persons.

There are two general forms of sign language— traditional sign language and signs that are unique to local governments. Traditional sign language is of value because it has greater acceptance among professionals. It can be used in the physical education class, the special education class, and the home and after the hearing-impaired person has completed schooling. There are two ways in which signs may be used to communicate with the deaf. One is through finger spelling and the other is through a system involving signs and accompanying verbalization of information transmitted through the hands. Fig. 14-5 indicates examples of some of the basic survival signs needed by physical education teachers to communicate with hearing-impaired persons.

Finger Spelling

The basic alphabet can be learned in a short time. The dominant hand, held at shoulder level with the palm out, spells the letters. If one loses a letter one should continue interpretation, since the remaining letters may suggest the total word. Fig. 14-5 shows the alphabet position.

Signing

Most signs are for concepts and ideas rather than for words. Pointing, motioning, demonstrating, and signaling are perfectly acceptable.[2] A foundation for communication with hearing-impaired individuals can be developed through study of *A Basic Course in Manual Communication.*[13] Fig. 14-6 indicates some specific signs for physical education.

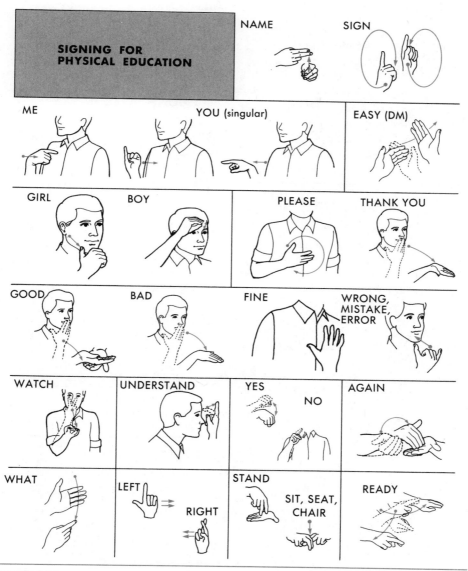

FIGURE 14-5
Survival signs.
(Reprinted with permission from the Journal of Physical Education, Recreation, and Dance, May 1978, pp. 20-21, a publication of the American Alliance for Health, Physical Education, Recreation and Dance, 1900 Association Drive, Reston, Va. 22091.)

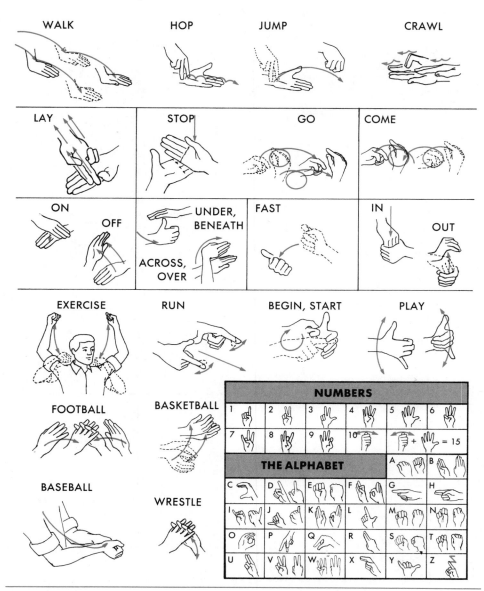

FIGURE 14-6
Specific signs for physical education.
(Reprinted with permission from the Journal of Physical Education, Recreation, and Dance, May 1978, pp. 20-21, a publication of the American Alliance for Health, Physical Education, Recreation and Dance, 1900 Association Drive, Reston, Va. 22091.)

Hearing Aids

Hearing aids amplify sound and are effective for conductive deafness. They can be worn in one or both ears. Some of the modern hearing aids are wireless transmitter receivers that operate on the same principle as a walkie-talkie and may be worn on the chest.

A number of hard-of-hearing children are enrolled in regular physical education classes, and adaptation in instructional techniques should be made for optimal learning. Many hard-of-hearing children wear hearing aids. If this is the case, it may be best to remove the aids when vigorous physical activity is scheduled. However, once the hearing aid is removed, the students are handicapped in audition and learning, particularly through the verbal medium, so that instructional adjustments are necessary. Judgment should be made concerning the removal of the hearing aid. The nature of the activity is usually the basis of such judgment. Active games involving body contact may require the removal of the hearing aid.

Excessive moisture corrodes batteries that operate hearing aids. Therefore, they should not be placed in damp grass or places of high humidity such as indoor swimming pool areas.

One adjustment that can be made easily is to place the children close to the instructor so that greater amplification of speech is received. A second adjustment that may help is for the instructor to keep the face in view of the hard-of-hearing children.

When one sensory avenue to gathering of information is impaired, it is necessary to rely more on other senses. In the case of children with learning loss, visual aids are of great significance in instruction. Visual demonstations, blackboard work, films, and slides are important instructional aids for the deaf. To get the attention of the class, waving the hands or turning off and on lights has proven effective in some instances.

TEACHING STRATEGIES

There are several teaching strategies that can be used to communicate effectively with hearing-impaired children. These relate to the teacher-learner position, intensity of the commands, interaction of teachers with hearing aids, and special attention to the environment. The following guidelines may assist physical education teachers in communicating with the hearing impaired.

1. Position yourself where the deaf child can see your lips; do not turn your back on the child and talk (for instance, writing on the blackboard).
2. When out of doors, position yourself so that you, rather than the deaf child, faces the sun.[16]
3. Use only essential words or actions to transmit messages.
4. Use visual attention-getters.
5. Make sure that the teaching environment has adequate lighting.
6. Allow the child to move freely in the gymnasium in order to be within hearing and sight range.
7. Encourage the use of residual hearing.
8. Coordinate the method (oral, total communication) that your school uses.
9. Reinforce all efforts to master speech.

Considerable individual differences exist among the deaf and hard-of-hearing regarding their response to various stimuli, and these differences must be taken into consideration. For example, persons with tinnitus (ringing in the ears) are highly sensitive to noise and vibration and may not perform well in a noisy facility such as the gymnasium. Deaf children with impaired semicircular canals, which affect balance, should not climb to high places. Also, some children with hearing loss should not participate in activity where there is excessive dampness, dust, or change in temperature.

Principles of Adapting Physical Activity

The same principles for adaptation described for the blind can be applied for adapting physical activity for the hearing impaired. In review they are (1) use of residual hearing and senses, (2) modification of the instructional environment, (3) use of special aids, (4) use of special techniques,

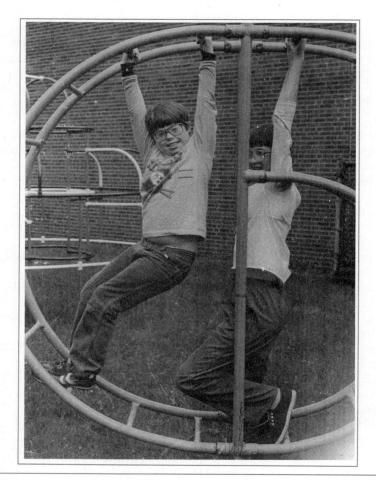

FIGURE 14-7
Movement activity on playground equipment may be restricted because of impairment of the semicircular canal.

(5) use of special feedback, and (6) use of peer assistance. Below is a chart outlining the application of those principles to the hearing impaired.

1. Use of residual senses
   a. Use visual signing.
   b. Use visual demonstration of skills to be taught.
   c. Use tactile and kinesthetic cues if necessary.
   d. Use the residual hearing.
   e. Provide audiovisual feedback.

2. Use and care of aids
   a. Use the appropriate hearing aid.
   b. Remove hearing aids before entering the pool area.

3. Instructional environment
   a. Avoid excessive noise in the instructional environment.
   b. Position self so there is effective communication.

4. Special instructional techniques and considerations
   a. The special system of communication.

b. Head should remain above water when swimming.
c. Underwater swimming is usually contraindicated.
d. Diving, which involves an impact between the water surface and the hearing mechanism, should be avoided.
5. Feedback
a. Provide audiovisual feedback.

Greater specificity for the modification of tasks to specific individuals can be developed within the context of these principles.

Implications for Physical Education

The objectives of a physical education program for hard-of-hearing children are the same as those for normal children. However, loss of hearing, which impairs the ability to communicate effectively with others, is a great social handicap. Therefore, an objective that should be given priority is the provision of opportunity for social interaction through games with other students. Activities in physical education for deaf and hard-of-hearing persons are similar to those in the regular program, and although deaf and hard-of-hearing persons may function well in regular programs, there is an obvious need for special and compensatory attention to those who are deaf to fulfill the objectives of the physical education program.

At the preschool and early elementary school levels, suggested activities for the deaf are those that develop basic motor skills and rhythm activities. Percussion instruments such as cymbals, triangles, drums, and tambourines are valuable for rhythm activities, because they are capable of producing vibrations to which the deaf child can respond.

Deaf and hard-of-hearing children do not, as a rule, need a set of activities that differs from that of typical children. However, assessment should be conducted to determine possible physical underdevelopment and poor motor coordination. If some children have these deficiencies, the program should be designed to remedy or ameliorate them. The physical education program for persons who are deaf or hard-of-hearing should provide for developmental activities.

DEAF-BLIND CHILDREN

Deaf-blind children have loss of both vision and hearing. They are considered to have less than 20/20 vision for a field of 20 degrees or less. In addition, they have a loss of hearing of 25 decibels or more. Thus they are often unable to be educated in class for the deaf or the blind.

Deaf-blind children have problems similar to those of the blind and the deaf. However, their problems are exponential rather than additive. There is practically no foundation for communicative ski.ls. Residual sight, hearing, or both can be the basis of communication. If there is no residual sight or hearing, communication is then made kinesthetically through the hands.

ATHLETIC OPPORTUNITIES FOR THE DEAF

There are opportunities for the deaf to participate in athletic competition in the postschool years. The American Athletic Association for the Deaf has approximately 14,000 members. This organization promotes state, regional, and national basketball and softball tournaments and prepares athletes for participation in the World Games for the Deaf. More than 150 local groups are affiliated with AAAD.

PARENT EDUCATION

Parent participation in the education of a child who has a hearing loss is very important. Many parents who face rearing a child with a severe hearing impairment have little knowledge of what they can do. After the child is in school, it is important for the parents to know how the child's hearing is developing, how skills in physical education are progressing, and how certain aspects of the school program can be extended to the home. There is general agreement that parent educational programs are necessary and that orientation is an essential part of any program for the child with impaired hearing.

SUMMARY

Physical educators are concerned primarily with the extent to which the hearing loss affects ability to participate in physical and sports activity. Classification of hearing loss is often based on the location of the problem within the hearing mechanism. Conductive losses interfere with the transferral of sound along the conductive pathway of the ear. Sensorineural problems are usually confined to the inner ear.

The electric audiometer is the most refined instrument for the detection of hearing loss. However, informal methods such as the watch tick test, coin clink test, and whisper test may be used in the absence of sophisticated equipment and for survey purposes. The results of formal testing are measured in decibel loss. Loss of 0 to 25 decibels is not significant, while loss of more than 90 decibels represents a severe handicap.

Methods of communication may be oral, manual, or total. Hearing aids amplify sounds and are effective for conductive deafness. Considerations for effective communication by teachers of the deaf during instruction are teacher-learner position, intensity of the commands, interaction with hearing aids, and special attention to the environment. Other considerations for adapting activity for the hard-of-hearing are appropriate use of residual hearing, care of hearing aids, adaptation of the instructional environment, visual feedback, and other special instructional techniques. Athletic opportunities should be provided for the hearing impaired so that attained skills may be expressed to further develop motor skills, physical fitness, and personal and social characteristics outside of the physical education class.

REVIEW QUESTIONS

1. What are the different categories of deafness?
2. What are the indicators of hearing loss that can be observed by the physical education teacher while teaching a class?
3. List informal methods that a physical educator might use to determine whether a student has a hearing loss.
4. What are some behavioral characteristics of hearing-impaired children?
5. Discuss three different methods of communicating with deaf persons.
6. Discuss the practical application of signing to communicate with hearing-impaired persons.
7. What are some teaching strategies that can be used with deaf persons?
8. What specific application of principles for the hearing impaired can be made in physical activity?

STUDENT ACTIVITES

1. Impaired hearing can be found in persons of any age. Survey your community to locate agencies that provide services to persons who have hearing impairments. What types of services are available? How do these differ from services provided by the public schools?
2. Simulate an interaction with a deaf person. Communicate to the person, through signs, the method of performing a physical education task.
3. Talk to a teacher of the deaf to determine the method of communicating with the deaf. Has the teacher used all three methods? Which method has been most effective with specific groups of deaf persons?
4. Observe hearing-impaired children participating in a physical education class. What teaching strategies were employed by the teacher? What adaptations were made to accommodate the hearing-impaired person in activity? What were the behavioral characteristics of the hearing-impaired children?
5. Talk with two physical educators from two different schools about how to improve the social acceptance of children with impaired hearing. What suggestions did they offer? What have they tried in the past that has worked?

REFERENCES

1. Cratty, B.J.: Adapted physical education for handicapped children and youth, Denver, 1980, Love Publishing Co.
2. Eichstaedt, C., and Seiler, P.J.: Signing: communicating with hearing impaired individuals in physical education, J. Phys. Educ. Rec. **49**:19-21, 1978.
3. French, R., and Jansma, P.: Special physical education, Columbus, Ohio, 1982, Charles E. Merrill Publishing Co.
4. Hallahan, D.P., and Kaufman, J.M.: Exceptional children, Englewood Cliffs, N.J., 1982, Prentice-Hall Inc.
5. Hoeman, H.W., and Briga, J.S.: Hearing impairments. In Kaufman, J.M., and Hallahan, D.P., editors: Handbook of special education, Englewood Cliffs, N.J., 1981, Prentice-Hall Inc.
6. Jensema, C.J., Karchmer, M.A., and Trybus, R.J.: The rated speech intelligibility of hearing impaired children: basic relationships and detailed analysis, Washington, D.C., 1978, Gallaudet College Office of Demographic Studies.
7. Kalakian, L.H., and Eichstaedt, C.B.: Developmental adapted physical education, Minneapolis, 1982, Burgess Publishing Co.
8. Kirk, S.A., and Gallagher, J.J.: Educating exceptional children, ed. 3, Boston, 1979, Houghton Mifflin Co.
9. Knobloch, H., and Pasamanick, B.: Developmental diagnosis, New York, 1974, Harper & Row, Publishers Inc.
10. Meadow, K.D.: Development of deaf children. In Heatherington, E.M., editor: Review of child development research, vol. 5, Chicago, 1975, Chicago University Press.
11. Meyen, E.L.: Exceptional children and youth, Denver, 1978, Love Publishing Co.
12. Moores, D.F.: Educating the deaf: psychological principles and practices, Boston, 1978, Houghton Mifflin Co.
13. O'Rourke, T.J.: A basic course in manual communication, Silver Springs, Md., 1973, National Association of the Deaf.
14. Schmidt, S., and Dunn, J.M.: Physical education for the hearing impaired: a system of movement symbols, Teaching Exceptional Children *12*:99-102, 1980.
15. Seaman, J.A., and DePauw, K.P.: The new adapted physical education: a developmental approach, Palo Alto, Calif. 1982, Mayfield Publishing Co.
16. Sherrill, C.: Adapted physical education and recreation, ed. 3, Dubuque, Iowa, 1985, Wm. C. Brown Co., Publishers.

SUGGESTED READINGS

American Alliance for Health, Physical Education, Recreation, and Dance: Physical education, recreation and sports for individuals with hearing impairment (annotated bibliography), Boston, Va., 1976 American Alliance for Health, Physical Education, Recreation, and Dance.

Birch, J.: Hearing impaired children in the mainstream, Reston, Va., 1975, Council for Exceptional Children.

Davis, H., and Silverman, R.: Hearing and deafness, New York, 1978, Holt, Rinehart & Winston.

Geddes, D.: Motor development profiles of preschool deaf and hard-of-hearing children. Percent. Mot. Skills *46*:291-294, 1978.

Methods of communication currently used in the education of deaf children, London, 1976, Royal National Institute for the Deaf.

Nix G.W.: Mainstream education for hearing impaired children and youth, New York, 1976, Grune & Stratton Inc.

Pennella, L.: Motor ability and the deaf: research implications, Am. Ann. Deaf **124**:366-372, 1979.

Riekehof, L.L.: The joy of signing, Springfield, Mo. 1980, Gospel Publishing House.

Wisher, P.: Dance for the deaf. In Sherrill, C., editor: Creative arts for the severely handicapped, Springfield Ill., 1979, Charles C Thomas, Publisher, p.p. 105-111

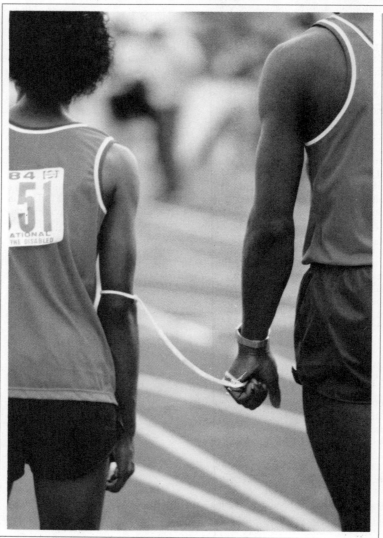

CHAPTER 15

Stewart Halperin

Visual Impairments

OBJECTIVES

♦ Know the nature of visual defects.

♦ Know the general characteristics of children with limited vision.

♦ Know principles and methods for adapting physical activity for the blind.

♦ Know how to design and manage the instructional environment.

♦ Know how to select appropriate activities for the blind.

♦ Know how to integrate physical education instructional programs with recreational opportunities in the community.

V isual disorders considered here are usually permanent. Children with visual disorders represent a unique challenge to the physical educator, because in addition to their visual impairments they usually demonstrate developmental lags. Many of these children have not had opportunities to physically explore the environment during their early years. As a result, intact sensorimotor systems are not stimulated adequately and motor development and physical fitness levels suffer. Low vitality and perceptual-motor development lags often prevent the children from participating in activities not contraindicated by the primary visual disorder.

For a child to qualify for special services in physical education, the visual handicap must adversely affect the child's physical education performance. Children with visual disorders who qualify for adapted/developmental physical education programs demonstrate one or both of the following:

1. A visual handicap that, even with correction, adversely affects the child's educational performance; the term includes both partially seeing and blind children

2. Concomitant hearing and visual impairments, the combination of which causes such severe communication and other developmental and educational programs that the child cannot be accommodated in special educational programs solely for deaf or blind children

CONTINUUM OF DISABILITY

Children with visual impairments must be approached in accordance with their own unique educational needs. All blind and partially sighted children should have a full evaluation as to the degree of visual loss.

A child who has a loss of vision may also be impaired in the function of mobility and may be less able than typical children in motor abilities. There is a great need for blind children to be provided with opportunities, through adapted physical education, that will compensate for their movement deficiencies.

Children with loss of vision are, for educational purposes, classified as blind (those who are educated through channels other than vision) or

317

partially sighted (those who are able to be educated, with special aids, through the medium of vision, with consideration given to the useful vision they retain). Blindness is determined by visual acuity and is expressed in a ratio with normal vision in the numerator and actual measured vision in the denominator; for example, 20/30 vision means that the eye can see at the distance of 20 feet what a normal eye can see at 30 feet. The legally blind are described as those who have a visual acuity of 20/200 or less in the better eye after maximum correction or who have a visual field that subtends an angle of 20 degrees or less in the widest diameter.

There are varying degrees of blindness. If a person is not totally blind, it is still possible to make functional use of whatever vision remains. Some blind persons have little residual vision and are unable to perceive motion and discriminate light. These individuals are at the upper end of the continuum of blindness. Some blind persons, however, are capable of perceiving distance and motion, whereas others possess these capabilities and are also able to travel with the use of residual vision.

The point to be stressed is that when a person is considered blind, it does not necessarily mean that the majority of the activities in a typical physical education program must be ruled out. Rather, a person's capacity for specific activity depends on the degree of blindness as well as available skill.

The term *partially sighted* refers to persons who have less than 20/70 visual acuity in the better eye after correction, have a progressive eye disorder that will probably reduce vision below 20/70, or have peripheral vision that subtends an angle less than 20 degrees. The visual acuity of a child is one consideration for participation in physical activity. Physical and psychological adjustments should be made for persons who lose sight as a result of injury or operations. Such injury may result in eye anomalies that necessitate reeducation of abnormal eyes. Each child must be considered according to his or her ability to function, regardless of the nature or degree of the visual handicap. In some instances a child's vision

may fall within the normal range, but the child may have progressive eye difficulties or a disease of the eye or body that seriously affects vision.

The residual vision of blind and partially sighted handicapped athletes may be related to the amount of assistance they need to participate. It may also be related to the quality of performance. Therefore, to provide equity in competition, classifying the competitors is based on the amount of sight. The United States Association for Blind Athletes (USABA) classification system of legally blind athletes is as follows:

1. Class A—totally blind; possess light perception only, have no visual acuity or see less than 3 degrees in the visual field
2. Class B—visual acuity no better than 20/400 or those with 3 to 10 degrees in the visual field; can see hand movement
3. Class C—visual acuity 20/399 through 20/299 or those with 10 + to 20 degrees in the visual field

INCIDENCE

It is difficult to assess the incidence of blindness and partial vision because of the differing definitions of blindness and the problems that exist in identification. Consequently, dependable statistics on the incidence of blindness in the United States are lacking, although there is a growing awareness that a greater incidence of blindness and vision impairment exists than had been believed previously. It is estimated that 0.1% of the population is visually handicapped. A considerable number of children with visual defects are not categorized as either blind or partially sighted. Estimates indicate that approximately 20% of elementary school children and 30% of high school students have some visual defect.

CAUSES

The underlying causes for visual loss include diabetes, accidents and injuries, poisoning, tumors, and prenatal influences such as rubella and syphilis. Several defects may cause degeneration of vision, such as the following:

♦ Refractive errors such as myopia, hyperopia, and astigmatism
♦ Structural anomalies such as cataracts
♦ Infectious diseases of the eyes
♦ Impaired muscle function of the eye such as strabismus and nystagmus

Refractive errors are a function of the internal ciliary muscles of accommodation, which increase the curvature of the lens. *Hyperopia,* or farsightedness, is a condition in which the light rays focus behind the retina, causing an unclear image of objects closer than 20 feet from the eye. The term implies that distant objects can be seen with less strain that can near objects. *Myopia,* or nearsightedness, is a refractive error in which the rays of light focus in front of the retina when a person views an object 20 feet or more away. *Astigmatism* is a refractive error caused by an irregularity in the curvature of the cornea, so that portions of the light rays from a given object fall behind or in front of the retina. As a result, vision may be blurry.

Nystagmus is another common visual abnormality. It involves rapid movement of the eyes from side to side, up and down, in a rotatory motion, or a combination of these.

In addition to the internal muscles of the eye mentioned previously, there are six muscles attached to the outside of each eyeball that control movement. Singular binocular vision involves coordinating the separate images that enter each eye into a single image in the visual cortex of the brain. When the two eyes function in unison, the images entering each eye are matched in the visual cortex, and binocular fusion results. If, however, the supply of energy to the extraocular muscles is out of balance, the eyes do not function in unison. When this occurs, the movements of one eye deviate from those of the other eye, and the separate images entering through each eye do not match in the visual cortex. The amount of visual distress experienced because of mismatched images *(strabismus)* depends on the degree of deviation of the eyes and the ability of the central nervous system to correct the imbalance.

The two most prevalent dysfunctions of external visual muscle control are heterotropias and heterophorias. *Heterotropias* are manifest malalignments of the eyes during which one or both eyes consistently deviate from the central axis. As a consequence, the eyes do not fixate at the same point on the object of visual attention. When the eyes turn inward, such as with crossed eyes, the condition is called *esotropia;* when one or both eyes turn outward, it is called *exotropia.* Hypertropia is the name given to the condition when one or both eyes swing upward; the term *hypotropia* is used when one or both eyes turn downward. Tropias always create depth perception difficulties.

Heterophorias are tendencies toward visual malalignments. They usually do not cause serious visual distress because when slight variations in binocular fusion occur in the visual cortex, the central nervous system tends to correct the imbalance between the pull of the extraocular muscles. However, after prolonged use of the eyes, such as after reading for several hours, the stronger set of muscles overcomes the correction and the eyes swing out of alignment. An individual becomes aware of the malalignment when the vision of the printed page begins to blur. Phorias, like tropias, are named for the direction the eye tends to swing (*eso-* means in, toward the nose; *exo-* is a lateral drift; *hyper-* means up; and *hypo-* refers to down). Phorias create depth perception difficulties only after the correction is lost.

Several visual abnormalities are acquired or hereditary.

Term	Description
Albinism	A hereditary condition in which there is a lack of pigment in the eyes; may include light sensitivity and require dark glasses
Cataract	Opacity of the normally transparent lens
Glaucoma	Increased pressure of the fluid inside the eye, which causes visual loss; associated with decreasing peripheral vision
Retinitis pigmentosa	Degeneration of the retina that produces gradual loss of peripheral vision
Retrolental fibroplasia	Visual impairment caused by oxygen during incubation of premature babies

TESTING VISUAL IMPAIRMENT

Vision tests are extremely important to identify and remedy vision disorders and to facilitate the education of visually handicapped persons. A widely used test of vision is the Snellen test, which is a measure of visual acuity. This test can be administered with expediency to a child by nonprofessional personnel and is applicable to young children. The Snellen chart can aid detection of myopia, astigmatism, higher degrees of hyperopia, and other eye conditions that cause imperfect visual images. However, the chart primarily measures central distance visual acuity. It does not give indications of near-point vision, peripheral vision, convergence ability, binocular fusion ability, or muscular imbalance. A thorough vision screening program must include tests supplementary to the Snellen test. Other visual screening tests that may provide additional information are the Massachusetts Vision Test, the Keystone Telebinocular Test, and the Orthorator Test.

Limitations in peripheral vision constitute a visual handicap, particularly in some activities involving motor skills. Consequently, knowledge of this aspect of vision may assist the physical educator in determining methods of teaching and types of activities for the visually impaired child. Peripheral vision is usually assessed in terms of degrees of visual arc and is measured by the extent to which a standard visual stimulus can be seen on a black background viewed from a distance of about 39 inches when the eye is fixed on a central point.[4]

It is difficult to evaluate the results found on a given test of vision because two persons with similar vision characteristics on a screening test may display different visual behavior physically, socially, and psychologically. Although objective screening tests of vision are important, it is suggested that daily observations be made to supplement the screening tests. Daily observation for symptoms of eye trouble has particular importance in the early primary years. Detection of visual handicaps early in development enables early intervention, which maximizes skill development. Symptoms that might indicate eye disorders and might be observed by the physical educator are included in the following list:

1. Eyelids that are crusted and red, on which sties or swelling appear
2. Discharge from the eyes
3. Lack of coordination in directing vision of both eyes
4. Frequent rubbing of the eyes
5. Inattention when sustained visual activity is required or when looking at distant objects
6. Body tension
7. Squinting
8. Forward thrust of the head
9. Walking overcautiously
10. Faltering or stumbling
11. Running into objects not directly in the line of vision
12. Failure to see objects readily visible to others
13. Sensitivity to normal light levels
14. Inability to distinguish colors
15. Difficulty in estimating distances
16. Bloodshot eyes

Some blind persons have accompanying mental retardation. These individuals may exhibit self-stimulatory behavior, or *blindisms*, such as rocking the body or head, placing fingers or fists into the eyes, flicking the fingers in front of the face, and spinning the body around repetitiously. These behaviors provide vestibular, tactile, or visual stimulation.

Within the last few years new techniques for evaluating vision and assisting individuals with visual disorders have been made available through low vision clinics. Generally, people whose best corrected vision is 20/70 or less or whose visual field is restricted to 30 degrees or less are considered to have low vision and are most likely to benefit from low vision services.

CHARACTERISTICS

There are widespread individual differences among visually limited persons. However, certain characteristics appear more often than in sighted persons. Some of the characteristics that have implications for physical education are the following:

- There is loss of vision but wide variations of residual vision.
- There are significant problems in mastering complicated movement patterns.
- Physical fitness scores are below those of sighted peers.
- Posture is often poor. There is no visual model to emulate.
- Physical growth and maturation may be impaired because of limited opportunities for movement.
- There is a tendency toward obesity caused by a sedentary life-style.
- Development of the ability to balance is impaired.
- Fundamental motor patterns and skills are below normative performance.

Developmental Factors

Vision loss has serious implications for the general development of motor, academic, intellectual, psychological, and social characteristics. The blind infant has little motivation to hold the head up because of lack of visual stimulation, so in the formative stages of postural development (head control) blind children are behind normative expectations. In many instances intervention with training programs and adaptive measures is necessary to meet the developmental needs of the maturing child with a loss of vision. It is important to have some knowledge of how the child with vision loss may develop physically, socially, and psychologically so that the physical educator can be alert to cope with needs that may arise.

Evidence indicates that blind pupils in the public schools are educationally retarded as compared with their sighted peers of the same chronological age.[1] Possible reasons are that blind

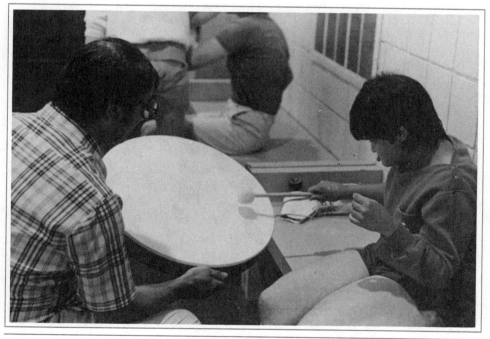

FIGURE 15-1
A drum provides auditory feedback to the motor movement.
(*Courtesy Verland Foundation, Inc.*)

children may have a maladjustment at the onset of blindness, making it difficult to stay abreast of sighted peers. Physical educators must be alert to detect educationally retarded blind children. They must not be misguided by grade placement but must assess and meet the physical, motor, and social needs of each child.

Physical activity is essential for optimum child growth and development. Through movement experiences children with vision losses acquire a better understanding of themselves, others, and the world around them. However, limited vision restricts physical motor activity, which in turn limits the range and variety of experiences the children may encounter. They then become less effective in meeting the demands of the environment. Opportunities for manipulating toys and objects are extremely important in the early life of

blind children because it is through touch and feeling, rather than through vision, that they learn about the physical world.

Providing an environment in which children with vision impairments can develop optimally is a great challenge. Blind children are often slower to learn skills such as walking, talking, prehension, feeding, and socialization unless they are given help in developing these traits.

Norris and Brody[6] found that blind children showed delayed mastery of motor responses in tasks requiring fine motor coordination. There is impressive evidence that fine motor coordination develops with fluency only after the children have had experiences in gross motor activity. This indicates a need to provide environmental experiences for both gross and fine motor activities. Planned physical experiences are required for

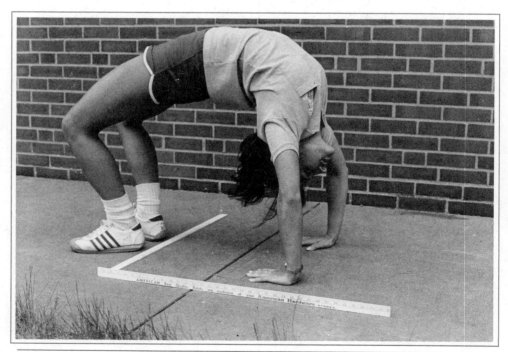

FIGURE 15-2
Many physical activities do not require the use of vision.

young blind children to counter slower rates of motor and physical development as compared with children who have normal vision.

Perceptual Development

Children with limited vision use other sensory abilities better as a result of increased attention to them in attempts to learn about and cope with the environment. A sighted person might be unaware of particular auditory stimuli, whereas a blind person might attach great significance to them.

These children need to use full proprioceptive, auditory, haptic, and space perception. Each form of perception contributes to the ability of the blind child to adapt to the environment. The proprioceptors can enable a blind person to maintain balance. Balance experience is acquired through different and unusual body positions. The proprioceptors are stimulated if the tasks become sequentially more difficult. Behavioral programs constructed in such a manner that balance is challenged will usually stimulate the proprioceptors and develop the balancing mechanism. Proprioceptive awareness can also be developed by adding small weights to the body, the added weight requires a differential movement.

Space Perception

Early visual experience of spatial relations establishes a method for processing information that affects cognitive and motor learning. Blind persons often cannot perceive the relationship of objects to each other in space. They also have an impaired ability to relate themselves to objects in space. Therefore the auditory, vestibular, kines-

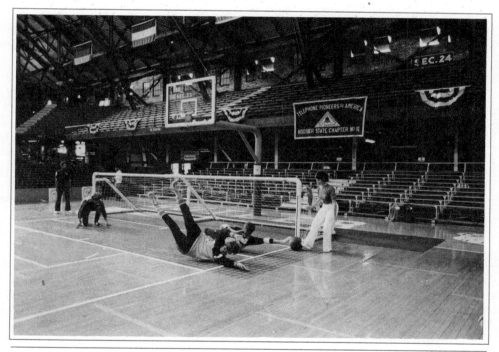

FIGURE 15-3
The Denmark team tries to push the bell ball (auditory stimuli) out of bounds.
(*Courtesy Eugenia Kreibel, International Sports Organization for the Blind.*)

thetic, and tactile senses are used to establish spatial relationships.

Auditory stimuli help the person determine the direction and distance of objects and thereby establish a spatial relationship between the object and the blind person. Beep balls, audible goals, and bell balls (used for goal ball) are special devices to develop perception of objects in space.

Psychological and Social Adjustment

The emotional and social characteristics of the visually limited vary according to the individual. Blind students may have personality problems as well as physical incapacities. Research available regarding the social maturity of blind children reveals that, in general, they receive significantly lower social maturity scores than do sighted children.[3] Physical education programs may well be an important medium for enhancing the social maturity of blind children.

Psychological and social adjustment of the blind cannot be separated from the attitudes with which the nondisabled view them. The lack of respect of one's peers may create a need for a disproportionate amount of social and emotional adjustment not only to blindness but also to their peers. The correlates of maladjustment are to be found in deficiencies of respect accorded the individual, rather than a lack of visual experience.

The uphill battle for social adjustment of the blind requires special attention; sighted persons acquire social habits through imitation, but the blind need direct instruction in everyday social adjustment. The emotional and social climate of the physical education class can be structured so that blind children are able to function comfortably at their own levels and establish wholesome social relationships. Lack of individualized instructional procedures can contribute to frustration by creating situations that accentuate, rather than minimize, differences.

Mobility

One of the greatest problems caused by blindness is impeded mobility. Success in school and at work in later years depends on mobility. By contributing to the independence of blind persons, it leads to opportunities for physical, social, and psychological development.

A mobility training program in a gymnasium or playing area greatly increases independence and thus the ability to perform in a physical education program. Orientation and training programs should help the persons cope with physical surroundings effectively. Training programs should also foster successful interaction with peers as well as with the physical facilities and equipment. It must be remembered that some blind persons have enough vision to travel about, known as *travel vision*. The individual capabilities of each child should be assessed to determine the extent of the mobility training program.

THE PHYSICAL EDUCATION PROGRAM

The physical education teacher may be requested to instruct a class in which visually limited children are integrated with the regular class, to instruct a class composed solely of visually limited children, or to instruct classes of multihandicapped children.

There is a growing awareness that similarities are greater than differences when visually limited children are compared with seeing children. Therefore integration of visually limited children with their nonhandicapped peers should be instituted to meet the new federal mandates of placement of all handicapped children in the least restrictive environment (regular class, if possible). Such placement emphasizes the positive aspects of the children and minimizes differences.

In the past it was not uncommon for children with limited vision to be referred to and placed in residential schools. However, with the implementation of P.L. 94-142 a countertrend has grown to bring instructional aids into resource rooms and regular classrooms of community schools. This practice has created a number of service delivery alternatives for least restrictive placement. Reynolds and Birch[7] indicate the following cascade system for placement of children with visual handicaps:

1. Regular class
2. Regular class with assistance by vision consultant
3. Regular class with consultation and itinerant instruction (orientation and mobility training)
4. Adapted physical education conducted by specialist; children attend part time
5. Self-contained adapted physical education class
6. Residential schools for the blind

The itinerant teacher is a specialist who possesses specific skills to work with children of limited vision. They team with regular classroom teachers on behalf of visually handicapped children. For more information concerning the duties of this type of teacher, refer to Moore and Peabody.[5]

The Teacher

The physical education teacher must be able to respect individuals who have atypical vision. Furthermore, attention should focus on the abilities, as well as the deficits, of visually handicapped children for the purpose of creating an environment conducive to optimal growth. An assessment of the needs, abilities, and limitations of visually limited children is necessary, with subsequent programs development according to defined needs. This is a challenging task for a teacher; however, it has been pointed out by many good teachers that instructing the visually limited has enabled them to do a better job with typical children because it was necessary to plan more carefully when working with the former group.

Some suggested considerations prerequisite to effective education of the visually limited child are as follows:

1. Skilled observation of motor performance and behavioral characteristics of individuals and of group participants
2. Recognition of differences in the manner in which the visually limited child learns, as compared with the typical child, followed by appropriate adaptive methodology
3. Understanding of the growth and development of physical and social competence
4. Knowledge of appropriate curricula and methods in physical education for the visually limited

Physical Education Needs

Loss of vision, by itself, is not a limiting condition for physical exercise. A considerable amount of developmental exercises of muscular strength and endurance can be administered to such children. Through developmental exercise the visually limited child develops qualities such as good posture, graceful body movement, and good walking and sitting positions. Furthermore, physical education programs develop and maintain a healthy, vigorous body with physical vitality and good neuromuscular coordination. In addition to physical benefits, the physical education program contributes to social-emotional outcomes such as security and confidence and acceptance of the handicapped by their sighted peers.

The ultimate goal of the class atmosphere for children with vision losses is to provide experiences that will help them adjust to the seeing society in which they live. The selection and method of experiences in the physical education program are critical. These experiences should not be overprotective to the extent that growth is inhibited; rather, the experiences should provide challenge yet remain within the range of the children's capabilities for achieving skill objectives.

The problems that confront the teacher regarding successful emotional and psychological adjustment of the visually limited involve both visually limited children and nondisabled children. Guidelines for achieving the goal of adjustment for these teachers follow:

♦ Provide opportunities for participation and enjoyment in new experiences
♦ Provide IEPs in which the children are free to grow and develop at their own rates
♦ Find ways in which they can best contribute to the groups that are satisfying to them
♦ Help them become acquainted with their physical surroundings

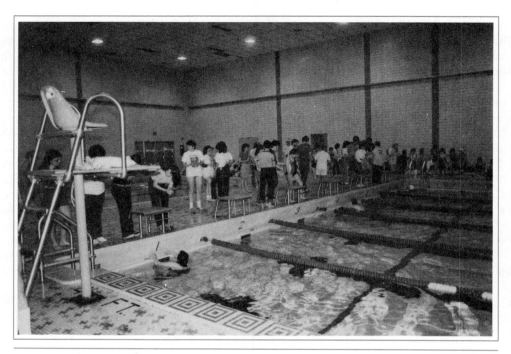

FIGURE 15-4
Blind children can be integrated into programs that individualize instruction.
(Courtesy Western Pennsylvania Special Olympics.)

Physical education teachers working with children who are visually handicapped should attempt to minimize the stereotyped manner in which the visually limited child receives an education and should encourage nonhandicapped children to accept their blind peers on a personal basis. The development of such attitudes of the nonhandicapped supports the principle of normalization of the handicapped.

Adapting Methods and Activities

Children with limited vision are capable of participating in numerous activities; however, the degree to which participation is possible depends on each child's particular abilities. It is recommended that there be available broad curriculum areas at appropriate levels of development to accommodate each child. Visually handicapped children may represent a cross section of any school population with regard to motor abilities, physical fitness characteristics, and social and emotional traits. The purpose of adapting methods and activities for the visually limited is to provide many experiences that sighted children learn primarily through visual observation. A goal of group activity in which a child with limited vision participates is to assign a role to the child that can be carried out successfully. It is undesirable for the child to be placed in the positon of a bystander.

Adaptation of the physical education program for visually limited individuals should provide confidence for them to cope with their environment by increasing their physical and motor abilities. It should also produce in them a feeling of acceptance as individuals in their own right. To achieve these goals, the program should include adaptation of the general program of activities, when needed; additional or specialized activities, depending on the needs of the child; and special equipment, if needed.

The physical educator who administers activities to children with limited vision should take special safety precautions. Some considerations that may enhance the safety factor in physical education programs for the visually limited are:

1. To secure knowledge, through medical records and observation, of the child's limitations and capabilities
2. To orient the child to facilities and equipment
3. To provide special equipment indicating direction, such as guidelines in swimming and running events, deflated softballs

TEACHING STRATEGIES

The visually limited child must depend on receiving information through sensory media other than vision. Audition is a very important sensory medium of instruction. Another sensory medium that can be used is kinesthesis through manual guidance and movement of the body parts administered by an instructor or another student. This provides comprehension of body position and body action. The blind child has little understanding of spatial concepts such as location, position, direction, and distance; therefore skin and muscular sensations give meaning to body position and postural change in motor activity. The manual guidance method (accompanied by verbal corrections) is often effective in the correction of faulty motor skills, since two senses are used for instruction. A technique that has met with some success in the integrated class is for the teacher to use the blind child in presenting a demonstration to the rest of the class by manually manipulating the child through the desired movements. This enables the visually limited child to get the tactual feel of movement, and instruction to the sighted class members is not deterred. Providing information, rules, and tests in braille for advance study of a class presentation may enable the visually limited child to better understand the presentation.

Developing Socialization Skills

One of the chief problems to be confronted in the social and psychological adjustment of the visu-

ally limited person is the lack of opportunity for social participation with sighted persons. Recreational opportunities are a possible outlet for making social contact with the sighted population and also provide self-expression for the visually limited individual (Chapter 9).

Because of the great visual content included in the components of certain games, some skill activities are more difficult to adapt to the visually limited than are others. In the case of the more severely handicapped, participation in the more complex activities may be extremely difficult to modify. However, the skills comprising a game can be taught, and lead-up games with appropriate modifications are usually within the child's grasp. Some adaptations of basic sports skills follow:

Activity	Modification
Archery	Pegs in the ground for stance
Running	Ropes for guidance
Swimming	Ropes that designate the swimming lane
Swimming	Swimming pool with nonslip bottom
Softball	Concrete or sand for base paths
Softball	Concrete bases slightly raised above base path
Softball	Different texture of ground or floor when near a surface that could result in serious collision
Class management	Environment that is ordered and consistent
Class management	Reference points that indicate the location of the child in the play area
Class management	Auditory cues to identify obstacles in the environment
Class management	Tactile markings on the floor
Class management	Rings or ropes that hang from the ceilings to indicate student's location
Class management	Boundaries of different texture

Cognitive Instruction

Communication of information and testing of knowledge are part of physical education instruction. Accommodations must be made for the visually impaired during the communication of the physical education program:

- Large print letters and numbers can be perceived by many partially sighted persons.
- Use braille, a shorthand for tactile reading. Dots in a cell are raised on paper to indicate letters, numbers, punctuation, and other special signs.
- Make better use of listening skills and position students where they can hear instructional information best. This may be directly in front of the instructor.
- Substitute kinesthetic (manual) guidance for vision when components of skills are to be integrated in space and time.
- Encourage the use of residual vision during the cognitive communication process between instructor and blind student.
- Arrange seats to accommodate range of vision.
- Design appropriate light contrasts between figure and ground when presenting instructional materials.
- Be alert to behavioral signs and physical symptoms of visual difficulty in all children.

There are several considerations that physical educators must make to effectively accommodate blind children in the diverse activities and environments where instruction takes place. It is beyond the scope of this book to compile all these adaptations. The application of principles of accommodation may help the physical educator to teach a wide variety of activities. Some suggested principles follow:

- Design the instructional environment to accommodate the individual.
- Introduce special devices, aids, and equipment to assist the individual.
- Use special instructional techniques to accommodate the individual.
- Introduce precautionary safety measures to meet the individual's needs.
- Provide special feedback for tasks to facilitate learning.
- Employ nonhandicapped peers to assist with instruction.
- Train the individual for mobility and understanding of the environment.

Instructional Environment

The instructional environment for the blind should be safe and familiar and possess distinguishing landmarks. As a safety precaution, play areas should be uncluttered and free from unnecessary obstructions.[1] Blind children should be thoroughly introduced to unfamiliar areas by walking them around the play environment before they are allowed to play.

Environmental characteristics can be amplified. For instance, gymnasiums can be well lighted to assist those who possess residual vision. Boundaries for games can have various compositions, such as a base or path of dirt and concrete or grass for other areas. Brightly colored objects are easier to identify. Also, equipment may be designed and appropriately placed to prevent possible injuries. For instance, two swings on a stand are safer than three. A third swing in the center is difficult to reach without danger when the other two swings are occupied. Attention to the safety and familiarity of environment specifically designed for the blind represents some degree of accommodation.

There are two parts to the management of safe environments. One is the structure of the environment, and the other is the teacher's control of the children as they participate in the environment. Following are suggestions to ensure safe play.

- Alter the playing surface texture (sand, dirt, asphalt); increase or decrease the grade to indicate play area boundaries.
- Use padded walls, bushes, or other soft, safe restrainers around play areas.
- Use brightly colored objects as boundaries to assist those with residual vision.
- Limit the play area.
- Limit the number of participants in the play area.
- Play in slow motion when introducing a new game.
- Protect the eyes.
- Structure activities commensurate with the blind child's ability.
- Protect visual aids such as eyeglasses.

♦ Select safe equipment.

♦ Structure a safe environment.

♦ Instruct children to use the environment safely.

The following material indicates the application of safety principles:

Principle	Safety Measure
Protection of aids	Protect all body parts; spotting in gymnastics
	Protect eyeglasses
Safe equipment	Use sponge ball for softball, volleyball, many projectile activities
Structure of safe environment	Check play areas for obstacles and holes in ground
Activity according to ability	Avoid activities that require children to pass each other at high speeds
	Close supervision of all potentially dangerous activity

Designing a safe environment is important. Equally important is instructing children with limited vision to use the environment safely. Sherrill[8] has suggested some techniques for teaching safe use of playground equipment. Safety instruction in play environments for blind young children is particularly important because of their unawareness of the distance from the ground when on elevated play apparatus. The children should demonstrate safe play on all the equipment by (1) pumping a swing while sitting, (2) walking a hand ladder, (3) climbing to the top of an 8- to 14-foot slide and sliding down feet first, (4) playing simple games on the jungle gym, and (5) using the seesaw safely with a companion.

Auditory Aids

Distance in space for the visually limited is structured by auditory cues. Therefore, it is desirable to structure space with these cues. For instance, a sighted partner may ride a bicycle with a piece of cardboard attached to the bike wheel. A noise is made when it touches the spokes.

Auditory aids can be built into the equipment that is a part of the game. For instance, in the game Jump the Shot "It" rotates a flat piece of metal attached to a rope from the center of a circle composed of players. The piece emits a sound as it travels along the ground and thus informs the participants of its whereabouts.

Audible balls emit beeping sounds for easy location. They may be the size of a basketball, soccer ball, softball, or playground ball.[2]

Audible goal locators are motor-driven noisemakers. They can indicate the position of backboards in basketball, goals in soccer, and the height and position of a net in volleyball and badminton. Furthermore, they can be used to identify dangerous objects in the environment and boundaries.

Activities that can be conducted to develop space perception through the use of auditory aids in the environment are to:

1. Walk a straight line. Measure the distance of deviations over a specific distance. Use an audible device to provide initial assistance for direction and then fade the device.

2. Face sounds made at different positions. The intensity and duration of the sound can make the task more or less difficult.

3. Reproduce pathways and specific distances just taken with a partner.

Auditory information in the environment is invaluable for positioning children with limited vision appropriately in activity environments.

Special Devices, Aids, and Equipment

Equipment, aids, and devices that enhance participation of the blind in physical activity should provide information about the environment. Beep baseball and goal ball are two competitive sports for the blind. Each sport requires special equipment that enables knowledge of the whereabouts of the ball. The beep baseball is a regular softball with a battery-operated electronic sound device. This special equipment tells the blind person where the ball is at all times because of continuous sound. Other special equipment is the bases, which are plastic cones 60 inches tall with a speaker that makes continuous sound installed in each base.

A goal ball is constructed with bells inside it.

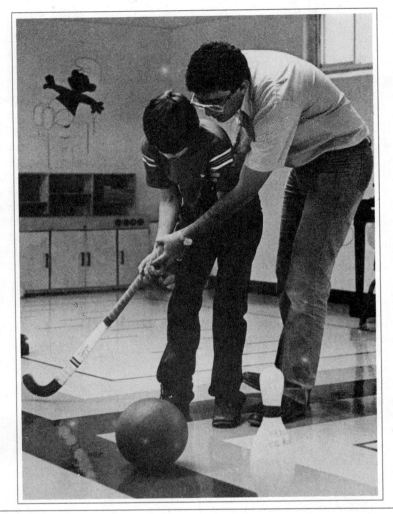

FIGURE 15-5
Kinesthetic aids and tactile information communicate instructional intent and circumvent the need for vision to receive information.
(Courtesy Children's Rehabilitation Center, Butler, Pa.)

When the ball moves, the bells help the players locate the ball. One of the skills of the game is to roll the ball smoothly to reduce auditory information (less sound from the bells) to make it more difficult for blind players to locate it. Following are other devices, aids, and techniques that can be used to accommodate the blind in physical activity:

Activity	Device, Aid, or Equipment
Swimming	Flotation to increase buoyancy
Gymnastics	Safety belt
	Soft mat to protect the performers

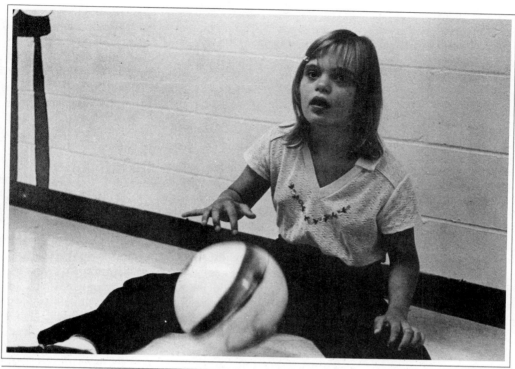

FIGURE 15-6
Tactile, kinesthetic information through hand contact with the ball and auditory feedback from the ball bouncing enables successful activity without the use of vision.
(Courtesy Children's Rehabilitation Center, Butler, Pa.)

Special Instructional Methods

The application of special methods requires astute observation of the characteristics of each blind student. A list of special methods follows:

♦ Give clear auditory signals with a whistle or megaphone.
♦ Instruct through manual guidance.
♦ Use braille to teach cognitive materials before class.
♦ Encourage tactual exploration of objects to determine texture, size, and shape.
♦ Address the child by name.
♦ Individualize instruction and build on existing capabilities. Do not let the child exploit visual limitations to the extent of withdrawing from activity or underachieving in motor performance.
♦ Use the sensory mode that is most effective for specific learners (tactile, kinesthetic, haptic, auditory) (Fig. 15-6).
♦ Manage the instructional environment to minimize the need of vision. Use chains where children touch one another. Participate from stationary positions. Establish reference points where all persons return for instruction.
♦ Instructional strategies should match the nature of the task. Games of low organization are an important part of elementary school

physical education programs. The games that require the least modification are those in which there is continuous contact with the participants, such as tug of war, parachute activity, end man tag, ring around the rosy, hot potato, over and under relay, wheelbarrow races.

Fundamental motor skills and patterns are essential prerequisites for successful and enjoyable participation in recreational sport activities. Some of these activities are running, jumping, throwing, and striking. They involve coordinated movements. Traditional instruction involves presentation of a visual model through demonstration of the whole task. Pupils then attempt to reproduce this task. However, children with limited vision must receive information from other senses.

Special Task Feedback

Blind children need to know the effects of their performance on physical tasks because they receive little or no visual feedback. Task feedback must come from other sensory modes. For example, buzzers or bells can be inserted inside a basketball hoop to inform the person when a basket is made. Gravel can be placed around the stake for horseshoes to indicate accuracy of the toss. Peers can also give specific verbal feedback on tasks that involve projectiles. Effective feedback is an important reinforcing property to be incorporated into physical activity for the blind.

Peer Assistance

Nonhandicapped peers can assist the handicapped child with instruction in integrated settings. The nature of the assistance depends on the nature of the task. Peer assistance in providing feedback to task success is one application of peer assistance. Blind persons may choose to have sighted guides. Kalakian and Eichstaedt[3] indicate that, for safety in travel skills, a blind person should grasp the guide's upper arm, above the elbow, with the thumb on the outside and the fingers on the inside of the guide's arm. Both student and guide hold upper arms close to the

body. When approaching doorways or objects, the guide moves the entire arm behind the back so blind students understand to walk directly behind the guide. Verbal cues inform the blind student when there are stairways and curbs. When nonhandicapped children provide such assistance, it is necessary to manage their time so as not to impede their own education.

Mobility Training

Mobility training is an adaptive technique that applies to blind children and children with limited vision. It enables them to learn about their physical play areas. Mobility training increases their confidence in moving with greater authority and provides greater safety while they are participating. It is a valuable way to enhance participation in the physical education program.

Orientation and training programs should help the persons cope with physical surroundings effectively. Training programs should also assist successful interaction with peers as well as with the physical facilities and equipment. Remember that some blind persons have travel vision. The individual capabilities of each child should be assessed to determine the extent of the mobility training program.

COMMUNITY-BASED ACTIVITIES

Several activities and equipment contribute to physical and motor fitness of children with limited vision: weight lifting, Universal gym equipment, isometric exercises, stationary running, the exercise bicycle, and the rowing machine. All these require simple environments and can easily be generalized to physical fitness programs in the home and community.

One of the purposes of physical education for the blind is development of skills that can be used in interscholastic athletics, intramurals, or for leisure in the community after formal schooling. Therefore activity should be community based. Such considerations for program development are sanctioned by Section 504 of the Rehabilitation Act of 1973. Clearly, there are to be equal opportunities for participation in extracurricular activities for the handicapped to the same extent as the nonhandicapped. Therefore opportunities for sports participation outside the schools should be integrally linked with the physical education program in the public schools. Such considerations for extension of extracurricular activities to the blind involve identification of activities that are available in the community.

USABA Activities

The United States Association for Blind Athletes (USABA) is an organization that sponsors national championships every year. Such high-level competition is an incentive for blind persons to engage in training regimens from which there are personal and physical benefits. Blind persons who participate in competitive activities such as those sponsored by the USABA may reach goals in both the sport and personal development.

Several activities sponsored by USABA are related to leisure activities. Thus the competition can serve participants in two ways—for athletic competition and for participation in leisure activities in the community. Some of the activities that are a part of international competition and that can be expressed as a recreational skill in the community are listed below:

Activity	Skill
Track running event	Physical fitness program
Cycling	Physical fitness and recreational program
Weight lifting	Physical fitness programs and body building
Sailing	Recreational aquatics
Crew rowing	Rowing a boat for fishing and boat safety
Competitive diving	Recreational swimming and diving
Archery	Recreational shooting at archery ranges
Swimming	Recreational swimming in community pools
Downhill and cross-country skiing	Recreational skiing in selected communities where the resources are appropriate

Other activities that are less community based recreational activities but provide opportunities to develop personal and social skills through participation are field events in track, wrestling, and gymnastics. Specific events in gymnastics and track and field are floor exercise, balance beam, uneven bars, vaulting, all-around competition, 60- or 100-meter dash, 200-, 400-, 800-, 1500-, 3000-, and 10,000-meter runs.

Goal Ball

Goal ball is a game that originated in Germany for blind veterans of World War II to provide gross motor movement cued by auditory stimuli (a bell ball). It is now played under the rules of the International Sports Organization for the Disabled.

The purpose of the game is for each team of three persons to roll the ball across the opponent's goal, which is 8.5 m (9¼ yards) wide for men and 7.5 m (about 8 yards) wide for women. A ball is rolled toward the opponent's goal. The entire team attempts to stop the ball before it reaches the goal by throwing the body into an elongated position. The ball is warded off with any part or the whole body. Games last 10 minutes with a 5-minute halftime. All players are blindfolded.

Many of the principles of accommodating visual impairment have been incorporated into this game. Examples of the application of these principles follow:

Instructional environment to accommodate the individual	The boundaries are made of rope so they can be detected by the players.
Special aids and equipment	Elbow and knee pads are provided to the players so they are not hurt when the body hits the floor or lunges to stop the ball. Bells are placed in the ball so the rolling ball can be heard en route to the goal.

Special instructional techniques	Kinesthetic movement of the body is required to instruct the players how to lunge to block the ball.
Precautionary safety measures	Pads and mats can be placed at the end of the gym where the goals are. The sidelines should be clear of objects.
Special feedback to facilitate learning	A piece of tin or materials that make sounds can be placed at the goal so players know when a goal has been scored rather than successfully defended.
Nonhandicapped peers to assist instruction	Nonhandicapped persons can provide feedback as to whether the movements of the game have been successfully achieved.
Train the individual to understand the environment	The individuals should be trained to know where the goal ball training area is within the gym and how to enter and leave the gymnasium.

SUMMARY

Children with visual disorders vary in functional ability to participate in physical activity. Partially sighted persons have less than 20/70 acuity, and a blind person has 20/200 or less. There are several abnormalities of vision. Some associated with curvature of the lens are myopia, hyperopia, and astigmatism. Nystagmus, tropias associated with difficulties in depth perception, and heterophorias concern visual malalignment.

Visual impairments may be identified by the Snellen test or other visual screening tests. They may also be identified by observing abnormal eye conditions, motor movements, and visual discrimination. Low vision clinics offer comprehensive evaluations and assistance to individuals with visual disorders.

Vision loss has serious implications for motor, intellectual, psychological, and social development. Vision loss early in life may delay mastery of motor responses, which can affect other areas of development. Planned physical experiences may counter maldevelopment in other areas.

Training programs in mobility increase the degree of independence of the blind. Accompanying direct instruction to develop travel vision and motor skills are techniques for adaptation. This may be accomplished by modifying activity and instructional environments and introduction of special aids, devices, or equipment.

Persons with visual disorders should be trained with self-help or recreational skills that can be used in the community. This may enable participation in some of the community sport programs for the blind and visually limited.

REVIEW QUESTIONS

1. Compare the movement capability of a child with slight loss of vision with that of a child who is totally blind.
2. List the classification system for severity of blindness used by the United States Association for Blind Athletes.
3. Indicate the estimated incidence of visually handicapped persons.
4. List some causes for loss of vision.
5. Discuss the consequence of loss of vision on the development of physical and social skills.
6. List some general characteristics of persons with limited vision that impair physical performance of skills.
7. Discuss problems and solutions for the social adjustment of the visually disordered in integrated and special physical education classes.
8. List ways in which activities and environments could be modified to include the visually impaired in physical activity.

STUDENT ACTIVITIES

1. There are organizations designed to serve parents of blind children. Contact a local or a national organization to learn the purpose of these groups. Do they provide information about the blind? Serve as advocates for parents? What should physical education teachers know about these organizations?
2. Talk with an adult who is blind. Ask about the ways in which blindness affects physical activity. Ask about the person's school experiences in physical education. Ask what the person would like as an outcome of a physical education program. Was the person mainstreamed into regular physical education classes?
3. There are several ways of adapting instruction and the environment to accommodate persons with visual disorders. Select three activities and indicate how you might modify the activity, environment, or equipment.
4. Talk with a physical education teacher who has taught blind children. Ask how the visual disorders were identified after assessment.
5. Presume you are blind. Design an instructional program for yourself. Simulate the blindness with a blindfold and make the necessary adaptations.

REFERENCES

1. Fait Dunn, H.: Special physical education, ed. 5, Philadelphia, 1984, W.B. Saunders Co.
2. Greaves, J.R.: Helping the retarded blind, Int. J. Blind 23:164-164, 1953.
3. Kalakian, L.H., and Eichstaedt, C.B.: Developmental adapted physical education, Minneapolis, 1982, Burgess Publishing Co.
4. Luria, A.: Higher cortical functions in man, ed. 2, New York, 1980, Basic Books, Inc.
5. Moore, M.W., and Peabody R.L.: A functional description of the itinerant teacher of visually handicapped children in the Commonwealth of Pennsylvania, Pittsburg, 1976, School of Education, University of Pittsburg.
6. Norris, M.S., and Brody, R.H.: Blindness in children, Chicago, 1957, University of Chicago Press.
7. Reynolds, M., and Birch, J.: Teaching exceptional children in all America's schools, Reston, Va. 1977, Council for Exceptional Children.
8. Sherrill, C.: Adapted physical education and recreation, ed. 3, Dubuque, Iowa, 1985, William C. Brown Co., Publishers.

SUGGESTED READINGS

American Foundation for the Blind, Inc.: Directory of agencies serving the visually handicapped in the United States, New York, 1980,

Barraga, N.: Visual handicaps and learning, Belmont, Calif., 1976, Wadsworth Publishing Co.

Beaver, D.P., editor: Official National Sports Development Committee Athletic Handbook, Beach Haven Park, N.Y., 1978, United States Association for Blind Athletes.

Blackhurst, A.E., and Berdine, W.H.: An introduction to special education, Boston, 1981, Little Brown and Co.

Buell, C.E.: Physical education and recreation for the visually handicapped, Washington, D.C., 1974, American Alliance for Health, Physical Education, and Recreation.

Cox, R.L.: A program for able pre-college students who are blind, Kappa Delta Pi Rec. 15:101, 108, April 1978.

Cratty, B.J.: Movement and spatial awareness in blind children and youth, Springfield, Ill., 1971, Charles C. Thomas, Publishers.

Eichstaedt, C.B.: Signing, Journal of Phys. Ed. and Recreat. 49:19-21, May 1978.

George, C., and Patton, R.: Development of an aerobics conditioning program for the visually handicapped, J. Phys. Ed. Recreat. 46:39-40, May 1975.

Hill, E., and Purvis, P.: Orientation and mobility techniques: a guide for the practitioner, New York, 1976, American Foundation for the Blind.

Kalakian, L.H., and Eichstaedt, C.B.: Developmental adapted physical education, Minneapolis, 1982, Burgess Publishing Co.

Kearney, S., and Copeland, R.: Goal ball, J. Phys. Ed. Recreat. 50:24-26, Sept. 1979.

Mandell, C.J., and Fiscus, E.: Understanding exceptional people, St. Paul, 1981, West Publishing Co.

Martin, G.J., and Hoben, M.: Supporting visually impaired children in the mainstream: the state of the art, Reston, Va., 1977, Council for Exceptional Children.

Tait, P.: Behavior of young blind children in a controlled play session, Percept. Motor Skills, 34:963-969, June 1972.

CHAPTER 16

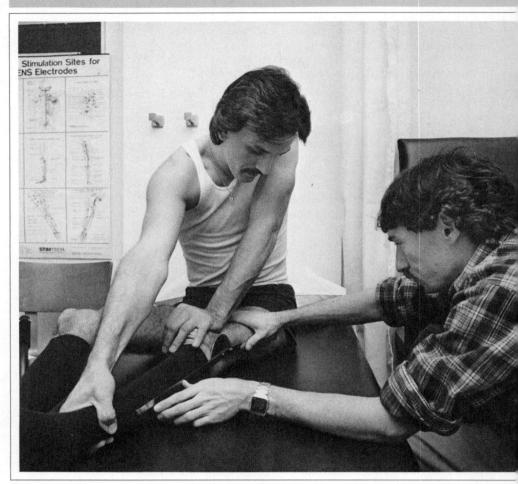

H. Armstrong Roberts

Posture and Body Mechanics

OBJECTIVES

♦ Know the values of good posture.

♦ Assess postural deviations of the foot and ankle, knee, pelvis, upper back, lumbar region of the spine, scapula, and head and neck.

♦ Select appropriate activities to ameliorate diagnosed postural deficiencies.

Good posture might be defined as a position that enables the body to function to the best advantage with regard to work, health, and appearance. An individual's posture, in a large measure, determines the impression that he or she makes on other persons. Good posture is socially valued, whereas poor posture is socially devalued. Thus it is extremely important for handicapped persons to have valued postural patterns to minimize difference so they appear more normal.[6] Good posture gives the impression of enthusiasm, initiative, and self-confidence, whereas poor posture often gives the impression of dejection, lack of confidence, and fatigue. We know that faulty posture does not necessarily indicate illness; however, we also know that good posture and body mechanics help the internal organs assume a position in the body that is favorable to their proper function and that allows the body to function most efficiently. Good posture should not be confused with the ability to assume static positions in which the body is held straight and stiff and during which good alignment is achieved at the sacrifice of the ability to move and to function properly. Possibly, good body mechanics would be a better term to use in describing the proper alignment and use of the body during both static and active postures.

Body mechanics is the proper alignment of body segments and a balance of forces so as to provide maximum support with the least amount of strain and the greatest mechanical efficiency.[3] There is general agreement that the human body operates best when its parts are in good alignment while sitting, standing, walking, or participating in a variety of occupational and recreational types of activities. There is no such thing as a normal posture for an individual. Certain anatomical and mechanical principles have been developed over the years that aid physicians, therapists, and physical educators in the identification of faulty body mechanics and posture.[2] Application of these principles helps individuals keep their bodies in proper balance with as small an expenditure of energy as possible and with the minimum amount of strain.

The center of gravity of the human body is located at a point where the pull of gravity on one side is equal to the pull of gravity on the other side. This center of gravity (higher in men than in women) falls in front of the sacrum at a point ranging from approximately 54% to 56% of the individual's height when standing. The center of gravity is changed any time the body or its segments change position.

In the upright standing position, the human

body is relatively unstable. Its base of support (the feet), is small, whereas its center of gravity is high; and it consists of a number of bony segments superimposed on one another, bound together by muscles and ligaments at a large number of movable joints. Any time the body assumes a static or dynamic posture, these muscles and ligaments must act on the bony levers of the body to offset the continuous downward pull of gravity.

Whenever the center of gravity of the body falls within its base of support, a state of balance exists. The closer the center of gravity is to the center of the base of support, the better will be the balance or equilibrium. This has important implications for the individual both in terms of good posture and as it relates to good balance for all types of body movement. The body is kept well balanced for activities in which stability is important, whereas it may be purposely thrown out of equilibrium when movement is desired, speed is to be increased, or force is to be exerted on another object.[1,3]

As the human being matures, balance for both static and dynamic positions becomes more automatic. An individual develops a feel for a correct position in space so that little or no conscious effort is needed to regulate it and attention can be devoted to other factors involved in movement patterns. This feeling for basic postural positions as well as for dynamic movement is controlled by certain sensory organs located throughout the body. The eyes furnish visual cues relative to body position. The semicircular canals of the inner ear furnish information on body equilibrium. Receptors in the tendons, joints, and muscles also contribute to the individual's ability to feel the body's position in space. The loss or malfunction of any of these sense organs requires that major adjustments be made by the individual to compensate for its loss.

CAUSES OF POOR POSTURE

There are many causes of poor posture and poor body mechanics, including environmental influences, psychological conditions, pathological conditions, growth handicaps, congenital defects, and nutritional problems. Any one of these may have an adverse effect on the posture of the growing child, the adolescent, or the adult. Extended periods of time are needed to establish good body mechanics.[4] The habits of poor posture cannot be overcome with a few minutes of daily exercise. The neuromuscular system must be given thorough reeducation so that positions and movements are conscious and subconscious routines.

Poor posture that contributes to incorrect muscle development, tension, spinal deviations, lower back disorder, poor circulation, and unattractive appearance overcome through specific muscle training and reorientation of postural habits.

Pathological conditions often lead to functional and structural posture deviations. Some of these are faulty vision and hearing, various cardiovascular conditions, tuberculosis, arthritis, and neuromuscular conditions resulting in atrophy, dystrophy, and spasticity. Growth handicaps include weaknesses in the skeletal structure and in the muscular system, growth divergencies, fatigue, and glandular malfunctions. Congenital defects include amputations, joint and bone deformities, spina bifida, clubfoot, and the like. Nutritional problems include underweight, overweight, and poor nourishment.

PROCEDURES FOR POSTURAL DEVELOPMENT

There are specific procedures that can be employed to improve posture. The first step is to assess the individual's posture to determine deficiencies in mechanical alignment. The deficiencies are usually expressed in the form of a clinical postural disorder such as kyphosis or lordosis. The second step of the process of postural education is to identify the muscles that need to be strengthened or improved for flexibility to develop efficient mechanical alignment. The third step is to structure the appropriate activity at

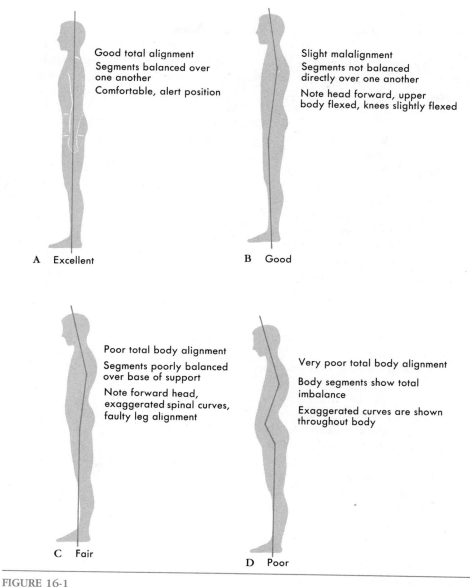

A   Excellent

Good total alignment

Segments balanced over one another

Comfortable, alert position

B   Good

Slight malalignment

Segments not balanced directly over one another

Note head forward, upper body flexed, knees slightly flexed

C   Fair

Poor total body alignment

Segments poorly balanced over base of support

Note forward head, exaggerated spinal curves, faulty leg alignment

D   Poor

Very poor total body alignment

Body segments show total imbalance

Exaggerated curves are shown throughout body

FIGURE 16-1

Four-figure system for rough assessment of posture is used to identify students in need of a more discriminating type of posture examination.

the person's present level of performance and conduct an individualized postural education program.

POSTURAL ASSESSMENT

The first step in development of a postural education program is to assess each person to determine whether there is a need for postural programs. There are two major types of screening. One is group screening and the other involves individual assessment. Group screening may be done by having a group of children move in a circle and then respond to changes in direction while the teacher observes from the center of the circle.[5] Group techniques may also be used to assess sitting posture. The other major type of screening involves individual assessment of each child by the teacher. There are several types of individual postural assessment. The focus of our discussion is on individual assessment techniques.

Plumb Line Test

The plumb line test is used to assess posture because it allows comparison of body landmarks with a gravity line. The plumb line can be hung so that it falls between the person being examined and the instructor. The vertical line is used as a reference to check the student's anteroposterior and lateral body alignment. Certain surface landmarks on the body that align with a gravity line of the human body have been located by kinesiologists and engineers. These surface landmarks can be used as points of reference in conducting examinations designed to see how well the body is balanced and how well its segments are aligned in the upright position.

Lateral View

From the lateral view (showing anteroposterior deviations), starting at the base of support and working up the body, the gravity line should fall at a point about 1 to 1½ inches anterior to the external malleolus of the ankle, just posterior to the patella, through the center of the hip at the approximate center of the greater trochanter of the femur, through the center of the shoulder (acromial process), and through the earlobe.

Viewed from the front or rear, the spinal column should be straight. However, when the spine is viewed from the side, or lateral view, curves normally exist in various vertebral segments. The cervical spine is slightly hyperextended, stretching from the base of the skull to about the top of the thoracic vertebrae. The spine is flexed throughout the area of the thoracic vertebrae and hyperextended throughout the area of the lumbar vertebrae, and the sacral curve is flexed. These curves are present in the spinal column to help the individual maintain balance and to absorb shock, and they should be considered normal unless they are exaggerated.

Anterior View

From the anterior view (showing lateral deviations), the gravity line should fall an equal distance between the internal malleoli and between

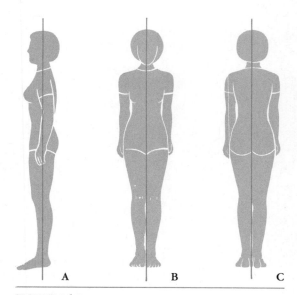

FIGURE 16-2
Plumb line tests. **A,** Lateral examination. **B,** Anterior examination. **C,** Posterior examination.

the knees; should pass through the center of the symphysis pubis, the center of the umbilicus, the center of the linea alba, the center of the chin, and the center of the nose; and should bisect the center of the upper portion of the head.

Posterior View

The landmarks to be checked in the posterior examination (showing lateral deviations) would include the same points as those checked in the anterior examination in the region of the ankle and the knee, the cleft of the buttocks, the center of the spinous processes of the spinal column, and the center of the head.

Recording Data

There are several ways in which data from a plumb line test can be recorded. A widely accepted assessment system has been adopted in the New York State Physical Fitness Test. Three

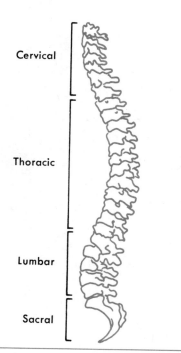

FIGURE 16-3
Normal spine.

sets of pictures represent three different and sequential levels of postural fitness. One sequence of pictures represents model posture, a second sequence represents devient posture, and a third sequence represents marked discrepancies from normal posture. The observer views the student according to plumb line testing procedures and for each picture on the evaluation sheet asks the question, "Which picture does the person being tested most look like?" The posture profile has various numbering systems. Some are ranked on a 10, 5, 1 scale, with 10 being good/model, 5 deficiency, and 1 marked deficiency. Other grading scales are 5, 3, 1 and 7, 5, 3. The scoring system is used to assign a number to the postural condition of the person observed. These numbers can be total for a postural index. However, the treatment plan must be derived from an evaluation of the specific anatomical part of the body that is misaligned. Usually, diagnosed deficiencies reflect a clinical postural disorder that is caused by tight or weak muscles. The target muscle groups must be identified and specific types of activity must be assigned to meet the unique problem of the specific postural deficiency.

A posture examination is much more meaningful to the student and far more useful to the teacher if the findings are carefully recorded by the examiner (especially during review of the material obtained in the examination prior to setting up an exercise or activity program or when doing a reevaluation of the pupil several months after the original examination). The examination form must provide space for the instructor to record the findings of the examination quickly and accurately. Provisions should be made for recording the severity of each of the conditions identified in the examination. The findings of successive examinations can also be recorded on the same form.

Posture Screen

Another form of posture testing may be done with a posture screen. The posture screen is a grid of vertical and horizontal lines that can be used as reference points to evaluate all segments of the

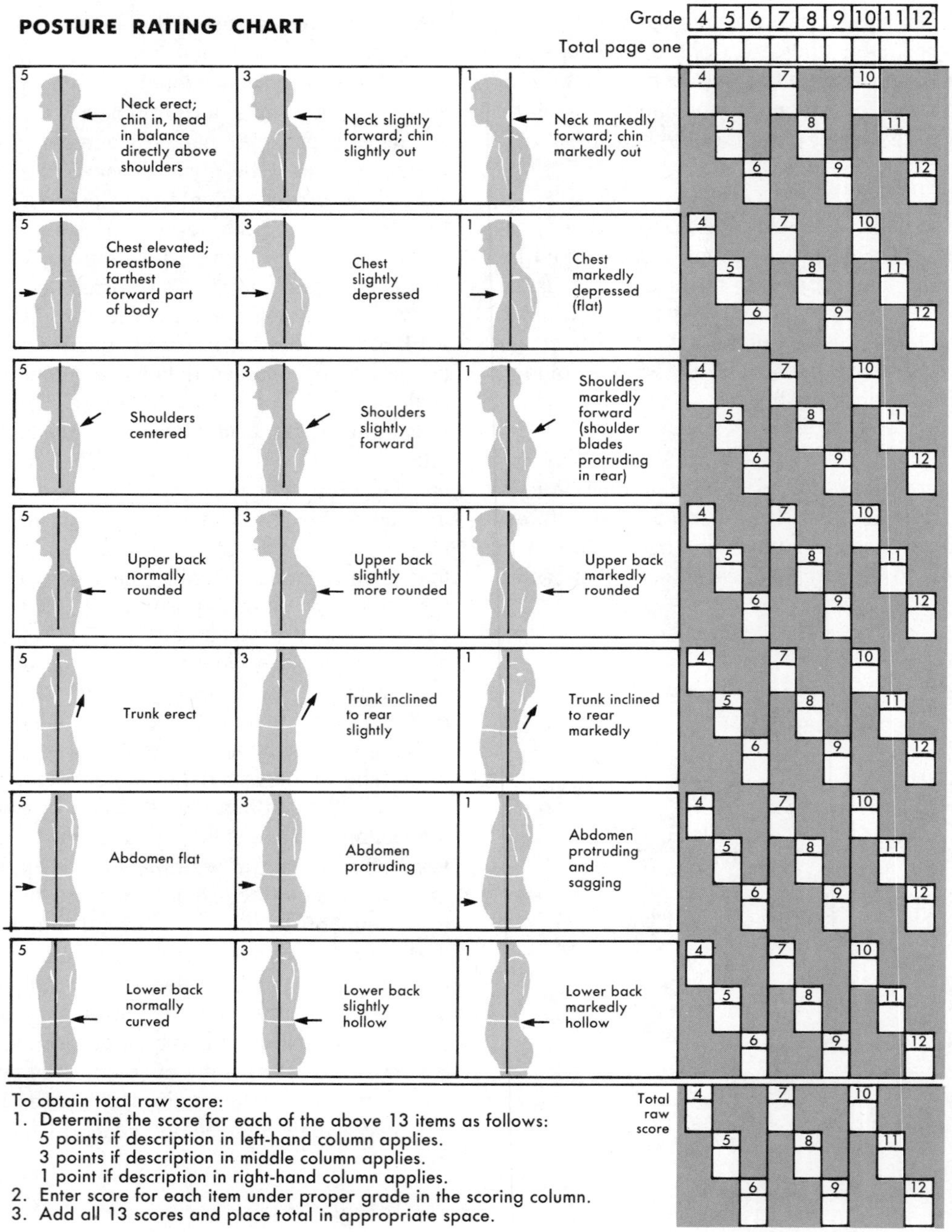

FIGURE 16-4

A lateral postural survey chart.

(Courtesy New York State Education Department.)

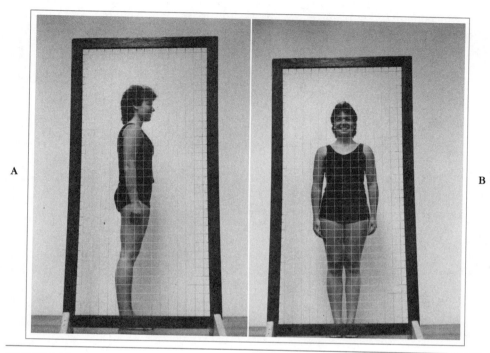

FIGURE 16-5

A, Lateral, and **B,** anterior, postural assessment with use of a screen.

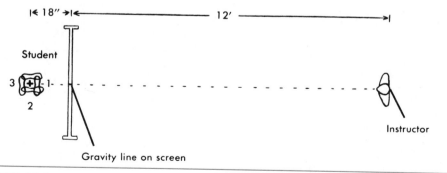

FIGURE 16-6

Alignment of posture screen as viewed from above. *1,* Anterior; *2,* lateral; *3,* posterior.

body in relationship to each other. It consists of a rectangular frame mounted on legs so that it stands upright and laced with string so that a 2-inch-square grid pattern (4- and 6-inch squares are recommended by some) crosses the frame. The vertical lines are parallel to a center (gravity) line and the horizontal lines are exactly at right angles to the gravity line. The color of the center line usually differs from that of the other strings. This makes the center line easy to identify and to use in comparison with the landmarks described previously.

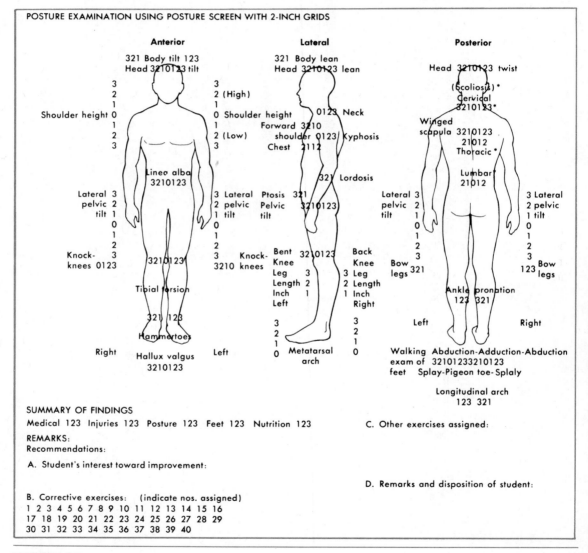

FIGURE 16-7
Data recording sheet for use with postural screen.

The posture screen should be checked for proper alignment with a plumb line to be sure that the gravity line is true and that the screen is also plumb when viewed from the side. It is then necessary to locate a point about 18 inches from the posture screen where the student will be centered properly behind the gravity line. The instructor determines this point moving to a position 10 to 15 feet away from the posture screen and standing in alignment with the center string while holding a plumb line out in front. Sighting through the plumb line and the center line of the screen, the examiner then marks a point on the floor 18 inches behind the screen. This point is in alignment with the instructor and the center line itself. Thus when the student stands behind the screen with the exterior malleoli of the ankles 1½ inches behind this point, it is possible to evaluate the posture from the anterior, posterior, and lateral views in relation to the center line of the screen.

A posture screen may be used to give quick, superficial screening examinations to identify students in need of special posture correction programs or it may be used to give very thorough examinations to students who have already been identified as requiring such programs. An example showing a three-way figure with the proper labels and with numbers to indicate the severity of the conditions discovered is shown in Fig. 16-7. With this kind of prepared examination form, the instructor can very quickly identify deviations observed through the posture grid and can record them by drawing a diagonal line through the number that indicates the severity of the condition (first degree, slight; second degree, moderate; and third degree, severe). No other writing is necessary unless the instructor identifies a problem that does not appear on the chart or wishes to record special information. The same posture form can be used for successive examinations with different colored pencils used to indicate second, third, or fourth examinations. In this way, improvement can be shown through the use of the cumulative record.

Anterior View

The student is instructed to stand directly behind the posture screen with the internal malleoli of the ankles placed 1½ inches behind and an equal distance from the mark on the floor. This will place the student in the proper position so that the surface landmarks of the body will fall in correct alignment in relation to the center (gravity) line of the screen. The student is then instructed to stand as he or she would normally. The instructor should take a position about 10 to 15 feet away from the posture screen and in direct line with the center line. The posture examination record can be mounted on a clipboard held by the examiner, or a lectern can be used to hold the forms so as to facilitate recording the findings. Since the feet serve as the base of support, it is important to examine the student from the base of support upward in checking for proper body alignment. Specific examinations for the foot, ankle, and leg will be covered in later sections of the chapter.

The feet should be checked to see if they are pointed straight forward or are toeing in or out. The longitudinal arch should be higher on its medial side than on its lateral side. The inner and outer malleoli should be about equal in prominence. The ankles and knees should be straight, with the kneecaps facing directly forward when the feet are held in the straight forward position. The height of the kneecaps should be even. The gravity line passes midway between the ankle bones, between the knees, and directly through the umbilicus, the linea alba, the center of the chin, and the center of the nose.

The symmetry of the sides of the body must then be checked. Any abnormal curvature or creasing on one side of the trunk (not found on the other side) should lead to more careful examination to determine whether a lateral sway or tilt of the body or a lateral curvature of the spine exists. Lateral spine curvature must be checked if any deviations in the position of the umbilicus exist or if there are any apparent differences in the depth of the sides of the chest. With boys, the

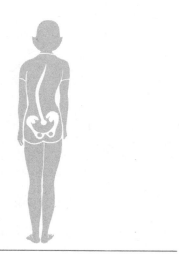

FIGURE 16-8
Lateral pelvic tilt.

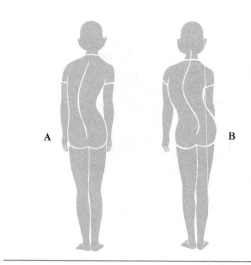

FIGURE 16-9
Scoliosis. **A,** Total left C curve. **B,** Regular S curve.

nipple levels are compared, and with both boys and girls the heights of the creases made where the arms join the body should be checked to be sure that the two creases on either side are symmetrical. It is also necessary to check to see if one arm hangs closer to the trunk than the other (Fig. 16-9). The shoulder height must be checked to see if the shoulders are level. If the pelvis is found to have a lateral tilt or if a high or low shoulder is noted, the student is then checked for lateral curvature of the spine. Although lateral curvatures do not occur with all the previously noted conditions, these types of conditions may serve as possible indicators of such a problem. The examiner next checks the head position to be sure that it aligns with the gravity line and to determine if there is any twisting of the head and neck. Finally, the total body should be viewed to determine whether it is being held in good alignment and balance and whether any lateral tilts of the total body exist.

Posterior View

The student is instructed to assume the same position in relation to the posture screen as in the anterior examination, except that the back is now turned to the screen—that is, with the inner ankle bones over the marker on the floor. The posterior examination gives the instructor an opportunity to double-check many of the conditions noted from the anterior view and to make an evaluation of certain other conditions that cannot be checked during the anterior view examination.

The gravity line passes directly up through the center of the spinous processes of each of the vertebrae, bisecting the head through its center. The posterior view is the best view for detecting scoliosis (rotolateral curvature). If a lateral curvature exists, further examinations should be made to see if there is any rotation or torque in the pelvic girdle. The degree of lateral deviation and the amount of rotation should be checked. The posture card indicates all the areas where lateral deviation of the spine could be present and provides a place to record the degree of severity. If scoliosis is suspected, the examiner can make the evaluation of the spinal column more meaningful by marking the posterior surfaces of the spinous processes of the vertebrae with a skin pencil so that the curves can be observed more accurately. The sides of the trunk are also checked as they were in the anterior view for any

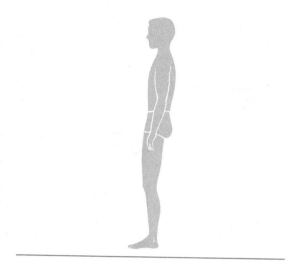

FIGURE 16-10
Posterior overhang.

abnormal unilateral curvatures and for any creases or bulges on one side only, which would indicate the presence of a tilt or of a lateral spinal curve.

The shoulder blades (or scapulae) are viewed from the posterior aspect to determine whether they are flat against the rib cage, whether the medial borders have been pulled laterally in abduction, and whether the medial borders and the inferior angles project outward from the back of the rib cage (this condition is called winged scapula).

Lateral View

For the lateral (side) view, the student stands with the left side to the screen (the side facing the screen is the one shown on the posture examination form). One foot is placed on either side of the mark on the floor, with the inner malleolus about 1½ inches behind its center. Deviations in alignment and posture can readily be observed through the screen. Abnormalities in flexion and extension of the toes may be easier to see from the side than they were from the front. The lateral examination is used to verify conditions noted in other phases of the examination.

If the student has a total forward or backward lean of the body, alignment is basically correct at all joints except the ankle, where he or she is leaning too far forward or backward. In this case, the examiner will find that the reference points become progressively farther out of alignment with each segment from the foot to the head. If the alignment is correct at the ankle and at the shoulder, but the center of the hip is too far forward, the individual has a total body sway. If the hips are too far back, the individual has a distorted position of the low back and buttocks. If the alignment is correct at the ankle, knee, and hip but the shoulder and the head are positioned too far back, the student has what is called a posterior overhang (Fig. 16-10). It is quite easy to identify these various conditions when the body landmarks are viewed in relation to the gravity line of the posture screen (Fig. 16-5). The amount of deviation is ascertained by judging the distance the affected body parts are out of alignment against one of the vertical lines. It is usually easier to evaluate these landmarks if the student places a finger on each of them so that the examiner can see them more easily.

The vertebral spine should then be checked throughout its length for what would be termed its normal curvatures. The two conditions that are noted in the region of the lower back are excessive hyperextension in the lumbar spine, a condition called lordosis, and too little curve in the lumbar spine, known as flat low back. When the lumbar spine goes into a flexion curve, it is called lumbar kyphosis. This is not observed frequently, however. Usually associated with these lower back conditions are a forward pelvic tilt (with lordosis) and a backward pelvic tilt (with a flat low back). Abdominal ptosis is often associated with these conditions, especially lordosis. Ptosis refers to a relaxation of the lower abdominal muscles with forward sagging of the abdomen often accompanied by misplacement of the pelvic organs. The degree of severity of this deviation must be judged subjectively.

In the region of the chest and shoulders, the normal curvature of the spine is one of mild flexion. The abnormal condition that would be looked for in the thoracic spine is an excessive amount of flexion, which in its severest form is called humpback. Any abnormal increase in flexion is known as kyphosis. Kyphosis is often associated with flattening of the chest and rib cage and, frequently, with deviations in the alignment of the shoulder girdle, called forward shoulders and winged scapula. Although these four conditions are often found in the same individual, they do not necessarily occur together. The winged scapula, mentioned in the discussion of the posterior examination, should be checked again from the lateral position to determine whether the inner border projects to the rear and whether the inferior angle projects outward from the rib cage. The degree of deviation in forward (round) shoul-

ders is judged subjectively and is related to how far forward of the gravity line the center of the shoulder falls.

The most common condition found in the region of the neck is a forward position of the cervical vertebrae accompanying a forward head. An abnormal amount of hyperextension in the cervical or neck vertebrae exists when the individual has attempted to correct a faulty head position by bringing the head back and the chin up.

In all the examinations described previously, the instructor must be alert to the possibility that one postural deviation often leads to or is the result of another. It is a pattern of the human body to attempt to keep itself in some semblance of a state of balance (homeostasis). Therefore, when one segment or various segments of the body be-

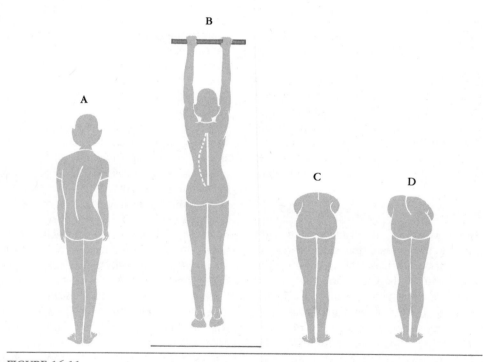

FIGURE 16-11

Test for functional-structural scoliosis. **A,** Left C-curve scoliosis. **B,** Hanging test for scoliosis. Note straight line indicates spinal position during hanging test. **C,** Adam's test showing functional scoliosis. **D,** Adam's test showing structural scoliosis.

come malaligned, it is customary for the body to attempt to compensate for this by throwing other segments out of alignment, thus obtaining a balanced position. An example of this would be the individual with lordosis who compensates with kyphosis and forward head. The individual with a simple C-shaped scoliosis curve in the spine may compensate for this with a complex S-shaped curve (an effort to return the spine and thus the body to a state of balance).

Tests for Functional or Structural Conditions

Several tests may be used to determine whether spinal curvatures are functional (involving the muscles and soft tissue) or structural (involving the bones). Postural deviations that are the result of muscle and soft tissue imbalance often disappear when the force of gravity is removed. Structural posture deviations have gone beyond the soft tissue stage, with involvement of the supportive bones and connective tissue, and are not eliminated by the removal of gravitational influences.

Prone Lying Test

The prone lying test is designed to check anteroposterior or lateral curves of the spine. Functional curves disappear or decrease when the student assumes the prone position on a bench, a table, or the floor.

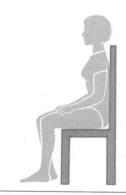

FIGURE 16-12
Good sitting posture.

Hanging Test

The hanging test has the same uses as the prone lying test. The individual hangs by the hands from a horizontal support. Functional curves disappear or are decreased in this position (Fig. 16-11, B).

Adam Test

The Adam test is used to determine whether a lateral deviation of the spine (scoliosis) is functional or structural. The student assumes a normal standing position, then gradually bends the head forward, continuing with the trunk until the hands hang close to the toes. The instructor stands a short distance behind the student and observes the student's spine and the sides of the back as the student slowly bends forward. If the spine straightens and if the sides of the back are symmetrical in shape and height, the scoliosis is considered functional (Fig. 16-11, C). Corrective procedures should be started under the direction of a physician.

If the spine does not straighten and if one side of the back (especially in the thoracic region) is more prominent (sticks up higher) than the other as the student bends forward, the scoliosis is judged to be structural (Fig. 16-11, D). In structural cases, the rotation of the vertebrae accompanying the lateral bend of the spine causes the attached ribs to assume a greater posterior prominence on the convex side of the curve. This curve does not disappear in the Adam test after changes occur in the bones of the spinal column. Structural cases must be cared for by an orthopedist.

Sitting Posture

The position of the body while sitting is similar to the position of the body while standing—that is, the head is held erect, the chin is kept in, normal anteroposterior curves are maintained in the upper and lower back, and the abdomen is flat. The hips should be pushed firmly against the back of the chair. The thighs should rest on the chair and help support and balance the body. The feet should be flat on the floor or the legs comfortably crossed at the ankles. The shoulders should be relaxed and level with the chest kept comfortably high.

Moving Posture Tests

Many persons have been critical of static posture evaluations for the following reasons:

1. Students are likely to pose in this type of examination.
2. Students may use it to obtain visual cues to correct faulty posture.
3. It does not indicate the student's habitual standing posture.
4. No attention is given to posture and alignment as they would relate to student's movements in activities.

For these reasons it is wise to include, as a part of the total posture examination, certain phases in which the students are actually in motion and during which they may or may not know that they are being examined. This may be accomplished in several different ways. One is to deploy the class for exercise, observing them as they perform during the exercise program and when they remain in a standing or sitting position between exercises. To enable the examining teacher to identify students with major deviations and to record this, either the instructor must know all the students by name or by a number or the students must be removed from the group as posture deviations are noted. Their names should then be taken so that the posture deviations noted are recorded for the proper students.

Another technique that can be used to evaluate posture and body mechanics during movement is to have the students gather in a large circle (with the teacher standing at the center or periphery of the circle) and then walk, run, or do various kinds of activities as they move continuously around the circle. The teacher or therapist identifies the children who are in special need of posture correction, removes them from the circle, and records their names along with the appropriate information regarding their posture deviations. As a part of each of these two types of examinations, especially if they are given in lieu of any type of static examination, the students should also assume a normal standing position with the teacher evaluating posture from the front, lateral, and rear views.

Walking Posture

The basic position of the body in walking is similar to that of the standing posture, but all parts of the body are also involved in moving through space. The toes face straight ahead or toe out very slightly as the leg swings straight forward. The heel strikes the ground first, with the weight being transferred along the lateral side of the bottom of the foot. The weight is then shifted to the forward part of the foot and balanced across the entire ball of the foot. The step is completed with a strong push from all the toes. The upper body should be held erect with the arms swinging comfortably in opposition to the movement of the legs. The head is held erect with the chin tucked in a comfortable position. The chest is held high, the shoulder blades are flat against the rib cage, and the shoulders are held even in height.

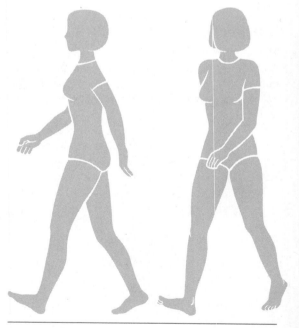

FIGURE 16-13
Good walking posture.

Persons with deviations in their sitting, standing, or moving posture and body mechanics should receive special attention so that correction of these problems becomes a part of their IEPs. Suggestions for corrective and preventive measures, for measurement, and for program adaptations are presented in this chapter as a part of the discussion of each deviation.

GUIDELINES FOR TESTING POSTURE

Gathering information on the postural characteristics of students requires many decisions. Some guidelines for testing posture follow:

1. Determine the method of posture evaluation (group or single subject).
2. Select a feasible assessment instrument (posture screen, comparative checklist, plumb line).
3. Determine a data collection procedure (notes, numerical scoring system).
4. Require children to wear as little clothing as possible during the examination.
5. Keep posture assessment equipment in correct working condition.
6. Use the correct testing procedures.
7. Have the same person administer the test on successive times.
8. Record all information accurately and indicate the date the test was given.
9. Determine accurately the location of landmarks used in measurement if they are a part of the evaluation process.
10. Standardize evaluation procedures and provide a written description of these procedures so that they can be followed on each occasion by any examiner.
11. Determine whether disorders are functional or structural.

POSTURAL DEVIATIONS: CAUSES AND CORRECTIONS

The first step for conducting a postural education program is assessment of the present level of postural functioning. If there is need of intervention,

activities need to be selected to remedy specific postural disorders. Usually weakening or lack of flexibility of specific muscle groups contributes to a specific postural disorder. Correction then involves strengthening the weak muscles and increasing flexibility of the tight muscles. Daniels and Worthingham[1] provide detailed procedures

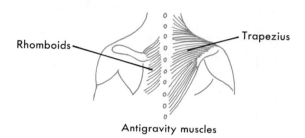

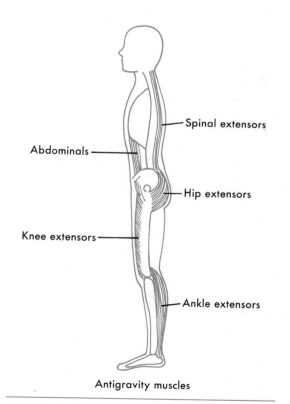

FIGURE 16-14
Antigravity muscles involved in maintaining erect posture.

for assessing the functional level of muscles that may contribute to poor posture. Procedures for strengthening weak muscles are described in Chapter 17. Garrison and Read[3] suggest that flexibility training for tight muscles is enhanced under the following conditions:

1. The stretch is carried out to the point of moderate pain.
2. There is application of increased effort at regular intervals.
3. It is done slowly and under control without development of momentum.
4. Movement of the body part proceeds through the full range.

The following sections include discussions of specific conditions as well as exercises to assist with the remediation of each condition. This should provide adequate information for teachers and therapists to plan IEPs for participants (handicapped or nonhandicapped) in their programs.

Foot and Ankle

Postural deviations of the foot and ankle can be observed while the student is standing, walking, or running. The evaluation of the foot should be made by observation from the anterior, lateral, and posterior views and should involve examination of both walking and static positions. The number of persons with deviations of the foot is large at all age levels, and the number of persons who have foot pain increases with increasing age. Muscles and joints of the foot and ankle become weakened from age and misuse. Pain associated with faulty mechanics in the use of the feet also begins to occur with increased age. The good mechanical use of the feet throughout life plus other factors such as good basic health, maintenance of a satisfactory level of physical fitness, proper choice of shoes and socks, and proper attention to any injury or accident to the foot should serve as preventive measures to the onset of weakness of ankles and feet in later life.

The foot consists of a longitudinal arch that extends from the anterior portion of the calcaneus bone to the heads of the five metatarsal bones.

The medial side of the longitudinal arch is usually considerably higher than the lateral side, which, as a general rule, makes contact throughout its length with the surface on which it is resting (Fig. 16-15, A to C). This is particularly true when the body weight is being supported on the foot. The longitudinal arch is sometimes described as two arches, a medial arch and a lateral arch, extending from the anterior aspects of the heel to the heads of the metatarsal bones. However, it is most frequently described as one long arch that is dome shaped and higher on the medial side than on the lateral side. On the forepart of the foot, in the region of the metatarsal bones, a second arch can be distinguished that runs across the forepart (ball) of the foot. This arch, called the transverse or metatarsal arch, is slightly dome shaped, being higher at the proximal ends of the metatarsal bones than at the distal ends. It often is considered a continuation of the dome-shaped long arch described previously, and thus we have just one dome-shaped arch of the foot (Fig. 16-15, D and E).

There is substantial agreement about the need for correct structures and placement of the bones, the importance of the strong ligamentous bands that help hold the bones in place to form the arches of the foot, and the need for good muscular balance among the antagonist muscles that support the foot. All these factors have an important effect on the position of the foot under both weight-bearing and non–weight-bearing conditions. A foot is considered strong and functional when it has adequate muscle strength (especially the posterior tibial muscle and the long flexor muscles of the toes) to support the longitudinal arch, when the bones have strong ligamentous and fascial bindings, and when the small intrinsic muscles are developed sufficiently to maintain proper strength of the arch in the metatarsal region.

In addition to considering the structure of the foot and ankle, it is also necessary to consider other factors such as the range of movement in the foot and ankle, the support of the body by the foot and ankle, and the effect that various posi-

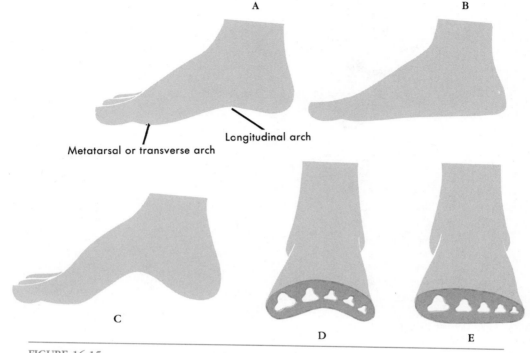

FIGURE 16-15

Arches of the foot. **A,** Normal foot. **B,** Pes planus. **C,** Pes cavus. **D,** Cross section of normal metatarsal arch. **E,** Flat metatarsal arch.

tions of the foot, ankle, knee, and hip have on the mechanics of the foot itself. A consideration of the various movements possible in the foot and ankle, together with a description of the terms used to describe these movements, should help clarify the discussion of deviations of the foot and ankle.

The ankle joint is a hinge joint and therefore only dorsiflexion and plantar flexion are possible. The numerous articulations between the individual tarsal bones and between the tarsal and metatarsal bones allow for inversion, eversion, abduction, and adduction of the foot.

Movements of the foot are as follows:

♦ *Dorsiflexion:* Movement of the top of the foot in the direction of the knee
♦ *Plantar flexion:* Movement of the foot downward, in the direction of the sole

♦ *Inversion:* Tipping of the medial edge of the foot upward, or varus (walking on the outer border of the foot)
♦ *Eversion:* Tipping of the lateral edge of the foot upward, or valgus (walking on the inner border of the foot)
♦ *Adduction:* Turning of the whole forepart of the foot in a medial direction (toeing-in)
♦ *Abduction:* Turning of the forepart of the foot in a lateral direction (toeing-out)
♦ *Pronation:* Combination of tipping of the outer border of the foot in a toeing out (eversion with abduction)
♦ *Supination:* Combination of tipping of the inner edge of the foot upward and toeing in (inversion with adduction)

It should also be remembered that it is possible to turn the foot into toed-in and toed-out po-

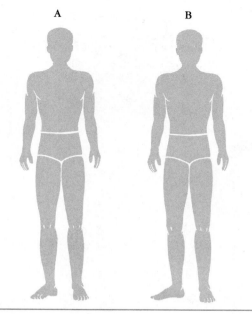

FIGURE 16-16
Abduction of the foot and leg. **A,** Abduction of the foot.
B, Toeing-out resulting from outward rotation of the hip
joint. Note difference in position of patella.

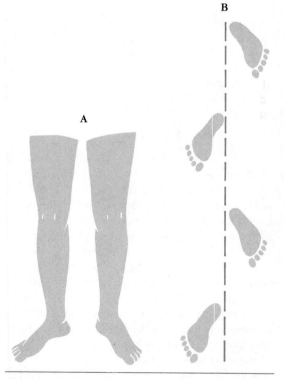

FIGURE 16-17
Improper walking. **A,** Toeing-out and walking across
medial border of the foot. **B,** Footprints show outward
rotation, or splayfoot position, while walking.

sitions by rotating the lower leg when the knee is bent and by rotating the whole leg at the hip when the knee is straight. Thus when an individual toes in or toes out while walking or standing, the examiner must determine whether this is the result of a foot deviation or a rotation of the leg. Many foot and ankle deviations are closely linked to alignment problems occurring in the leg above the ankle.

Pes Planus

Pes planus, or flatfoot, is a lowering of the medial border of the longitudinal arch of the foot. The height of this side of the longitudinal arch may range from the extremely high arch known as *pes cavus* to a position in which the medial border lies flat against the surface on which the individual is standing. When this side of the foot is completely flat, the medial border of the foot may even assume a rather convex appearance (Fig. 16-15, *A* to *C*). Pes planus may be the result of faulty bony framework, faulty ligamentous pull across the articulations of the foot, an imbalance in the pull of the muscles responsible for helping to hold the longitudinal arch in its proper position, or racial traits. The specific cause may often be linked to improper alignment of the foot and leg and to faulty mechanics in the use of the foot and ankle.

When the foot is held in a toed-out (abducted) position while standing and walking, there is a tendency to throw a disproportionate amount of body weight onto the medial side of the foot, thus causing stress on the medial side of this arch. Over a period of time, this stress may cause both a gradual stretching of the muscles, tendons, and ligaments on the medial aspect of the foot and a tightening of like structures on the lateral side. When the individual walks with the foot in the abducted position these factors are again accentuated, and in addition there is a tendency for the individual to rotate the leg medially in order to have it swing in alignment with the forward direction of the step. When the leg is swung straight in line with the direction of travel and with the foot toed-out, the individual walks across the me-

dial side of the foot with each step (Fig. 16-17). This not only weakens the foot but also predisposes the individual to a condition called tibial torsion. Since the individual is walking with the leg in basically correct alignment but with the foot abducted, malalignment results. Thus it will be found that when the legs and kneecaps face straight forward, the feet are in the abducted position, and when the feet are parallel to one another, the kneecaps are facing in a slightly medial direction (tibial torsion). This may produce strain and possibly cause a lowering of the medial side of the longitudinal arch.

Correction of pes planus must involve a reversal of the factors and conditions just described. The total leg from the hip through the foot must be properly realigned so that the weight is balanced over the hip, the knee, the ankle, and the foot itself. The antagonist muscles involved must be reoriented so that those that have become stretched (tibial muscles) are developed and tightened and those that have become short and tight (peroneal muscles) are stretched; thus the foot is allowed to assume its proper position. The muscles on the lateral side of the foot must be stretched (peroneal group). The gastrocnemius and soleus muscles, which sometimes become shortened in the case of flatfoot, exert an upward pull on the back of the calcaneus bone, thus adding to the flattening of the arch. These muscles must also be stretched whenever tightness is indicated. The major muscle group that must be shortened and strengthened is the posterior tibial muscle group, which is extremely important in terms of supporting the longitudinal arch, along with help from the long and short flexor muscles of the toes. The individual must also be given foot and leg alignment exercise in front of a mirror in order to observe the correct mechanical position of the foot while exercising, standing, walking, and otherwise using the feet (Figs. 16-18 to 16-20).

Such activities as walking in soft dirt, on grass, or in sand with the foot held in the proper position can do much to help strengthen the foot and realign it with the ankle and hip. Emphasis here should be on walking straight over the length of

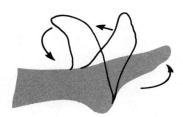

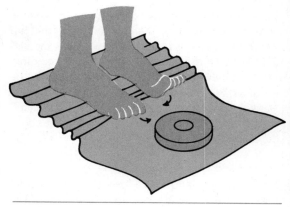

FIGURE 16-18
Foot circling.
Specific for: Metatarsal arch and toe flexors
Beneficial in: Flexibility and strength of the foot and ankle and longitudinal arch
Starting position: Sitting on bench with knees extended, shoes off, and toes pointed
Actions
1. Circle foot inward; toes extended.
2. Circle foot upward; toes extended.
3. Circle foot outward; toes extended.
4. Circle foot downward; toes flexed.
5. Repeat actions 1-4.

FIGURE 16-19
Building mounds.
Specific for: Metatarsal arch and toe flexors
Beneficial in: Flexibility and strength of intrinsic muscles of the feet
Starting Position: Sitting on a bench, feet directly under the knees, toes placed on the end of a towel.
Actions
1. Grip the towel with the toes.
2. Pull toward the body; both feet work together and build mounds; heels remain on floor.
3. Repeat movements until the end of the towel is reached.
Measurement: The amount of weight that is placed on the towel and the distance over time the weight travels

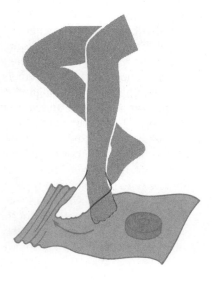

FIGURE 16-20
Foot curling.
Specific for: Metatarsal arch and toe flexors
Beneficial in: Flexibility and strength of foot and ankle and longitudinal arch
Starting position: With no shoes or socks, sitting on a bench, knees straight, heels rest on bench/mat/floor
Actions
1. Circle foot inward with toes flexed.
2. Circle foot upward with toes extended.
3. Circle foot outward; extend toes.
4. Circle foot downward while flexing toes.
5. Repeat, making full circles with the feet.
Contraindications: Should never be used for students with hammer toes
Measurement: Circumference of the circle and repetitions over time

the foot and placing the heel down first, with the weight being transferred along the outer border of the foot and with an even and equal push-off from the forepart of the foot and the five toes. In actual practice, the great toe should be the last toe to leave the surface on the push-off.

Pes Cavus

Pes cavus is a condition of the foot in which the longitudinal arch is abnormally high. This condition is not found as frequently in the general population as is pes planus. If the condition is extreme, the student is usually under the special care of an orthopedic physician. Special exercises are not usually given for the high arch unless the person has considerable associated pain, requiring special corrective procedures recommended by the physician (Fig. 16-15, C).

Pronation of the Foot

Since the ankle joint is a hinge joint allowing only plantar flexion and dorsiflexion, pronation of the ankle—as it is sometimes called—is actually a condition of pronation of the foot. As described previously, this is a combination of abduction and eversion of the foot. Since pronation involves eversion, the medial border of the foot is lowered because it is in the flat longitudinal arch. The forward part of the foot is also abducted, a condition caused by a shifting of the calcaneus bone downward and inward. (The reverse of this condition,

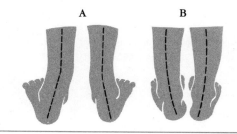

A   B

FIGURE 16-21
Faulty foot and ankle positions. **A,** Foot and ankle pronation. **B,** Supinated foot.

one that involves inversion and adduction of the forepart of the foot, is called supination of the foot.) Correction of pronation of the foot is similar to that described for pes planus or flatfoot.

Metatarsalgia

Two types of metatarsalgia may be recognized in a thorough foot examination. The first is a general condition involving the transverse (metatarsal) arch, in which considerable pain is caused by the pressure of the heads of the metatarsal bones on the plantar nerves. The second type, Morton's toe, is more specific.

General metatarsalgia. General metatarsalgia may be caused by undue pressure exerted on the plantar surface. This pressure ultimately causes inflammation and therefore pain and discomfort. Its causes relate to such factors as wearing shoes or socks that are too short or too tight, wearing high-heeled shoes for long periods of time, and participating in activities that place great stress on the ball of the foot. The mechanism of injury may result in stretching of the ligaments that bind the metatarsophalangeal joints together, therefore exerting pressure on the nerves in this area. Correction involves the removal of the cause, if this is possible, and the assignment of special exercises to increase flexibility of the forepart of the foot. Exercises are then assigned to strengthen and shorten the muscles on the plantar surface, which may aid in maintaining a normal position in the metatarsal region. The physician may prescribe special shoes or suggest that an arch support or metatarsal bar be worn to support the metatarsal region of the foot to help reduce pain.

Morton's toe. Morton's toe, often called true metatarsalgia, is more specific than the general breakdown of the metatarsal arch described previously. The onset of true metatarsalgia is often abrupt and the pain associated with it may be more intense than that found in general metatarsal weakness. In true metatarsalgia the fourth metatarsal head is severely depressed, sometimes resulting in a partial dislocation of the fourth metatarsophalangeal joint. The abnormal pressure on the plantar nerve often produces a neuritis in the area, which in turn causes intense pain and disability. Treatment consists first of the removal of the cause of the condition. The orthopedic physician will advise which procedure will follow this. Another type of Morton's toe is characterized by the presence of a second metatarsal bone longer than the first metatarsal bone.

Hammer toe

In hammer toe the proximal phalanx of the toe is hyperextended, the second phalanx is flexed, and the distal phalanx is either flexed or extended. The condition often results from congenital

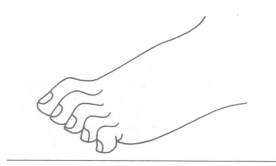

FIGURE 16-22
Hammer toe.

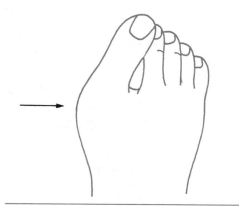

FIGURE 16-23
Hallux valgus.

causes or from having worn socks or shoes that are too short or too tight over a prolonged period of time (Fig. 16-22). Tests must be made to determine whether the condition has become structural. If the condition is functional in nature and the affected joints can be stretched and loosened, corrective measures may be taken to reorient the antagonist muscle pull involved in this deviation. The first step, however, must be the removal of the cause, and in severe cases an orthopedic physician should be consulted relative to special bracing, splinting, or operation for correction of this condition.

Hallux Valgus

A faulty metatarsal bone or shoes or socks that are too short, too narrow, or too pointed can cause a deviation of the toe known as hallux valgus. In this condition the great toe is deflected toward the other four toes at the metatarsophalangeal joint (Fig. 16-23). Correction of this condition must involve consultation with a physician. If the foot is not properly aligned and is toeing-out excessively, remedial measures should be taken to correct this alignment in order to prevent a further aggravation of hallux valgus.

Knee and Leg

Three conditions involving the knee and the upper and lower leg may be noted when a student

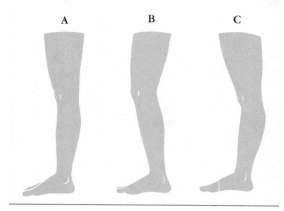

FIGURE 16-24
The knee. **A,** Normal. **B,** Bent (flexed). **C,** Hyperextended.

is examined from the anterior or posterior view. Bowlegs and knock-knees are recognized from either of these two views, whereas tibial torsion is more easily identified from the anterior view.

Other common deviations of the knee consist of hyperextension (genu recurvatum) and hyperflexion. The normal position of the knee is straight but not stiff. The student can correct forward or backward knee by realigning the pull of the muscles that control its flexion or extension and by readjusting to the proper position of the leg (Fig. 16-24). Bent knee and backward knee are often associated with flat lower back and lordosis of the lumbar spine, respectively.

Bowlegs (Genu Varum)

Bowlegs can be identified by examining a student with a plumb line, by comparing alignment of the leg with one of the vertical lines of the posture screen, or by having the student stand with the internal malleoli of the ankles touching and the legs held comfortably straight. In the last of these three tests, if a space exists between the knees when the malleoli are touching, the individual may be considered to have bowlegs. Unless this

is either a functional condition in the young child (which may be outgrown) or a condition related to hyperextension of the knees and rotation of the thighs in order to separate the knees, corrective measures ordinarily must be prescribed by an orthopedic physician. The student can correct hyperextension and rotation of the knees by assuming the correct standing position and developing proper balance in the pull of the antagonist muscles of the hip and leg (Fig. 16-25, C).

Knock-knees (Genu Valgum)

Knock-knees can be identified as described in the section on bowlegs; however, in this case, when the inner borders (medial femoral condyles) of the knees are brought together, a space exists between the internal malleoli of the ankles. Knock-knees may be related to pronation of the ankle and weakness in the longitudinal arch. Correction involves realignment of the antagonist muscles of the leg and foot, which control proper alignment (Fig. 16-25, B). This usually involves development of the outward rotators of the thigh and shortening and tightening of the structures that traverse the medial side of the leg at the knee; those on

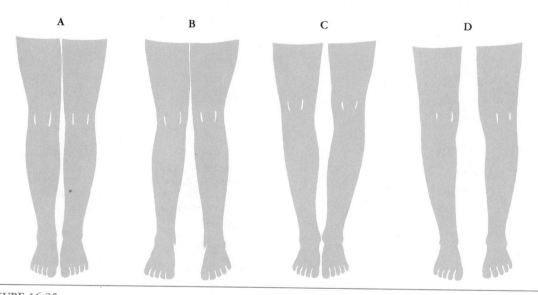

FIGURE 16-25
Leg alignment. **A,** Normal. **B,** Knock-knees. **C,** Bowlegs. **D,** Tibial torsion.

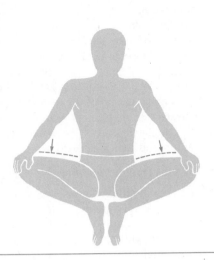

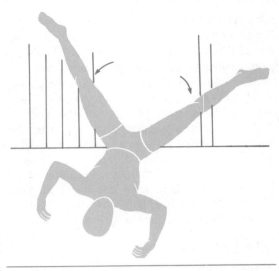

FIGURE 16-26

Hip stretching.
Specific for: Hip adductors
Beneficial in: Knock-knees
Starting position: Sitting, soles together, hands on inner surface of abducted knees
Actions
1. Push the knees toward the floor.
2. Release the pressure.
3. Repeat 1 and 2.
Measurement: The distance between the outer portion of the knee and the floor

FIGURE 16-27

Hip stretching.
Specific for: Hip adductors
Beneficial in: Knock-knees
Starting position: Lying on back, legs at right angle to trunk, and resting against a wall, arms reverse T
Actions
1. Lower the legs (abduct) as far as possible, with the knees straight.
2. Return the legs to the original position.
Measurement: The distance between the inner portion of the heels

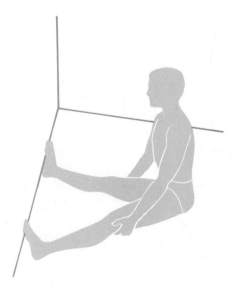

FIGURE 16-28

Hip stretching.
Specific for: Hip adductors
Beneficial in: Knock-knees
Starting position: Sitting, facing a wall, legs adducted, feet propped against the wall at right angle, hands beneath knees, knees straight
Actions
1. Bend forward with spine extended; pull trunk with arms.
2. Relax and return to starting position.
3. Repeat 1 and 2.
Measurement: (1) The distance between the inner portion of the heels; (2) distance the head is from the wall

the lateral side should be stretched. Correction of this condition also involves realignment of the foot, ankle, and hip. Knock-knees also may be related to tibial torsion.

Tibial Torsion

Tibial torsion, or twisting of the tibia, is identified by examination of the student from the anterior view. When the feet are pointed straight ahead, one or both of the kneecaps face in a medial direction, or when the kneecaps are facing straight forward, the feet are rotated in a toed-out position (Fig. 16-25, *D*). Correction of this condition involves realignment of the total leg, with emphasis being placed on the regions of the ankle, knee, and hip. The outward rotators of the hip and the thigh must be developed, whereas muscles on the medial and lateral sides of the foot and ankle must be stretched and strengthened to obtain proper alignment.

Trunk, Head, and Body
Pelvic Tilt

The normal pelvis is inclined forward and downward at approximately a 60-degree angle when a line is drawn from the lumbosacral junction to the symphysis pubis. Any variation in this angle with the pelvis tipping (tilting) downward and for-

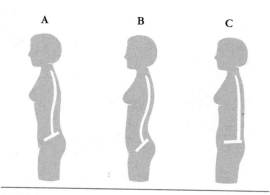

A   B   C

FIGURE 16-29
Pelvic positions. Note position of spine as pelvic position changes. **A,** Normal. **B,** Forward (downward) pelvic tilt. **C,** Backward (upward) pelvic tilt.

ward would usually result in a greater curve of the lumbar spine; by the same token, a variation in the angle with the pelvis tipping upward and backward would tend to produce a flatness in the lumbar area. Since the sacroiliac joint is basically an immovable joint and only a minimum amount of motion takes place at the lumbosacral joint, pelvic inclination and lumbar spinal curves are closely linked (Fig. 16-29). Since exaggerated spinal curves may limit normal motion in the lower back, both lordosis and flat low back require special attention.

A lateral pelvic tilt, in which one side of the pelvis is higher or lower than the other side, can be observed during anterior and posterior posture examinations. The examiner can evaluate these conditions by marking either the anterosuperior iliac spines or the posterosuperior iliac spines of the ilium and then observing their relative height through the grids of a posture screen. The examiner can also evaluate the height of the pelvis by placing his or her fingers on the uppermost portion of the crest of the ilium and by observing the relative height of the two sides of the pelvis. A lateral pelvic tilt may result from such things as unilateral ankle pronation, knock-knees, bowlegs, a shorter long bone in either the lower or upper portion of one leg, structural anomalies of the knee and hip joint and deviations in the pelvic girdle, or scoliosis. Before an exercise program for lateral pelvic tilt is initiated, the cause of the condition must be determined by a physician, who may then suggest either symmetrical or asymmetrical exercises to realign the pelvic level. The position of the pelvic girdle as viewed from the anterior or posterior view has very definite implications for the position of the spinal column as it extends upward from the sacrum. A lateral tilt of the pelvis will be reflected in the spinal column above it, since the sacroiliac and the lumbosacral joints are semi-immovable. The resulting lateral spinal curvatures are discussed in the next section of this chapter. Lateral tilt of the pelvis may also be related to a twisting of the pelvic girdle itself. This is a complicated orthopedic problem involving both hip joints, the legs, and the vertebral column. Such cases should be referred to the orthopedic physician for treatment and for advice relative to a special exercise program.

Lordosis

Lordosis is an exaggeration of the normal hyperextension in the lumbar spine. It is usually associated with tightness in the lower erector spinae (sacrospinalis), iliopsoas, or rectus femoris muscle group and either weakness or stretching of the abdominal muscles. Correction of this condition would therefore necessitate stretching and loosening of the lower erector spinae (Figs. 16-30 to 16-35), the iliopsoas (Figs. 16-36 to 38), and the rectus femoris muscles, together with assignment of exercises designed to shorten and tighten the abdominal muscle group (Figs. 16-39 to 16-44). It may also be important to develop control of the gluteal and hamstring muscle groups, which can exert a downward pull on the back of the pelvis. The development of the gluteal and hamstring muscle groups can help the individual assume a correct position while stretching, while exercising, and even while in the static standing position, but these muscles must be relaxed when the individual wishes to walk, move, or run. It is then necessary for the abdominal muscles to hold the front of the pelvis up and to maintain the desired curvature in the lower back. A condition called ptosis (visceroptosis) is often associated with a forward pelvic tilt and lordosis. This condition is characterized by sagging of the lower abdominal muscles and protrusion of the lower abdominal area. It can also be corrected by shortening, tightening, and strengthening of the abdominal muscle groups. *Text continued on p. 369.*

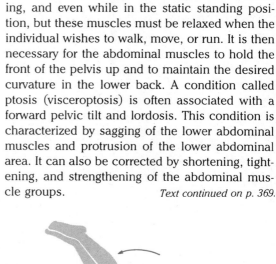

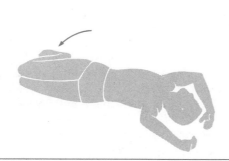

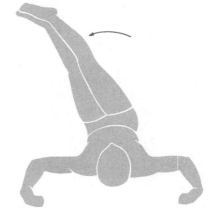

FIGURE 16-30
Spine mobilization.
Specific for: Mobilize the lower spinal area
Beneficial in: Lordosis
Starting position: Hook-lying, arms reverse T, knees flexed fully
Actions
  1. Raise both knees until thighs are vertical and shoulders flat.
  2. Lower knees to one side until they touch the floor.
  3. Repeat actions 1 and 2; legs do not fall but are controlled throughout movement.
Measurement: Repetitions over time
Sequence: Increase the distance below the hip where knees are to touch floor/mat; the closer to the hips the more difficult

FIGURE 16-31
Spine mobilization.
Specific for: Mobilize the lower spinal area
Beneficial in: Lordosis
Starting position: Lying on back
Actions
  1. Flex the knees to the chest.
  2. Straighten the knees, keeping the legs as high as possible.
  3. Lower both legs toward the floor.
  4. Return the legs to the vertical position on one side at hip level or as high as possible.
  5. Repeat 3 and 4.
Measurement: Repetitions over time
Sequence: The distance the heels strike the floor from the hips; the farther away from the hips, the easier the task

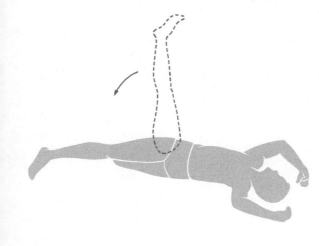

FIGURE 16-32

Spine mobilization (single leg).

Specific for: Mobilize the lower spinal area

Beneficial in: Lordosis

Starting position: Lying on back, arms reverse **T**

Actions

1. Flex one leg to a right angle.
2. Move the flexed leg so foot touches the floor on the opposite side of the body at *hip level.*
3. Return the leg to a vertical position; keep thorax as flat as possible.
4. Lower the leg to the original position.

Measurement: Repetitions over time

Sequence: Foot hits floor at lower levels down the leg

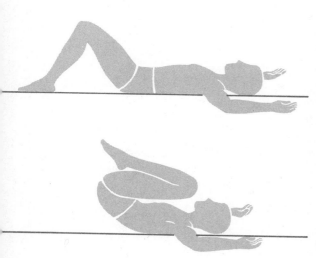

FIGURE 16-33

Knee-chest curl.

Specific for: Ptosis, lordosis, and developing abdominal strength

Beneficial in: Development of hip flexors and stretch of spinal extensors

Starting position: Lying on back with knees bent at right angles, feet flat on floor, arms straight out from shoulders, elbows bent 90 degrees, palms up

Actions

1. Bring knees toward chest by pulling with the abdominals. Curl spine segment by segment off the mat; knees touch chest or shoulders.
2. Return to starting position.
3. Repeat 1 and 2.

Measurement: Number of repetitions and distance the knees are from the chin

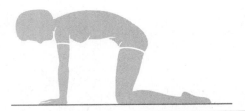

FIGURE 16-34
Mad cat.
Specific for: Lordosis and abdominal muscles
Beneficial in: Dysmenorrhea, arms, shoulders, shoulder
girdle, and low back stretch
Starting position: Kneeling on all fours
Actions
1. Hump low back by tightening abdominal and
   buttocks muscles.
2. Lean forward by bending arms until forehead
   touches the floor.
3. Repeat 1 and 2.
Measurement: The number of repetitions and the height of
the middle of the lumbar region of the spine from the
floor

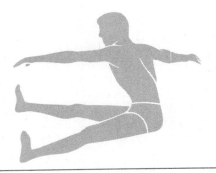

FIGURE 16-35
Arm windmill.
Specific for: Mobilizing the spine
Beneficial in: Lordosis
Starting position: Sitting position, arms out
Actions
1. Rotate the trunk at the lumbar region.
2. Rotate the trunk in the opposite direction.
Measurement: The number of degrees of rotation

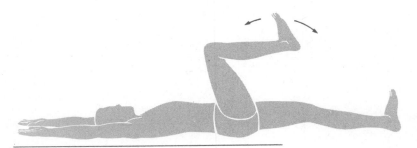

FIGURE 16-36
Specific for: Hip flexors
Beneficial in: Lordosis
Starting position: Hook-lying, arms reverse **T**
Actions
1. Flex one knee to the chest; maximal flexion.
2. Extend the opposite leg so it rests on the plinth.
Measurement: Distance the back of the knee is from the
plinth

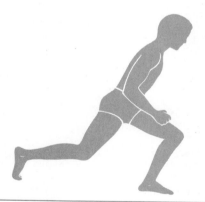

FIGURE 16-37
Stretch hip flexors.
Specific for: Hip flexors
Beneficial in: Lordosis
Starting position: Back-lying diagonal position on the
 table, outside leg hangs over the edge of the table
Action: Hold flexed knee to chest.
Measurement: Distance heel is from the floor; program
 should be built with a table a specified distance from
 the floor

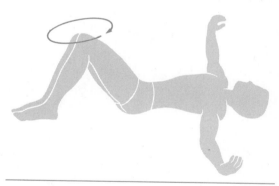

FIGURE 16-38
Lunges.
Specific for: Hip flexors
Beneficial in: Lordosis
Starting position: Kneeling, hip and knee of one leg flexed
Actions
  1. Lean trunk forward against thigh.
  2. Slide resting knee back as far as possible.
Measurement: The distance between heel of flexed leg
 and knee of rear leg; height of hip from the floor

FIGURE 16-39
Knee circles.
Specific for: Abdominals
Beneficial in: Lordosis
Starting position: Hook-lying, arms reverse T
Actions
  1. Flex the knees until the thighs are vertical and
   shoulders flat.
  2. Make circles with the knees, keeping heels close to
   the thighs.
Measurement: Repetitions
Sequence: Increase the radius of the circle to make the
 task more difficult

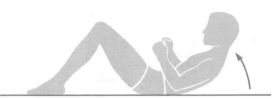

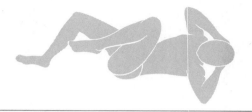

FIGURE 16-40
Abdominal curl.
Specific for: Ptosis (protruding abdomen), lordosis, and developing and shortening abdominals
Beneficial in: Forward pelvic tilt
Starting position: Lying on back, elbows at side of body and bent at 90 degrees, knees flexed, feet flat on floor
Actions
   1. Curl body forward: low back flat on mat, elbows at side bent 90 degrees
   2. Uncurl slowly and with control.
Measurement: Repetitions; the height of the nose from the floor on the sit-up
Note: In all leg raising or trunk raising from the backward lying position, the student should exhale or count aloud as legs or trunk are raised to relieve intraabdominal pressure and strain.

FIGURE 16-41
V sits.
Specific for: Abdominals
Beneficial in: Lordosis
Starting position: Hook-lying, hands behind neck
Actions
   1. Simultaneously flex one thigh toward chest and touch knee with opposite elbow so they contact at waist level.
   2. Repeat to other side.
Sequence: Reach farther with the elbow and less with the opposite knee
Measurement: Repetitions over time

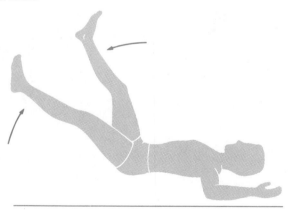

FIGURE 16-42
Straight-legged pedal.
Specific for: Abdominals
Beneficial in: Lordosis
Starting position: Back-lying, hands grasp table
Actions
   1. Flex one leg to a right angle.
   2. Simultaneously lower raised leg and raise other; pause at the end of each sweep.
   3. Repeat
Measurement: (1) Number of repetitions over time; the fewer the better; (2) the distance the legs are raised from the table

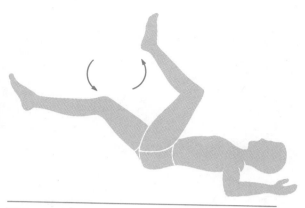

FIGURE 16-43

Bicycle.

Specific for: Abdominals and lumbar extensors

Beneficial in: Lordosis

Starting position: Hook-lying, arms in reverse T

Actions

1. Move knees to chest with low back and neck flat.
2. Extend legs upward with knees straight.
3. Flex knees and move to chest.
4. Lower flexed knees to table.

Increase difficulty: Abduct and adduct the legs when they are in extended positions.

Measurement: Repetitions over time

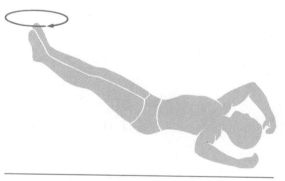

FIGURE 16-44

Leg circle (straight).

Specific for: Abdominals

Beneficial in: Lordosis

Starting position: Back-lying, legs flexed at hips, knees straight

Actions

1. Make circles with both feet; shoulders flat and heels together.
2. Repeat.

Measurement: Repetitions over time

Sequence: The distance the circles are from the floor/mat and the radius of the circle make the task more difficult.

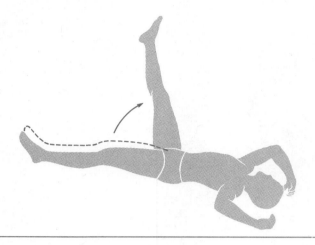

FIGURE 16-45
Leg raise (straight).
Specific for: Knee flexors (hamstrings)
Beneficial in: Flat back
Starting position: Back-lying, arms reverse **T**
Actions
1. Raise the leg with knee straight and no rotation of the thigh.
2. Return to the starting position.
3. Repeat 1 and 2.
Measurement: The distance the posterior surface of the ankle is from the iliac crest
Equipment: Feedback apparatus
Placement: Strings are in line with the iliac crest.

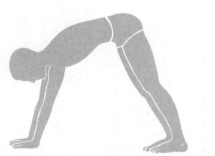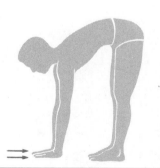

FIGURE 16-46
Walk hands to feet.
Specific for: Hamstrings
Beneficial in: Flat back
Starting position: Standing
Movement to desired position: Lean forward and rest weight on the hands with knees straight
Action: Move the hands toward the feet; heels of hands on the floor/ground and knees straight; heels on floor.
Measurement: Distance between the heel of the hands and the toes

Flat Lower Back

A flat lower back condition can develop when the pelvic girdle is inclined upward at the front, thereby decreasing the normal curvature of the lumbar spine. Often associated with this condition are tightness in the hamstring and gluteus maximus muscles, stretching of iliopsoas and rectus femoris muscles, and weakness in the lumbar section of the erector spinae muscle group. The student can correct a flat back by stretching and increasing the length of the hamstring (see opposite page), and gluteal muscles and by developing, shortening, and tightening the iliopsoas, rectus femoris, and erector spinae muscle groups.

In the correction of both lordosis and flat low back, the individual student must learn to feel what it is like to stand with the body in the correctly aligned position. It is helpful for the student to stand sideways to a regular or three-way mirror and observe the body in the correct mechanical position. A gravity line painted on the mirror or a plumb line hung down the length of the mirror will assist the student in realigning the body.

Kyphosis

Kyphosis is an abnormal amount of flexion in the dorsal or thoracic spine. An extreme amount of kyphosis is called humpback. This condition ordinarily involves weakening and stretching of the erector spinae and other extensor muscle groups in the dorsal or thoracic regions, along with shortening and tightening of the antagonist (pectoral) muscles on the anterior side of the chest and shoulder girdle. Its correction is effected primarily through stretching of the anterior muscles of the chest and shoulders, which allows the spinal extensor and shoulder girdle adductor muscle groups to be developed, strengthened, and shortened in and thus to pull the spine back into a more desirable position. Forward (round) shoulders, flat chest, and winged scapula are often associated with kyphosis.

Forward (Round) Shoulders

Forward shoulders is a condition involving an abnormal position of the shoulder girdle. This

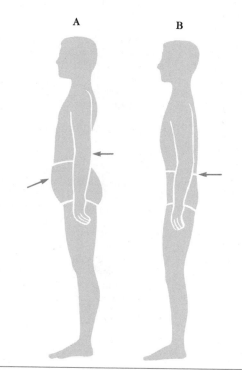

FIGURE 16-47
A, Ptosis and lordosis. **B,** Flat back.

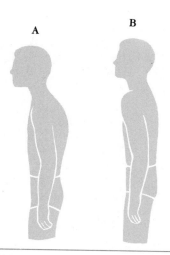

FIGURE 16-48
A, Kyphosis. **B,** Forward or round shoulders.

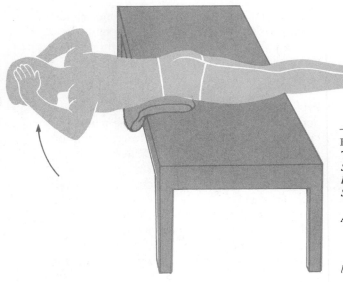

FIGURE 16-49

Trunk raises.

Specific for: Thoracic extensors

Beneficial in: Kyphosis

Starting position: Prone lying, trunk hanging over the edge of a table, hands behind neck

Actions
1. Raise trunk to a horizontal position.
2. Lower the trunk so head is supported on a chair.
3. Repeat.

Measurement: (1) number of repetitions, (2) amount of weight placed on head, (3) distance of the repetition (distance between chair and table)

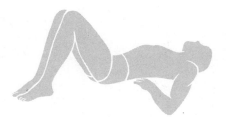

FIGURE 16-50

Neck, back, and shoulder flattener.

Specific for: Forward head, cervical lordosis, kyphosis, forward shoulders, and lordosis

Beneficial in: Pelvic tilt

Starting position: Lying on back, knees drawn up, arms at sides with palms down

Actions
1. Inhale and expand chest as nape of neck is forced to mat by stretching tall and pulling chin toward chest.
2. Flatten small of back to mat by tightening abdominal and buttocks muscles.
3. Neck and back are flat on mat. Fingers cannot pass under neck. As it becomes easier to flatten back, the exercise may be made more difficult and more beneficial by gradually extending legs until the low back cannot be maintained in a flattened position.

Measurement: Number of repetitions

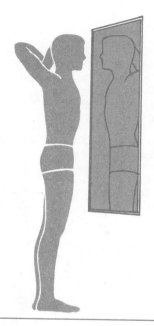

FIGURE 16-51

Neck flattener at mirror.

Specific for: Forward head, kyphosis, forward shoulders, lordosis, and shoulder development

Beneficial in: Total anteroposterior postural deviations

Starting position: Standing tall in front of mirror, head up, chin in, elbows extended sideward at shoulder level, fingertips behind base of head

Actions

1. Draw head and neck backward vigorously as fingers are pressed forward for resistance and elbows are forced backward (flattening upper back). Inhale.
2. Flatten low back by tucking the pelvis by tightening the abdominals and hip extensors.
3. Hold; exhale; return to starting position. (Student can stand facing the mirror or with side of body toward mirror to check body position and to correct either anteroposterior or lateral posture deviations.)

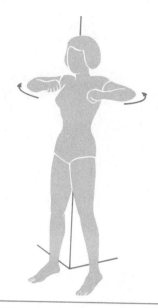

FIGURE 16-52

Breaking chains.

Specific for: Forward shoulders

Beneficial in: Kyphosis, flat chest, forward head, lordosis, and shoulder development

Starting position: Standing, with back against corner of post or sharp edge of corner of a room, feet 6 inches apart; place fists together in front of chest with elbows at shoulder level

Actions

1. Pull fists apart, keeping elbows at shoulder level; pinch shoulder blades together.
2. Inhale.
3. Tuck pelvis and press low back to wall as close as possible.
4. Hold position for 10 seconds.
5. Repeat.

Measurement: Repetitions

Caution: Keep abdomen and buttocks tight and maintain body in starting plane during the exercise; when lordosis is present, the exercise may be done in sitting position with legs crossed in tailor's position.

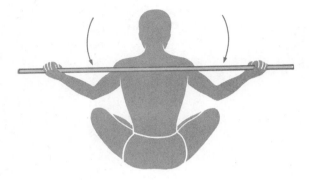

FIGURE 16-53
Pectoral stretch (wand).
Specific for: Pectorals
Beneficial in: Round shoulders
Starting position: Sitting, grasp wand with hands, arms
   extended overhead
Actions
   1. Lower the wand to the shoulders; good extension of
      neck and spine by flexing arms.
   2. Return the wand to the starting position with arms
      straight.
Measurement: Distance between the inner portions of the
   hands

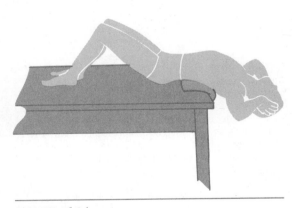

FIGURE 16-54
Pectoral stretch (lying).
Specific for: Pectorals
Beneficial in: Kyphosis
Starting position: Back-lying, hands behind the neck, edge
   of a table across the base of the scapula
Actions
   1. Simultaneously lean trunk back and down toward
      the floor, adduct the scapula, and extend the
      cervical spine.
   2. Relax to the starting position.
   3. Repeat.
Measurement: The distance the elbows are from the floor;
   the program should be developed with specific
   measurement of the height of the table

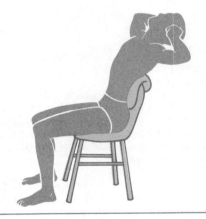

FIGURE 16-55
Pectoral stretch (sitting).
Specific for: Pectorals
Beneficial in: Kyphosis
Starting position: Sitting in a chair, hands behind the neck
   (touch head)
Actions
   1. Simultaneously lean trunk backward, extend upper
      spine, adduct the scapula, and pull arms backward.
   2. Relax to starting position.
Measurement: The distance the elbows are from the
   ground/floor

condition usually exists when the anterior muscles of the shoulder girdle (pectoral muscles) become shortened and tightened and the adductor muscles of the shoulder girdle (rhomboid and trapezius muscles) become loose, weak, and stretched. It is often associated with a flat chest and kyphosis. The basic means of correction of this condition are to stretch and loosen the anterior muscles of the chest shoulder girdle and to develop, strengthen, and shorten the adductor muscles of the shoulder girdle.

The student with kyphosis or forward shoulders should also practice standing and sitting in good alignment in front of a mirror to get the feeling of what is is like to hold the body comfortably in proper balance. When the correct position becomes easy and natural, the student will no longer have to rely on the mirror and the visual cues associated with its use.

Kypholordosis

Kypholordosis is a combination of kyphosis in the upper back and lordosis in the lower portion of the spine. Often one of these deviations is a compensation for the other and involves the body's attempt to keep itself in balance. Correction of kypholordosis consists of the same basic principles involved in correcting the individual conditions described previously; however, time can often be saved in the exercise program by assigning certain exercises that are beneficial for the correction of both conditions.

Flat Upper Back

A flat upper back is the opposite of a kyphotic spine and involves a decrease or absence of the normal anteroposterior spinal curve in the dorsal or thoracic region. Stretching of the posterior muscles of the upper back allows the antagonist muscles on the anterior side of the body to be developed and shortened and thus is beneficial for this condition.

Winged Scapula

Winged scapula is a condition that involves the abduction or protraction of the shoulder blades (the medial border of the affected scapula being farther from the spinal column than normal). Projection of the medial border of the scapula posteriorly and protrusion of the inferior angle are other concomitants of this condition (Fig. 16-57). Winged scapula is very common among children,

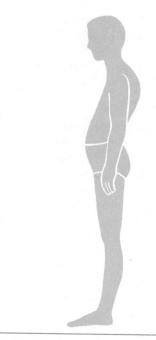

FIGURE 16-56
Fatigue slump with kypholordosis.

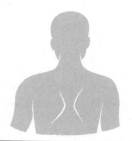

FIGURE 16-57
Winged scapula.

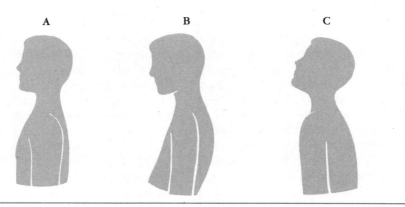

FIGURE 16-58
A, Normal head position. **B,** Forward head. **C,** Cervical lordosis.

who exhibit it especially when their arms are raised forward to the shoulder level. This results from lack of shoulder girdle strength; ordinarily, the condition will be outgrown as the children begin to participate in hanging and climbing activities for the development of the muscles of the shoulder girdle. In adolescents and young adults the condition involves unequal pull on the antagonist muscles of the shoulder girdle; corrective measures may be necessary. In general, the procedure would be to stretch and loosen the anterior muscles of the shoulder girdle and to develop the adductors of the scapula, involving both the trapezius and the rhomboid muscles. Developmental exercises for the serratus anterior muscle also are necessary, since it has a major responsibility for keeping the scapula in the correct position flat against the rib cage.

Forward Head

Forward head is one of the most common postural deviations. It often accompanies kyphosis, forward shoulders, and lordosis. Two factors are involved in analyzing the causes of forward head and correcting it. The extensors of the head and neck are often stretched and weakened because of the habitual malposition of the head (Fig. 16-58). Correcting this condition involves bringing the head into proper alignment, with the chin tucked so that the lower jaw is basically in line with the ground and so that it is not tipped up when the head is drawn back. This involves reorientation of the head and neck so that the individual knows what it feels like to hold the head in the correct position. The antagonist muscles involved must be reeducated to hold the head in a position so that the lobe of the ear approximates a position in line with the center of the shoulder.

Cervical Lordosis

Cervical lordosis may result from an attempt to compensate for other curves occurring at a lower level in the spinal column or from incorrect procedures in attempting to correct a forward head. The spinal extensors are often tight and contracted so that the head is tilted well back and the chin is tipped upward (Fig. 16-57, C). As in the case of forward head, a reeducation of the antagonist muscles and the proprioceptive centers involved is necessary so that the lower jaw is held in line with the ground. In the correction of cervical lordosis and forward head, the student must learn to assume the proper position and must exercise in front of a mirror in order to recognize this position.

Posterior Overhang (Round Swayback)

In posterior overhang, the upper body sways backward from the hips so that the center of the shoulder falls behind the gravity line of the body. To compensate for this position, the hips and thighs may move forward of the gravity line, the head may tilt forward, and the chest may be flat. Correction of posterior overhang involves reorientation of the total body so that its several parts are returned to a position of alignment. The student is instructed to work in front of a mirror and align the body with a gravity marker on the mirror. As an alternative, the instructor may check and correct the student's posture. The exercise program includes reeducation of the antagonist muscles to enable the student to return the body to a position of balance. The muscle groups needing special attention are the abdominal muscles, the antagonist muscle groups responsible for anteroposterior alignment of the tilt of the pelvis, the adductor muscles of the shoulder girdle, and the extensor muscles of the upper spine. The student must stand tall, with chin tucked and abdomen flat, to correct this condition.

Scoliosis

Scoliosis is rotolateral curvature of the spine. When viewed from the front or from the rear, a scoliotic spine has a curvature to one side; in advanced stages it may curve both to the left and to the right. Scoliotic curves are ordinarily described in relation to their position as the individual is being viewed from the rear. A curvature is described as a simple C curve to the left or right. In a more advanced stage compensation above or below the original curve may occur, and the resulting curvature is described as a regular S curve or a reverse S curve. Examples of scoliotic curves are shown in Fig. 16-60.

Initially, a lateral deviation of the spine may involve only a simple C curve to the left or right in any segment of the spine, depending on the cause of the problem, the resulting change in soft tissues, and the pull of the antagonist muscles. These curves are often functional in nature and thus are correctable through properly assigned stretching and developmental exercises under the guidance of a physician. Untreated spines often become progressively worse, involving permanent structural changes.

Scoliosis is often caused by asymmetry of the body. Lateral pelvic tilt, low shoulder, asymmetrical development of the rib cage, or lateral deviation of the linea alba may be a cause or effect of rotolateral curve of the spine. Evidence of this would be found in one or more of the following body changes:

1. When the thoracic vertebral column is displaced laterally, the rotation of the vertebral bodies is in the direction of the convexity of the curve.
2. Lateral bending of the spine is accompanied by a depression and protrusion of the intervertebral discs on the concave side, with a greater separation between the sides of the vertebrae on the convex side of the lateral curve.
3. There is an imbalance in the stability and pull of the ligaments and muscles responsible for holding the vertebral column in its normal position. Muscles and ligaments on the concave side become tight and contracted, whereas those on the convex side become stretched and weak. Muscle atrophy may occur.
4. Changes in the rib cage involve flattening and depression of the posterior aspects of the ribs on the concave side, with a posterior bulging of the ribs on the side of the convex spinal curve. The opposite is true of the anterior aspect of the chest. There the ribs on the concave side are prominent, whereas they are flattened or depressed on the convex side.

During the past several years, orthopedic physicians have stressed the importance of identifying and treating scoliosis in young children between the ages of 9 and 14 years. Early detection by physical education teachers, therapists, and nurses and immediate referral to a physician who

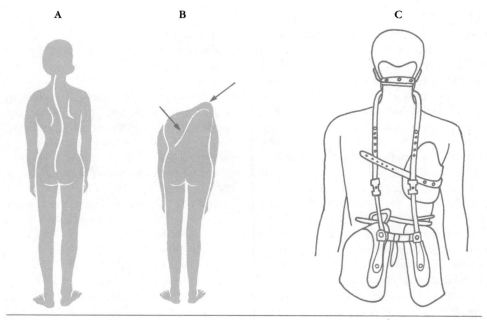

FIGURE 16-59
Scoliosis. **A,** Rotolateral curve. **B,** Rotation viewed from Adam's position. **C,** Milwaukee brace.

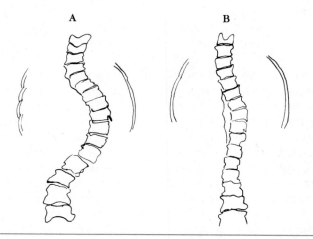

FIGURE 16-60
Severe scoliosis. **A,** Before surgery. **B,** After surgery and corrective procedures.

specializes in scoliosis treatment may prevent permanent deformity in many of these young persons.

The treatment of scoliosis is rather specific, depending on the cause of the condition and the resulting changes in the spinal column. Students with scoliosis must be referred to an orthopedist for examination and recommendations relative to stretching and developmental exercises, which may be either symmetrical or asymmetrical in nature. Some orthopedic physicians believe that the treatment of scoliosis should be very specific and indicate the types of asymmetrical exercises to be performed by the student. Others subscribe to the theory that the cause of scoliosis should be eliminated if possible, but that only symmetrical types of exercise should be assigned for this condition.

Since scoliosis is very complicated and difficult to diagnose and treat, it is necessary for the adapted teacher or therapist to rely on the advice of the physician concerning the types of activities and exercises that should be prescribed for the student. Since lateral spinal curves are accompanied by a certain amount of rotation of the spine, a great deal of skill is required to diagnose and treat the condition correctly. Recommendations relative to types of games, sports, and activities should therefore be made by the examining physician.

Treatment may consist of use of casts or braces (Fig. 16-59, C) combined with a special exercise program assigned by the physician. Exercise programs without the cast or brace are not usually recommended. Cases that are not discovered early may require operation with spinal fusion or the insertion of rods along the vertebral column to straighten the severely curved spine (Fig. 16-60).

Physicians at the Los Angeles Orthopedic Hospital and the Orange County Orthopedic Hospital in California have successfully treated large numbers of children and have spearheaded campaigns to provide for early diagnosis of this serious problem.

Treatment of patients with severe scoliosis may include any or all of the following:

1. Removal of the cause, if possible
2. Assignment of symmetrical exercises, especially for the abdomen, back, and hip regions
3. Mobilization of tightness in soft tissue in the trunk, shoulder girdle, and hip region
4. Assignment of asymmetrical exercises to tighten muscles on the convex side of the curves on the recommendation of an orthopedic physician
5. Recommendation of traction of the spine by the physician
6. Assignment of exercises to increase the strength, anteroposterior balance, and alignment of the spine
7. Specific prescription of any derotation exercises by the physician

Physical educators who specialize in adapted physical education and specialists in therapeutic recreation should inform those teaching regular physical education, the school nurse, and other health-related personnel of the importance of early screening of young persons to detect scoliosis and other body mechanics problems. The students can then be involved in preventive programs under the guidance of a physician who specializes in the diagnosis and care of scoliosis and other serious orthopedic problems.

Shoulder Height Asymmetry

It is rather common for an individual to have one shoulder higher or lower than the other. This condition usually results from asymmetrical muscle or bone development of the shoulder girdle or lateral curvature in the spinal column. Correction of an abnormal curve in the spine may result in the return of the shoulders to a level position, although special exercises may be required in the process. When the cause is faulty muscle development, correction is a relatively simple matter of developing the strength of the weaker or higher side and stretching the contracted side. This also involves a reorientation of the student's feeling for the correct shoulder and body alignment. Exercises for a low or high shoulder should be performed in front of a regular or three-way mirror to

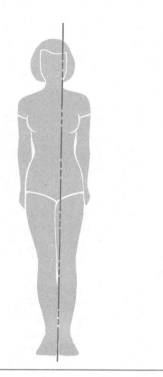

FIGURE 16-61
Body tilt.

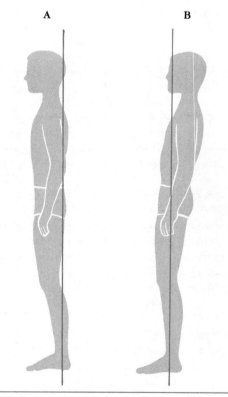

FIGURE 16-62
Total body forward **(A)** and backward **(B)** leans (plumb line test).

enable the student to recognize the position of the body when it is being held in proper alignment.

Head Tilt or Twist

When viewed from the anterior or posterior view, the head may be either tilted directly to the side or tilted to the side with a concomitant twisting of the neck. In either case, it is necessary to reorient the student to the proper position of the head. Often, deviations in the position of the head and neck are compensatory for other postural deviations located below this area. The correction of these conditions involves reorientation to the proper position of the head. This entails reeducating the antagonist muscles responsible for holding the head in a position of balance, plus reorienting the student in terms of holding the head in the correct position, which will activate the appropriate proprioceptive centers and balance organs. The exercise program for correction of the condition should be rather specific in terms of the muscle groups that are stretched and developed. Moreover, the student should practice the exercise program standing in front of a mirror so that he or she can visualize the correct position and develop the feeling of holding the head in correct alignment.

Body Tilt

Another deviation that may be noted in the anterior and posterior posture examinations is a problem of body alignment in which the total body is tilted to the left or right of the gravity or plumb line (Fig. 16-61). Standing with the body tilted to the side causes increased strain on the bones, joints, and muscles and may result in compensation being made to bring the body back into a position of balance over its base of support. Often, this compensation results in the hips and shoulders being thrown out of alignment, leading to the development of lateral curvature in the spine. Correction of this condition involves an analysis of the causative factors of the tilt, such as unilateral flatfoot, pronated ankle, knock-knee,

or short leg. On the other hand, standing out of balanced alignment may be habitual with the student. Before correction of the lateral body tilt can be accomplished, unilateral deviations must be corrected. Specific suggestions for the correction of a weak foot, ankle, or knee are contained in another section of this chapter. Together with these specific corrective measures, exercises should be given to the student for body tilt. Exercises and activities that involve the symmetrical use of the total body and that will help the student learn to stand with body in correct alignment and balance are needed. Exercising in front of the mirror will give the student a visual concept of the feeling of standing with the body in a balanced position, which should help to effect a correction of a lateral tilt of the body.

Body Lean

When viewed from the side, the total body may lean a considerable distance either forward or backward of the line of gravity. When the total body is in good alignment but leans forward or backward from the ankle so that the lobe of the ear is positioned either anterior or posterior to the gravity line, the condition is considered to be a total body lean (Fig. 16-62). If the body lean is not corrected, as the individual attempts to compensate for the lean and bring the body back into a balanced standing position, the body often will be transferred into one or more of the postural conditions discussed previously. Correction of the forward or backward lean of the total body is primarily a matter of reorientation of the proprioceptive centers of the body to enable the individual to feel when the body is in correct alignment in the standing position. Checking the forward or backward deviation of the body against a gravity line or a plumb line hung vertically before a three-way mirror is an excellent way for the student to recognize the feel of standing with the body in the correct position. Symmetrical exercises can then be assigned so that the student can develop the flexibility and strength necessary to hold the body in correct alignment.

SUMMARY

Good posture contributes to the well-being of the body and gives the impression of enthusiasm and self-confidence. There are good postures for sitting, standing, and walking. Antigravity muscles that are weak and stretched and reciprocal muscles that shorten are often the functional causes of poor posture. The procedure for ameliorating poor posture is as follows: (1) know the model of good posture, (2) assess the individual against the model of normal posture for deficiency, (3) identify the specific muscles that need to be strengthened or loosened, and (4) conduct the IEP to develop the deficient muscles. The specific areas to be assessed for postural abnormalities are the foot, ankle, leg, hips, anteroposterior aspect of the spinal column, lateral aspect of the spinal column, shoulders, and head and neck. Tests and measurements can be used in adapted physical education to evaluate improvement, aid in instruction, determine whether body parts are properly aligned, and motivate students to work toward correction of body malalignment. Some of the tests and measurements traditionally used in adapted physical education programs are not highly valid or reliable but may still be of some use in identifying deviations, helping the instructor explain malalignments to students, and motivating students to work toward self-improvement. If any or all of these values are obtained from testing, it should be a worthwhile part of the total program. The data thus obtained are used to formulate specific performance objectives for each person and to aid in the development of the IEP.

The physician and the physical educator may diagnose and prescribe physical activity for school-age children with postural disorders. If a physician diagnoses a postural disorder and prescribes treatment, this should be noted in the child's school health record. All activity that has been contraindicated by the physician should be noted by the physical educator. Under these conditions there should be close communication between the physical educator and the physician.

When postural conditions are of structural origin, surgical techniques can usually improve mechanical alignment. Thus remedies for postural conditions that are structural in nature are under jurisdiction of the medical profession. On the other hand, postural conditions caused by soft tissue and functional defects may respond to physical fitness programs to increase strength and flexibility of specific muscles as directed by physical educators. Postural education regarding functional disorders requires specially designed instruction to meet the postural needs of children as set forth in IEPs. In accordance with regulations for engaging "related services," if children do not respond or benefit from the postural education programs, they should be referred to a physician.

REVIEW QUESTIONS

1. What are the values of a postural education program?
2. What are the positions from which posture may be evaluated?
3. Can you list some deviations of the foot and the ankle? What activities might be used to ameliorate the conditions?
4. What are some disorders of the legs? How would one go about correcting the deficiencies?
5. Can you describe lordosis and identify activities that may remedy the condition?
6. Can you describe postural deviations of the upper back and scapula and indicate activities that may assist in correcting the muscles which contribute to the deficiencies?
7. How would you treat abnormal postural conditions of the head and neck?
8. Can you describe the different scoliotic curves and suggest activities to treat the disorders?
9. Can you describe tests to determine deviations of the foot and ankle, leg, pelvis, and spine?
10. How would you determine whether a postural deviation is structural or functional?

STUDENT ACTIVITIES

1. Examine a peer for postural deficiencies and indicate activities that may assist the individual to better his or her posture.
2. Visit a home for the aged and assess the posture of some of the clients. Analyze each segment of the body in terms of good alignment and indicate appropriate activities for the individual.
3. Teach your peers some postural activities. Specify the manner in which the activities are to be performed and identify the muscles that are to benefit from the activity.
4. Visit a teacher who conducts a postural education program. Are there individual postural education programs and postural objectives for each child? Do the activities that children are performing match the assessment information?
5. Have three persons evaluate an individual's postural fitness. Indicate differences and agreement on the evaluation of each of the areas of the postural assessment.

REFERENCES

1. Daniels, L., and Worthingham, C: Muscle testing: techniques of manual examination, Philadelphia, 1982, W.B. Saunders Co.
2. Fairbanks, B.L.: Vigor and vitality, Salt Lake City, 1982, Hawkes Publishing Inc.
3. Garrison, L., and Read, A.K.: Fitness for every body, Palo Alto, Calif., 1980, Mayfield Publishing Co.
4. Miller, D.K., and Allen, T.E.: Fitness: a lifetime commitment. Minneapolis, 1982, Burgess Publishing Co.
5. Sherrill, C.: Adapted physical education and recreation, ed. 2, Dubuque, Iowa, 1985, Wm. C. Brown Co., Publishers.
6. Sherill, C.: Posture training as a means of normalization, Ment. Retard. **18:**135-138, 1980.

SUGGESTED READING

Daniels, L.: Therapeutic exercises for body alignment and function, ed. 2, Philadelphia, 1977, W.B. Saunders Co.

CHAPTER 17

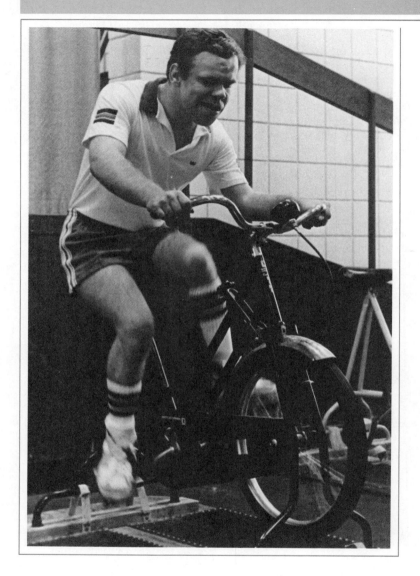

Physical Development

OBJECTIVES

♦ Know the causes of poor physical fitness and the purposes of physical fitness programming.

♦ Know how to determine a unique physical fitness need.

♦ Know the difference and relationships between abilities and skills.

♦ Know the physical and motor fitness taxonomy and psychomotor taxonomy.

♦ Know how to construct a progressive resistive exercise program and an interval training program.

♦ Understand the problems associated with overweight, underweight, and obesity.

♦ Understand the problems of physical fitness in the elderly.

One of the objectives of physical educators is to develop in their students the physical characteristics necessary to perform the activities of daily living without undue fatigue. Furthermore, the outcome of the development of these physical characteristics is the ability to perform motor skills competently.

The physical and motor underdevelopment and low vitality of handicapped persons constitute a major concern of physical education. Chronically ill persons with debilitating conditions are particularly prone to poor physical vitality and development. Persons with cardiorespiratory conditions such as chronic bronchitis and various heart defects also tend toward poor physical fitness and are a special challenge to the physical education instructor. Handicapped children as well as normal children often lack the physical and motor abilities prerequisite to successful participation in sports and the activities of daily living. This chapter includes a discussion of physi-

cal and motor fitness and special problems demonstrated by undernourished, obese, and elderly persons.

DEFINITION

It is important for handicapped children to move as efficiently as possible. To move efficiently a person must possess both physical fitness and motor fitness. Physical fitness is maintaining appropriate levels of muscular strength, joint flexibility, muscular endurance, and cardiovascular endurance to carry out everyday activities. Motor fitness is achieving the agility, balance, and coordination levels necessary to perform tasks and skills such as running, jumping, playing basketball, and playing soccer. Both physical fitness and motor fitness are important prerequisites to participation in movement activities, therefore both must be considered when programs for handicapped individuals are being developed.

THE FITNESS CONTINUUM

There are three purposes of physical fitness: to promote and maintain health, to develop prerequisites for functional motor skills for independent living, and to develop prerequisites for sport and leisure skills.

According to Falls, Baylor, and Dishman,[4] health-related fitness refers to those aspects of physiological and psychological functioning that are believed to offer protection against degenerative conditions such as obesity and coronary heart disease. Also, health-related fitness includes the ability to maintain proper postural alignment.

Physical fitness for the purpose of performing daily living, sport, and leisure skills refers to developing and maintaining levels of stength, flexibility, and muscular and cardiovascular endurance to contribute to the agility, balance, coordination, and stamina needed to participate in those tasks.

Severely handicapped persons need to develop physical fitness to be able to lift the head, roll over, maintain a sitting position, and achieve

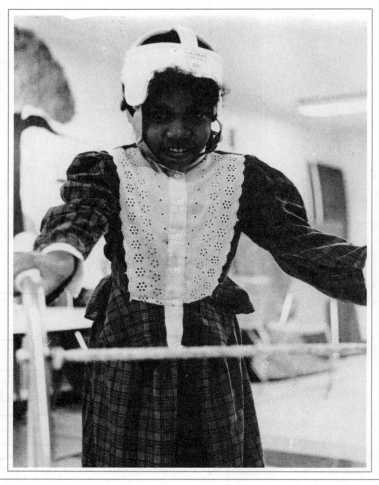

FIGURE 17-1
A handicapped child uses a walker for support because of a lack of strength in the legs.
(Courtesy Children's Rehabilitation Center, Butler, Pa.)

range of motion in the joints. For less severely handicapped individuals, development of physical fitness can contribute to the ability to walk, engage in sports, or swim.

Because a person needs basic levels of physical fitness before agility, balance, and coordination can be developed, it can be said that physical fitness is prerequisite to motor fitness. Once minimal levels of physical fitness are achieved, development and use of motor fitness can contribute to additional physical fitness development. That is, once an individual begins to use agility, balance, and coordination in daily living activities and games and sports, physical fitness levels continue to rise.

FACTORS CONTRIBUTING TO POOR FITNESS

There are several factors that contribute to poor physical and motor fitness. Low physical fitness levels are caused by obesity, asthma and other chronic respiratory problems, susceptibility to infectious diseases including the common cold, poor nutrition, inadequate sleep, and a life-style that does not include physical exercise.

Low motor fitness levels can result from abnormal reflex development; delayed vestibular function; poor vision; delayed cross-lateral integration, spatial awareness, body image; and any other factor that limits the ability to move efficiently.

Before a physical educator can decide how best to improve physical and motor ability, present levels of performance must be determined through evaluation.

EVALUATING PHYSICAL AND MOTOR FITNESS

The full evaluation of a handicapped child's physical and motor fitness requires comprehensive as-

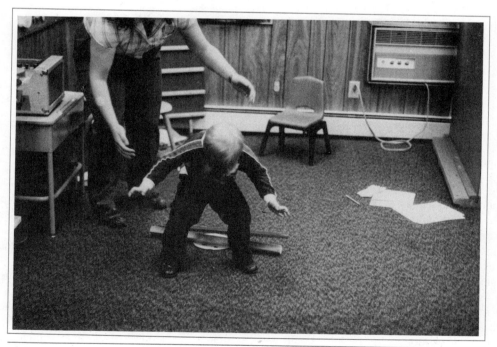

FIGURE 17-2
A child vault-jumps over two sticks a specific distance apart, which is commensurate with his ability.

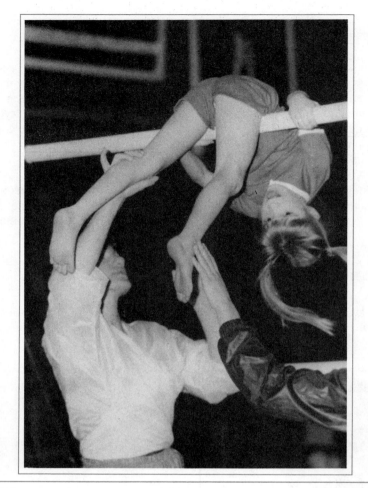

FIGURE 17-3
Pulling one's body over a bar for a gymnastics task requires practice and many physical and motor ability prerequisites.

sessment of ability areas identified through research (see Chapter 4). One does not just measure strength as a single entity. Rather, one measures the strength of specific muscle groups such as the knee extensors, elbow flexors, or abdominal muscles. In the same manner, when flexibility is evaluated it is necessary to determine range of motion at specific joints in the body. A severe loss of strength in any muscle group or limited range of motion in any joint could seriously affect the attainment of specific daily living or sport skills. Thus a full evaluation of physical education needs would involve assessing the strength of major muscle groups, range of motion of many joints, and factors that affect cardiovascular efficiency.

The procedures for determining educational needs have been previously described. In review, an educational need is determined by identifying a discrepancy between an individual's performance on a physical or motor fitness task and normative expectations for that task. For example,

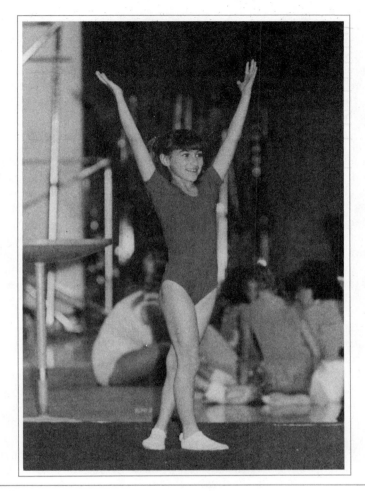

FIGURE 17-4
A child has just completed a gymnastics routine, which requires sound development of physical and motor prerequisites.

if the normative expectation of a 6-year-old child's long jump is 60 inches, but the child can only jump 45 inches, then long-jumping ability needs to be developed. Thus full evaluation to determine the unique needs of an individual is based on discrepancy between actual performance and normative performance.

It should be obvious that there is seldom enough time or personnel in a school system to comprehensively assess every child. Therefore, the physical educator usually only samples some

physical and motor fitness components. Which components are measured is usually determined one of two ways. Either a specific test (such as the Health-Related Physical Fitness Test or the Bruininks-Oseretsky Test of Motor Proficiency) is administered, or test items that measure specific aspects which contribute to a given daily living or motor skill are selected and administered.

The ultimate purpose of preevaluation in the areas of physical and motor fitness is to determine which activities will meet the unique needs of the handicapped child. The procedures to be employed for determining the needs in the areas of physical and motor fitness are as follows:

1. Identify motor skills to be taught in the physical education program that can be expressed as recreational skills and activities of daily living for independence in the community.
2. Select physical and motor fitness areas associated with the skills needed for independent living in the community.
3. Identify levels of physical and motor fitness necessary for independent recreation and activities of daily living in the community.
4. Test for present levels of educational performance in physical and motor fitness domains.
5. Compare the child's performance with normative community standards to determine whether there is sufficient discrepancy to indicate an educational need.
6. If it is determined that there is a need in an identified domain, then ascertain present levels of educational performance on tasks related to the domain and postulate short-term instructional objectives.

TESTS OF PHYSICAL CONDITION

Most exercise tests for an evaluation of physical work capacity, or more specifically maximal oxygen uptake, are based on a linear increase in heart rate with increased oxygen uptake or workload. However, all predictions from submaximal tests should be done with caution. When persons of different age groups are included, some sort of correction factor must be included, since the maximal heart rate declines with age.[1] Even when the tests are carried out under strictly standardized conditions, the methodological error in a prediction of the maximal aerobic power is considerable (standard deviation 10% to 15%). However, the tests can be applied as a valuable screening tool for the evaluation of the functional capacity of the oxygen-transporting system; they

may provide a useful method for selecting the best, the worst, and the average performances of persons from a group.

Objective tests to determine the effect of training on different functions are both important and desirable. Such tests may be an aid in the development of the program, and they encourage the individual to continue training. The submaximal bicycle ergometer test is a simple, inexpensive, and reliable test. In longitudinal studies it is an advantage to apply a test in which variations in body weight do not complicate the choice of workload, and in this connection the bicycle ergometer is superior to treadmill or step tests. At the very least, indirect measurements (or prediction) can give an indication of the person's physiological fitness for endurance-type work, and periodic retesting can give an indication of improvement. Such evaluation also constitutes a strong motivational tool for the participants.

A maximum heart rate can be determined from standard tables, and then exercise prescriptions can be started somewhere below the 60% level and gradually increased. The prescription of exercise follows certain basic guidelines that are applicable to all individuals regardless of age, state of health, or functional capacity. To be meaningful, the exercise prescription must include the type(s), intensity, duration, and frequency of physical activity. The task of exercise prescription is much more difficult for sedentary persons, older persons, persons with risk factors. Thus for each person the degree of risk associated with exercise involves (1) the severity of the exercise relative to the habitual intensity of exercise performed, (2) age, (3) functional capacity, (4) health, (5) individual risk factors, and (6) symptoms.

The target level for training is defined as the level at which or below which progressive abnormalities occur. Target levels for training should be used only as guidelines and must be adjusted for each subject individually with the aid of clinical observations and response to the initial effort test to arrive at an "actual" target level. This ac-

TABLE 17-1

Energy expenditure in METs during stepping at different rates on steps of different heights

Step height		Steps per minute			
Centimeters	Inches	12	18	24	30
0	0	1.2	1.8	2.0	2.4
4	1.6	2.1	2.5	2.9	3.7
8	3.2	2.4	3.0	3.5	4.5
12	4.7	2.8	3.5	4.1	5.3
16	6.3	3.1	4.0	4.7	6.1
20	7.9	3.4	4.5	5.4	7.0
24	9.4	3.8	5.0	6.0	7.8
28	11.0	4.1	5.5	6.7	8.6
32	12.6	4.4	6.0	7.3	9.4
36	14.2	4.8	6.5	8.0	10.3
40	15.8	5.1	7.0	8.7	11.7

From American College of Sports Medicine: Guidelines for graded exercise testing and prescription, Philadelphia, 1975, Lea & Febiger.

tual target level may vary from day to day, depending on daily fluctuations in the subject's other activities.

One MET is the equivalent of a resting oxygen consumption, which is approximately 3.5 milliliters per kilogram per minute. METs during exercise are determined by dividing work metabolic rate by resting metabolic rate. The MET cost of treadmill work depends on body weight, but the MET cost of bicycle ergometry is independent of body weight. The intensity of the exercise may be prescribed by METs or by heart rate.

PROGRAMMING FOR PHYSICAL AND MOTOR FITNESS

Once the unique physical and motor fitness needs of a handicapped individual have been determined, the teacher has several programming alternatives from which to select. The most popular techniques for developing physical and motor fitness are circuit training, progressive resistance exercises, and interval training.

Circuit training involves setting up a series of exercise stations to fulfill specific deficiencies. Progressive resistance exercise programs are de-

signed to develop muscular strength. Interval training consists of running, swimming, rope skipping, and bicycle riding for the purpose of improving circulorespiratory endurance. The physical educator should select the training technique that best meets the unique needs of the students in the physical education program.

Circuit Training

Circuit training has the potential to fulfill specific diagnosed areas of deficiencies among students through the selection of carefully arranged exercises. Each numbered exercise in a circuit is called a station. There can be many stations throughout a particular gymnasium, with persons of varying deficiencies routed to the exercise stations appropriate to the specific deficiency. The circuit training system is extremely adaptable to a great variety of situations and has the potential to meet individual differences within a particular class. The advantages of a circuit training system in developing subaverage physical and motor factors are (1) that it can cope with most diagnosed deficiencies, (2) that it has the potential of applying the progressive overload principle, and (3) that it enables a large number of performers to

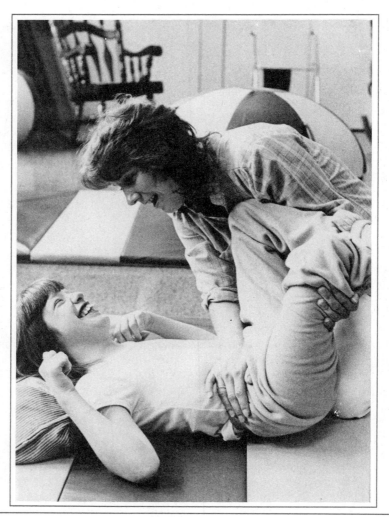

FIGURE 17-5
Stretching activities increase extent flexibility at the hip to improve walking gait.
(Courtesy Children's Rehabilitation Center, Butler, Pa.)

train at the same time and yet meets the individual needs of each performer.

Circuit training usually involves the introduction of a time element into exercise, which often forces the participant to perform at submaximal levels. However, this need not be entirely the case. Each performer can be assigned a specific circuit for a prescribed number of repetitions at each station. If a person wishes to develop both cardiovascular and strength variables, the load may be of submaximal nature so that the person may continuously engage in exercise while moving from station to station. However, if the strength component is a more desirable outcome, then fewer repetitions with more weight should be achieved before the person moves to the next

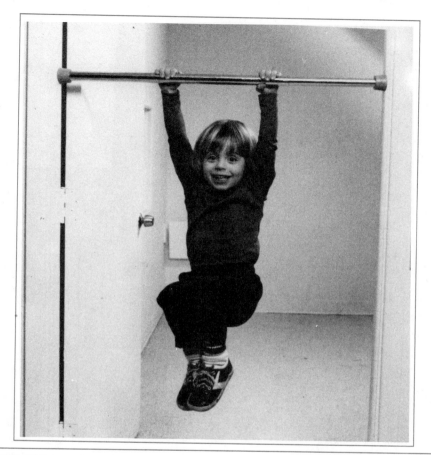

FIGURE 17-6
A child develops abdominal fitness on a doorway gym bar.
(Courtesy Childcraft Education Corporation.)

station. After one circuit lap has been completed, it is at the discretion of the instructor to move the student through a second or third lap, depending on the total dosage desired for a given student. The advantages of the circuit system are as follows:

1. It is adaptable to a number of varying situations.
2. It can be used by 1 or 100 persons and fits almost any time requirements.
3. It assures progression.
4. It allows a person to always work at his or her present capacity and then progress beyond that.
5. It provides a series of progressive goals, which is a powerful motivating force.
6. It may use variables such as load, repetition, and time and consequently it may develop motor and physical characteristics that have been identified as deficient by diagnostic testing.
7. It has the possibility of providing a vigorous bout of exercise in a relatively short period of time.

Name of exercise	Developmental levels*				
	I	II	III	IV	V
	Wt.	Wt.	Wt.	Wt.	Wt.
Two arm curl	40	50	55	60	65
Military press	50	60	65	70	75
Deep knee bends	70	80	85	90	95
Dead lift (straight leg)	70	80	85	90	95
French curl (or dip) with dumbbell	10	15	20	25	30
Situps (time)	--	--	--	--	--
Bench step-ups (time)	--	--	--	--	--
Bench press	55	60	65	75	85
Lateral raises (dumbbell)	5	10	15	20	25
Pushups (time)	--	--	--	--	--

*When 10 repetitions are reached, advance to the next developmental level.

FIGURE 17-7

A suggested circuit training program.

8. It can provide any number of stations to meet any identifiable need.
9. The student knows what must be done because of the construction of an individual program.

Regardless of the system of training used in the developmental program, it should always be kept in mind that the primary goal of the system is to meet the individually diagnosed needs of each child in the program through planned progressive exercise. If this principle is applied, chances are that the program will be beneficial to the physical and motor development of the child. Fig. 17-7 shows the implementation of a circuit program. This circuit program consists of 10 different exercises at separate stations, each performed according to a prescribed number of repetitions and load. It must be remembered that there are as many stations possible as there are exercises or

areas of subdevelopment. The illustration shows five different levels at each station, permitting four steps of progression. Individuals subjectively select a starting level, and when a criterion of 10 repetitions is reached they move to the next level. Progression depends on the ability to meet a set number of repetitions, which will enable the persons to move on to the next progressive level. At each station, it is desirable to place on the wall a card naming the exercise and showing the five levels of performance. The load and number of repetitions should be initially selected to meet the capabilities of the average students in the class; however, from this point weights are adjusted to determine students' present levels of performance so that short-term instructional objectives can be determined. Also, it must be remembered that it is not necessary for all students to participate at each of these 10 stations. Therefore, students may

PROGRESSIVE RESISTANCE EXERCISE PROGRAM

	Maximum Weight Lifted Once	Maximum Weight Lifted 10 Times	3 Sets 10 Times each (½ max.)	3 Sets 10 Times each (¾ max.)	3 Sets 10 Times each (max.)
Bench press (pounds)	60	50	30	45	50
Leg press (pounds)	100	90	50	75	90
Arm curl (pounds)	60	50	30	45	50

USE OF TARGET TIMES FOR THE SIT-UP*

Day	Progression of Repetitions
First 3 days	10
Fourth day	11
Fifth day	12
Sixth day	13
Seventh day	14
Eighth day	15

*Target time: sequence of 10 to 15 repetitions of the sit-up in 20 seconds.

be routed to four, five, or six stations according to their needs as compared with normative performance. Any station may be devised that meets a physical or motor need of children, and a progressive program may be established.

Progressive Resistance Exercises (DeLorme program)

Progressive resistance exercises are used widely in rehabilitative settings and athletics. They can be used to activate most muscle groups of the body. As the strength of the muscle group in-creases, progressively heavier weights are used. The progressive resistance technique of DeLorme, based on knowledge of the individual's ability level, entails the following three procedures:

1. Determine maximal resistance that can be lifted 10 times (10 RM).
2. Determine the maximal resistance that can be lifted one time (1 RM). Three sets (10 RM) are performed as follows:
   a. Ten repetitions at ½ 10 RM (half the maximal resistance determined in procedure one)
   b. Ten repetitions at ¾ 10 RM (three-fourths the maximal resistance determined in procedure one)
   c. Ten repetitions at 10 RM (the maximal resistance determined in procedure one)
3. Increase the 10 RM as determined by increases in the 1 RM.

An example of a progressive resistance exercise program is presented above.

Interval Training

Interval training involves short periods of exercise with a rest interval in between. This training technique can be applied to most activities that require endurance. The interval training prescription should be planned for each student individually. A typical interval training prescription for one day is represented on p. 393. Target times are used as motivation to encourage all-out performance.

Sherrill lists six components of an interval training program. They are as follows[9]:

1. *Set:* The work interval and the rest interval. An ITP [interval training program] may have any number of sets.
2. *Work interval:* A prescribed number of repetitions of the same activity under identical conditions. Work intervals may involve optimum number of sit-ups or push-ups within a prescribed number of seconds.
3. *Rest interval:* The number of seconds or minutes of rest between work intervals during which the student recovers from fatigue for the next set of repetition. During the rest period the student should walk rather than sit, lie, or assume a stationary position.
4. *Repetitions:* The number of times the work interval is repeated under identical conditions.
5. *Target:* The best score that a student can make on the prescribed activity. Target times are usually determined by present levels of performance from data sheets.
6. *Goals:* A statement made by the student of the score he thinks he can attain in a particular activity. All-out effort is often motivated after the first few weeks by prescribing a behavioral goal.[12]

Older children may be guided in developing individual exercise sessions comprised of sets that reflect their own levels of aspiration. Presumably, the child will be more motivated to accomplish a goal established by himself or herself than one imposed by an adult.

In keeping with the overload principle, the exercise sessions become increasingly more demanding each week.

The following list of procedures may help the adapted physical education specialist in planning each IEP.

1. Test each student individually to determine the present level of performance.

2. Organize the children for performance based on test data.
3. Develop specific behavioral objectives for each individual.
4. Explain the principle of interval training to the group and establish a card file where the students may pick up their individualized interval training prescriptions at the beginning of each physical education period.
5. Review data to determine if behavioral goals are being met and readjust programs if necessary.

Exercise Prescription by METs

The peak and average intensity of exercise may be estimated by determining 90% and 70% of the individual's functional capacity. Thus for a person with a maximum functional capacity of 8 METs, intensity would be calculated as follows:

$$\text{Peak conditioning intensity} = 0.9 \times 8 = 7.2 \text{ METs}$$
$$\text{Average conditioning intensity} = 0.7 \times 8 = 5.6 \text{ METs}$$

There is an alternate method that sets a sliding scale for estimating the average conditioning intensity.[3] The sliding scale allows for the variability resulting from known differences in the intensity that can be tolerated by persons with different functional capacities. The baseline intensity is set at less than 60% of the functional capacity in METs.

METs may be estimated from the workload performed (see Table 17-1) or by calculation of oxygen intake from measurements of minute ventilation and expired gas composition. Either estimate of METs may be used effectively in exercise prescription.

In supervised exercise programs, it would appear that the greatest hazard might likewise lie in the subject's activity above and beyond that which is appropriate for him or her at any given time. Associated with this hazard are potential errors in the exercise prescription that call for inappropriately excessive levels of activity. This factor is controllable with proper supervision of the training sessions.

Progressively greater restrictions need to be placed on exercise regimens for untrained persons. This frequently means that, in the beginning, subjects are trained at paces that are less demanding than those they themselves might choose. The initial workout should not exceed 2 or 3 METs for a sedentary person, with 1 MET as the increment of step size.

Intensity of Exercise

The most difficult problem in designing exercise programs is the prescription of the appropriate exercise intensity. The percentage of functional capacity a given individual is able to sustain for a given conditioning period is quite variable. Consideration must be given to the fact that the capacity for performing routine or conditioning work is relatively lower in persons with low functional capacities (6 METs or less) than it is in those with high functional capacities. One report[1] indicates that reasonable estimates for exercise prescription are that during conditioning sessions, peak efforts should not exceed 90% of functional capacity and average intensity should approximate 70% of functional capacity. The duration can then be set empirically on the basis that the participant recovers fully.

In the early stages of a conditioning program precise control of effort is necessary to ensure that participants do not create difficulty by expending too much effort, and peak efforts may need to be lowered to less than 60% of functional capacity and then gradually increased. These controls continue to be useful at all stages of a conditioning program because they enable the participant to expend the most energy per unit of time. Furthermore, improvements, plateaus, or regressions in performance can be evaluated quickly and efficiently.

Target Levels for Training

Exercise prescriptions are determined primarily according to the heart rate and electrocardiographic response to the initial effort test. The purpose of the initial exercise test is to determine the target level for training and to provide a basis for future comparative fitness measurements.

Patterns of exercise for persons with abnormal heart rate or electrocardiographic responses do not differ greatly from those for persons without such symptoms, except for the factors that determine peak severity. For subjects who respond normally to exercise tests, the factors would include a predetermined heart rate; for those who respond abnormally, these would include the level at which progressive abnormality occurs (for example, some untoward event occurs and thus places an upper limit on exercise). As work capacity increases, exercise programs are changed to challenge the individual and thus the target range is increased.

PRINCIPLES AND TRAINING

An adaptation to a given load takes place gradually; in order to achieve further improvement, the training intensity must be increased. However, there is no linear relationship between the amount of training and the training effect. For instance, 2 hours of training each week may cause an increase in maximal oxygen uptake by 0.4 liter per minute. The rate and magnitude of the increase vary from one individual to the next. It is important to ascertain what amount of training may produce a satisfactory result. Less effort is demanded to maintain a reasonable degree of physical condition than to attain it after a period of prolonged inactivity. Since maximal oxygen uptake and cardiac output can be attained at a submaximal speed, this lower speed is probably optimal as a training stimulus. As pointed out, even workloads demanding only a submaximal oxygen uptake improve the physical condition for untrained individuals. Principles for physical fitness training are as follows:

♦ *Individual differences:* Every student's IEP should be based on specific assessment data, which indicate the unique needs for alleviating deficits in prerequisites for self-sufficient living.

- *Overload/shaping principle:* Increases in strength and endurance result from small increments of workload greater than present ability. Overload can be achieved in the following ways:
  1. Increase in the number of repetitions or sets
  2. Increase in the distance covered
  3. Increase in the speed with which the exercise is executed
  4. Increase in the number of minutes of continuous effort
  5. Decrease in the rest interval between active sessions
  6. Any combination of the above.
- *Maintenance or development of physical fitness:* Training sessions can be used to maintain or develop physical fitness. The data on

the frequency of the training will indicate whether the training results maintain or develop physical fitness levels.
- *Physical fitness for a purpose:* Values gained from exercises should be relevant to development of functional skills of health components. Exercises are highly specific; they need to be done at intensity levels commensurate with the ability of the student.
- *Active/voluntary movement:* Benefits are greatest when the exercise is active (done by the student) rather than passive (done by the therapist or teacher). When the student performs the activity, it is possible to provide behavioral measurement and apply learning principles from research and demonstration.
- *Recovery/cool-down:* Students with dyspnea (breathlessness, breathing difficulty) should

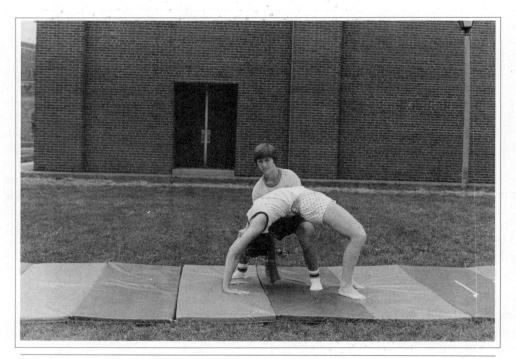

FIGURE 17-8
A student performs an activity that may develop extent flexibility of the lumbar region of the spine.

not lie or sit down immediately after high-intensity exercise. This tends to subvert return of blood to the heart and cause dizziness. Cool-down should entail continued slow walking or mild activity.

♦ *Warm-up:* A few minutes of warm-up exercises using movements specific to training should precede high-intensity exercise sessions or competitive games. Warm-up is particularly important for persons with chronic respiratory problems or cardiovascular conditions. Warm-ups should emphasize stretching exercises that facilitate range of motion (flexibility) rather than ballistic (rhythmic bouncing) exercises.

♦ *Contraindications:* Physical educators should know what exercises or activities are contraindicated for each individual. This information may be obtained from medical records.

♦ *Task analysis of activity:* Physical educators should know how to task analyze exercises to determine which specific muscles should be exercise targets. A principle often used in adapting exercises is *leverage;* the shorter the lever, the easier the exercise. For instance, straight leg lifts from a supine position to develop or assess abdominal strength are very difficult since the body (as a lever) is in its longest position. By doing bent-knee leg lifts, the body lever is shortened and the exercise is made easier.

♦ *Sequence of activity:* Reduction of lever length usually makes a task less difficult and enables sequencing in activities where the body or its parts move against gravity from a prone position. For instance, bending at the waist or knees makes a push-up less difficult.

SELECTED FITNESS PROBLEMS

As mentioned earlier in this chapter, the problems of underdevelopment and low physical vitality are closely associated with a great number of organic, mental, physiological and emotional problems discussed throughout this book. However, three major problem areas transcend the others—namely, malnutrition, anemia, and aging.

Malnutrition

The term *malnutrition* means poor nutrition, whether there is an excess or a lack of nutrients to the body. In either instance the malnourished individual has relatively poor physical fitness and has other serious disadvantages.

It is important that the cause of physical underdevelopment be identified. One cause of physical underdevelopment may be a lack of physical activity, which, consequently, does not provide opportunity for the body to develop its potential. However, some children are physically underdeveloped partially because of undernutrition. When a person's body weight is more than 10% below the ideal weight indicated by standard age and weight tables, undernutrition may be a cause. Tension, anxiety, depression, and other emotional factors may restrict a person's appetite, causing insufficient caloric intake and weight loss. Impairment in physical development may also ensue. In culturally deprived areas, individual diets may lack proper nutrition as a result of insufficient food, idiosyncrasy, and loss of appetite caused by some organic problem. Proper nutrition and exercise go hand in hand in growing children. One without the other may cause lack of optimal physical development. The role of the physical educator in dealing with the underweight person is to help establish sound living habits with particular emphasis paid to proper diet, rest, and relaxation. The student should be encouraged to keep a 5-day food intake diary, after which, with the help of the teacher, a daily average of calories consumed is computed. After determining the average number of calories taken in, the student is encouraged to increase the daily intake by eating extra meals that are both nutritious and high in calories.

Overweight

Many persons in the United States are overweight. Obesity, particularly in adults, is considered one of the great current medical problems because of its relation to cardiovascular and other diseases. The frequency of overweight among patients with angina pectoris, coronary insufficiency, hypertension, and coronary occlusions is considerable.

Overweight may be defined as any excess of 10% or more above the ideal weight for a person, and obesity is any excess of 20% or more above the ideal weight. Obesity constitutes pathological overweight that requires correction. Several factors must be considered in determining whether a person is overweight. Among these are gender, weight, height, age, general body build, bone size, muscular development, and accumulations of subcutaneous fat.

In the past there has not been sufficient attention given to the diagnosis of overweight among many children in our society. The incidence of overweight among children in our schools has been estimated at 10% or more—a rate of such significance that attention to prevention and remediation should be provided by public school doctors, nurses, and health and physical educators.

Overweight persons have a greater tendency than normal or underweight individuals to contract diseases of the heart, circulatory system, kidneys, and pancreas. They also have a predisposition to structural foot and joint conditions because of their excess weight and lack of motor skill to accommodate the weight.

The basic reason for overweight is that the body's food and calorie consumption is greater than the physical activity or energy expended to utilize them. Consequently, the excess energy food is stored in the body as fat, leading to overweight. In many instances overeating is a matter of habit. Thus the body is continually in the process of acquiring more calories than are needed to maintain a normal weight.

Overweight and obesity have many causes. Among them are (1) caloric imbalance from eating incorrectly in relationship to energy expended in the form of activity; (2) dysfunction of the endocrine glands, particularly the pituitary and the thyroid, which regulate fat distribution in the body; and (3) emotional disturbance.

There is impressive evidence that obesity in adults has its origin in childhood habits. There seems to be a substantial number of overweight adults whose difficulty in controlling their appetite stems from childhood. The social environment may have some influence on obesity. In the preschool years, thinness rather than obesity is the general developmental characteristic of children. However, during the early school years and up to early adolescence, children seem susceptible to excess fat deposition.

A belief prevalent among some authorities is that a great portion of obesity is caused by emotional problems. They theorize that children at the age of 7 years are particularly susceptible to obesity from overeating in order to compensate for being unhappy and lonely. Evidently eating may give comfort to children. This particular period is significant because it is when children are transferring close emotional ties from the family to peer relationships. In the event that children do not successfully establish close friendships with other children, they feel alone. Therefore, a compensatory mechanism of adjustment is eating, which gives comfort. Eating may also be used as a comfort when children have trouble at home or at school.

Adverse Effects of Obesity

Obese children, in many instances, exhibit immature social and emotional characteristics. It is not uncommon for obese children to dislike the games played by their peers, for obesity handicaps them in being adept at the games in which their peers are adequate. These children are often clumsy and slow, objects of many stereotyped jokes, and incapable of holding a secure social position among other children. Consequently, they may become oversensitive and unable to defend themselves and thus may withdraw from healthy play and exercise. This withdrawal from activity decreases the energy expenditure needed to maintain the balance that combats obesity.

Therefore, in many instances obesity leads to sedentary habits. It is often difficult to encourage these children to participate in forms of exercise that permit great expenditure of energy.

Obesity may be an important factor as children form ideas about themselves as persons and about how they think they appear to others. The ideas that they have about themselves will be influenced by their own discoveries, by what others say about them, and by the attitudes shown toward them. If the children find that their appearance elicits hostility, disrespect, or negative attention from parents and peers, these feelings may affect their self-concept. Traits described by their parents and peers may affect their inner feelings and may be manifested in their behavior, for children often assess their worth in terms of their relationships with peers, parents, and other authority figures.

When children pass from the child-centered atmosphere of the home into the competitive activities of the early school years, social stresses are encountered. They must demonstrate physical abilities, courage, manipulative skill, and social adeptness in direct comparison with other children of their age. The penalities for failure are humiliation, ridicule, and rejection from the group. Obesity places a tremendous social and emotional handicap on children. Therefore, educators should give these children all possible assistance and guidance in alleviating or adjusting to obesity.

Evaluating Obesity

There are many ways that overweight or obesity can be determined; some of these are highly technical methods requiring sophisticated equipment, whereas others are relatively simple but less valid. One of the least recommended means of measuring fatness is comparison of data about the individual with normative age, gender, and height/weight tables. These tables do not normally allow for the person who may have a preponderance of muscle tissue in place of fat or for those with wide frames or heavy skeletal structures. The most accurate method of determining fatness that can easily be used by the adaptive physical educator is the direct application of anthropometric measures.

The Pryor method predicts body weight based on an individual's skeletal structure. By ascertaining the diameter of the chest at the nipple line and the width of the pelvis at the iliac crest and then comparing these measurements with the height and age of the individual, a predicted weight is determined. Fig. 17-9 shows the Pryor method for predicting weight for boys 2 to 6 years of age.[7]

Skin fold measurement provides a simple and accurate method of assessing quantitatively the fat content of the human body. The skin fold caliper is applied to locations on the body where a fold of skin and subcutaneous fat can be lifted between the thumb and the forefinger so that it is held free of the muscular and bony structure. The skin fold caliper has become an evaluation tool for universal comparison of fat fold measurements. The accepted national recommendation is to have a caliper designed so as to exert a pressure of 10 grams per millimeter on the caliper face. The surface area to be measured should be in the neighborhood of 20 to 40 millimeters. The recommended method is to pinch a full fold of skin and subcutaneous tissue between the thumb and forefinger, at about 1 centimeter from the site on which the caliper is to be placed, and then to pull the fold away from the underlying muscle. The calipers are then applied to the fold about 1 centimeter below the fingers so that the pressure on the fold at the point measured is exerted by the faces of the calipers and not by the fingers. The handle of the caliper is then released and a recording is made to the nearest 0.5 millimeter. The recording should be made 2 or 3 seconds after the caliper pressure is applied.

Although the skin fold at the triceps site has been thought by many authorities to adequately represent total body fat, it is advisable, for the greatest accuracy, to take measurements at several additional body sites. It is common practice

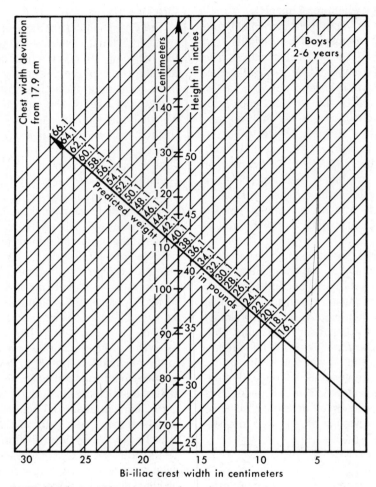

1. Find bi-iliac width at bottom of graph.
2. Follow the vertical channel indicated, up to standing height.
3. Take nearest slant axis to predicted weight.
4. Correct for chest width if necessary. (Go up 1 unit or down 1 unit for each centimeter that the chest measurement exceeds or falls short of the mean at the top of the graph.)

FIGURE 17-9
Pryor method to predict weight.

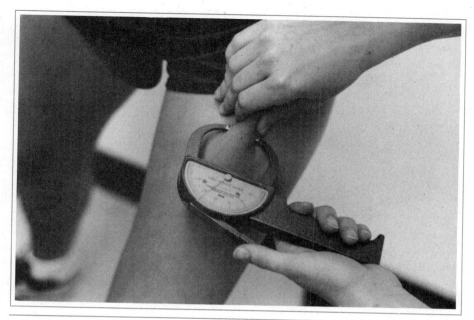

FIGURE 17-10
Technique for skinfold measurement.

to use four sites to study body content of 13- to 34-year-old persons: the biceps, triceps, subscapular, and suprailiac areas. A method of taking skin fold measurements is as follows:

1. The subject is seated.
2. Only measurements of the right side are taken.
3. The biceps area is measured over the midpoint of the muscle while the forearm is resting on the subject's thigh.
4. The triceps area is measured at a point half the distance between the olecranon and acromion process while the arm is hanging down.
5. The subscapular region can be measured just below the hip and to the lateral side of the inferior angle of the scapula.
6. The suprailiac region can be measured just above the iliac crest at the midaxillary line.

Programming for the Obese Child

Since overweight children often cannot perform the activities of the physical education program efficiently, it is not uncommon for them to dislike many of these activities. As a result of their inability to participate in the program, they are often the objects of practical jokes and disparaging remarks made by other children. In such an environment obese and overweight boys and girls become unhappy and ashamed and often withdraw from the activity to circumvent emotional involvement with the group. The physical educator should attempt to create an environment that will enable the obese child to have successful experiences in the class, thus minimizing situations that could degrade the child's position as a person of worth. The physical educator is also challenged with regard to developing the attitudes of the nonhandicapped majority. Consequently, proposing to the class the acceptance of children who are different is an important and worthwhile goal of the physical educator.

There can be no one program for the remediation of children who are overweight. It is necessary that the true cause of the problem be found. When the cause of overweight or obesity is

TABLE 17-2
Obesity standards for white Americans

Age (years)	Skin fold measurements (mm)*	
	Men	Women
5	12	14
6	12	15
7	13	16
8	14	17
9	15	18
10	16	20
11	17	21
12	18	22
13	18	23
14	17	23
15	16	24
16	15	25
17	14	26
18	15	27
19	15	27
20	16	28
21	17	28
22	18	28
23	18	28
24	19	28
25	20	29
26	20	29
27	21	29
28	22	29
29	23	29
30-50	23	30

Modified from Seltzer, C.C., and Mayer, J.: Postgrad. Med. **38**:101-107, 1965.
*Minimum triceps skin fold thickness indicating obesity. Figures represent the logarithmic means of the frequency distributions plus one standard deviation.

TABLE 17-3
Measurements required to determine total skin fold thickness at four skin fold sites (biceps, triceps, subscapular, and suprailiac)

Body Build	Skin Fold Measurement (mm)			
	Men	Women	Boys	Girls
Thin				
Mean	24.0	31.2	22.4	33.3
Standard deviation	7.1	6.3	5.3	9.5
Intermediate				
Mean	34.7	39.9	29.7	36.2
Standard deviation	15.7	10.0	7.6	8.8
Plump and obese				
Mean	57.2	66.0	43.2	49.0
Standard deviation	21.4	22.7	13.2	13.6

Modified from Durnin, J.V.G.A., and Rahaman, M.M.: Br. J. Nutr. **21**:681-689, 1967.

5. A program of exercise within the capacity of the child to increase energy expenditure in order to balance the caloric intake
6. Disruption of sedentary ways of living

It is sound reasoning in combating obesity and overweight to attempt to change living patterns in terms of physical activity and diet rather than to go into crash programs for fast reduction of weight. The habits of everyday living are of longer range than the crash programs, and more value will be accrued by a change in life-style in the long run.

Obese or overweight students should be guided into activities that can be safely performed and successfully achieved. This will tend to encourage them to participate in more vigorous activities. Some of the activities that can be used to combat obesity are general conditioning exercises, jogging, dancing, rhythmical activities, swimming, and sports and games. Much can be done for these children with personal individual guidance, encouragement, and selection of the proper developmental experiences.

Weekly weigh-ins in which a certain number of pounds is scheduled to be lost in a given week provide program incentives. Sustained reduction

known, there are several avenues available for treatment:
1. Control of the diet by reduction of caloric intake
2. Medical treatment in the case of a glandular dysfunction
3. Counseling when emotional causes are at the root of the problem
4. Counseling on the consequences of obesity to the total personality

TABLE 17-4

Percentages of fat corresponding to the total of skin fold measurements at four sites (biceps, triceps, subscapular, and suprailiac)

Total Skin Fold Measurement (mm)	Body Fat (%)			
	Men	Women	Boys	Girls
15	5.5	—	9.0	12.5
20	9.0	15.5	12.5	16.0
25	11.5	18.5	15.5	19.0
30	13.5	21.0	17.5	21.5
35	15.5	23.0	19.5	23.5
40	17.0	24.5	21.5	25.0
45	18.5	26.0	23.0	27.0
50	20.0	27.5	24.0	28.5
55	21.0	29.0	25.5	29.5
60	22.0	30.0	26.5	30.5
65	23.0	31.0	27.5	32.0
70	24.0	32.5	28.5	33.0
75	25.0	33.5	—	—
80	26.0	34.0	—	—
85	26.5	35.0	—	—
90	27.5	36.0	—	—
95	28.0	36.5	—	—

From Durnin, J.V.G.A., and Rahaman, M.M.: Br. J. Nutr. **21:**681-689, 1967.

may afford opportunities for establishing permanent patterns for exercise and eating. The value of the weigh-in is that it projects a precise goal for the student to achieve each week. Furthermore, the exercise program in which the student engages should be progressive. Exercises based on calculated energy expenditures are initiated with slight progression ensured in the program with each successive day of attendance. Suggested activities are walking, jogging, bicycle riding, rope jumping, swimming, stair and hill climbing, and stepping up on and down from a bench.

Heart Conditions

There are several prerequisites to effective use of exercise treatment programs for persons who have heart conditions. Some of them are as follows:

1. A classification sequence in which diagnosed patients can be placed
2. Evaluation procedures to determine the level of the individual's functioning and activity capability
3. Individual prescriptions of activity for each person
4. Objectives and goals for each person

Prior to entering an activity program, the participants should be medically screened and then informed of the benefits and risks of such a program. Information should be provided both on the effects of training and fitness on cardiovascular function and on potential risks. It may be wise to make a brochure that answers some of the questions individuals may have about the program.

Cardiovascular Assessment

Cardiovascular assessment is an essential feature of the total exercise program. It is important that contraindications for cardiac conditions be identified. These may be ascertained through physical examinations, chest x-ray films, biochemical assays, metabolic tests, and electrocardiograms. As a rule, these tests will detect cardiac murmurs, arrhythmias, hypertrophy, intraventricular blocking, hypertension, congenital anomalies, diabetes, hypercholesterolemia, heavy smoking, signs of myocardial insufficiency, and other risk factors. In addition, it is advisable to test, under dynamic conditions, the physiological parameters that indicate the current functioning ability of the individual. Steady state of the heart rate during bicycle ergometer exercise and recovery rate from step or treadmill tests are not enough, in and of themselves, to furnish an adequate index of the initial level of the individual's physical condition.

It is important that goals be set prior to the initiation of the activity program in order to facilitate measurement of progress. The goals that the programmer may project are increases in the parameters of measurable functioning (oxygen uptake) and the behavioral capability to produce greater amounts of activity as a result of progression through the program. When objectives are set for

BEHAVIORAL STATEMENTS FOR DEVELOPMENT OF PHYSICAL AND MOTOR FITNESS

Many physical and motor fitness tasks are measurable. Usually, if measure can be incorporated into a task, performance difficulty can be prescribed for the individual learner. Below are statements that involve physical and motor tasks requiring specifications of measurement to be ascribed to the tasks. Many handicapped children will be able to participate in these tasks at their ability level if objectives are sequenced.

1. Walk a specified distance at a heart rate of 120 beats per minute.
2. Jog and walk alternately 50 steps for a specified distance.
3. Run in place lifting the foot a specified distance from the floor a specified number of times for a specified period of time.
4. Run in place 100 steps in a specified amount of time.
5. Run a specified distance in a specified period of time.
6. Perform a modified push-up a specified number of times.
7. Perform a modified chin-up a specified number of times.
8. Climb a rope a specified distance in a specified amount of time.
9. Perform knee dips to a specified amount of flexion in the knee a specified number of repetitions.
10. Perform toe raises with a specified amount of weight a specified number of repetitions.
11. Perform prone lift of a specified weight a specified number of repetitions.
12. Perform a sit-up (modified if necessary) a specified number of repetitions; sit-up difficulty can be modified by performance on an incline where gravity assists with the sit-up.
13. Lift a ball of specified weight with the soles of the feet a specified number of times.
14. Perform a specified number of dips on the parallel bars (lower and raise the body by straightening and bending the arms) with a specified amount of weight attached to a belt. If one dip cannot be done reduce the range of motion of the dip.
15. Perform arm curls with a specified weight and a specified number of repetitions.
16. Perform a prone arch (hands under the hips in prone position) in which the hands and feet are moved a specified distance from one another.
17. Curl the toes and pick up a specified number of pencils or sticks of the same size; move them a specified distance to a target of a specified size over a specified time frame.
18. Perform a wrist roll in which a rope of specified length has a weight of specified pounds attached to it a specified number of repetitions over a specified time frame.
19. Perform toe curls with a towel with the heels flat on the floor; bunch up the towel under the feet and put a weight of a specified number of pounds on the towel a specified distance from the toes.
20. Perform a wrist curl in which the wrist is over the edge of a table or a chair, then bend and straighten the wrist holding a weight of a specified amount a specified number of repetitions.
21. Jump and reach a specified height.
22. Throw a medicine ball of specified weight from a sitting position a specified distance.
23. Perform back extensions from a prone position, so the low back reaches a specified height a specified number of repetitions over a specified amount of time.
24. From a standing position with the knees straight, bend forward at the hips and measure the distance the tips of the fingers are from the floor. If the person can touch the floor, place a book or object on the floor and measure the distance the fingers are below the surface of the object on which the student is standing.
25. Run a specified distance over a specified period of time.
26. Run around a hoop 4 feet in diameter a specified number of times over a specified time frame.
27. Leap over a rope placed at a specified height.

BEHAVIORAL STATEMENTS FOR DEVELOPMENT OF PHYSICAL AND MOTOR FITNESS—cont'd

28. Leap over two lines on the floor that are a specified distance apart.
29. Step up and then down on a bench of a specified height a specified number of repetitions over a specified time frame.
30. Run in a figure 8 fashion around a specified number of cones set a specified distance apart a specified number of times during a specified time frame.
31. Perform a shuttle run in which the parallel lines are a specified distance apart a specified number of trips in a specified amount of time.
32. Jump with two feet successively in each of four quadrants formed by two lines crossing at right angles a specified number of repetitions over a specified time frame.
33. Perform a specified number of squat thrusts (from a stand, bend the knees and place the hands on the floor, throw the legs back return the legs to the squat position, stand erect and repeat) during a specified time frame.
34. Run in place so one foot strikes the floor a specified number of times over a specified time frame.
35. Stand on one foot for a specified number of seconds.
36. Stand on sticks of specified width for a specified number of seconds.
37. Walk on a balance beam of specified width for a specified number of steps.
38. Walk backward on a balance beam of specified width for a specified number of steps.
39. Balance a bean bag on the head and walk a specified distance.
40. Balance a bean bag on the head and hop a specified number of times over a specified distance.
41. Run, skip, leap, and gallop specified distances over time with a bean bag on the head.
42. Stand on stilts that are a specified distance above the ground a specified period of time.
43. Walk on stilts which are a specified distance above the ground a specified distance in a specified period of time.
44. Walk backwards on stilts which are a specified distance above the ground, a specified distance over a specified time.
45. Stand on one foot and on a stick/beam of specified width, raise the free leg to the rear a specified height, and hold for a specified amount of time.
46. From a kneeling position on one knee and with one hand on a beam of known width, lower the head a specified distance from the beam and raise the leg a specified distance from the floor.
47. Walk with an eraser on the top of the head on a beam of specified width a specified distance without letting the eraser fall off the head.
48. Using stilts walk a specified distance in a specified time frame and stay within a pathway of a specified width.
49. Balance on one foot and bring the toe of the other foot to a point a specified distance from the forehead.
50. On a beam of specified width and length perform the following tasks: (a) Hold the left foot at toes with the right hand behind the right knee, move the left knee a specified distance from the beam and return. Perform the task a specified number of consecutive times. (b) Raise the left leg forward with the knee straight, bend the right knee and lower the seat a specified distance from the beam, and return to a stand.
51. From a standing position on one or two feet move the left knee a specified distance from the floor with out losing balance. Grasp the left foot with the right hand behind the right leg. Repeat on opposite side a specified number of times.
52. Run the 5000-yard dash in a specified amount of time.

an exercise program, it should be possible to measure progress toward them.

Physical Training and Coronary Heart Disease

The goal of training is to achieve physical fitness conducive to good cardiovascular function and good health. The desired level of fitness should be attained in orderly fashion, usually at a restrained rate of progress. This is necessary if programming is to be beneficial for persons who possess great variability in cardiovascular functioning.

Recently, a number of deaths have been reported for persons undertaking currently popular "do-it-yourself" jogging programs. The high incidence of death in the natural course of programming, regardless of the level of physical activity, makes it impossible to exclude all possibility of death from any regimen. It would therefore be unreasonable to discontinue programs for which the incidence of death or myocardial infarction is not increased. Instead, specific steps must be taken to educate subjects and professional staffs in the proper application of activity. The statement made by the American Heart Association's Committee on Exercise emphasizes this by stating that "for the sedentary individual there is serious risk in the sudden unregulated and injudicious use of strenuous exercise. But it is a risk that can be minimized and perhaps even eliminated through proper preliminary testing and the individualized prescribing of exercise programs."[1] To clarify the term *risk* the following definitions are suggested:

1. Persons at risk or at high risk are those who have a few, a majority, or all of the established risk factors pointing toward the potential development of coronary heart disease. An exercise testing and conditioning program, properly supervised, should prove useful in reducing those risks.
2. If used freely, the term *risk* or *high risk* is synonymous with *hazard,* indicating potential danger of unhealthy occurrences when individuals are physically stressed.

Before a sedentary person begins unrestricted exercise, he or she should have a thorough medical examination to exclude contraindications. This should include orthopedic, respiratory, and cardiovascular evaluation as well as assessment of physical fitness. Other sources[2] offer details of contraindications to exercise testing.

Potential Hazards in Exercise Prescriptions

Some factors or practices frequently associated with physical training sessions of normal persons should be specifically prohibited for or used with extreme caution by persons with cardiac conditions. Close supervision is essential until the patient and the physician have been educated as to the pattern, progression, and regression of abnormalities and a study has been made of the coronary arterial circulation. Improvements in workload tolerance may be associated with gross changes in the anatomy of the coronary arterial system, as characterized by coronary arteriograms.

Features that constitute additional stresses to the cardiovascular system, and that therefore should be avoided, are as follows:

1. It is well known that thermal stress (extremes of heat and cold) can evoke considerable strain in humans.
2. Sudden death during snow shoveling is caused by a combination of the effects of cold exposure and sudden severe effort in an unconditioned subject. Care should be taken to be preconditioned, enter the cold gradually, keep the chest covered, and intersperse work with rest periods.
3. The ingestion of fluids at extreme temperatures is known to produce cardiac arrhythmias, but fluids are needed to prevent dehydration.
4. Large meals tend to divert a greater portion of the cardiac output to mesenteric vascular beds.

Guidelines for Exercise Testing and Prescription

When properly prescribed, physical activity is beneficial, since it maintains or increases functional capacity and may modify some risk factors associated with atherosclerotic disease. Initial prescription, including upper limits of exertion and subsequent modifications, can be safely determined from knowledge generated from repeated graded exercise tests given under medical supervision. The attainment and maintenance of functional capacity and workloads commensurate with ability are of concern to professionals, particularly for individuals considered at risk from an injudicious increase in their physical activity levels.

Fitness is relative, and therefore training must be individualized. The subject's symptoms can be useful in assessing limitations in physical training.

In summary, the minimal amount and type of exercise required to achieve optimal physical fitness and to protect against lethal coronary attacks need to be better delineated. There is also a need to demonstrate whether physical reconditioning after a coronary attack actually reduces the propensity to recurrence and prolongs life. The hazards as well as the benefits of carefully supervised exercise programs need to be ascertained, but there is much evidence to suggest that the potential benefits far exceed the hazards. More discrete guidelines and criteria are needed to delineate the indications and contraindications and to ensure safety and efficacy.

Aging

The science that studies aging is called gerontology, whereas the field of geriatrics is concerned more specifically with diseases and management of old age.[2]

Aging is relative. Chronological age is a poor indicator of the stage of a person's total development. Aging per se does not progress or decline at an even rate. There is great variability in anatomical, physiological, and psychological aging. Consequently, a person may have a chronological age of 50 years, the heart and arteries of a person aged 30 years, and the mental vitality of a person aged 25 years.

Therefore, aging must be considered a dynamic biological process of growth and development and not merely degeneration or organic regression. Physiological aging, in general, produces a loss of the essential functioning and the gradual degeneration of organs. The collagenous substances within the connective tissues of the body (such as tendons and ligaments) become hardened and inelastic. Organs that undergo aging lose their ability for normal nutrient and metabolic transfer between the cellular structures and blood. Microscopic degeneration resulting in cellular death progresses to organs and subsequently to an entire organ system. Senescence occurs when the death rate of cells is greater than the rate of their reproduction.

Problems in Aging

The cardiovascular system is vital to the normal functioning of the entire body. Aging affects cardiovascular efficiency and subsequently results in alterations in the rate and efficiency of oxygen nutrient utilization. Connective tissue and fat content increases with age, within inner surface membranes and cavities of the heart. The senile heart moves from an oblique position to a more upright position. Valves become inelastic, resulting in a tendency toward dilation and muscular incompetency in the heart, with subsequent arrhythmia. Coronary arteries become thickened at their innermost lining (intima). Blood vessels, particularly arteries, display aging by their inelasticity and thinning muscular walls. Stretched arteries become more twisted in their courses. Degeneration and the collection of fat deposits further weaken artery walls. After structural arterial change comes a functional increase in systolic blood pressure and a decrease in diastolic pressure. The aging person's lungs gradually become inelastic, smaller, and in general less viable. Chest excursion may be hampered by the rigidity of the thorax as a result of the calcification of cartilaginous tissue. An inability to inhale or expand the chest fully produces lowered vital capacity and a decreased breathing capacity.

With senescence come a number of musculoskeletal changes, primarily degeneration and atrophy of muscle fibers and resultant strength loss, cartilage calcification, and softening of bony structures through absorption of mineral matter (osteoporosis). Changes also occur in joints, resulting in articular degeneration and eventually arthritis. Disuse of joints is the reason given for accentuated osteoporosis and muscular atrophy. Evidence indicates that strength diminishes very slowly during the mature adult period and then declines more rapidly after the fifth decade.

Gross brain size diminishes with age; microscopic studies show degeneration of the nerve ganglion cells as well as the highly specialized supporting elements of the nervous system. Anderson and Langton[2] indicate that an increase in cerebrospinal fluid, a thickening of dura mater, and a decrease in metabolism occur with brain atrophy and cellular degeneration. Such alterations are manifested in slower learning and motor responses, an inability to visually accommodate near points (presbyopia), and a decrease in auditory acuity.

Organs of internal secretion, such as thyroid, pituitary, and adrenal glands, start a definite regression as aging progresses. Body functions controlled by the endocrine glands, such as basal metabolism rate and resistance to infection, decline with age. Also the reproductive organs degenerate rapidly and cease to function at about 50 years of age for women and 65 years of age for men. Advancing age brings with it a decrease in androgenic hormones and increases in the speed of atrophy of muscular tissue and internal organs. The following is a summary of the basic findings of scientific investigation on the changes produced in aging:

1. An increase in connective tissues
2. A gradual loss of connective tissue elasticity
3. A disappearance of nervous system cells
4. A reduction of normal cells
5. An increase in the amount of fat
6. A decrease in the ability to use oxygen
7. A decrease in blood volume while resting
8. A decrease in vital lung capacity
9. A decrease in muscle strength
10. A decrease in the amount of hormones and endocrine excretion

All adults are affected to some degree by the aging process. A number of factors cause an individual's aging process to be either atypically slow or prematurely fast—namely, heredity, general adaptation to stress, and life-style. An individual's constitutional inheritance affects the aging process because it passes on deficiencies or the predisposition for certain diseases. Heredity also helps determine an individual's ability to adapt to life's stresses.

As aging progresses, there is increased susceptibility to tissue deterioration. In general, the most common degenerative diseases are considered to be those of the heart, arteries, and kidneys. Anderson and Langton[2] describe arteriosclerosis, hypertension, nephritis, and heart disease as the degenerative quartet, arteriosclerosis, cancer, arthritis, rheumatic disorders, nervous diseases, and mental breakdowns are considered the most prevalent aging disorders.

Many authorities have attributed premature aging and degenerative diseases, primarily in the area of the cardiovascular system,[2,4] to American living practices. A cause has not been singled out, but rather there appears to be a multitude of causes. The main ones might be listed as hypoactivity, overweight, excessive cigarette smoking, and stress.

Each year more than 100,000 Americans die of some major disease of the heart and/or blood vessels, and many more are permanently disabled by such disease. This number accounts for about one half of the deaths that occur annually in the United States. Besides cardiovascular disease, the adult population suffers from untold orthopedic, emotional, and metabolic disorders that may be attributed directly or indirectly to contemporary life-styles.

Exercise and Aging

To prevent involution, atrophy, and ultimate cellular and organ death, tissue stimulation must occur. Exercise is a factor capable not only of ameliorating the processes of involution and atrophy but also of reversing them, which in turn promotes the process of self-renovation at the molecular level in organs of the elderly. Planned progressive exercise can produce such positive gains as increased strength and skeletal muscle hypertrophy, hypertrophy of the heart with the resultant training effect of decreased heart rate, increased ability to expend energy, more efficient use of oxygen, greater vital capacity, and improved body suppleness from increased joint mobility. Activity can maintain the anabolic protein-building qualities of muscle strength. Many physically active older persons express a higher level of vitality, ability to sleep, mental capacity, and desire for socialization than do their sedentary counterparts.

To offset many of the problems of premature aging, preventive conditioning programs have been emerging in the United States primarily in YMCAs, colleges, universities, municipal recreation departments, and private organizations. However, the government, insurance companies, and industries have been slow to respond to this need because of a lack of concrete evidence that preventive measures can be applied to the subfit adult. In these supervised programs adults can remedy or offset the debilitating influences of inactivity.

As discussed previously, aging progresses at varying speeds in different persons and in different organs within the same person. However, the organ system that should be of the greatest concern to the average American today is the cardiovascular system.

Huttinger[8] has indicated that physical activity is a key for delaying the aging process. Indeed, he reports that men in their sixties and seventies possess the capability of achieving percentages of improvement in the functional use of the heart and lungs and have a physical work capacity comparable to that of young men. The decline in physical work capacity is normally from 9% to 15% during the ages 45 to 55 years. There is impressive evidence that through a program of endurance with running and swimming at sufficient intensity of maximum oxygen uptake, the normal decline in work capacity was forestalled. Thus the use of systematic exercise as an intervention technique to retard the onset of aging of the cardiovascular system appears to have merit.

There is speculation as to just how much development can be achieved in motor and physical fitness in aged persons. The full benefits to be expected from physical education programs that are systematically implemented by trained personnel are as yet unknown. However, aged persons, whether handicapped or not, should receive systematic instructional programs consisting of positive developmental objectives in areas of physical and motor fitness.

It has been pointed out that the fit individual has the ability to deliver oxygen to the body as it is required. On the other hand, an unfit person experiences a greater energy demand than physical capacity to deliver it.

Research studies and clinical observations point to the fact that regular physical activities may contribute to fitness by preventing obesity and by decreasing the possibility of premature coronary heart disease.

Most authorities agree that the benefits of exercise to the cardiovascular system are as follows:

1. Improved oxygen economy of the heart
2. More effective parasympathetic and sympathetic inhibitory counterbalances
3. Slower heart rate at rest and less acceleration during effort
4. Faster heart deceleration after exercise
5. Reduction of peripheral blood vessel resistance
6. Increased residual blood volume of the heart
7. Improved coronary blood flow as a result of increased collateral capillarization of heart muscle
8. Prolongation of coagulation time and a lowering of the serum cholesterol level

Although there are signs that exercise may be beneficial to the cardiovascular system, proof must come through further research. Studies have attempted to obtain definitive information from programs designed to intervene actively in living patterns of postcoronary disease patients or persons who are considered high-risk subjects, as determined by an electrocardiograph stress test. Such tests are administered by a cardiologist, who determines whether there are ischemic heart changes after exercise. Test results serve as a useful index for the amount of exercise in which an individual can safely engage.

IMPLICATIONS FOR PHYSICAL EDUCATION

Physical education has emerged with new importance as awareness of the deleterious effect of inactivity on the sedentary adult population has increased. Through the efforts of many disciplines, the public is beginning to realize that proper exercise can be a deterrent to many characteristics of premature physiological aging as well as to their concomitant diseases.

Research and studies have resulted in new concepts about the type of physical fitness activities best suited for adults. Continuity of well-planned activities can serve as a preventive conditioner. Isotonic exercise is preferable to isometric exercise, particularly for persons with a history of cardiovascular disease. Isometric exercise may result in irregular heartbeats, premature ventricular contractions, and abnormally fast heartbeats in heart disease patients.

A multidisciplinary approach has resulted from medicine's concern for permature cardiovascular disease and the positive effects of proper exercise. The physician, physical educator, applied physiologist, and many other professionals are lending their skills to help solve the problem of lack of physical fitness among adults. With the implementation of many medically oriented adult physical education programs, there is an increased need for trained teachers of adapted physical education who understand the problems and needs of the adult population. establishing individual physical education programs for adults is one of the greatest challenges of our times.

SUMMARY

There are three purposes of physical and motor fitness: to promote and maintain health, to develop prerequisites for maximal performance of daily living skills, and to develop prerequisites for leisure and sport skills. Each person possesses a unique composition of physical and motor abilities and therefore should be assessed and provided with an individual physical and motor fitness program. Activity programs should be constructed so that the physical and motor fitness tasks can be adapted to the ability level of each learner. Progressive resistance exercise programs are desirable for the development of strength, while interval training programs are desirable for the development of endurance. Circuit training can be used to develop a wide range of performance levels.

Physical and motor fitness programs are beneficial as deterents to obesity and the aging process. Weight control is a product of energy expenditure and balanced caloric intake. Therefore, the amount of exercise is an important factor in the control of obesity. Elderly persons tend to be less capable of general motor functioning than younger persons. The physical prerequisites of physical and motor fitness may retard physiological and functional degeneration of the motor systems and enable longer periods of self-sufficient living for elderly populations.

REVIEW QUESTIONS

1. Describe the three types of physical fitness programs.
2. What are the causes of low physical fitness?
3. How would one determine a unique physical fitness need for an individual for functional skill?
4. What are the characteristics that distinguish a physical skill from a physical ability, and what is the relationship between the two?
5. Name seven physical and motor fitness abilities.
6. What are five psychomotor abilities that are prerequisites to motor skills?
7. Construct a progressive resistive exercise and interval training programs.
8. Evaluate and design a program for persons who are overweight.
9. What are the problems involved in physical fitness programs with the aged?

STUDENT ACTIVITIES

1. Administer a physical fitness test to determine the strengths and weaknesses of a handicapped child, another student, or yourself. Have a test for each of the physical and motor fitness abilities.
2. Select a person with poor physical fitness and determine the activities that might assist in raising the level of fitness.
3. Identify a task that is heavily loaded with physical and motor fitness prerequisites. Identify the physical and motor fitness abilities of a student at specific body parts that, if programs were developed, would facilitate performance of the skill.
4. Construct a progressive exercise for a person who has specific strength deficits or an athlete for a specific sport skill.
5. Design an interval training program for yourself or a friend.
6. Write a paper on the causes of and procedures for correcting overweight and underweight.

REFERENCES

1. American College of Sports Medicine: Guidelines for graded exercise testing and prescription, Philadelphia, 1975, Lea & Febiger.
2. Anderson, C.L., and Langton, K.: Health principles and practice, ed. 6, St. Louis, 1970, The C.V. Mosby Co.
3. Clarke, H.H.: Development of muscular strength and endurance, Physical Fitness Research Digest, Series 4, No. 1, Washington, D.C., 1973, President's Council on Physical Fitness and Sports.
4. Falls, H., Baylor, A., and Dishman, R.: Essentials of Fitness, New York, 1980, W.B. Saunders Co.
5. Hettinger, T.: Physiology of strength, Springfield, Ill., 1961, Charles C Thomas, Publisher.
6. Huttinger, P.A.: A key for delaying the aging process, Swimmer Magazine, 2:36-41, Feb./March 1979.
7. Pryor, H.B.: Charts of normal body measurements and revised width-weight tables in graphic form, J. Pediatr. 68:615-631, 1966.
8. Rarick, L.: Cognitive-motor relationships in the growing years, 50:180-181, 1980.
9. Sherrill, C.: Adapted physical education and recreation, ed. 3, Dubuque, Iowa, 1985, Wm. C. Brown Co., Publishers.

SUGGESTED READINGS

Cooper, K.: Aerobics, New York, 1970, Bantam Books Inc.
DeVries, H.: Physiology of exercise, ed. 3, Dubuque, Iowa, 1980, Wm. C. Brown Co., Publishers.
Miller, D., and Allen, T.: Fitness: a lifetime commitment, ed. 2, Minneapolis, 1982 Burgess Publishing Co.
Williams, S.: Nutrition and diet therapy, ed. 4, St. Louis, 1981, The C.V. Mosby Co.

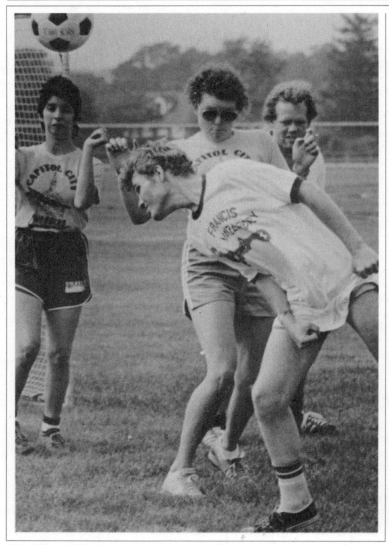

CHAPTER 18

United Cerebral Palsy Associations, Inc.

Other Conditions

OBJECTIVES

♦ Understand the effect of diet and activity on dysmenorrhea.

♦ Know three exercises that can be used to reduce most dysmenorrhea.

♦ Know the value of exercise for diabetics.

♦ Understand how kidney disorders and inguinal hernias affect exercise prescriptions.

♦ Identify three infectious diseases and their effects on physical performance levels.

♦ Know the characteristics of an anemic person.

The Education for All Handicapped Children Act included "other health impaired" as a category of students who might qualify for special physical education services. In the law "other health impaired" persons are defined as those with "limited strength, vitality or alertness, due to chronic or acute health problems such as a heart condition, tuberculosis, rheumatic fever, nephritis, asthma, sickle cell anemia, hemophilia, epilepsy, lead poisoning, leukemia, or diabetes, which adversely affects a child's educational performance."[17] Some of these conditions are discussed in other sections of this text. The conditions that are included under the law discussed in this chapter are diabetes, kidney disorders, and tuberculosis. Other conditions that can affect a child's performance in physical education are included, such as menstruation and dysmenorrhea, hernia, pneumonia, streptococcal infections, encephalitis, meningitis, and anemia. A description of each condition, causes, and programming suggestions are discussed.

MENSTRUATION AND DYSMENORRHEA

Menstruation is a complex process that involves the endocrine glands, uterus, and ovaries. The average menstrual cycle lasts for 28 days. However, each woman has her own rhythmic cycle of menstrual function. The cycle periods usually range from 21 to 35 days, but they may occasionally be longer or shorter and still fall within the range of normality.

The average total amount of blood lost during the normal menstrual period is 3 ounces; however, a woman may lose from 1½ to 5 ounces.[15] This blood is replaced by the active formation of blood cells in bone marrow and consequently does not cause anemia. On occasion, some women may have excessive menstrual flow, and in this event a physician should be consulted. The average menstrual period lasts 3 to 5 days, but 2 to 7 days may be considered normal. The average age of onset of menstruation is 12.5 years, although the range of onset may be from 9 to 18 years.

Dysmenorrhea, or painful menstruation, is a common occurrence among some girls and women. The ratio may be as low as 1:4 among college women, indicating that it is the exception rather than the rule. It has been estimated that only 20% to 30% of cases of dysmenorrhea are a result of organic causes such as ovarian cysts, endocrine imbalance, or infections. Most of the causes are of functional origin such as poor posture, insufficient exercise, fatigue, weak abdominal muscles, or improper diet.

Diet and Its Effects on the Menstrual Period

Many women are unaware of the effects dietary habits can have on their degree of comfort during the onset of their menstrual flow. During this age of fast foods saturated with salt, the modern woman needs to understand how her diet choices can influence her comfort during the menstrual period. With such knowledge many women can reduce the painful discomfort of dysmenorrhea. Reduction of pain is directly associated with the amount of salt stored in the body.

Approximately 1 week prior to the onset of the menstrual period the body begins storing sodium chloride. When this storing process begins, a woman craves salt. If she yields to the craving for salt at that time in her cycle, a whole series of events occur that result in abdominal bloating, which increases the pain associated with the first 2 days of the menstrual flow.

What occurs is that when salt intake is increased, it tends to move into and be held by the body tissues. The salt stored in the body tissues draws water towards those tissues, thereby upsetting the osmotic balance in the body. Much of the water that is drawn into the tissues is pulled from fecal matter moving through the large intestine. When large amounts of water are removed from the fecal mass, the mass begins to harden and its progress is slowed. Thus the net result of increasing salt intake 1 week prior to the onset of the menstrual period is bloating from stored water and accumulating fecal material. This increased congestion presses against nerves in the abdominal and lower back area and causes pain.

The entire chain of events can be avoided (or markedly reduced) if, 1 week prior to the onset of her menstrual flow, a woman will decrease (or at least not increase) salt intake and, at the same time, increase water and roughage (raw celery,

carrots, apples) intake. By following these simple guidelines a woman can preserve the osmotic balance of water in the body, and softness and progress of the fecal mass through the large intestine can be maintained. Regular movement of the fecal mass results in reduction of the amount of bloating associated with the menstrual period. Reduced bloating and faithful adherence to exercises described later in this chapter will relieve most of the pain associated with menstruation.

Physical Activity during the Menstrual Period

In a study of problems associated with menstruation, Nolen[12] indicated that postural deficiency may be responsible for some discomfort not only during the menstrual period but also on other days. She found that when posture was improved and good physical condition was achieved, the menses did not incapacitate girls for physical education or recreational programs.

Gilman's findings[8] indicate that activity during the menstrual period has proved helpful in the correction of dysmenorrhea. According to Clow and Sanderson,[5] many girls have discovered that if they do not have some form of exercise prior to and on the first day of their period, they may have pain.

A number of studies report the effect of exercise on menstruation. Runge[15] studied 107 college girls who trained 15 hours each week and found that in a majority of the cases activities continued during the menstrual period did not affect performance ability. Forty-five percent showed a decrease in performance either during menstruation or immediately before the onset of flow. The findings of these studies seem to indicate that menstruation affects women differently. It is suggested that menstruation does not necessarily prohibit exercise during flow, but there are exceptions to the rule.

The consensus in the literature would seem to be that excuse from physical education activity because of normal menstruation would be unwarranted.

The question has been raised as to whether

girls and young women should refrain from swimming during the menstrual cycles. Phillips, Fox, and Young[13] conducted a survey among gynecologists and other physicians to determine their points of view on this issue. The menstrual period was divided into three phases: the premenstrual period (3 or 4 days prior to the actual onset of the menses), the first half of the menstrual period and the second half of the menstrual period. The consensus among the physicians and gynecologists was that restriction from participation in vigorous physical activity, intensive sports competition, and swimming during all phases of the menstrual period were unwarranted for girls who are free of menstrual disturbances. However, with regard to the first half of the menstrual period, some physicians advised moderation with limited participation in intensive sport competition. The reason for moderation during the first half of the menstrual period is that the flow is heavier during the first 2 or 3 days and some women experience cramps during the first 2 days. Restrictions increase for women with premenstrual discomfort as the severity of the discomfort increases.[14]

Anderson[1] conducted a study on swimming and exercise during menstruation. This study showed that the incidence of discomfort associated with menstruation was lower for an active group of competitive swimmers than for girls who did not participate in swimming activities. Also of interest is the study by Astrand et al.[2] of the training of 30 champions who swam a distance of 6000 to 6500 meters each week. They found no evidence that the strenuous swimming regimen caused menstrual disturbances.

The conclusion reached after review of studies on the effects of physical activity on menstruation is that, for the most part, excuse from physical education class because of the menstrual cycle is not warranted. Social, professional, and athletic schedules cannot be adjusted to each woman's menstrual cycle. It is also realized that many girls and women experience discomfort with menstruation. However, by continuation of activity through the cycle, the impact of menstrual discomfort experienced often decreases.[2]

Exercises for Dysmenorrhea

The question has often been asked as to what effects exercise has on dysmenorrhea. Studies indicate that women previously suffering from moderate or severe cases of dysmenorrhea showed a decrease in severity of cramps after performing prescribed abdominal exercises for 8 weeks. These exercises, prescribed for women who had no organic causes for dysmenorrhea, provided relief of congestion in the abdominal cavity caused by gravity, poor posture, poor circulation, or poor abdominal muscle tone. Physical activity also assists relief of leg and back pains by stretching lumbar and pelvic ligaments in the fascia to minimize pressure on spinal nerves. Undue muscular tension may also have a bearing on painful menstruation; therefore, relaxation techniques and positioning of the body, accompanied by heat from a heating pad on the lower back area, may relax tensions and consequently lessen the pain. Other relaxation techniques and exercises may also be used to reduce tension in the body (see Chapter 8).

Women who suffer from dysmenorrhea may benefit from a daily exercise program designed to alleviate this condition. The exercises should provide for improvement of posture (especially lordosis), stimulation of circulation, and stretching of tight fascia and ligaments. The exercises discussed here are suggested to alleviate the symptoms of dysmenorrhea.

Fascial Stretch

The purpose of fascial exercise is to stretch the shortened fascial ligamentous bands that extend between the lower back and the anterior aspect of the pelvis and legs. These shortened bands may result in increased pelvic tilt, which may irritate peripheral nerves passing through or near the fascia. The irritation of these nerves may be the cause of the pain. This exercise produces a stretching effect on the hip flexors and increases mobility of the hip joint[3] (Fig. 18-1). To perform the exercise, the woman should stand erect, with the left side of her body about the distance of the bent elbow from a wall; the feet should be to-

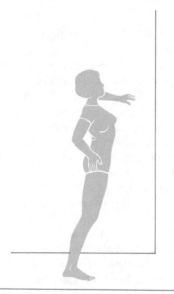

FIGURE 18-1
Fascial stretch.

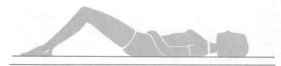

FIGURE 18-2
Abdominal pumping.

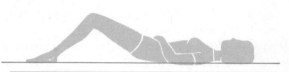

FIGURE 18-3
Pelvic tilt with abdominal pumping.

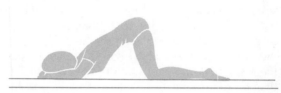

FIGURE 18-4
Knee-chest position.

gether, with the left forearm and palm against the wall, the elbow at shoulder height, and the heel of the other hand placed against the posterior aspect of the hollow portion of the right hip. From this position, abdominal and gluteal muscles should be contracted strongly to tilt the pelvis backward. The hips should slowly be pushed forward and diagonally toward the wall and pressure should be applied with the right hand. This position should be held for a few counts, then a slow return should be made to the starting position. The stretch should be performed three times on each side of the body. The exercise should be continued even after relief has been obtained from dysmenorrhea. It has been suggested that the exercise be performed three times daily. To increase motivation the girls should record the number of days and times they perform the exercise.

Abdominal Pumping

The purpose of abdominal pumping is to increase circulation of the blood throughout the pelvic region. The exercise is performed by as-

suming a hook-lying position placing the hands lightly on the abdomen, slowly and smoothly distending the abdomen on the count of one, then retracting the abdomen on the count of two, and relaxing (Fig. 18-2). The exercise should be repeated 8 to 10 times.[12]

Pelvic Tilt with Abdominal Pumping

The purpose of the pelvic tilt with abdominal pumping is to increase the tone of the abdominal muscles. In a hook-lying position, with the feet and knees together, heels 1 inch apart, and hands on the abdomen, the abdominal and gluteal muscles are contracted. The pelvis is rotated so that the tip of the coccyx comes forward and upward and the hips are slightly raised from the floor. The abdomen is distended and retracted. The hips are lowered slowly, vertebra by vertebra, until the original starting position is attained (Fig. 18-3). The exercise is to be repeated 8 to 10 times.

Knee-chest Position

The purpose of the knee-chest exercise is to stretch the extensors of the lumbar spine and strengthen the abdominal muscles. The exercise is performed by bending forward at the hips and placing the hands and arms on a mat. The chest is lowered toward the mat, in a knee-chest position, and held as close to the mat as possible for 3 to 5 minutes[9] (Fig. 18-4). This exercise should be performed once or twice per day.

DIABETES

Diabetes mellitus is a chronic metabolic disorder, the basis of which is the inability of the cells to use glucose. The diabetic person's body is unable to burn up its intake of carbohydrates because of a lack of insulin, which is produced by the pancreas. The lack of insulin in the blood prevents the storage of glucose in the cells of the liver. Consequently, blood sugar accumulates in the bloodstream in greater than usual amounts.

Combs, Hale, and Williams[6] indicate that there are 4,000,000 persons with diabetes in the United States. It has been estimated that approximately 65,000 new cases of diabetes develop each year and that approximately 4,750,000 persons presently residing in the United States, who are now free of diabetic symptoms, will develop diabetes during their lifetime. About 10% of the recorded cases occur among children.[14] However, there is greater prevalence of diabetes with increasing age; approximately half the people who are afflicted with the disease are over the age of 60 years. Furthermore, there is evidence that maternal diabetes may contribute to a greater prevalence of diabetes among children. Kogan[10] indicates that diabetic mothers have malformed children 10 times more frequently than do nondiabetic mothers.

Teachers should be aware of the symptoms of diabetes in order to help identify the disease if it should appear in any of their students, since early identification and treatment promise the best hope. Symptoms of diabetes include infections that may be slow to heal, fatigue, excessive hunger, itching, impairment in visual acuity, excessive urination and thirst, and skin afflictions such as boils, carbuncles, ulcers, and gangrenous sores.

The etiology of diabetes is, as yet, unknown. This condition may be caused by too much food, infection, resistance to insulin, injury, surgical shock, pregnancy, or emotional stress.[16] There seem to be hereditary predispositions for the acquisition of the disease. Also, 70% to 90% of diagnosed diabetics have a history of obesity as a result of having a high fat and carbohydrate content in their diets. Endocrine imbalances, mental trauma, and sedentary living also appear as precipitating factors in the onset of diabetes.

Although the symptoms mentioned may be important in identifying diabetes, the most reliable method of detecting the disorder is urinalysis.

Characteristics

Overweight is one of the best-known characteristics of diabetic persons, particularly in adults. Reducing to normal weight often brings about definite improvement in a diabetic condition. Another characteristic of diabetic persons is susceptibility to infection. Therefore, it is suggested that care and prompt treatment be exercised in the event that abrasions, blisters, cuts, or infections occur in physical education activities. Still another complication the physical educator should be cognizant of is a condition called *insulin shock*. This condition occurs when the glycogen stored in the liver is depleted. The patient develops general muscular weakness, mental confusion, vertigo, profuse sweating, trembling, and either a pale or a flushed face. If there is a rapid decrease in glycogen, symptoms progress to epileptic-like convulsions. When the warning symptoms appear, the patient should eat or drink something containing sugar.

Treatment

It is important that the physical educator understand diabetes treatment procedures so that cooperative efforts with the medical profession can enhance the total development of the child. Effective control of diabetes solely by diet and oral medication has long been sought. Progress toward this objective has been made in recent years through the development of therapeutic drugs that have the properties of insulin. However, another factor is important in the control of diabetes. Participation in exercise functions like insulin in that it burns glucose so less insulin is needed to convert it to glycogen for storage. Many individuals with diabetes take insulin orally; however, some still require insulin injections that are usually self-administered with a hypodermic needle. Also important in the treatment of diabetes is the psychological adjustment patients must make. In addition, patients must undergo regular health checkups and have periodic urinalyses recorded by medical personnel. They must also realize that the condition still is not curable, although it can be controlled. By adjusting to the disciplines placed on them by the physician, diabetic persons can expect to live lives as long and productive as those of nondiabetic persons.

Insulin Shock and Diabetic Coma

In dealing with diabetic persons the physical educator should be aware that a life-and-death situation can arise from too much or too little insulin. With an inadequate dosage of insulin, the early stages of insulin shock involve lassitude, uneasiness, loss of appetite, unquenchable thirst, and excessive urination. As the demand for insulin becomes greater, symptoms of vomiting, dizziness, and even a diabetic coma may result. A coma and shock condition can also occur from the opposite state of too much insulin. Insulin shock or hypoglycemia may cause a loss of consciousness and eventually, if unchecked, a comatose state. When the diabetic coma is compared with insulin shock, certain differences are apparent; insulin shock occurs rapidly, the patient's skin is moist and pale, there is seldom nausea, and the breath does not smell sweet as in cases of diabetic coma.

Exercise and Diabetes

Physical exercise is an important aspect in controlling diabetes. Before the discovery of insulin

in the late 1920s, diabetes was controlled primarily through diet and mild exercise. Although scanty, studies conducted before the discovery of insulin show that the number of deaths from diabetes was higher among the group of persons whose occupations were of a sedentary nature than among those with more physically active jobs. From these findings, it might be inferred that exercise is a variable in the longevity of the diabetic. Exercise has been considered so valuable to diabetic persons that it should be looked on as a duty and incorporated into their daily lives. Walking and mild exercise were thought to be of sufficient value. The findings of Yahraes[18] suggest that there might be a relationship between exercise and efficient control of diabetes.

Diabetes does not prevent persons from improving their physical fitness through exercise. Zankle[19] demonstrated that it is possible, through exercise, to increase the Rogers physical fitness index. Furthermore, Engerbretson[7] found that daily insulin dosages for diabetic patients could be reduced when accompanied by exercise. Also, control of the diabetes improves during the period of training. In addition, the motor fitness of an experimental group subjected to exercise increased during the training period, whereas the motor fitness of a nonexercising control group decreased.

Regular exercise programs are of value to children with diabetes, for exercise may help to stimulate pancreatic secretion as well as contribute to overall body health and assist in maintaining optimal weight, which is a problem for many diabetics. The child with diabetes can participate, in general, in the activities of the unrestricted class. However, in many cases, diabetic patients are more susceptible to fatigue than their nonhandicapped peers. Therefore, the physical educator should be understanding in the event the diabetic cannot withstand prolonged bouts of more strenuous exercise.

Programming for the Diabetic Student

School medical records should be examined in an effort to identify children with diabetes as well as other conditions that may impair their education. After the identification of such students, programs of exercise should be established (with medical counsel) according to the needs of each student. The limits to the activity each diabetic child can perform vary. Continuous evaluation must be made to determine the capabilities and limitations of each diabetic child in the performance of physical and motor activity. The physical education program for the diabetic child, as all other physical education programs, should follow specific progressive sequences ranging from light to intense and simple to complex with regard to the development of physical characteristics and motor skills. It is suggested that the initial capability of the child be identified precisely so that no exercise will be prescribed that is more intense or difficult than the child's capabilities permit. Such a situation could be physiologically and psychologically damaging and might retard the child's receptivity to subsequent activity. The setting most suitable for the child with diabetes is a regular physical education class. In the event that the condition warrants adaptation of exercise and games, these adaptations should be made. The social values accrued from participation with peers seem to far outweigh the possible slight stigma that may be placed on the child because of the adaptations in the physical education program.

KIDNEY DISORDERS

The kidneys and their related structures are the primary organs for excretion in the body, for they remove nitrogenous wastes and various other substances. In addition, the kidneys eliminate water and help control the water content and osmotic pressure of the blood. They eliminate excess salts to keep proper salt concentration in the blood and control acid-base balance by secreting an excess of either acid or alkaline residues. Thus the kidneys play an important role in the maintenance of health.

The rate of kidney secretion is influenced by the pressure of the blood passing through the kidneys. Strenuous and vigorous exercise may cause the blood pressure to increase, thus augmenting the rate of urine excretion. Under conditions of vigorous exercise or high temperature, there is a loss of water and salts. In the event that the salt loss is great, the water content in the tissues will be decreased and the restoration of normal levels of salt will be difficult to achieve. Therefore, in the case of kidney disorders, vigorous exercise may be contraindicated. However, the best procedure to follow with a person who has a kidney disorder is to implement the recommendations of the physician with respect to dosage, duration, and intensity of exercise.

Perhaps the most prevalent kidney disorder that occurs in children and young adults is chronic nephritis. This disorder often follows acute infections such as scarlet fever, tonsillitis, diphtheria, and even colds. The symptoms for chronic nephritis may be pain in the lumbar region of the spine, fever, frequent and painful urination, and the presence of blood in the urine. If a student has such a disorder, vigorous exercise is usually contraindicated because chronic nephritis usually yields to rest, proper medical care, and, in some instances, antibiotic treatment.

Brooks and Brooks[4] indicate that "hollow-back posture" may sometimes interfere with normal kidney function and produce albumin in the urine. Also, severe and prolonged chilling of the body, especially after vigorous exercise, may cause congestion and injury to the kidneys. Precaution is particularly important if the child already has a kidney disorder.

A child who has contracted chronic nephritis should take part in programs of physical education within the current limits of functioning. However, the treatment and activities to be included in the program should be under the direction of the physician.

INGUINAL HERNIA

A hernia is a protrusion of an organ through an abnormal opening. The most prevalent site is the abdominal region. Millions of persons in the United States suffer from some type of hernia, and in the majority of cases the hernias are of the inguinal type. However, along with inguinal hernia, there is a high incidence of femoral and umbilical hernias. Generally, the inguinal hernia is more prevalent in males and occurs most often in childhood, whereas the femoral hernia is most prevalent in females.

The inguinal canal is found in the lower abdomen just above Poupart's ligament and serves as a passageway for the spermatic vessels and the vas deferens in the male and the round ligament in the female. It is about 1½ inches long, and extends downward and inward. The canal's internal and external openings are termed the internal and external abdominal rings.

There are two types of inguinal hernias—congenital and acquired. The congenital or direct hernia is primarily associated with the descent of the testes before birth and is often discovered soon after birth. Many congenital hernias close spontaneously with application of a truss, which is a mechanical device that aids in reducing the hernia by placing external pressure at the site; however, operation is the choice of many physicians for the congenital inguinal hernia.

The second type of inguinal hernia occurs between the ages of 16 and 20 years and is categorized as acquired or indirect. This is best described as a sac protruding through the internal inguinal abdominal ring. An incomplete hernia would still be in the inguinal canal, whereas a complete hernia extends past the subcutaneous external ring and descends into the scrotum.

The femoral hernia, unlike the inguinal hernia, is associated with the female sex. A portion of the lower intestine protrudes through the femoral ring that is provided for the femoral vessels leading to the upper thigh.

There are many reasons attributed to the occurrence of hernia. Some common congenital causes may be inherited weakness of the lower abdomen, faulty descent of the testes, or abnormal enlargement of the internal inguinal ring. An acquired hernia can stem from trauma (as from a blow or lifting a heavy object), pregnancy, or degeneration. In general, the anatomy of a hernia may be divided into three parts: the mouth, the hernial ring, and the body. The body of the hernia consists of a sac that protrudes outside the abdominal cavity, often containing a portion of the abdominal viscera.

An early symptom of the hernia is swelling in the area of the internal inguinal ring that expands while the abdomen is under strain and contracts under slight pressure (Fig. 18-5). Pain upon exertion may also be elicited in the region of the groin.

Besides causing discomfort and aggravation, the inguinal hernia can also be a serious threat to health. A number of complications may aggravate hernial conditions; these include infection, incarceration, and strangulation. The incarcerated hernia is an irreducible hernial sac. An incarcerated hernia, if not treated promptly, may become strangulated and result in tissue damage, severe pain, and shock.

The student with a hernial condition should be aware of the inherent dangers and should be encouraged to undergo corrective operation as soon as feasible. During the preoperative period, a restrictive physical education program must be afforded. Activities that produce extreme fatigue or intraabdominal strain (such as weight lifting, gymnastics, track and field, and breath-holding activities) must be avoided. Programming emphasis should be placed on proper body mechanics, mild to moderate exercises, and voluntary lower limb movement while sitting or prone.

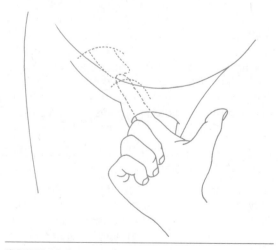

FIGURE 18-5
Palpating an inguinal hernia.

INFECTIOUS DISEASES

There are several infectious diseases that may be contracted by schoolchildren. In many cases, modification of activity is necessary to meet the temporary needs and abilities of these children. Some of the infectious diseases that may require the special attention of the physical educator are tuberculosis, pneumonia, streptococcal infections, infectious encephalitis, meningitis, and mononucleosis.

Tuberculosis

Tuberculosis is a disease of the lungs caused by the tubercle bacillus. Predisposing factors may include emotional or physical lowering of resistance, alcoholism, a chronic debilitating disease, poor nutrition and hygiene, or a combination of these factors.

No age group is exempt from the disease, but the greatest prevalence of tuberculosis is found among young adults and middle-aged persons.

It is difficult to identify tuberculosis. Perhaps the first indication that such an infection exists may come from a routine x-ray examination of the chest. However, other minor symptoms that may be associated with the onset of the disorder are fatigue, failure to gain weight during growth, low fever, cough, chest pain, and mild influenza.

There is great variability in degree, stage, and type of tuberculosis. Since each case of tuberculosis is different, there are many complex factors that must be resolved by the physician during treatment. Usually, complete bed rest is required in active cases until the disease can be brought under control. With the resumption of activities of daily living, general strength and endurance may be developed by means of progressive exercise. Also included in the treatment is a nutritious diet and activities that contribute to both physical and mental health. The child who is returning to school after an attack of tuberculosis is usually unable to engage in the unrestricted physical education program. The activities must be adapted to the child's present level of physical ability. Frequent periods of rest must be afforded so that the child will not become unduly fatigued. The physical education program for the child recovering

from tuberculosis should be under the direction of the physician.

The activity program should be mild at first and contain the element that all good programs contain, which is progression commensurate with the abilities of the afflicted person. Care should be taken to involve the student in activities that do not cause undue fatigue. The milder recreational activities such as swimming, archery, bowling, camping, and golf provide the student with opportunities for participation.

Pneumonia

Pneumonia is an infection of the air spaces of the lung. Usually, bacteria that cause pneumonia gain a foothold through the lowered resistance of a person. There are several types of pneumonia. Some of the most prevalent types are lobar, viral, bronchial, and foreign organism pneumonia.

Lobar pneumonia is often manifested by chills, fever, chest pain, coughing, shortness of breath, and inability to withstand fatigue. The temperature often reaches 104° to 105° F; consequently, bluish discoloration of the lips and skin occurs.

Viral pneumonia, which generally occurs in the younger and middle-aged groups, involves symptoms that are often difficult to identify because of gradual onset. On the other hand, pneumonia may also appear very abruptly after an upper respiratory tract infection. The most prevalent symptoms indicating viral pneumonia are generalized muscular pains and a slight cough. At times, however, the symptoms may be similar to those of the more explosive lobar pneumonia.

Bronchopneumonia occurs most often in children. The lungs are usually inflamed and there is often an inability to withstand fatigue. A cold is also present. Foreign organisms may also cause pneumonia, for they often precipitate a cough or low fever. In many instances, through the identification of the specific organism responsible for pneumonia, antibiotic treatment can control the disease effectively. An effort should be made to maintain a balanced, nutritious diet.

The physical educator should see that a child who has returned to school after an occurrence of pneumonia is not exposed to environmental conditions that would lower resistance and provoke another attack. Also, a progressive exercise program starting with activity at the student's present ability level, should be undertaken.

Streptococcal Infections

The streptococcal bacteria cause a wide variety of diseases that differ with regard to the portal of entry and the tissues on which the infectious agent acts. Some of the more important conditions caused by the streptococcal bacteria are scarlet fever and streptococcal sore throat such as tonsillitis and pharyngitis. Other diseases include mastoiditis, osteomyelitis, otitis media, impetigo, and other skin and wound infections.

Sources of the streptococcal infections are acutely ill or convalescent patients; discharges from the nose, the throat, and purulent lesions; or objects contaminated with such discharges. The transmission of the bacteria is by direct contact with the carrier, by indirect contact with objects handled, or by the spreading of droplets whereby the bacteria can be inhaled. Repeated attacks of streptococcal infections of the throat by different types of streptococci are frequent. It appears that neither active nor passive immunization against the *Streptococcus* organism itself can be accomplished satisfactorily.

When a student is recovering from a streptococcal infection, caution should be exercised with assignment to an unrestricted physical education program. The same procedures for implementing an exercise program for the person recovering from streptococcal sore throat are applicable to other illnesses: progressive exercise in accordance with the student's present abilities. Care must be taken to place the student in an environment that will not cause a lowering of resistance, thereby increasing vulnerability to recurring streptococcal infections. Streptococcal infections are particularly dangerous for children who have had rheumatic fever. Consequently, the fact cannot be overemphasized that a child who has been afflicted with rheumatic heart disease should be guarded judiciously against streptococcal infections, which could conceivably further

impair heart function. Antibiotic injections can be administered periodically to persons who tend to have recurrent streptococcal infections. This constitutes special risks in that the body may build an immunity to the antibiotic; however, for individuals who have had recurring rheumatic fever, antibiotic treatment may be necessary to avoid subsequent streptococcal infections that may prove damaging to the heart.

Infectious Encephalitis

Among the many forms of encephalitis, there are two major types—acute nonsuppurative encephalitis that follows or is a part of some infectious disease and the arthropod-borne viral encephalitis.

Nonsuppurative Encephalitis

Nonsuppurative encephalitis is an acute inflammatory condition of the brain that occurs as a result of complications of various infectious diseases and is characterized by some manifestation of cerebral dysfunction. The condition itself is not contagious, but it may complicate any acute infectious disease, even the common cold. Consequently, the cerebral symptoms may become more prominent than the primary disease. This form of encephalitis may attack persons of any age group, although children under 10 years of age are more frequently affected than adults.

Symptoms that may indicate acute nonsuppurative encephalitis are headache, visual disturbances (particularly double vision), vertigo, nausea, and general weakness. Observable symptoms may include change in sensory media and inattentiveness to ongoing activity. It is not uncommon to find symptoms such as convulsion, muscle twitchings or spasms, tremors, ataxia, and aphasia with the disease. Recovery from encephalitis is usually rapid and seemingly complete, but in many instances the nervous system is permanently impaired because of degenerative changes resulting from the disease.

Arthropod-borne Encephalitis

Although there are many forms of the athropod-borne viral encephalitis, all types produce an almost identical clinical picture. The symptoms that may be present are headache, tight hamstring muscles, stiff neck and back, fever, disorientation, stupor, coma, tremors, and spasticity. The symptoms may occur abruptly or may develop over a period of 1 week or more. When adults contract the disease, tendon and skin reflexes usually remain normal.

Programming for the Student with Encephalitis

The physical educator should be aware of changes that may occur in a student who has had infectious encephalitis. In many instances, particularly if there has been degeneration of the nervous system, the mental as well as the physical needs of the individual may be different upon return to class as compared with performance prior to the attack. The physical education teacher should know the limits of activity for each child and should be sensitive to adapting the activities so that the child may make a satisfactory adjustment to regular school activities. Characteristics that may be manifested after the attack are fatigue, impaired motor coordination, and a decrement of strength.

Meningitis

Meningitis is an acute contagious disease characterized by inflammation of the meninges of the spinal cord. The severity with which persons are attacked by the disease varies greatly. Epidemics of meningitis occur with greater frequency in rural areas as opposed to urban areas. The disease occurs at any age; however, 40% of meningitis cases occur in children under 10 years of age. There is also a great prevalence of meningitis in older children and young adults. Epidemics of meningitis are more prevalent in the winter and spring.

The onset of meningitis is usually abrupt and accompanied by severe headache and chills, followed soon by fever and vomiting. Other characteristics indicating the presence of the disease may be irritability, delirium, stupor, coma, convulsions, constipation or diarrhea, rash, infections of the ear such as mastoiditis or otitis me-

dia, difficulty in hearing, or eye conditions such as conjunctivitis, optic neuritis, diplopia, and strabismus. Other complications associated with meningitis are pneumonia, arthritis, hydrocephalus, cystitis, endocarditis, or pericarditis.

Many forms of meningitis can be classified within four major types. The main classifications are meningococcic meningitis, lymphocytic choriomeningitis, influenzal meningitis, and purulent meningitis. Each form needs to be diagnosed differentially for medical treatment.

Usually, the convalescent period for meningitis is not as long as for some other communicable diseases. It may be possible to involve the child more quickly in a graded program of activity than is possible in the case of other illnesses.

ANEMIA

Anemia is a condition of the blood in which there is a deficiency of hemoglobin, which delivers oxygen to body tissues. This deficiency of hemoglobin may be a result of the quantity contained in the red corpuscles of the blood or a reduction in the number of red corpuscles themselves.

The physical education teacher should be aware of the charcteristics that anemic persons display. In many instances, anemic persons appear to be pale because their blood is not as red as that of typical persons. Persons with anemia tire easily because of impaired oxidation in the muscles, and they also may become short of breath. Consequently, in many instances the rate of breathing is increased. As a rule, children with anemia become fatigued more easily than do typical children, are often unable to make gains in physical strength, and are impaired in learning motor skills.

Some of the symptoms that signify anemia are an increased rate of breathing, a bluish tinge of the lips and nails (because the blood is not as red), headache, nausea, faintness, weakness, and fatigue.

Causes

There are many diverse causes of anemia. Some of the main ones are (1) great loss of blood; (2)

decreased blood production within the system; (3) diseases such as malaria, septic infections, and cirrhosis; (4) poisons such as lead, insecticides, and arsenobenzene; and (5) chronic dysentery, intestinal parasites, and diseases associated with endocrine deficiency and vitamin deficiencies. Anemia is symptomatic of a disturbance that in many cases can be remedied. Inasmuch as there are several varieties of anemia, the method of treatment depends on the type of anemia present.

Types

There are several forms of anemia. Chlorosis, or iron deficiency anemia, is characterized by a reduced amount of hemoglobin in the corpuscles and usually occurs in young women at about the time of puberty. Anemia can be caused by excessive hemorrhage, in which case the specific gravity of the blood is reduced because there is a greater proportion of fluid in comparison with corpuscles in the blood. Occurring less often than chlorosis, pernicious anemia is characterized by a decrease in the number of red corpuscles. It can cause changes in the nervous system, along with loss of sensation in the hands and feet. In aplastic anemia, the red bone marrow that forms blood cells is replaced by fatty marrow. This form of anemia can be caused by radiation, radioactive isotopes, and atomic fallout. Certain antibiotics may also be causative factors. One prevalent type of anemia among blacks is sickle cell anemia.

Treatment

The various forms of anemia require different treatments. Chlorosis may be remedied by an increase in the amount of iron-bearing foods in the diet or by taking iron supplements. However, pernicious anemia requires the intramuscular injection of liver extracts. Aplastic anemia may be corrected by transplantation of bone marrow from healthy persons and by use of the male hormone testosterone, which is known to stimulate the production of cells by the bone marrow if enough red marrow is present for the hormone to act on.

Vitamin B is stored in the liver and released as required for the formation of red blood cells in the bone marrow.

Programming for the Anemic Student

The final decision regarding the nature of physical education activities for a child with anemia should by made by medical personnel. A well-conceived and supervised physical education program can be of great value to the child who has anemia. Exercise stimulates the production of red blood cells through the increased demand for oxygen. However, to be beneficial, an activity must be planned qualitatively with regard to the specific anemic condition. It is not uncommon for children who have anemia to be retarded in the development of physical strength and endurance. The alert physical educator should be able to assist in the identification of anemia and thus refer the student to medical authorities. Undiagnosed anemia may curtail motor skill and physical development and thus may set the child apart from peers in social experiences.

SUMMARY

Some other conditions in the law that qualify a student for special programming consideration are diabetes, kidney disorders, and tuberculosis. Additional conditions that may limit a student's strength, vitality, or alertness are menstruation and dysmenorrhea, hernia, pneumonia, streptococcal infections, encephalitis, meningitis, and anemia. The physical educator should understand the nature of each of these conditions, how the condition can affect a student's performance capability, and types of program modifications that best meet the needs of each student.

Most of the conditions discussed in this chapter require medical attention. When this is the case, it is advisable to consult with the student's physician to assure that the type of exercises and activities selected for the student will not aggravate the condition. In most situations mild exercise will benefit the student.

REVIEW QUESTIONS

1. What causes painful menstruation?
2. What diet changes might decrease pain during the first two days of menstruation?
3. What is the effect of activity during menstruation?
4. What are two exercises that can reduce dysmenorrhea?
5. What are four symptoms of diabetes?
6. What is the effect of exercise on glucose levels in the body?
7. How does exercise affect diabetic individuals?
8. What is the most prevalent kidney disorder in children and young adults?
9. What are the two types of inguinal hernias?
10. What activities should be avoided if a person has a preoperative hernia?
11. Name three infectious diseases and describe their effects on physical performance levels.
12. What are three characteristics of an anemic person?

STUDENT ACTIVITIES

1. Working with a partner, demonstrate the three exercises to reduce dysmenorrhea that are described in this chapter. Have your partner check the exercises for accuracy. Exchange roles.
2. Look through six recent issues on the *Journal of the American Medical Association*. List the articles that relate to the conditions described in this chapter. Read through some of the articles to see if exercise is mentioned as a possible way to relieve the condition.
3. Interview a diabetic person. Find out what type of medication the person takes and how often it must be taken. Ask if the person ever failed to take the medication and how they felt because of missing their dosage.
4. Interview a school nurse. Find out what percentage of the students in the nurse's school have the conditions discussed in this chapter.

REFERENCES

1. Anderson, T.W.: Swimming and exercise during menstruation, Health Phys. Educ. Rec. **36:**66-68, 1965.
2. Åstrand, P.O., et al.: Girl swimmers with special reference to respiratory and circulatory adaptation and gynaecological and psychiatric aspects, Acta Pediatr. [Supp.] **147:**1-71, 1963.
3. Billig, H.E., Jr., and Lowendahl, E.: Mobilization of the human body, Stanford, Calif., 1949, Stanford University Press.
4. Brooks, S.M., and Brooks, N.A.: Turner's personal and community health, ed. 16, St. Louis, 1983, The C.V. Mosby Co.
5. Clow, A.E., and Sanderson, M.: Effect of physical exercise on menstruation, Mind Body **30:**19-21, 1923.
6. Combs, B.J., Hale, D.R., and Williams, B.K.: An invitation to health, ed. 2, Menlo Park, Calif., 1983, Benjamin/Cummings Publishing Co.
7. Engerbretson, D.L.: The effects of internal training on the insulin dosage, sugar levels and other indexes of physical fitness in three diabetic subjects, Unpublished master's thesis, University of Illinois, Urbana, Ill., 1962.
8. Gilman, E.: Exercise program for correction of dysmenorrhea, J. Health Phys. Educ. Rec. **15:**377-381, 1944.
9. Kelly, E.D.: Adapted and corrective physical education, New York, 1965, Ronald Press Co.
10. Kogan, B.: Health, ed. 3, New York, 1980, Harcourt Brace Jovanovich Inc.
11. Mosher, C.D.: Dysmenorrhea, J.A.M.A. **62:**1297, 1914.
12. Nolen J.: Problems of menstruation, J. Health Phys. Educ. Rec. **36:**12, 1965.
13. Phillips, M., Fox, K., and Young, O.: Sports activity for girls, J. Health Phys. Educ. Rec. **30:**23-25, 1959.
14. Remein, Q.R., and Shields, F.A.: Diabetes fact book, Washington, D.C., 1962, United States Public Health Service.
15. Runge H.: Effects of bodily exercise on menstruation, J.A.M.A. **129:**68-72, 1928.
16. Schmitt, G.F.: Diabetes for diabetics: a practical guide, Miami, 1973, Diabetes Press of America Inc.
17. U.S. Department of Health, Education, and Welfare: Fed. Reg. **4:**42478, Aug. 23, 1977.
18. Yahraes, H.: Good news about diabetes, Public affairs pamphlet no. 138, New York, 1948, Public Affairs Committee, Inc.
19. Zankle, H.T.: Physical fitness index of diabetic patients, J. Assoc. Phys. Ment. Rehab. **10:**14-17, 1956.

SUGGESTED READINGS

Boyd, W.: A textbook of pathology, ed. 8, Philadelphia, 1970, Lea & Febiger.
Daniels, A.S., and Davies, E.A.: Adapted physical education, ed. 3, New York, 1975, Harper & Row, Publishers Inc.
Fait, H.F., and Dunn, J.M.: Special physical education, Chicago, 1984, Saunders College Publishing.
Seaman, J.A., and DePauw, K.P., The new adapted physical education: a developmental approach, Palo Alto, Calif., 1982, Mayfield Publishing Co.

PART FOUR

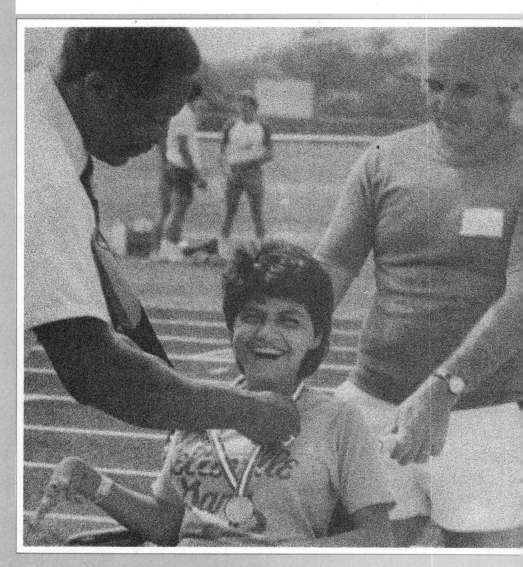

Organization and Administration

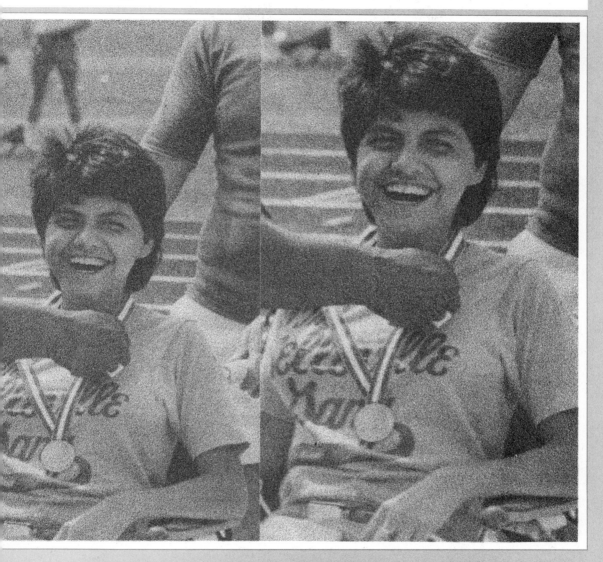

The roles of the adapted physical education teacher and other professionals and their contributions to the IEP are discussed in Chapter 19. Options for structuring physical education classes to best meet a variety of specific individual needs are presented. Types of equipment needed and ways to administer programs for students with disabilities are dicussed in detail.

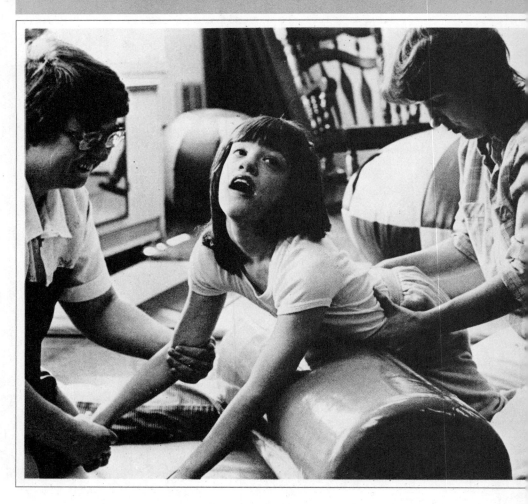

Multidisciplinary Staffing

OBJECTIVES

♦ Understand six provisions in P.L. 94-142 that concern necessary staffing for each student.

♦ Understand the types and roles of specialists who may occupy staff positions.

♦ Know how small school districts provide services for handicapped students.

♦ Know how children who need special services are identified.

♦ Understand what information is needed for the preliminary IEP staff meeting.

♦ Understand how often an IEP must be reviewed.

♦ Understand how often a handicapped student must be reevaluated.

Public Law 94-142 mandates that children with handicapping conditions be given every opportunity to function as normally as possible in the school setting. That is, the intent of the law is to ensure that children with handicapping conditions be given the same educational opportunity that their nonhandicapped peers enjoy. Early efforts to provide educational services in our schools were based on categorical labels; however, as more handicapped children entered the schools, it became increasingly apparent that these children had different needs. The heterogeneity of handicapped children made individualization of instruction a necessity. For this reason the requirement that an IEP be developed for each handicapped student who was experiencing adverse educational performance in the classroom, gymnasium, hospital or institution, or at home was built into the law. The law is very specific about how the IEP is developed and who takes part in the process. The process of developing the IEP is known as "staffing a student." The usual culmination of this process is the IEP meeting between school personnel and the student's parents or guardians.

Six provisions in the law that concern staffing a student follow:

1. The child must be identified by a physician or a psychologist as having a condition that impedes educational progress.
2. The parents must give informed consent for the child to be tested.
3. The child must be measured with tests that are valid and do not discriminate against the child (for example, you cannot give a test that includes verbal instruction to a child who is deaf and cannot read lips).
4. The child must be placed in the least restrictive environment, and that decision must be made by a multidisciplinary team.
5. The test results and proposed educational procedures must be reviewed with the parents (IEP meeting) and approved by them.
6. The parents have the right, under the law, to seek an independent evaluation.

Each of these provisions protects against inappropriate placement of the child in the school system. Although some schools attempt to comply minimally with the regulations, most schools

429

keep each child's best interest in mind throughout the evaluation and placement process.

PERSONNEL

The types of personnel involved with the educational process have increased dramatically since 1975. The variety and expertise of personnel available to students has never been greater. Specialists hired by school systems include school psychologists, psychometrists, speech therapists, audiologists, social workers, special educators, adapted physical educators, physical therapists, occupational therapists, music therapists, recreation therapists, and vocational counselors. Each of these disciplines plays a unique role in the educational process of children with handicapping conditions.

Educational Psychologist

The educational psychologist is concerned with cognitive learning problems and maladaptive behaviors that could interfere with a child's educational progress. Services offered by the educational psychologist include diagnostic evaluation (IQ, achievement, and emotional status testing), behavior modification, and in some cases psychotherapy and career counseling.

Psychometrist

In large school districts the role of administering and interpreting cognitive, achievement, and behavioral tests is filled by the psychometrist. In those school districts the educational psychologists limit their role to dealing with behavior management techniques.

Speech Therapists

These professionals evaluate and provide intervention programs to children with speech deficiencies or impediments. In addition to providing services to children, these professionals consult with teachers working directly with children and with parents of children who demonstrate speech problems.

Audiologists

In some school districts specialists in measuring hearing are on staff to provide routine and more extensive evaluation of hearing ability. In addition to testing, the audiologist can refer children for hearing device fittings or services that will improve the children's ability to pick up or process auditory information. Some school districts hire specialists who are trained in both speech and hearing disorders. Such specialists might be called communication therapists, speech correctionists, or speech pathologists. Regardless of the title, they deal with hearing, language comprehension, speech production, language expression, rhythm, and voice quality.[1]

Social Workers

Social workers are increasingly prevalent in school districts. These professionals must have an understanding of the broad spectrum of intraprofessional specialties and how they affect each student. Social workers often serve as the primary link between the school and the home. They gather information about the conditions and interpersonal relationships in the home, explore the personal effects of a disability, and evaluate the extent and quality of the disabled person's social contacts with friends and peers. The social worker's understanding of social and environmental pressures on a disabled person provide the multidisciplinary team with special insights that no other profession can.

Special Educators

Special educators are the supervisors or teachers who have direct contact with students in the classroom or special educational setting where academic lessons are conducted. These educators are in constant contact with the learner and have an opportunity to observe patterns of behavior and learning over extended periods. Because of their continued exposure to specific learners, they often have a greater understanding of an individual's style of performance than do those who have minimal contact with the student.

Adapted Physical Education Teachers

These professionals are physical educators with specialized training in evaluating, designing specialized physical and motor programs, and teaching the child with a handicapping condition. By law they are to provide *direct* services to children who have disabling conditions that interfere with the ability to move and develop motor skills.

Physical Therapists

Physical therapists evaluate and treat physical impairments through the use of various modalities. Some devices that bring about a healing or rehabilitative response from the patient are deep heat (diathermy, ultrasound), superficial heat (infrared heat, hydromassage), cryotherapy (cold therapy), electrical muscle stimulation, massage, mobilization techniques, and specific exercises for affected muscles and joints. The physical therapist may also instruct the learner in the use of braces, wheelchairs, crutches, and prosthetic appliances and in activities of daily living. As a related service physical therapy *should not* substitute for physical education. Rather, this profession should be called on to provide testing, consulting, and rehabilitation treatment that will better enable the student to function in the physical education class.

Occupational Therapists

Occupational therapists traditionally have worked with patients to improve functional living and employment skills to improve the patient's psychological outlook as well as foster self-sufficiency and occupational independence. More recently, occupational therapists have been trained to evaluate and design intervention programs for individuals believed to have sensory integration deficits. Like physical therapists, they are classified as a related service providers, and their services *should not substitute* for physical education. These professionals can be called on to provide testing, consultation, and habilitation treatment to enable students to function more ably in the physical education class.

Music Therapists

These therapists use music as a recreational, creative, and therapeutic medium to produce physiological, psychological, and emotional responses from individuals with handicapping conditions. Music can serve as an important therapeutic adjunct to the total rehabilitation program.

Vocational Counselors

Vocational counselors have a broad knowledge of handicapping conditions, the habilitative process, and the needs of the disabled. Persons with physical, mental, or emotional handicaps are guided by vocational counselors as they develop their capacities and abilities for employment.

Each of these professionals brings a special expertise to the school setting; however, not all these individuals are found in every school district. When a school district is limited in size or resources, rather than hire all these experts, the school district may rely on a special education center to provide such services. These centers are called by different names in different states. In Kansas the term *cooperative special education center* is used. In Michigan the title *intermediate school district* is given to centers that provide specialized services. In Texas *regional special education center* is used. In every case the purpose of the center is to house a group of professionals trained to deal with the special problems of the handicapped. In small school districts that use centers, several schools within the district are assigned to one center. When centers are not available, school districts either hire their own specialized personnel or refer children to hospitals or private practitioners for testing and recommendations.

Regardless of the arrangement used to ensure that handicapped students receive adequate appraisal and programming, the process of staffing the child is very similar in most school districts.

The first step in the process is to identify the child with special needs.

IDENTIFYING THE CHILD WITH SPECIAL NEEDS

Children who have serious handicapping conditions are identified as needing special services before they reach school age. When children are identified before they enter the formal school setting, they often have a history of receiving professional help from as early as birth. Children who have received services early in life arrive at school with a large portfolio that includes assessment and intervention information. Generally, they offer no surprises other than that they perform at higher levels than do children who did not have the benefit of early intervention programs.

Children with less apparent disabling conditions are often not so fortunate. Even with the active searches that have been conducted by Child Find programs, sooner or later every school district discovers a child who is entitled to, and should receive, special services. These children are eventually classified as educable mentally retarded, learning disabled, or emotionally disturbed. It is not until the child enters the formal schooling years that deficits and an inability to keep up with other children are recognized. These children are first identified by school personnel. Most often the classroom or physical education teacher is the first to become aware of these children's learning problems.

The physical educator can pick up on disabling conditions of specific children early in the school year if he routinely administers screening tests to all children in the physical education class. However, whether the teacher administers a test or not, as children participate in activities with their classmates the slow developing children soon become apparent.

In both the case of severely handicapped children and children with less apparent conditions the school principal assumes the major responsibility for ensuring that the child receives appropriate services. The principal is contacted either by the parents or other professionals who have been providing services to the severely disabled child or by a teacher who first suspects a child is not performing to the standards expected in the classroom or gymnasium.

Once the principal has been notified, a preliminary meeting is usually scheduled. This initial meeting includes a minimum of educational professionals. The personnel involved are the principal, the teacher, and the educational psychologist; however, a social worker and possibly a director of special education might also attend. The child's learning problems and special needs are discussed, and then the parents are contacted for their approval to test the child. If the parents agree to the recommendation that their child be evaluated, one member of the professional staff is designated as the coordinator of the proposed testing. The coordinator then makes arrangements with each of the professionals who is to test the child and follows up to see that the testing is carried out. If during the testing procedure it becomes apparent that additional opinions are needed, the coordinator is contacted and the recommendations are made. The coordinator and principal discuss the recommendations and decide whether to follow through with the suggestions. The physical educator should keep in mind that, when the school recommends professional opinion not available in the school district be sought, the school is responsibile for paying the bill. In large school districts where many professionals are on staff and in school districts that subscribe to services offered by special education centers, there may be no cost for the additional testing. When there is no cost to the school district, it is relatively easy to receive permission for the additional testing. However, in school districts where professional services are limited and services have to be purchased from private practioners or hospitals, the decision might be to disallow additional testing.

Whether services of the related therapies are available or not, the adapted physical educator should administer as comprehensive an evaluation as possible. If the physical education teacher suspects problems beyond his expertise, then permission should be requested to provide additional testing. The situation can be very delicate and requires good judgment in trying to serve the child while being as thorough and professional as possible.

Whatever the case, it is important to determine accurate levels of educational performance when evaluating the student because during the next meeting goals, objectives, and alternative educational strategies will be discussed. Therefore, to best prepare for reporting on the student, all these procedures should be completed *before* the preliminary IEP staff meeting.

THE PRELIMINARY IEP STAFF MEETING

Ideally, the preliminary IEP staff meeting should be attended by each individual who tested the child, the coordinator, the principal, and the classroom teacher. Unfortunately, this is not always possible. Often, because of time limitations, not all the people who actually tested the child can attend every meeting. The argument is made that it is neither expedient nor necessary for all evaluators and teachers to be present if those who do attend can interpret the test results. The adapted physical education teacher who finds himself in this situation should be certain that the person making the physical education report understands what the evaluation results were and why it is important to follow the physical education recommendations.

On a more positive note, many school districts do recognize the value of having the professionals who evaluated the child present at the preliminary IEP staff meeting. In these cases the meeting proceeds as follows.

1. The principal or coordinator gives general background on the child, including the reason the child was referred for testing and the professionals included in the overall evaluation.

2. Each evaluator then gives a concise report that includes the name of the tests administered, the results of the testing (including strengths and deficits demonstrated by the child), and the goals and objectives that should be set for the child. Whenever possible, it is important to tie the physical education findings to results found by other evaluators (for example, poor balance often can be tied to fine motor delays, visual problems can be tied to reading difficulties, poor self-concept can be associated with motivational problems in the classroom).

3. An open discussion among the people present at the meeting usually is the next step. During this discussion all the needs of the child and alternative methods for meeting these needs are explored. At this point the true multidisciplinary nature of the meeting should surface. Each professional must be willing to recognize the value of the services that other professions have to offer, as well as the value of her own expertise. The knowledgeable physical educator will understand and appreciate services that can be provided by the various therapies; however, she must also recognize that many activities in physical education can accomplish the physical and motor goals of the child in an interesting, novel fashion unique to the discipline.

4. Agreement must be reached among the professionals in attendance about which of the child's needs are most pressing and which goals and objectives take precedence over others. When contributing to these decisions, the physical educator should focus on the present level of educational performance evidenced by the child in the physical and motor areas. If through testing the child was found to have basic level deficits such as reflex abnormalities, vestibular delays, or range of motion limitations the physical educator does not believe can be included in the physical education program activities, referral to a related therapy may be the best recommendation. Such a recommendation does not mean the child should not or cannot participate in some type of physical education class. It simply means that the related therapies should focus on the immediate low level deficits while the child continues to participate in a physical education program that is designed to reinforce the intervention programs pro-

vided by the other services. None of the related therapies should replace physical education; however, they could be used to help the student take a more active role in the physical education class.

5. Alternative placements are discussed and agreed on. Once again, physical educators should remember that their services are valuable, regardless of the child's demonstrated functioning levels.

IEP STAFFING

Once the staff members who participate in the preliminary IEP staff meeting have explored the student's present levels of educational performance and discussed possible goals, objectives, and alternate programs or placements that will meet the child's needs, the parents are contacted by the principal or coordinator to meet with the entire multidisciplinary team or representatives of the team. P.L. 94-142 states that the following participants must be involved in the IEP staffing[2]:

♦ One or both of the child's parents
♦ When appropriate, the child
♦ The child's teacher
♦ A representative of the school, other than the child's teacher, who is qualified to provide or supervise the provision of special education
♦ Other individuals at the discretion of the parents or school

During the IEP staff meeting findings and recommendations of the team are discussed with the parents, and parental approval is sought. If the parents agree with the recommendations of the team, they sign the form, and the placement and programs are initiated. If the parents do not agree with the recommendations of the team, alternative solutions must be explored until the parents are satisfied with the school's efforts. If agreement between the team and the parents cannot be reached, the parents may seek the opinion of an outside agency. Although disagreement is not appealing to a school team, it is the parents' right to ask for due process.

If the parents do not agree wih the recommendations of the staff, there is an appeal process that should be followed. Some of these cases end in formal litigation (in federal court or an office of civil rights); however, most are resolved before such a step is taken.

An additional provision in the law is that personnel who contribute to the student's IEP must reconvene at least once yearly to review and revise it (Section 121a.343 [d]) and reevaluate at least once every 3 years (Section 121a.543 [b]).[2]

Throughout the entire process of testing and staffing the adapted physical educator should strive to be as helpful, thorough, and professional as possible. Often, when acceptance of the physical educator's recommendations seems impossible, patience and perseverance will win out. To be accepted and heard by other professionals we must remain calm, stick to presenting the facts, and be willing to overlook belittling comments that simply reflect others' lack of knowledge about the depth and importance of physical education. We are important, we have a unique dimension to contribute to students' lives, and we can make a dramatic difference in the quality of life for handicapped people.

SUMMARY

P.L. 94-142 mandates that handicapped children who demonstrate adverse educational performance must be tested and that the test results and recommendations by a professional team be approved by the parents of the child. The disciplines involved with the evaluation of the child include school psychologists, psychometrists, speech therapists, audiologists, social workers, special educators, adapted physical educators, physical therapists, occupational therapists, music therapists, vocational counselors, and administrative personnel. The number of professionals involved with the evaluation and staffing depends on the needs of the students and the resources of the school district.

The adapted physical education teacher should play a major role in the evaluation and staffing of students demonstrating adverse physical education performance. Related therapies should be involved in the evaluation and staffing only if they have something unique to contribute to the motor and physical evaluation and program.

Ideally, the preliminary IEP staff meeting should be attended by each individual who tested the child plus other professional educators; however, often one professional will be appointed to present another's test results and recommendations. During the preliminary IEP staff meeting the tests administered, results of the testing, and goals and objectives are discussed. After that discussion agreement is reached about which goals and objectives are most important and the appropriate placement that should be made.

In the actual IEP staffing the parents meet with the entire multidisciplinary team or representatives of the team. The team's findings and recommendations are discussed with the parents, and parental approval is sought. If the parents agree with the recommendations, the placement and programs are initiated. If the parents do not agree with the team's recommendations, the parents may appeal the case.

A student's IEP must be reviewed yearly and reevaluated at least once every 3 years.

REVIEW QUESTIONS

1. What six provisions that relate to staffing a student are included in P.L. 94-142?
2. What types of specialists could be involved in staffing a student?
3. Describe the functions of at least five specialists who might be involved in testing or staffing a student.
4. Under what circumstances should a related service such as physical or occupational therapy be involved in testing a handicapped child?
5. How do small school districts provide testing services for handicapped students?

STUDENT ACTIVITIES

1. Interview a school principal or a director of special education and find out how the school or district conducts preliminary and actual IEP staffings. Who makes the original referral? Who is involved with testing the referred child? Which professionals are present during the preliminary IEP staffing? What role does physical education have in testing and staffing handicapped students?
2. Contact the parents of a handicapped student. Find out how their child was originally identified as having a handicap and what type of testing and staffing was done for their child. Ask the parents if the recommendations the school made were satisfactory.
3. Interview an adapted physical education teacher and find out what role she plays in testing and staffing handicapped students in her school.

REFERENCES

1. Seaman, J.A., and DePauw, K.P.: The new adapted physical education: a developmental approach, Palo Alto, Calif. 1982, Mayfield Publishing Co.
2. U.S. 94th Congress, Public Law 94-142, Nov. 29, 1975.

SUGGESTED READINGS

Christopolos, F., and Valletutti, P.J., editors: Interdisciplinary approaches to human services, Baltimore, 1977, University Park Press.
Howell, K.: Inside special education, Columbus, Ohio, 1983, Charles E. Merrill Publishing Co.

CHAPTER 20

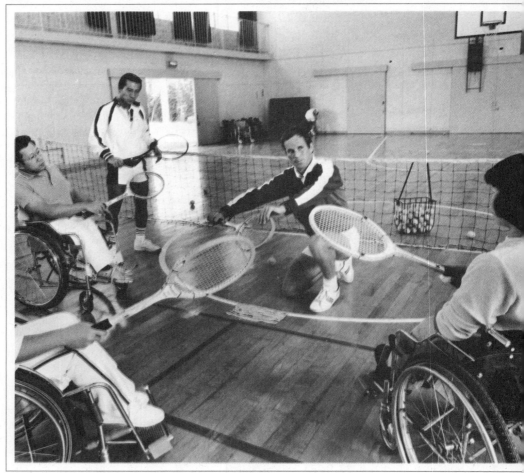

Photo by Bruce Haase, Peter Burwash International

Class Organization

OBJECTIVES

♦ Demonstrate knowledge of different ways of teaching physical education and organizing curriculum skills and information.

♦ Know how to set up a learning station to conduct an IEP and arrange the physical environment.

♦ Use peer and cross age tutors in an individualized learning system.

♦ Effectively group students.

♦ Monitor pupil performance and progress.

♦ Manage instructional time efficiently and compose a daily plan.

Adapted physical education classes can be organized for instruction in several different ways. Throughout the United States factors such as the number of days physical education is offered each week, the time allowed for the activity phase of the program, whether the adapted physical education program is integrated with the regular physical education program, the availability of specially trained teachers, and special facilities and equipment vary widely. The special abilities and the preferences of the supervisor and teachers also can influence the type of program offered.

The various types of classes require different formats of organization. They include (1) regular class with handicapped children mainstreamed with nonhandicapped children, (2) handicapped-only classes in which there are 10 to 20 mild to moderate handicapped students, and (3) small classes that contain 1 to 10 severely and profoundly handicapped students. Each group of children requires different types of class organization. Furthermore, other variables relevant to

class organization besides the nature of the handicap are (1) the age of the learners, (2) the tasks to be learned, and (3) incentive for learning the tasks.

In each of these situations the physical education teacher must adapt instruction, manage behavior, and promote social acceptance of handicapped children. Furthermore, the teacher is responsible for arranging and managing the total instructional environment in physical education. It is important to choose the type of class organization that will enable students to progress to the best of their abilities in physical education activities.

SPECIAL EXERCISE AND ACTIVITY PHASE

Many students in adapted physical education need special exercises to help them correct or prevent disabilities or to improve their physical fitness or their perceptual-motor abilities. Exercise and activity programs can be conducted by

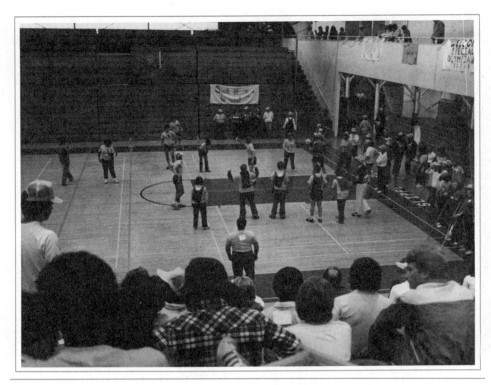

FIGURE 20-1
A class of moderately mentally retarded persons in line to participate in a game.
(Courtesy Western Pennsylvania Special Olympics.)

using a combination of the following methods of instruction.

Organizing Individual Activity

Adapted classes can be organized for instruction so that each student has an individual exercise and/or activity program. This method is implicit in the IEP of P.L. 94-142. Through the use of self-instructional and evaluative standard teaching sequences children in the early elementary school years can participate in individual exercise programs. The major advantage of this method is that students have programs specifically planned to meet their needs and interests. The exercises, the number of repetitions, the amount of resistance used, the rest periods, and the special equipment needed are all assigned to enable students to meet predetermined objectives. Students can be

strongly motivated to work toward correction or improvement of their disabilities in this type of class. Some teachers may find that controlling a group of 20 to 25 students who are all working on individual programs is more difficult than class control of students who are all doing the same program simultaneously. However, the advantages of having each student engage in an individual program of activities outweigh such problems. Preparation of individual programs is time consuming, but certain shortcuts can be used to enable the teacher to prepare these individual programs in a minimum amount of time.

Organizing Group Teaching

A class organized formally for exercises and other selected activities is one in which all students perform the same activity at the same time, usually under the direction of the teacher or a student leader. However, each student performs to his or her present level of educational performance on the specific instructional task. This type of program lends itself well to the instruction of younger children in elementary school or to the instruction of boys and girls who cannot accept the responsibility of an individual program. The advantages of this type of organization are that it gives teachers good control of the class and allows them to observe the performance of all the students more adequately than if they were watching 20 students, each doing something different. A disadvantage of this system is the lack of opportunity to give individually assigned activities to students with special needs. The use of special types of equipment is also more difficult, since each student must have his or her own piece of apparatus in the formal plan.

Homogeneous Grouping

A third method of class teaching involves the organization of an adapted physical education class into homogeneous groups based on similarities in the type of exercise and activity program needed. Students in need of anteroposterior posture correction might be grouped together to perform the same exercises (at their own ability levels), another group might work on foot exercises, and another group might do special adapted activities and exercises for perceptual-motor growth. These groups of students might remain the same throughout the class period or they might change to allow for more flexibility in the programs. Dependable students can lead and motivate those with less interest and drive. The teacher can also take advantage of assigning some individual types of programs and still have adequate supervision because of the several homogeneous groups that perform their programs together.

Combined Method

Many teachers prefer to use a combination of the preceding types of class organization to meet the individual needs of the students, to provide for some small group activities and some individual exercise and activity sessions during which the teacher more directly controls the amount of work done.

This combination plan might be organized as follows:

5 minutes: Formal warm-up consists of all students doing the same exercises under the leadership and direction of the teacher or a student leader.

5 minutes: Students are divided into homogeneous groups according to their needs and perform three activities or exercises with the members of their group under direction of a student leader.

10 minutes: Each student performs five exercises or activities specifically assigned to him or her, doing the number of repetitions assigned and recording progress on the exercise card. (Activities using special equipment can be assigned here, since students are able to take turns in the use of special pieces of apparatus.)

5-10 minutes: Games, relays, and contests are organized and led by the teacher, finishing with formal dismissal of the class, if desired.

Activities for Daily Living and Instructional Aides

Whether teachers use the individual or the group method of class organization, additional help is always needed, especially with more severely handicapped persons. Both paid aides and volunteer help are needed to instruct and carry out the activities of daily living.

There must be considerable inservice training for these important members of the instructional staff. Parents, high school and college students in training to become teachers, and members of the PTA and other service groups often serve as volunteers to enrich the individualized program.

Allocation of Time for Components of the Program

The sports phase of an adapted physical education class can be organized in several different

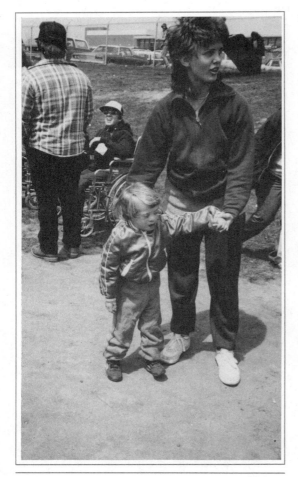

FIGURE 20-2
A volunteer assists a child during Special Olympics.
(Courtesy Western Pennsylvania Special Olympics.)

ways, depending on the general plan for adapted physical education in the school, how it is coordinated with the regular physical education program, the availability of regular and special facilities and equipment, and the background and skill of the teacher in charge.

Often the special class in adapted physical education has, as a part of its yearly program, a certain amount of time scheduled for adapted sports and games. This can be organized in one of the three following ways:

1. A part of each period is devoted to team sport or lifetime sport games.
2. From 1 to 3 days of each week are set aside for these activities.
3. A period of 1, 2, or more consecutive weeks is blocked out for an activity. There can be as many of these blocks of time for sports activities during the semester as are deemed desirable.

Some teachers have found that the first method, in which up to 15 minutes of each class period is devoted to games and sports (usually after the exercise portion of the class is finished), serves as a good motivation device, keeping interest at a high level in the exercise and sports parts of the program. Time, of course, is a limiting factor in this type of organization, tending to rule out sports and games that require extensive preparations, equipment checkout, instruction, or travel to a specialized location for the activity. This method is often used in elementary school classes and, to some extent, in junior high classes.

Where 1 to 3 days a week are set aside for the adapted sports program, activities that require more time, organization, and instruction can be included. Almost any game or sport can be modified so that handicapped students can participate. Junior and senior high school classes are often organized in this fashion. This type of schedule enables the teacher to keep interest high in the exercise and sports programs throughout the year. It also gives the student an opportunity to work on a special exercise program continuously throughout the semester or year without having to stop the exercise routine for an extended period to participate in various sports and games.

Some teachers prefer to organize the adapted sports portion of the class into blocks of time for instruction and activity. This type of program might consist of 4 weeks of swimming, 4 weeks of a team sport, 4 weeks of exercise, and 4 weeks of an individual sport. Thus student and instructor attention and interest can be focused on one activity at a time. If the regular physical education

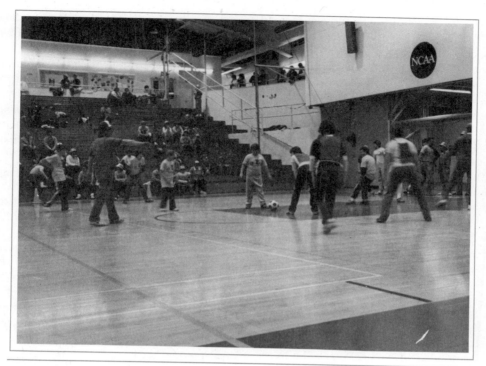

FIGURE 20-3
Handicapped and nonhandicapped play in a game of indoor soccer.
(Courtesy Western Pennsylvania Special Olympics.)

classes are scheduled on the block system, it is usually easier to obtain facilities and equipment for the adapted physical education classes if they, too, are scheduled for a single activity for a block of time.

However, inasmuch as each parent has the prerogative to participate in the planning of the child's program, great flexibility must be built into the program. A considerable portion of the physical education program must be individualized so that each child may engage in the specific activities that have been written into the IEP with the approval of the parents.

Handicapped Students in Regular Classes

Some IEPs require that students in adapted physical education join a regular physical education class for their work in sports and games. This is in keeping with the concept of mainstreaming. By joining this regular group for various types of activities during the year, handicapped children can learn culturally relevant social behaviors that hopefully will generalize to a normal society in the postschool years. A free interchange between handicapped and nonhandicapped children can do much to eliminate any feeling of stigmatization on the part of the student who is placed in a special class. Physical education teachers who instruct handicapped children in the regular class need skills for the conduct of individualized instruction and for the development of attitudes of the nonhandicapped that are conducive to acceptance of individual differences.

Coeducational Classes

Many schools are attempting to offer adapted physical education classes to their students on a coeducational basis with varying degrees of success. These programs might be most successful at the elementary school and college levels. At the secondary school level students are especially peer conscious and are sometimes apprehensive about coeducational physical education. Even in the regular classes it would take a strong teacher with excellent backing from the other teachers and the administration to break down some of the traditional feelings associated with a coeducational program.

If feasible, there are several advantages to be found in the conduct of a coeducational adapted physical education program. They include the following:

- ◆ The best teacher, male or female, can be used to administer and teach in the program.
- ◆ In small schools this would increase the flexibility in student scheduling.
- ◆ The arbitrary division of the class because of the sex of the individual student is discouraged.
- ◆ The majority of teachers are trained in corrective or adapted physical education in coeducation classes and thus are prepared to direct such programs.

The major problems associated with the coeducational class occur in the examination and the exercise phases of the program. Having a male teacher and a female teacher present during the initial posture and the other examinations and having the students wear appropriate apparel during both the examination and the exercise phases of the progam should minimize these two problems. The traditional pattern of having completely separate classes for boys and girls in both regular and adapted physical education is rapidly being replaced by more coeducational classes. Well-conceived organization and administration of coeducational programs do much to promote quality physical education for the handicapped.

COORDINATING THE LEARNING ENVIRONMENT

The physical education teacher must have considerable management skills to coordinate the learning environment. Stephens[10] outlines six classroom elements that teachers should consider:

1. Demographics: the group's composition
2. Physical environment: the use of the play area and its surroundings
3. Time: the amount of time available each week for the program
4. Student motivation: ways in which students are reinforced for performance
5. Provision for interacting: mixing students among peers and the teacher
6. Differentiating instruction: the extent to which and how the instruction is individualized

Physical education teachers must be able to cope with individual differences of their students. It is no longer desirable for physical education teachers to stand in front of a class and instruct all pupils on the same task and expect that they will all be successful and learn at the same rate. The need for individualized instruction requires that the teacher be a facilitator and manager of learning. This requires that in regular classes where children are mainstreamed, peers must be trained to assist those who need help. In many handicapped-only classes the physical education teacher may need to train special education teachers, their aides, and volunteers to effectively manage all the children. An effective class structure consists of learning stations, with adult teacher aides and peer or cross-age tutors (faster learners or children who are older) in assistance. Children then move to appropriate stations and learn skills appropriate to their needs. This requires that much of the planning for programming and reviewing student progress, teacher plans, and development of material must be done before class. Under these conditions effective learning is contingent on excellent classroom organization, planning, and management.

PEER TEACHERS AND MODELING

One's peers are powerful facilitators of learning. Once instruction becomes specific, it is not difficult for students to learn what it is they are to do and then communicate information to their peers. The peer instruction or modeling can be done by either handicapped or nonhandicapped children.[8] Prerequisites for peer or cross-teaching are student knowledge of what is to be done and ability to communicate and evaluate peer performance of the activity. Such instructional activity is what Mosston[6] calles *reciprocal teaching.* Sherrill[8] indicates that peer and cross-teaching encourages the acceptance of the handicapped by the nonhandicapped when nonhandicapped children are the peer instructors. The PEOPEL Project (Physical Education Opportunity Program for Exceptional Learners) is nationally recognized. This organization has effectively used peer teachers.

Role of Peer Teachers

Peer teachers can be indispensible to organizations of individualized learning environments. They can assume several responsibilities that contribute to class management and record keeping of progress in physical education, such as setting up and storing equipment before and after class, collecting data on self and others, and assisting with the instruction of peers.

Setting Up Equipment

It is not difficult for a teacher to manage equipment if there is to be mass instruction in group activity. However, if learning stations are to be set up, which requires considerable equipment to accommodate individual differences at each station, assistance from pupils is desirable. Certain measurements, such as those which indicate distance from targets and evaluation of jumping and throwing, objectify learning on tasks. Therefore it is imperative that the physical education teacher request and be provided with assistance from trained students to help with instruction and classroom management. Assignments can be made for specific children to carry out specific responsibilities. Diagrammed and posted floor layouts are valuable aids to students in setting up the learning situations.

Data Collection

Conduction of the IEP requires that instructional decisions be made from a data base. Often it is not feasible for the teacher to collect the data. Peer teachers can accomplish the task when there are sequences of written objectives. The students, under these conditions, need to know how the instructional objectives are performed and when the objectives have been mastered. The data can then be recorded. The pupil in question can collect this type of data or pupils can collect the data on one another.

Data on positive and negative social behavior of children are valuable for conducting programs and should be recorded. Peer teachers can help here too. Masking tape can be placed on the wrist as a recording format and peers can record data on the tape (see Chapter 7).

Cross-Age Tutors

Cross-age tutors are usually honor students who are released from school or are scheduled with younger and slower learning children. They serve for a short time and usually feed back information about errors in task performance and student collection of data. Tutors need to be thoroughly familiar with the programming if their assistance is to be valuable. Research indicates that third grade children are capable of correcting one another's movement errors. However, in a structured behavioral program that uses stick figures to represent objectives kindergarten students and trainable mentally retarded children can learn to self-instruct; by first grade some can feed back information to peers.[7,13]

LEARNING STATIONS

Learning stations are areas in the facility where activity is conducted to achieve specific objectives. Often stations are used to improve skills through behavioral programming. Learning stations vary in number, nature of the learning task, or permanency of the assignment. Playing a game may be considered a learning station.

Once learning stations have been established,

it is necessary to manage each student at the stations during the entire class period so the unique learning needs of each child can be met. Several systems can be used to assign students to stations that meet their learning needs:

- Rotation: Every student participates at every learning station.
- Free movement: Students have individualized programs and move to the learning stations at their own discretion.
- Structured movement: Students are assigned to stations that meet their learning needs and spend a specified amount of time at each station. There is a period when all students move to stations to start other activities.

Each of these systems requires a particular degree of skill management by the physical education teacher. The rotation system requires initial assignment of students to groups with accommodation for specific learners. The groups are rotated after a specified time frame. Free movement rotation may be necessary when IEPs are provided for each student. This management system enables students to participate in activities that meets their unique needs. Therefore it is unlikely that any two students will be assigned to the same learning stations. Each student manages himself with respect to time. Structured movement requires that the teacher make individual schedules of participation for each child. Under these conditions rotation is structured so each child participates in necessary activities in a structured manner. The younger the child and the more severe the handicap, the greater the need for structured movement.

Characteristics

Most learning stations have a set of general characteristics. Minimum requirements for most learning stations are that they be a designated area for participation, that they include specific learning activities designed to meet an educational need, and that equipment is related to the physical activity.

Learning systems involving behavioral programming and structured movement require more elaborate designs. Additional items might be (1) lines and targets needed to specify the conditions of the objectives, (2) measuring instruments, such as time clocks and tapes, (3) program cards (chart) with all of the behavioral objectives, (4) labels to indicate the number of the station, and (5) a data sheet on which progress can be recorded. Each learning station should be designed to maximize the independence of each learner and to enable peer teachers and cross-age teachers to assist with the instructional process.

Advantages

Some advantages for using learning stations to conduct individualized programming are included in the following list:

- The number of students at any learning station at a specific time can vary.
- Learning stations can accommodate persons with differing skill levels.
- The length of time one spends at a learning station can vary.
- The nature of the activity is specified so other persons can assist with instruction.

Learning stations need not be used all the time. Many of the activities, such as games, require the entire group; in this case the use of learning stations is undesirable. However, to accommodate the unique physical education needs of children with diverse skill and ability levels, group instruction alone will not suffice.

Grouping Students

When skills and abilities are the focus of instruction, learning stations can accommodate individual differences. However, the skills are often utilized in the form of a group game. When populations of handicapped and nonhandicapped are diverse, techniques are needed to coordinate groups of students so that activity in games can be mutually beneficial. Some of the questions that need to be answered when selecting groups for specific activities are:

1. Does the learner have the prerequisite skills to play the game?
2. If there are deficient skills, what modifications can be made for participation?

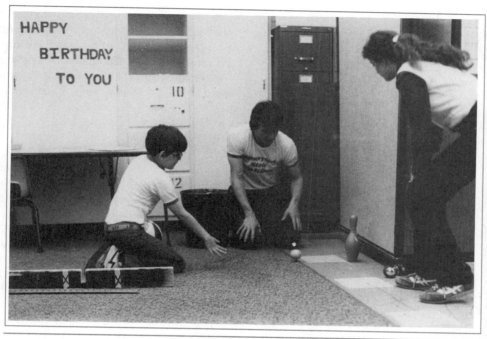

FIGURE 20-4
Learning stations require specific equipment that matches programmed activity to achieve stated objectives.

3. Does the learner know the rules?
4. Does the learner have the social discipline to play the game without impairing the benefits of other participants?
5. What is the maximum size of the group?
6. What is the minimum number of persons who should participate in the group?

No hard rules can be given for the selection of participants for a group. In the final analysis professional judgments are needed by the physical education teacher to decide the composition of a group formulated to achieve a specific educational purpose.

GENERALIZATION OF INSTRUCTIONAL SKILLS TO THE COMMUNITY AND SPORTS ORGANIZATIONS

The activities and skills learned in the physical education class should generalize and be applicable to community activity. Therefore the gen-

eral nature of physical activity should represent, to the greatest extent possible, the sports and skills being taught in a regular class or sports currently being played in the community.

Special Olympics and other sports organizations for individuals with disabling conditions comprise many sports. Each sport is conducted during a particular time of the year. Interscholastic events of sports organizations provide an opportunity for widespread participation. Therefore the selection of the physical education content should take into consideration linkage with culminating sports events in the community that relate directly to the instructional skills.

MONITORING PERFORMANCE

There are two general phases of instruction—presenting new material and practicing what has been learned from the presentation to improve performance. During practice, methods should be

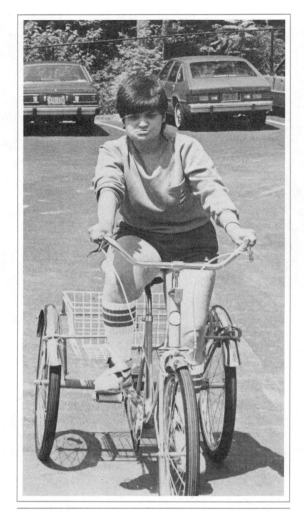

FIGURE 20-5
Adapted bicycle activity can be used to attain mobility in natural community environments.
(Courtesy Verland Foundations, Inc.)

been performed correctly. This works well with students who have a history of failure, since a behavioral shaping program ensures more success than failure.[5] In behavioral programming learners progress at their own rate through small, incremental steps that build on previous learning.[3]

MONITORING PROGRESS

It is necessary to monitor the progress of handicapped children in the acquisition of objectives listed on the IEP according to the nature of the activity and the type of instructional approach. If standardized normative-referenced tests are used, testers must be trained to measure continuous instructional progress and learning outcomes before the post test is given. Then it can be decided whether the programming is effective. If behavioral hierarchical programming is used, progress can be monitored daily. However, in the event that the students participate in self-instructional and evaluative activity, these student skills must also be monitored to verify the validity of progress. If student data collection proves invalid (unsuccessful), a peer teacher or the regular teacher conducts the monitoring test.

The acquisition of cognitive objectives such as rules of the game and strategies can be reported from written/oral tests or checklists designed to evaluate participation (see Chapter 5). Clearly, the progress of each child should be monitored to determine whether programming is effective. If it is not effective, it should be changed.

MANAGING INSTRUCTIONAL TIME EFFICIENTLY

Physical education teachers often have limited time with their handicapped students. To maximize benefits, class time should be managed efficiently by establishing a daily schedule for each class. Mercer and Mercer[5] indicate that schedules tell what activities will occur and when they will occur; also, schedules divide the class periods into time blocks and ascribe specific amounts of

incorporated into instruction to monitor student performance. Self-instructional behavioral programs (Chapter 5), in which the learner performs alone, enable students to receive feedback from performance and practice independently without the assistance of the teacher. This frees the teacher from direct instruction. When objectives are specific, students know when the task has time to the activities. Highest priority activities should be given to instructional activity. Noninstructional activities should be kept to a minimum. They suggest the following:

♦ Move from definite to flexible schedules.
♦ Alternate highly preferred with less preferred activities.
♦ Plan for leeway time.
♦ Provide a daily schedule for each student.
♦ Provide a variety of activities.

It is usually best to keep the activity periods short. The more mature the learner, the longer the activity period. The schedule should be shared with students and assistive personnel, and the format should be consistent from day to day.

Time on Task

Efficient class organization requires that students be managed so they are on task a considerable portion of the class period. Long lines where children wait for their turn to participate is an unacceptable situation. Develop a system to control the frequency of an individual's positive response.

Dead time is that portion of the class when students are not working to achieve objectives of the instructional program. Children may be active, but the instructional tasks may be irrelevant or detrimental to learning. For instance, participation in an activity that is well within the capability of the learner has little benefit. Activity reinforcers, where children participate in tasks of interest that do not contribute to objectives, are also dead time. The two dimensions of time on task are percentage of time spent learning a task and the qualitative aspects of the learning experience.

ORGANIZING THE INSTRUCTIONAL ENVIRONMENT

The instructional environment of a physical education class facility comprises the procedures, materials, and equipment used by the teacher to improve pupil achievement. The teacher selects the curriculum, manages the individual learning of students, and sets up the delivery systems for instruction and improved performance of the skills. The management structure directly affects social conduct as well as student achievement in motor skills. Students actively involved in appropriate instruction are less likely to exhibit behavioral problems.

Functional Arrangement of Space

The physical environment is made up of space and equipment. The nature of the physical environment and how it is arranged can affect behavior[9] and exerts great influence on performance of students. Weinstein[12] concludes that classroom characteristics affect attitudes and social behavior.

The arrangement of students in relation to one another can affect social behavior and thus acquisition of motor skills. Peers influence one another in both positive and negative directions. If students have an adverse effect on one another (act out or disrupt class), they should be separated. The physical environment of the class facility can be arranged in many ways to promote successful pupil achievement.

Classroom space should be divided into performance areas or zones to accommodate routine activities and tasks.[5] Stowitschek, Gable, and Hendrickson[11] suggest that when planning the arrangement, teachers consider typical storage needs for materials and equipment and procedures for distribution and collection of equipment and student work.

In some gyms small group instructional areas are set up for specific subjects or activities. For example, in classrooms that use learning stations, there may be separate areas for physical fitness, perceptual-motor skills, and science. These areas can be used by the teacher for direct instruction or by students for independent performance in programmed activity.

In addition to instructional areas, each student should have an individual work space. A separate storage area may be needed if there is a considerable amount of equipment. Some teachers set up a specific area where students pick up their work for the day and return their score sheets.

Free times or recreational areas are common for leisure activities such as games, records, and tapes. Time in this area may be used as a reinforcement for appropriate behavior, completed work, or accurate performance. It is also possible to designate a time-out area to which students can be removed for inappropriate or disruptive behavior.

The relationship between different areas within the gymnasium should be carefully planned by considering the following important factors:

- *Convenience:* Store equipment, supplies, and materials near where they are used.
- *Movement efficiency:* Make traffic patterns direct; discourage routes that lead to disruptions (for example, students distracting others when turning in assignments or moving to activities).
- *Density:* Arrange students so that personal space is preserved; avoid crowding.

Once classroom space is arranged, the teacher should not consider it permanent. New arrangements should be tried as often as necessary to increase the effectiveness of the learning environment.

Safe and Barrier-Free Environment

A primary concern with any environment is the safety of the students. Students with physical and sensory disabilities require special precautions. For example, objects and other clutter on the playing surfaces are hazards for students with balance problems or poor eyesight. Students with mobility problems may need accommodation to participate in active games, and deaf students may need visual cues to react in emergency situations.

Another major consideration is *access* to the gymnasium. Many of the newer school buildings are designed to be barrier free; that is, *architec-*

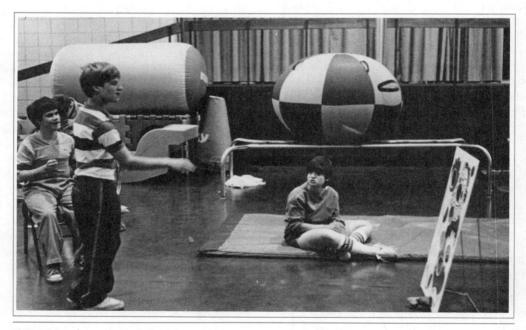

FIGURE 20-6

This environment provides measurement of success on a throwing task. Specific objectives enable a class to be organized efficiently at the ability level of each learner.
(Courtesy Verland Foundation, Inc.)

tural barriers are removed to allow disabled individuals entry to and use of the facility. Elevators and ramps are available, stairs have handrails for persons with crutches or canes, doorways are wide enough to allow entry of wheelchairs, and bathroom facilities are specially designed. Drinking fountains, lockers, vending machines, trash cans, towel dispensers, and telephones are accessible to persons in a wheelchair. However, it may be necessary to make more modifications for disabled students. The environment of the classroom should also be barrier-free. The room should be arranged to allow easy travel to and from showers.

Organization of Curricular Skills and Information

Even though the scope and sequence of the regular curriculum are usually well specified, the teacher can arrange the skills and information in different ways. The traditional organization is by sports skills and prerequisites. This structure is most apparent at junior and senior high levels. At the elementary level skills and abilities may also be divided into different areas, such as posture, physical fitness, fundamental motor skills and patterns, and perceptual-motor activities.

Severely handicapped individuals who cannot self-instruct need to be *grouped for instruction.* Students are most often grouped homogeneously. Students with similar ability, at similar levels, or with similar skills are placed in one group. For example, an entry level test might be given to pinpoint each student's current instructional level and the results used to form instructional groups. *Skill-specific groups* are those made up of students who require instruction in the same skill area. This type of homogeneous grouping, although temporary because skill needs change, is the most effective means of individualizing instruction.

Heterogeneous groupings can also be used for instruction. Smith, Neisworth, and Greer[9] point out that in this type of group, lower functioning students are provided with models if higher functioning children are also in the class.

Flexible grouping is the practice of using several kinds of grouping formats at different times; this allows all students to interact with one another. Although skill-specific grouping remains the most effective for the purpose of instruction, several of the other methods suggested by these authors may be appropriate. Examples are groups of students with common interest, grouping by choice, proximity grouping, alphabetical grouping, and grouping by counting off.

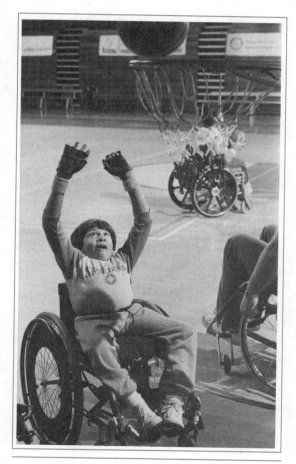

FIGURE 20-7
A child engages in self-instruction on a basketball shooting task.
(Photo by Wendy Parks; courtesy National Foundation of Wheelchair Tennis.)

Instructional Materials

Preplanned learning materials are essential for conduction of the IEP. These take the form of task-analyzed materials, recording instruments, assessment instruments, and audiovisual packages. Examples of these preplanned materials are included in Chapters 3 to 7. These learning materials must be managed so that the individual needs of the learner are served.

Guidelines for Selection

Several different types of instructional aids can be introduced into the physical education classroom to instruct handicapped children, such as (1) audio tapes, (2) books, models of skill sequences, (3) filmstrips, (4) slides, (5) overhead transparencies, (6) motion pictures, and (7) videotapes. Each of these media has different attributes, which should be considered in the selection of the materials. Some of these attributes are motion, pacing, random access, sign type, and sensory mode. Appropriate selection of instructional aids should consider the instructional objective to be achieved in relation to the specific attributes of the media.

Instructional Attributes of Media

The question to be answered by those who select instructional materials is "Which aid is best suited to help handicapped children attain physical education objectives?" A description of the specific attributes of media follow:

Motion: Film and videotape possess the attribute of showing motion. When motion is an attribute of the media there is a presentation of a total picture of the task or the instructional event.

Pacing: Pacing permits the teacher or the student to spend as much time on each piece of information as is desired. Written material such as books and models of skill sequences which are printed, belong to this category. Once films, videotapes, and audiotapes are set in motion they are uncontrolled.

Random access: Random access refers to the degree to which the student can go directly to any specific part of the instructional materials, such as printed matter.

Sensory mode: Most media used by teachers are transmitted through the ears or eyes. Educators of the blind find the tactile mode very useful and may make extensive use of three-dimensional models. Media for the blind should be auditory, and media for the deaf visual.

The utility of instructional materials and aids is a consideration in the selection process, as is the feasibility of acquisition and continued use. The following considerations apply:

- *Cost:* How expensive are the materials to purchase initially?
- *Accessibility:* Are the materials and equipment accessible to the children and teachers?
- *Training required to use the materials:* Are extensive training and skill required to use the materials?
- *Durability:* Are the instructional materials and related equipment easily damaged or are they durable?
- *Technical quality:* Is the technical quality of the materials and related equipment acceptable?

Microcomputers

An important new advance is the development of microcomputers. These small, self-contained computer systems consist of both hardware (or equipment) and system-operating software (or programs); they have many advantages over traditional computers—they are portable, relatively inexpensive, and easier to program.

Microcomputers can be used in the classroom for the management of information. Computers can keep track of student performance and do other nonteaching chores to free teacher time. For example, Dagnon and Spuck[2] report a computer-managed instructional system in which teachers are provided with achievement profiles, diagnostic reports, and grouping recommendations for each of their students. Computers are used to store IEP behavioral objectives and day-by-day progress of pupils. However, the use of sophisticated technology, when a simple explanation from the teacher would suffice, is not effective.

DAILY LESSON PLANS

The daily lesson plan is taken from the unit plan so that appropriate elements of implementation are followed and all essential topics and plans are included in the time scheduled for a given unit. Unit plans need not be rigidly followed. As student or class needs are discovered, the curriculum should be modified to meet these special circumstances.

In a similar way, a daily lesson plan should help teachers and students plan ahead for desired learning experiences. A typical lesson plan should include the following information:

1. Name (title of unit)
2. Subunit
3. Activities of the day
4. School level or grade
5. Date
6. Major objective(s) for the teacher
7. Procedures
8. Facilities and equipment necessary
9. Evaluation after completion of lesson

Some adaptations in planning may be necessary for severely handicapped persons. The suggested topics can be modified and the order changed if this will facilitate learning.

ITINERANT AND RESOURCE ROOM TEACHERS

An itinerant teacher moves from school to school to serve children with instructional problems in physical activities. The itinerant teacher usually helps teachers in the regular physical education class who serve the handicapped. However, these professionals may also aid elementary and special education teachers who are charged with the responsibility of meeting the physical education needs of handicapped children. A resource room teacher meets the instructional needs of teachers who have problems with handicapped children.

The physical educator may assume several roles in the capacity of delivering services to handicapped children. Whatever the role, it is clear that an organizational system needs to be developed that coordinates the efforts of aides, volunteers, and special and elementary classroom teachers who deliver services, and itinerant and resource room teachers if they are involved in the program.

GRADING (MARKING) IN ADAPTED PHYSICAL EDUCATION

A grade in any subject should promote educational goals and should reflect educational aims and objectives. For programs to be most effective, established objectives must indicate the desired goals of instruction so that they become the criteria on which grades are based. If they are valid criteria, successful measurement will result in valid evaluation. The grade, if one desires to translate behavioral performance, could reflect how well these criteria have been met.

The complexity of grading physical education classes is magnified when an attempt is made to evaluate the performance of students in an adapted class. The one common denominator among all the students is the mastery of individual performance objectives. If students are graded on the basis of how well they meet their objectives, a student with poor posture, a student with a cardiac disorder, and obese student, and a student who has just had surgery all can be properly evaluated for their grades in the class.

The following criteria might be applied to students to determine how well they have met objectives in the adapted physical education class:

1. *Performance:* standard of performance in reference to individual limitations, such as vigorous work on specific activities and pos-

ture exercise for obese students, control of the amount and intensity of work for cardiac and postoperative students

2. *Persistence:* accomplishment of individual performance objectives determined in the IEP

Suggestions for recording and computing the grade are as follows:

1. Since the grade may involve some subjective judgments on the part of the instructor, the student should be observed and graded many times throughout the semester (daily or weekly).

2. Numerical ratings (recorded on the exercise card and in the roll book) can be given to the student; in this way, the student and the instructor are always aware of the student's progress toward stated behavior objectives.

3. These numerical grades can be averaged and then should be considered, along with other factors that may influence the final grade (knowledge examinations and health factors, if they are considered), to determine the final mark for the semester.

4. Objective measurements should be used to test skill and knowledge.

SUMMARY

The nature and needs of handicapped children differ greatly. The size of the classes as well as the nature of the physical education content also differ. Therefore a number of considerations need to be taken into account in the formulation of the organization of classes to accommodate the individual needs of students. Some of these considerations are effective grouping of students for certain types of tasks, effective management of time, the physical environment, use of peer teachers, developing learning stations, and effective organization of the instructional environment. Flexible daily lesson plans should be developed to facilitate meeting the needs of all learners. Students should be graded on both performance and persistence as objectively as possible.

REVIEW QUESTIONS

1. What are some of the different types of class organization needed for physical education that serves all children in a range of physical activities?

2. What are the characteristics of a learning station that is capable of accommodating individual differences?

3. How can peer teachers and cross-age tutors help conduct IEPs for the handicapped?

4. What are some considerations for effectively grouping students for instruction?

5. What are some considerations for managing time effectively?

6. What are some considerations for arranging a sound physical environment?

STUDENT ACTIVITIES

1. Talk to a teacher who has used peer or cross-age tutors. Determine how they were selected, the nature of their training program, methods of communication between the teacher and the tutors, and the advantages and disadvantages of such an instructional system.

2. The development of technology provides many opportunities for upgrading practice in physical education. Indicate some of the technology that can be used and how it might be employed in the physical education class with the handicapped.

3. Test ideas such as learning stations and peer and cross-age tutors as they relate to mainstreaming handicapped children. This can be done in practice or hypothetically.

4. Vist a class and describe the organization. What would you do differently to more efficiently arrange the physical environment, manage instructional time, and effectively group students?

5. Set up a system for monitoring pupil performance and progress.

6. Set up a learning station.

REFERENCES

1. Berdine, W.H., and Cegelka, P.T. Teaching the trainable retarded, Columbus, Ohio, 1980, Charles E. Merrill Publishing Co.
2. Dagnon, C., and Spuk, D.W.: A role for computers in individualizing education, and it's not teaching, Phi Delta Kappan **58**:460-462, 1977.
3. Heron, T.E., and Harris, K.C.: The educational consultant: helping professionals, parents, and mainstreamed students, Boston, 1982, Allyn & Bacon.
4. Lewis, R.B., and Doorlay, D.H.: Teaching special students in the mainstream, Columbus, Ohio, 1981, Charles E. Merrill Publishing Co.
5. Mercer, C.D., and Mercer, A.R.: Teaching students with learning problems, Columbus, Ohio, 1983, Charles E. Merrill Publishing Co.
6. Mosston, M.: Teaching physical education, Columbus, Ohio, 1966, Charles E. Merrill Publishing Co.
7. Runac, M.: Acquisition of motor awareness related tasks between kindergarten and primary mentally retarded children through individually prescribed instruction, Master's thesis, Slippery Rock State College, 1971.
8. Sherrill, C.: Adapted physical education and recreation, ed. 3, Dubuque, Iowa, 1985, William C. Brown Publishers.
9. Smith, R.M., Neisworth, J.T., and Greer, J.G.: Evaluating educational environments, Columbus, Ohio, 1978, Charles E. Merrill Publishing Co.
10. Stephens, T.M.: Teachers as managers, Directive Teacher **2**(5):4, 1980.
11. Stowitschek, J.J., Gable, R.A., and Hendrickson, J.M.: Instructional materials for exceptional children, Germantown, Md., 1980, Aspen Systems Corp.
12. Weinstein, C.S.: The physical environment of the school: a review of the research, Rev. Educ. Res. **49**:577-610, 1979.
13. White, C.: Acquisition of lateral balance between trainable mentally retarded children and kindergarten children in an individually prescribed instructional program, Unpublished master's thesis, Slippery Rock State College, 1972.

SUGGESTED READINGS

French, R.W., and Jansma, P.: Special physical education, Columbus, Ohio, 1982, Charles E. Merrill Publishing Co.

Larsen, S.C., and Poplin, M.S.: Methods for educating the handicapped: an individualized education program approach, Boston, 1980, Allyn & Bacon.

Wiseman, D.C.: A practical approach to adapted physical education, Reading, Mass., 1982, Addison-Wesley Publishing Co.

CHAPTER 21

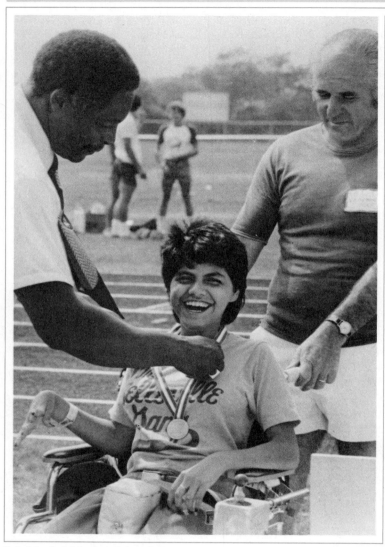

United Cerebral Palsy Associations, Inc.

Program Organization and Administration

OBJECTIVES

♦ Know the guiding principles of adapted physical education programs.

♦ Know the aims and goals of adapted physical education.

♦ Know how to organize an adapted physical education program.

♦ Know how to identify students who need adapted physical education.

♦ Know how to counsel students about their adapted physical education program.

No one type of adapted physical education program is suitable for all school levels or for all school districts. Possibly, this is why there is a very limited amount of material written about the organization and administration of physical education for the handicapped. Good organization and administration are essential if handicapped children are to be included in increasing numbers in our schools and colleges and if they are to grow and flourish at a time when educational costs are rising and when pressures exist to examine carefully the total curricular offerings at all school levels.

If one believes in the importance of providing worthwhile physical education programs for all students at all school levels, it is then equally important to offer athletic and extramural activities for gifted students, regular physical education and intramural sports for average students, and adapted physical education for handicapped students. Handicapped students, who probably need physical education and recreation experiences mores than do gifted or average students, have in the past been provided with inadequate experiences.

State and federal legislation, culminating in P.L. 94-142, should provide quality educational experiences in most states for handicapped persons from the ages of 3 to 21 years. Adapted physical education teachers at all school levels should plan to include special programs for the handicapped in their curricula to satisfy this mandate. Teacher education institutions must also include information on procedures to be followed for their students specializing in physical education and recreation so that they are prepared to teach classes and offer programs for all types of disabled persons in both adapted and regular physical education classes.

Adapted physical education is traditionally offered in one or more ways in districts across the United States. Prior to the signing of P.L. 94-142, many states provided adapted physical education classes for their handicapped students under a state-supported plan. Other plans were supported by the local school district, and still others were under the sponsorship of the county. Ideally, these various agencies should offer a cooperative program designed to meet the needs of all handicapped persons.

In the final analysis, each state, county, and local district must now face up to the problem of how best to meet their mandated obligation to the disabled student. In any case, the principles and objectives of such programs are similar to those for nonhandicapped students.

In 1951 the American Association for Health, Physical Education, and Recreation and the Joint Committee on Health Problems in Education of the American Medical Association and the National Education Association prepared an excellent set of principles that should prove worthwhile to persons interested in organizing, promoting, and evaluating programs of adapted physical education.

GUIDING PRINCIPLES OF ADAPTED PHYSICAL EDUCATION*

It is the responsibility of the school to contribute to the fullest possible development of the potentialities of each individual entrusted to its care. This is a basic tenet of our democratic structure.

1. There is need for common understanding regarding the nature of adapted physical education.
2. There is need for adapted physical education in schools and colleges.
3. Adapted physical education has much to offer the individual who faces the combined problem of seeking an education and living most effectively with a handicap.

Through adapted physical education the individual can: a) be observed and referred when the need for medical or other services is suspected; b) be guided in avoidance of situations which would aggravate the condition or subject him/her to unnecessary risks or injury; c) improve neuromuscular skills, general strength and endurance following convalescence from acute illness or injury; d) be provided with opportunities for improved psychological adjustment and social development.
4. The direct and related services essential for the proper conduct of adapted physical education should be available to our schools.

These services should include: a) adequate and pe-

riodic health examination; b) classification for physical education based on the health examination and other pertinent tests and observations; c) guidance of individuals needing special consideration with respect to physical activity, general health practices, recreational pursuits, vocational planning, psychological adjustment, and social development; d) arrangement of appropriate adapted physical education programs; e) evaluation and recording of progress through observations, appropriate measurements and consultations; f) integrated relationships with other school personnel, medical and its auxiliary services, and family to assure continuous guidance and supervisory services; g) cumulative records for each individual, which should be transferred from school to school.
5. It is essential that adequate medical guidance be available for teachers of adapted physical education.

The possibility of serious pathology requires that programs of adapted physical education should not be attempted without the diagnosis, written recommendation, and supervision of a physician. The planned program of activities must be predicated upon medical findings and accomplished by competent teachers working with medical supervision and guidance. There should be an effective supervision and guidance, and referral service between physicians, physical educators, and parents aimed at proper safeguards and maximum student benefits. School administrators, alert to the special needs of handicapped children, should make every effort to provide adequate staff and facilities necessary for a program of adapted physical education.
6. Teachers of adapted physical education have a great responsibility as well as an unusual opportunity.

Physical educators engaged in teaching adapted physical education should: a) have adequate professional education to implement the recommendations provided by medical personnel; b) be motivated by the highest ideals with respect to the importance of total student development and satisfactory human relationships; c) develop the ability to establish rapport with students who may exhibit social maladjustment as a result of a disability; d) be aware of a student's attitude toward his disability; e) be objective in relationships with students; f) be prepared to give the time and effort necessary to help a student overcome a difficulty; g) consider as strictly confidential information related to personal problems of the student; h) stress similarities rather than deviations, and abilities instead of disabilities.
7. Adapted physical education is necessary at all school levels.

The student with a disability faces the dual problem of overcoming a handicap and acquiring an education which will enable that person to take a place in society as a respected citizen. Failure to assist a student with problems may retard the growth and development process.

*Presented by permission of the Committee on Adapted Physical Education, American Alliance for Health, Physical Education, Recreation, and Dance.

Offering adapted physical education in the elementary grades, and continuing through the secondary school and college, will assist the individuals to improve function and make adequate psychological and social adjustments. It will be a factor in attaining maximum growth and development within the limits of the disability. It will minimize attitudes of defeat and fears of insecurity. It will help the student face the future with confidence.

Content areas for physical education for the handicapped are indicated in the regulations of P.L. 94-142. The objectives should represent definite behaviors that are attainable by students in the program; however, all students would not be expected to attain all the objectives. An adapted physical education program should be organized so that all students meet those objectives of importance to their particular needs and interests.

ESTABLISHING AN ADAPTED PHYSICAL EDUCATION PROGRAM

The legal obligations to handicapped children are different than those to nonhandicapped children. In the past adapted physical education programs have been developed to accommodate students who have temporary injuries (such as preoperative and postoperative cases), weak musculature, or problems with posture or body mechanics. Under the law many of these students are not considered handicapped. Schools may provide special programs for these students, but they are not obliged to do so. Students classified as handicapped by P.L. 94-142 are to be provided with IEPs in the least restrictive environment or the regular class, if possible.

School administrators are aware of the mandate to provide classroom instruction and vocational training for handicapped students, but frequently they do not understand that the same provisions must be made for physical education of their handicapped students. When an appropriate physical education program is not provided, it is imperative that steps be taken to bring the school curriculum into compliance with the law. Before an adapted physical education program can be established, three things must be accomplished. First, it is important to determine the

number and types of children classified as handicapped in the school or district. Second, school administrators must be made aware of the federal requirements. Third, the school or school district administration must agree to begin planning to provide appropriate physical education experiences for their handicapped students. A brief discussion of procedures for the first two of these steps and a more extensive discussion of the third step follow.

Determining the Number and Types of Handicapped Students

It is important to determine the number and types of handicapped children in the school system, because this information provides clues to the types of physical education programs needed. If only mildly mentally handicapped students are being served by the school or district, chances are their needs can be met through mainstreaming. However, if more seriously impaired students are enrolled, a separate adapted physical education program may be needed. The number of handicapped students and their conditions should be a matter of public record. This information should be available from the school psychologist, special education director, school principal, or superintendent. It is not necessary at this point to learn the names of the students. Data concerning their ages, number, and types of conditions should be gathered. If it is learned that handicapped students are enrolled in the school district, the next step can be undertaken.

Bringing Attention to the Problem

School officials' awareness of the need for inclusion of appropriate physical education can be increased through discussion of the situation with the principal, superintendent, and director of special education. If any of those administrators are unaware of the exact content of the law, they should be provided with a copy of the Education for All Handicapped Children Act.[7]* Their attention should be drawn to the specific sections of

---

*A copy can be obtained from the local library or from the U.S. Office of Education, Department of Education, 7th and D Sts. S.W., Washington, DC 20202.

the law that pertain to physical education. Arguments that occupational or physical therapists are meeting the physical education needs of the handicapped students and arguments that the law says that all handicapped students should be mainstreamed in physical education should not be accepted. The same provisions that are being made for classroom instruction of handicapped students apply to physical education. That is, whether or not a handicapped student needs a special physical education program must be determined through testing of the physical and motor functioning of the child.

If school administrators continue to ignore the need to provide appropriate physical education for handicapped students, assistance should be sought from other sources. Assistance can be obtained from the local, district, or state professional teachers' association and the Office of Special Education in the State Department of Education. Persistence may be necessary, but with enough effort the problem will be recognized as an important one. Once the school administrators recognize the need for appropriate physical education services, steps must be taken toward establishing a program.

Planning Programs

The most important step in providing appropriate physical education services for handicapped students is long-range planning. Programs that are carefully planned have a much greater chance of meeting the students' needs than do programs that are hurriedly put together. Thorough long-range planning involves (1) identifying an individual who will be responsible for the program; (2) appointing an advisory committee; and (3) having the supervisor and advisory committee survey the district to establish goals for the program, interpret the need for the program, secure support for the program, and agree on general policies for the program.

There should be a long-range plan of organization, whether a new program is being formulated or a well-established one is being evaluated and changes are being suggested for it. Responsibility for the program should be delegated to one person, usually a supervisor at the district level or a well-qualified teacher if the program will be limited to one school. In either case, this person should be aided by an advisory committee or council. This committee helps in such matters as establishment of policy, formation of long-range plans, selection and release of students (at the school level), and interpretation and promotion of the program.

Selecting the Supervisor

The person in charge of the program, together with the teachers, constitutes the program's most important single aspect. For this reason, the supervisor or teacher should be selected because of outstanding qualifications, including personality, experience, training, and knowledge of local, state, and federal regulations.

The traditional role of adapted physical education was to provide opportunities for handicapped persons to successfully participate in the activities of the physical education program. Today, there are two different aspects to the adapted physical education program—accommodating the handicapped child in handicapped-only classes and making provisions for the IEP in the regular class. The supervisor of physical education for the handicapped should be competent in both roles.

Interpersonal Skill

Interpersonal skill is a most important quality for a teacher and is doubly important for the supervisor-teacher of adapted physical education. The very nature of the position, involving as it does both teaching and administration, requires close contact with administrators, counselors, medical personnel, teachers, and students. Students with special needs require a superior teacher—one who can establish close rapport with students, teach effectively, and work diplomatically with physicians, nurses, administrators, and other teachers. These qualities are necessary for success in an adapted physical education program.

Experience

Prior teaching experience with competency for implementing the IEPs is a prerequisite for the person who assumes the leadership of an adapted physical education program. Techniques and procedures used in teaching special physical education vary somewhat from those used in teaching regular physical education classes. Generally, more individual teaching and counseling are done with the handicapped, and a close bond is established between teacher and pupil. Special skills and knowledge also are necessary to deal effectively with physicians, nurses, and other medical personnel.

Training

It is desirable that the person heading the adapted physical education program have, as minimum qualifications, special training in life and physical sciences, psychology, applied anatomy and physiology, and adapted physical education. Graduate training in adapted or corrective physical education, corrective therapy, or physical therapy would strengthen this background so

that expert leadership can be given to members of the adapted physical education teaching faculty and to students in the program.

Federal and state legislation has allowed for the expansion of educational programs for handicapped persons. To provide better instructional programs for these persons, teacher education institutions have had to expand their training programs. Special credentials, certificates, and degrees are granted to persons who complete advanced specialized programs, and internship or student teaching assignments should be part of such advanced training.

In 1980 a committee representing the Adapted Physical Education Academy, Therapeutics Council, and Unit on Programs for the Handicapped of the American Alliance for Health, Physical Education, Recreation, and Dance developed a statement on competencies for the specialist in special physical education. Those competencies are presented in Table 21-1.

TABLE 21-1
Competencies for the specialist in special physical education*

Competency	Specialist
1.0 Biological Foundations	
1.1 Kinesiology	Demonstrate proficiency in evaluating and analyzing motor performance in terms of motor dysfunction and in applying biomechanical principles that affect motor functioning to posture and to neurological, muscular, and other specific health needs.
1.2 Physiology of exercise	Demonstrate ability to design and conduct physical education programs for disabled individuals that adhere to sound physiological principles.
1.3 Physiology and motor functioning	Demonstrate the ability to apply an understanding of physiological motor characteristics for individuals with physical, mental, sensory, neurological, and other specific health needs to programs designed to improve the motor performances of these individuals.
2.0 Sociological foundations	
2.1 Sports, dance, play	Demonstrate ability to analyze the significance of sport, dance, and play in the lives of individuals with disabilities.
2.2 Cooperative/competitive activities	Demonstrate understanding of the potential for human interaction and social behavior occurring in cooperative/competitive activities for individuals with disabilities; cooperate with organizations that conduct adapted sport, dance, and play programs for individuals with disabilities.
2.3 Social development	Demonstrate understanding of the potential that sport, dance, and play provide for social interactions among individuals with or without disabilities.

*Adapted from a statement prepared by the Adapted Physical Education Academy, Therapeutics Council, and Unit on Programs for the Handicapped of the American Alliance for Health, Physical Education, Recreation, and Dance, 1980.

Continued.

TABLE 21-1
Competencies for the specialist in special physical education—cont'd

3.0 Psychological foundations

3.1 Human growth and development — Demonstrate ability to apply understanding of deviations in human growth and development and atypical motor development to assist individuals with physical, mental, sensory, neurological, and other specific health needs.

3.2 Motor learning — Demonstrate ability to apply principles of motor learning, including motivation techniques, to the teaching and learning of motor skills by individuals with disabilities.

3.3 Self-concept and personality development — Demonstrate ability to apply skills and techniques in the teaching of physical and motor skills to assist individuals with disabilities in overcoming attitudinal barriers that can affect interpersonal relationships and development of positive self-concept.

3.4 Management of behavior — Demonstrate ability to apply appropriate techniques for managing behavior, including techniques of motivation to enhance acceptable behavior and promote motor performance.

4.0 Historical and philosophical foundations

4.1 Historical development — Demonstrate understanding of the historical development of adapted physical education, including the role and significance of professional and voluntary organizations in the development of professional standards and ethics related to adapted physical education

4.2 Philosophical development — Demonstrate understanding of the philosophies of adapted physical education, current issues, and trends in adapted physical education and identify ways individuals with disabilities realize and express their individualities and uniqueness through physical education, sport, dance, and play programs.

5.0 Assessment and evaluation

5.1 Program goals and objectives — Demonstrate ability to develop instructional objectives that lead to fulfillment of physical education goals in psychomotor, affective, and cognitive domains by individuals with disabilities.

5.2 Screening and assessment — Demonstrate proficiency in using appropriate instruments to assess and interpret the motor performances of students with disabilities.

5.3 Evaluation — Demonstrate proficiency in applying appropriate instruments and evaluative procedures to determine student progress in adapted physical education.

6.0 Curriculum planning, organization, and implementation

6.1 Program planning — Demonstrate ability to plan individual physical education programs that are adapted to individual student need based on goals and objectives established by an interdisciplinary team.

6.2 Individual instruction — Demonstrate ability to implement appropriate physical education programs for individuals with disabilities based on each student's current level of performance using appropriate strategies, including task analysis techniques.

6.3 Program implementation — Demonstrate ability to function effectively as a member of an interdisciplinary team using appropriate techniques for facilitating interdisciplinary communication among all persons working with disabled individuals.

6.4 Safety considerations — Demonstrate understanding of scientific bases for specifically contraindicated exercises and activities, including transfer techniques for individuals with disabilities.

6.5 Health considerations — Demonstrate understanding of the effects of medication, fatigue, illness, posture, and nutrition on the mental, physical, and motor performances of individuals with disabilities.

Selecting the Advisory Committee

The advisory committee may be district-wide or may be set up to advise relative to the program at one particular school.

An advisory committee at the district level might consist of the school district physician, a key administrator at the district level, a district or school nurse, the supervisor of adapted physical education, a special education teacher or supervisor, and, possibly, a representative from each of the following groups:

1. Regular physical education teachers
2. Instructors who do not teach physical education
3. Parent-Teacher Association or other parents' group
4. Community groups closely associated with handicapped children

This advisory committee aids the supervisor in establishing and interpreting policy, fostering good public relations, procuring funds for the program, and dealing with physicians, nurses, and parent groups in the community.

An advisory committee at the school level has responsibilities similar to those of the district committee. It should advise and support the teachers of adapted physical education. It is concerned with interpretation of the program and with public relations at the school level. Members of this committee usually include the school physician, the school nurse, an administrator, teachers of adapted physical education, and one or more of the following persons: a teacher from an area other than physical education, a parent or Parent-Teacher Association member, a counselor, a student, the health coordinator, or a representative of the health education teachers.

The supervisor and the teachers of adapted physical education will find that the adapted physical education committee can give them invaluable aid in planning for and interpreting this special type of program. The members of these committees must therefore be selected with great care.

After the advisory committee has been selected, several tasks must be carried out under their direction. These include surveying the involved schools, establishing objectives, interpreting the program, securing support for the program, and agreeing on general principles that will be followed. A discussion of each of these tasks follows.

Surveying the Schools

A survey of a school or district must be conducted to determine what will be required to implement or improve an adapted physical education program and should include information about the following factors:

1. Availability of teachers and their background of education and experience
2. Time allotment necessary for the program
3. Cost of the program
4. Existing facilities and equipment and amount of additional space and supplies needed
5. Special problems concerning related services
6. Special problems involved in counseling these students and scheduling them for classes at special hours during the day

The caliber of the adapted physical education teacher is the single most important factor of those listed. Money, equipment, support from related service care providers, and other teachers all are important, but an enthusiastic, well-qualified teacher is a necessity. The teacher of physically, mentally, or emotionally handicapped children must not only be a good instructor, but also have the understanding and the ability to establish rapport with students who are seeking an education despite their disabilities.

Because the adapted physical education program involves special classes for only a portion of the total student enrollment of a school and because class size should often be limited to allow for considerable individual instruction, schedule problems sometimes result. School administrators and counselors must be convinced that students who have special needs should be scheduled for physical education class early in the selection of their class schedule. The IEP requires that each handicapped child receive instruction that meets his or her specific needs. Furthermore, the placement of the child (where the instruction is to take place) is cooperatively decided by the parents and the school. Therefore, the scheduling of handicapped children in physical education activity must be flexible.

An adapted physical education program does cost a school or school district additional money. Small classes, special equipment, a special room, and additional related services increase costs over what is spent on regular physical education classes. These costs need not be exorbitant, however. An excellent program can be provided with a minimum of special equipment and even without a special room if one is not available. To help meet the excess expenses, district, state, and federal funds should be made available for classes for handicapped students who have need for special attention in physical education.

Adequate equipment and a well-planned adapted physical education room facilitate positive teacher performance and add enjoyment to the program for the student. The teacher who has adequate facilities and equipment can do a better job of meeting the needs of the special student.

The school physician and the nurse play an important role in the adapted physical education program. The support and active backing of these persons are essential if a top-quality program is to be presented. The initial screening is often performed by medical and psychological personnel. This information indicates whether the child is handicapped and provides data concerning contraindicated activity for a specific handicapping condition. However, once the program is underway, revision of the program must be done with the cooperation of the parents and the persons providing the related services.

Considerable data substantiating the importance of providing physical education classes for all students enrolled in school, from kindergarten through college, have been gathered by local districts: the American Medical Association; the California Association for Health, Physical Education, and Recreation; the American Alliance for Health, Physical Education, Recreation, and Dance; and the President's Council on Physical Fitness. Publications recommending special programs of adapted physical education in our schools are numerous.[1-6,8] P.L. 94-142, discussed in Chapter 1, mandates the inclusion of equal educational opportunity for handicapped persons.

Establishing Program Objectives

The aim of physical education for handicapped persons is to aid them in achieving physical, mental, emotional, and social growth commensurate with their potential through carefully planned programs of regular and special physical education activities. Specific objectives are as follows:

- To help students correct conditions that can be improved
- To help students protect themselves and any conditions that would be aggravated through certain physical activities
- To provide students with an opportunity to learn and to participate in a number of appropriate recreational and leisure time sports and activities and to become self-sufficient in the community
- To help students understand their physical and mental limitations
- To help students make social adjustments and develop a feeling of self-worth and value
- To aid students in developing knowledge and appreciation relative to good body mechanics
- To help students understand and appreciate a variety of sports that they can enjoy as spectators

Government programs and state laws currently require that program administrators and teachers state their program goals in behavioral or performance terms. This provides for more accurate assessment and accountability of programs, teachers, and students. A meaningfully stated objective is one that succeeds in precisely communicating to the reader the writer's instructional intent. Performance objectives must include the following:

1. A statement of who is going to demonstrate (the performer)
2. A statement of what exactly is included (knowledge, skills, and behavior)
3. A statement of the conditions under which the performance will be done
4. A statement identifying the standard of achievement (how well or how much)
5. A statement indicating how the performance will be measured (with what instruments, used by whom)

Physical education programs are influenced by a number of practical factors that vary from district to district and even among schools located in the same district. These factors include community and administrative support, adequacy of the budget, available facilities and equipment, availability of qualified supervisory and teaching personnel, and student interest and support.

Thus based on sound aims and principles and conditioned by practical factors that may influence the curriculum of a school, physical education for the handicapped must be planned so that it operates most effectively for the students, teachers, and administrators of the particular school or district.

Interpreting the Program

Promoting an adapted physical education program in a school or school district requires excellence in program planning and teaching, demonstrating that positive results can be obtained through the conduct of a quality program.

Prior to the passage of P.L. 94-142, it was often necessary for the physical educator to promote programs for handicapped children. However, every handicapped child is entitled to physical education. Extensive child identification procedures were a part of P.L. 94-142 in the middle 1970s. Once the handicapped children were identified, they were comprehensively assessed in specific areas of educational need. Thus at present each local school district should have detailed data on the physical education needs of each handicapped child. These can be presented to school boards, administrators, parents' and

teachers' groups, and students to inform them of the need for and value of adapted physical education.

Securing Support for the Program

The support of five persons or groups of persons is essential if a school or school district is to have a quality program in adapted physical education. They are the administrator, the teacher, the related service personnel, the parents, and the student. The teacher's role has already been discussed, and the student's role will vary with the particular handicap involved.

The administrator. The support of the administrator is necessary if the program is to receive its share of district and school resources. The administrator can help by (1) giving enthusiastic support to the total program; (2) providing an adequate budget; (3) requiring adequately trained teachers; (4) supporting necessary student schedule changes; and (5) providing auxiliary services such as medical aid, nursing, transportation, and maintenance.

Related service personnel. Related service personnel play a very important role in physical education programs for handicapped persons. In addition to providing services that will help the children benefit from the program, they may also enhance the program by (1) interpreting the program to medical personel in the district, to parents, and to the total school population (Fig. 21-1); (2) handling or making referrals of students with special problems; and (3) fully informing the adapted physical education instructors of the students' conditions and recommending exercises and activities (Fig. 21-2).

The parents. Parents must be informed as to their children's level of developmental progress and the specific skills that they will be able to perform by the end of the year. Such information must be contained in a written document. Many schools provide the parents of each student with an information sheet or brochure that gives an overview of the general regulations of the physical education departments. It may also include information about the adapted program, its objectives, its activity offerings, and its admission and dismissal procedures. It should be described as an extension and an integral part of the total physical education program, open to any student in the school during a time of special need. The scope of the program can be described to the parents as including provisions for the following:

1. Physically, emotionally, or mentally handicapped persons
2. Persons with temporary injuries

3. Preoperative or postoperative patients
4. Persons convalescing from serious illness
5. Persons in need of special instruction to improve physical fitness or to ameliorate a postural problem

These matters can also be covered if the school provides an orientation day for parents or offers a special program during the year to inform the parents about the curricular offerings of each of the departments in the school. Another way to

A

```
                        YOURNAME HIGH SCHOOL
                       LONG BEACH, CALIFORNIA

        Alan Walters, M.D.

        Dear Dr. Walters,

            In order that we may better serve the health needs of our
        students, the Yourname High School wishes to acquaint the medi-
        cal profession with the service it is prepared to render through
        its physical education departments.

            As you know, physical education is required, by law, for
        all students attending high school in California.

            Classes for girls/boys are conducted by specially trained
        teachers and include special programs as follows:

        Posture and body          Preventive and corrective exercise pro-
           mechanics:             grams for feet, ankles, knees, spinal
                                  curvatures, and other postural problems.

        Weak musculature:         Developmental exercises and activities
                                  for the subfit student.

        Restricted activities:    Adapted sports and activities for those
                                  students in need of a limited activity
                                  program (cardiac, asthma, etc.).

        Pre- and post-            Special exercise programs as prescribed
           operative:             by the physician.

        Dysmenorrhea:             Counseling and exercise and activity
           (girls)                programs as advised by the physician.

        Rest:                     Quiet games and activities, relaxation
                                  techniques, or rest as prescribed.

            Classes are small and individual attention is given each
        student.  Your suggestions and your interest in this program
        are solicited.

                                  Sincerely yours,

                                  Marie Carol M.D.
                                  School physician

        Approved:  J. Officer
                   Principal
```

FIGURE 21-1

A, Letter to the private physician from the school doctor.

inform parents about the adapted program is through a form letter from the adapted physical education teacher (Fig. 21-1, *C*).

Agreeing on General Principles

The supervisor should develop general policies for the adapted physical education program and then discuss these with the advisory committee. These professionals, working together, should agree on how the students should be selected, classified, and scheduled. The combined experience of the supervisor and members of the advisory committee should provide clear-cut guidelines that will ensure smooth implementation of the program.

IMPLEMENTING THE PROGRAM

The selection of students for adapted physical education and their assignment to the proper type of activity are two very important phases of the program. Students with disabilities can be identified through physical examination, through observation in classroom or activity situations, and through special testing procedures that are administered by members of the physical education department.

Physical Examination

There are several purposes for giving each student in the school a physical examination. Ideally, the physical examination should identify pu-

Date _____

To: _____
               School physician

_____ High School

From: _____, M.D.

Subject: Recommendations re: Physical Education for my patient,

_____

Based on my examination of _____, his/her

physical education assignment should be as follows:

Diagnosis _____

Temporary _____ (How long) _____

All activities except (please list) _____

_____

Only the following activities (please list) _____

_____

Special exercises for (please list) _____

_____

Date _____ Signed _____, M.D.
                                    Personal physician

B

FIGURE 21-1—cont'd   *Continued.*
B, Letter from the private physician to the school.

```
                    YOURNAME HIGH SCHOOL

                PHYSICAL EDUCATION DEPARTMENTS

                            Date  Jan 15th

    Dear  Mr Hunter,
        Your  daughter/son  Michael      , by recommendation
    of  Alan Walter, M.D has been assigned to the Adapted
    Physical Education program because  of cardiac
    problems and poor posture
                                                        .

        Yourname High School's Adapted Physical Education program
    offers each student in the class an opportunity to either correct,
    improve, or compensate for physical or organic problems he might
    have.  Each student is given individual attention in accordance
    with the recommendations of a family doctor or a school physician.
    Every effort is made to make the time spent in this class safe
    and profitable for your child.

                            Sincerely yours,

    Approved:
    Chris Steffy, M.D.          David Walter Daniels
    School Physician            Adapted Physical Education Instructor

    - - - - - - - - - - - - - - - - - - - - - - - - - - - - - - -

        I would like to have a conference with the Adapted Physical
    Education Teacher.  Day _____ Time _____. (You
    may call for an appointment if you would prefer.)

                            Signed
                            _____
                            Parent or Guardian

    Telephone number: 437-0007
                      437-0707
```

FIGURE 21-1—cont'd
C, Letter to parents from the physical education instructor.

pils who have pathological conditions, provide teachers with information concerning students' growth and health status, and identify students who can benefit from the IEP. The examination must be sufficiently personalized to form a desirable constructive educational experience for the students and their parents and provide the examining physician-patient relationship.

It is more important that the examination be comprehensive and painstaking than that it be given annually. It is suggested that the examination be given to each pupil at least every third year. The usual pattern is to require an examination in the first grade and then every 3 years through the elementary, secondary school, and college years. Parents should be informed of any disabilities discovered at the discretion of the examining physician. The records of these exami-

LONG BEACH STATE COLLEGE

Division of Health, Physical Education, and Recreation

A PLAN OF COORDINATION BETWEEN THE DEPARTMENT OF PHYSICAL
EDUCATION AND THE STUDENT HEALTH SERVICE

Every entering or re-entering student will be given a medical examination by the student health service. At the conclusion of this examination, the student will be classified by the examining physician for physical education activities according to the classifications listed below.

Class A--No restrictions

Class B--Minor restrictions in activity where a student might be excused from one or two hazardous types of sports but would be cleared for all others.

Class C--Limited (adapted) physical education. The physician should state reason and briefly describe the types of exercises or activities that would benefit the student. Assignment to a special class might be necessary. Use code below where possible and indicate approximate length of time for restriction.

CODE

1) Output of energy to be reduced: Not to exercise severely enough to become much out of breath, nor long enough to become much fatigued. This class will include persons with heart disease, diabetes, severe asthma, hyperthyroidism, neurocirculatory asthenia, etc., or convalescing from recent illness.
2) Protect from physical trauma: Should be used for cases too severe or complicated to be safely handled under a simple "B" classification. Atrophied limbs, recurrent dislocations, damaged brains, and progressive high myopia are examples.
3) Avoid close contact with other students or with mats: Cases in which there is mildly infectious or a repulsive skin condition, such as severe acne or eczema. Infectious cases should be excluded from physical education entirely, until cured. Persons who have a C-3 classification should also be placed in a "B--no swimming" class.
4) Not to use legs more than necessary: For persons otherwise OK who have foot strain, varicose veins, old leg injuries, healed thrombophlebitis, and similar conditions, which are severe enough to cause them some trouble.
5) Epileptic: MUST BE KEPT OUT OF POOL AND OFF OF HIGH PLACES.
6) Adapt activity to some deformity: Students who are blind or deaf or who have amputated limbs are often not especially fragile, and do very well in many activities if given proper assistance.
7) Hernia: Avoid anything that causes increased intra-abdominal pressure, such as heavy lifting or straining, and anything else that causes pain at the site of the hernia.
8) Recommended for certain activity only. Specify.
9) Has some physical condition which, while not disabling, may be benefited by special corrective physical exercises. Examples are spinal curvatures, foot strain, certain recurrent dislocations, and general muscular underdevelopment.

ACCIDENT OR ILLNESS REQUIRING A CHANGE OF CLASSIFICATION

A student who becomes ill or is injured may require a change in medical classification. These students should report to the Student Health Service upon their return to school for a check-up by the attending physician who may or may not change the student's classification. If a change is necessary, the doctor should fill out form #HPER 20 which will be attached to the student's permanent record card in the Department of Physical Education. If no change is necessary, a re-admittance slip should be filled out to clear the student for full activity in physical education classes.

Physical Education instructors must not admit a student to an activity class unless the student has a medical classification card on file in the Physical Education office, nor should he admit a student to re-enter class if he has been ill, without either a "readmittance slip" or a "change of medical classification card."

The health and safety of each student at Long Beach State College can best be guaranteed by close cooperation between the Health Service and the Division of Health, Physical Education, and Recreation. Close observance of these procedures will make this possible.

FIGURE 21-2
Explanation of the code used on the medical report cards from the physician to the physical education department.

nations can then be forwarded to the counseling office of the school that the student will be attending the next year, thus facilitating program planning.

Some school districts are unable or unwilling to provide physical examinations. In this event each student should be required to present evidence to the school of an adequate examination from his or her own physician. There is considerable support for requiring an examination from the private physician rather than from the school physician, since the private physician should have a better longitudinal picture of the student's health or health problems.

The following policies should be instituted with regard to the physical examination;

- ♦ Information obtained by the school nurse should include the student's health history and records of vision and hearing tests, height and weight, and general posture and foot examinations.
- ♦ The physician's examination should include the heart (before and after exercise), lungs, blood pressure, abdomen, eye, ear, nose, throat, skin, glands, and posture.
- ♦ The student should be referred to the family physician by a specialist provided by the school district or to the city, county, state, or other public agencies for additional examinations by specialists when needed. These examinations could include psychological examinations, checkups for tuberculosis, or services of other medical specialists such as cardiologists and orthopedists. The service agencies concerned with crippled children and children who have cerebral palsy, neuromuscular disorders, asthma, heart disorders, diabetes, mental retardation, or other disabling conditions may be consulted as needed.

Examination Records

A comprehensive record card or file should be begun during the initial examination, and it should follow the student throughout the school years. Many school districts will not forward medical records to a new school district. Since the health record is of such vital importance, provisions should be made to make inexpensive photostatic copies of the record to forward to the new school with the academic records. The card should contain a record of all previous physical examinations, illnesses, immunizations, tests, injuries, referrals (and their findings), and defects (and their correction); the health history; and information relative to the assignment of students to special classes and activities in physical education (Fig. 21-4).

It is essential that the physical education department receive from the health office a written recommendation that provides the following information: student's full name, year in school, date of examination, classification for physical education activity, and nature of the IEP. The recommendation should be signed by the examining physician or by the nurse who transposes the information from the permanent medical record. This card is filed in the physical education department office. It is then the responsibility of each instructor to check that all students have had a physical examination and that they are enrolled in the types of activity that meet their physical education needs.

Methods of Identification

All handicapped children should be preevaluated in specific areas of physical education need. For most of these children, specific programming will be underway; however, there may be children who are not legally handicapped but who need special physical education programs. These children need to be identified so that special assistance can be provided. There are a number of ways for classroom teachers in the school—and specifically the teachers of regular physical education classes—to help identify students in need of special assistance.

Observation of Activities

Observation of the students in the classroom or on the athletic field will often disclose physical deviations which have been overlooked by the

Activity recommendations

Indicate body areas for which physical activities should be minimized, eliminated, or maximized.

	Maximized	Minimized	Eliminated	Both	Left	Right	Comments, including any medical contraindications to physical activities
Neck							
Shoulder girdle							
Arms							
Elbows							
Hands and wrists							
Abdomen							
Back							
Pelvic girdle							
Legs							
Knees							
Feet and ankles							
Toes							
Fingers							
Other (specify)							

Remedial

☐ Condition is such that defects or deviations can be improved or prevented from becoming worse through use of carefully selected exercise and/or activities. The following are remedial exercises and/or activities recommended for this student: (Please be specific.)

_____

_____

_____

_____

_____

_____

_____

_____

Signed _____ M.D.

Address _____

_____ Zip _____

Telephone No. (   ) _____

Date _____ , 19____

FIGURE 21-3

Physical education medical referral form approved and endorsed by the Committee on the Medical Aspects of Sports of the American Medical Association, 1975.

SECTION F	CORRECTIVE TEACHER'S NOTES		SECTION G	DOCTOR'S RECOMMENDATIONS	
Date		Signature	Date		Signature

SECTION H   PROGRAM EVALUATION

SECTION J   DISPENSATION OF CASE

	First Semester	Sig.	Second Semester	Sig.	Third Semester	Sig.
Case closed (date)						
Pupil to regular P.E.						
Recommended for further exercise						

LOS ANGELES CITY SCHOOL DISTRICTS
Auxiliary Services Division — Health Education and Health Services Branch
CORRECTIVE PHYSICAL EDUCATION HISTORY FOLDER

INFORMATION AND DIRECTIONS FOR USE OF THIS FOLDER

1. **WHAT IS THE PURPOSE OF THIS INSTRUMENT?** This folder has been prepared for the corrective physical education teacher to use during three semesters as a history record of pupil progress in corrective physical education.

2. **WHO IS TO FILL IT OUT?** This folder is to be filled out by the corrective physical education teacher in whose class the pupil is enrolled.

3. **WHEN IS THE FOLDER TO BE FILLED OUT?** The folder is to be filled out when the pupil first enters the class and each semester period during the time the pupil is enrolled in corrective physical education. Use additional folders when necessary.

4. **TO WHOM IS THE FOLDER TO BE SENT?** The folder is to be sent to the Corrective Physical Education Section of the Health Education and Health Services Branch.

5. **WHEN IS THIS FOLDER DUE?** Upon request. However, if the pupil transfers, the folder should be sent immediately to the Corrective Physical Education Section of the Health Education and Health Services Branch, with pupil's new address or school.

6. **DIRECTIONS FOR SECTION A.** Record date in appropriate column. Record body type as L (lithe), M (medium), S (stout). Record muscle tone as good or poor. Record items 4 to 9 inclusive according to degree using a 1 to 4 scale with 1 (little) and 4 (much). Record feet as N (normal), P (pronated), S (supinated), F (flat. Record leg alignment as N (normal), B (bowed), K (knock-knee). Record prominent abdomen as "yes" or "no." Record chest as N (normal), F (flat), P (pigeon). Record items 14 and 15 as "yes" or "no." Record items 16 through 20 as "yes" or "no"; if "yes," indicate whether left or right.

7. **DIRECTIONS FOR SECTION B.** Place in the appropriate space the photographs taken at the beginning of the first semester and at the end of the second and third semesters.

8. **DIRECTIONS FOR SECTION C.** Using a cloth or steel tape, record measurements in inches to the nearest quarter, and weight (including over or under) to the nearest pound.

9. **DIRECTIONS FOR SECTION D.** Describe all exercises planned by the corrective teacher for the pupil and list these according to the following code numbers, putting the appropriate number in the column for numbers:

   1. Specific individual exercises
   2. Relaxation exercises
   3. Coordination exercises
   4. Head and neck exercises
   5. General trunk exercises
   6. Lateral trunk exercises
   7. Foot and leg alignment exercises

10. **DIRECTIONS FOR SECTION E.** The information for this section should be obtained from the pupil's health record card after conferring with the health coordinator and school nurse if a secondary school, or with the school nurse and principal if an elementary school.

11. **DIRECTIONS FOR SECTION F.** This space is for the corrective teacher to use in recording pupil progress and significant information from home or other sources relative to the child's general health problems, including his feelings regarding his defects.

12. **DIRECTIONS FOR SECTION G.** Information for this section should be obtained also from the pupil's health record card or from the school doctor or private physician.

13. **DIRECTIONS FOR SECTION H .** This space is to be used by the corrective teacher to evaluate the corrective program of the pupil. Record significant developments that have been accomplished for the pupil within the corrective class.

14. **DIRECTIONS FOR SECTION J.** This space is for the corrective teacher to use to record the dispensation of the case, that is, when the pupil leaves the class, when the pupil is returned to regular physical education, or in case the pupil is recommended for more than the three semesters of corrective physical education.

CORRECTIVE TEACHER'S SIGNATURE	DATE
1.	
2.	
3.	

FIGURE 21-4
Sample cumulative folder.

physician and of which the students are unaware. Persons with posture deviation, slow learners in physical education activities, students with poor coordination or balance, and persons with limited strength and endurance may be in need of specially designed programs of exercise and activity to enable them to keep up with their peers in a regular physical education class.

Teachers, counselors, and the school nurse should also watch for the student who has a change of status because of illness or injury. The student should be transferred to an appropriate setting if necessary until the condition is corrected or the fitness level is raised sufficiently for the student to return to a regular class.

Physical Education Testing

There are a number of different tests that can be administered by the physical educator to aid in the identification of students with some form of physical disability. These tests, combined with the judgment of a qualified instructor, help screen the students who have special needs.

For selection of the test method, factors such as the following should be considered: the specialized training of the instructors, the number of qualified teachers in the physical education department, the space available, the number of students to be tested, when the examinations are to be given, the amount of time available, and the special testing and recording equipment available.

Individual examinations by one instructor or several instructors (station-to-station). There are two types of individual examinations that are commonly used in schools and colleges. In one type one instructor examines each student individually, covering all of the tests in the battery. In the other method several stations are set up with different trained personnel at each station, each responsible for administering one or more tests.

Individual examination by one instructor is usually used to evaluate thoroughly the specific problems of the student. It would involve the procedures described in more detail in other sections of this text. The instructor usually allows 6 to 10 minutes for each student's examination.

Individual examination by several instructors (station-to-station) can be very thorough or can be used to identify the most pronounced cases. These will be reexamined later with more care by the adapted physical education specialist. As many as six to eight stations are set up, either in a large room such as the gymnasium or in a series of small rooms, if they are available. Each instructor must be skillful in the administration of one or more tests, and the students move from one area to another to receive the complete examination. A typical station-to-station examination plan is shown in Fig. 21-5, *A*. Students come to the gymnasium properly dressed for the examination. They fill out the appropriate sections of their appraisal sheet, remove shoes and socks, and proceed to station one for anthropometric measurements and evaluation of nutritional status. Age, height, weight, body width, depth, fat measurements, and girth measurements may be taken. The student then proceeds to station two for an examination with the posture screen or plumb line. Station three is a moving (functional) body mechanics examination. The student walks, performs exercises, climbs steps, sits down in a chair, and the like while the instructor evaluates these movement patterns. The student next proceeds to station four for the foot examination. Here evaluation can be made with the podiascope, pedograph, plumb line, foot tracer, and other devices needed. Stations five to eight may be used for physical fitness, range of motion, relaxation, or perceptual-motor-tests, as described in the other chapters of this text. The adapted physical education specialist then reviews the total examination results and prepares the final summary evaluation, which will later be used to determine which students are in need of special attention, counseling, and placement in the least restrictive environment.

Group examinations. The IEP requires that instructional decisions be made from a data base. Therefore, it is important that expedient procedures be employed to collect such data. There are several ways to collect the data: (1) the instructor tests each student, (2) the instructor trains other persons to collect the data, (3) all

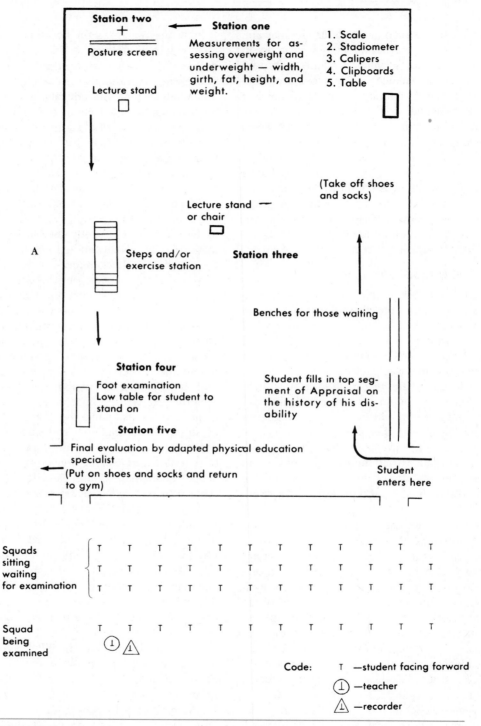

Station two
+
Posture screen

Station one
Measurements for assessing overweight and underweight — width, girth, fat, height, and weight.

1. Scale
2. Stadiometer
3. Calipers
4. Clipboards
5. Table

Lecture stand
☐

(Take off shoes and socks)

Lecture stand — or chair
☐

Steps and/or exercise station

Station three

Benches for those waiting

A

Station four
Foot examination
Low table for student to stand on

Student fills in top segment of Appraisal on the history of his disability

Station five
Final evaluation by adapted physical education specialist
(Put on shoes and socks and return to gym)

Student enters here

Squads sitting waiting for examination

T	T	T	T	T	T	T	T	T	T	T	T
T	T	T	T	T	T	T	T	T	T	T	T
T	T	T	T	T	T	T	T	T	T	T	T

B

Squad being examined

T	T	T	T	T	T	T	T	T	T	T	T

Code:
T —student facing forward
⊥ —teacher
△ —recorder

FIGURE 21-5
For legend see opposite page.

students are trained to test another person and the testing is done in pairs, (4) all persons are trained to test themselves and record the scores. The type of testing technique chosen depends primarily on the maturity of the students, the complexity of the task, and the difficulty of administering the test. An example of administering a postural evaluation for which the instructor trains others to help is provided.

The entire class is examined by having the students line up in regular (or a predetermined) squad formation. The students are then positioned so that the examiners will have room to pass along each squad and assess each student. The students' names will have been entered previously on a group examination form (Fig. 21-5, *B*) in the same order as they are arranged in squads. A recorder fills out the form as each student is observed. (This is usually conducted as a gross type of screening to identify students who need special programs to improve fitness, body mechanics, coordination, and the like. These students can be examined more carefully at a later date.) Each student is then checked, with the same procedure, from the side and posterior views. The postural problems most easily identified from each view are so indicated on the group examination form illustrated. The key to the abbreviations on the form is found on the back of the form (Fig. 21-5, *B*). Fitness and coordination can be similarly recorded.

Many other types of tests can be used to aid in identifying students who require special assistance. These tests are described in other parts of this text and in most standard texts on physical education tests and measurements. Some of the

C

ADAPTED PHYSICAL EDUCATION
GROUP POSTURE EXAMINATION CHECK SHEET

SAMPLE FORM

NOTE: Fold up bottom of page for explanation of symbols

	BODY			FEET			KNEES			PELVIS			ABD.	CHEST		SHOULDERS			SPINE			HEAD		
Check for dev. from Ant., Pos., or Side view																								
	A	S	A&P	A	A	P	A	S	S	A&P	S	S	S	S	S	S	P	A	P	S	S	S	S	A&P
	BB	L	T	L	M	Pro	TT	Hy	Bt	T	FT	BT	Pt	P	F	F	ScW	T	Sc	Lo	Ky	B	F	T
Name of Student																								
Able, Judy																								
Baker, Suzi																								

Examine total class from anterior, side and posterior views. Record your eval. of all conditions for each view as you check each student, i.e. check all students from front view and record the major deviations in appropriate columns, then side, then posterior views. (1°=slight, 2°=moderate, 3°=severe)

BODY
BB Body build
l Lithe
m Medium
h Heavy

L Body lean
T Body tilt

FEET
L Long arch
M Meta. arch
Pro Pronation

PELVIS
T Tilt
FT Forward tilt
BT Backward tilt

ABDOMEN
Pt Ptosis

SHOULDERS
F Forward
ScW Winged scap.
T Tilt

SPINE
Sc Scoliosis
Lo Lordosis
Ky Kyphosis

HEAD
B Back
F Forward
T Tilt (side)

KNEES
TT Tibial torsion
Hy Hyper-extended
B Bent

CHEST
P Pigeon
F Flat

FIGURE 21-5

A, Individual method (station-to-station) of conducting a posture and body mechanics examination. **B,** Group method of conducting a posture and body mechanics examination. **C,** Form used to record findings of the group examination. (The information on the bottom half of the illustration is on the back of the form and is used to indicate the meaning of the code letters on the front of the form.)

types of evaluations that should be included in the procedures previously described are the following:

1. Range of motion tests (goniometry, tracings)
2. Perceptual-motor tests
3. Relaxation tests (Jacobson, Rathbone, and Benson) (see Chapter 8)
4. Physical fitness evaluations (American Alliance for Health, Physical Education, Recreation, and Dance; Canadian Association for Health, Physical Education, and Recreation; Clarke and Clarke[1]; and President's Council on Physical Fitness)
5. Health or personal history of student (health, sleep, rest, relaxation, recreation, etc.)

Classification for Physical Education

The handicapped student should be placed in the physical education class that is most normalizing (least restrictive). This placement, as has been noted, is a cooperative arrangement made by the parents, child, and school personnel. A suggested system used in some schools and colleges combines simplicity with accuracy and thus facilitates the transfer of important information from the physician to the teachers (Fig. 21-2).

When the physician, the nurse, and the members of the physical education department are familiar with the information presented in the plan just described, rather detailed information can be forwarded by the examining physician to the physical education department by means of the code described. Busy physicians can therefore furnish more complete information to the physical education department and, specifically, to the adapted physical education instructor than would be possible if they had to write out complete descriptions of the students' conditions and make complete recommendations for their activity programs.

The adapted physical education teacher is often expected to be present during the physical examinations when they are conducted at the school. Although this is a time-consuming procedure, it provides an excellent opportunity for the examining physician and the teacher of adapted physical education to communicate. The physician can ask specific questions regarding the curriculum and can then approve exercises and activities more adequately. The physical education teacher can seek detailed information from the physician about the nature of the various disabilities and contraindicated activities. Understanding and free communication between the examining physician and the teacher are essential if the special needs of the child are to be adequately met.

Classification Code

In addition to indicating which students should be assigned to adapted physical education classes, the classification code has several other functions (Fig. 21-2). Students who are classified "A" are permitted to enroll in any physical education activity. This often clears them for all intramural and extramural sports. Boys and girls who participate in interscholastic athletic programs are usually given an additional yearly examination to clear them for competition in one or more of the sports activites.

A "B" classification indicates that the student has a disability that limits participation in one or two specific activities. Using the "B" classification to indicate that a student can participate in all physical education activities except one or two reduces the problem of assigning the student to the proper physical education class to one of clerically checking on enrollment in physical education. An example would be "Class B, no swimming." The counseling and physical education departments should be informed to eliminate swimming from the student's schedule.

A very limited number of students have in the past been restricted from all participation in physical education by the examining physician. The number of students in this group should diminish as the quality of the adapted physical education program improves. A good adapted physical education program should provide some type of activity for any student who is well enough to attend regular classes in the school. Students in need of such specialized programs are classified "C" by the physician and are assigned to an adapted physical education class. Their exercise and activity assignments are then planned by a physical education teacher with special training.

Teacher and Student Schedules

Because the adapted physical education class requires a teacher with special training, certain problems may develop in scheduling the classes of that teacher. In a small school, classes may be offered only one or two periods during the day. If more than one class is offered, it is advantageous to have them scheduled consecutively. This will facilitate opening the special adapted physical education room and providing the special equipment. These same advantages prevail for a single class if it is scheduled the first period in the morning, before or after lunch, or the last period in the afternoon.

Some important factors in student scheduling were discussed earlier in this chapter; however, there are additional matters that also should be considered. If the special exercise room, the pool, or the special game areas used by the adapted physical education classes are available only during certain periods of the day, the schedule should be arranged so that the adapted classes can be held in as many of these areas as possible during the course of the year. Often adapted classes are held in the gymnasium, the dance studio, or the gymnastic, weight-training, or wrestling room. When this is done, it should be a part of the master schedule of this particular facility. These rooms may be used in lieu of a special adapted room, or they may be used as a facility for one of the activities offered in the adapted sports and activity program.

The adapted sports and activity program can usually be quite flexible and can be organized to permit facilities to be used when they are not needed by the other physical education classes that meet during the same period. However, it is important that a block of time be provided for the adapted class for each activity area, including the pool, so that students in this program have a rich and varied experience in a wide range of physical education activities.

If possible, adapted physical education classes for the boys and girls should be coeducational classes or should be scheduled at the same time of day. Thus coeducational classes can be offered or coeducational activities can be arranged for the students in this program when the time and the activities permit.

Program Adaptations in Regular Physical Education

Students with minor disabilities or posture problems that are functional in nature may receive valuable assistance with their problems if the regular physical education instructor is notified of these conditions and a recommendation is made for a preventive program of exercises and activities. Students who need a special sport skill or activity may receive it in the regular class. As an example, a student may need special kicking drills in the swimming pool on a kickboard to strengthen a knee. With a little special help and planning, the regular instructor can make a substantial contribution to the specific educational needs of students who have certain physical deviations and who are mainstreamed in a regular physical education class.

Transfer of Students

One of the important features of a quality program of adapted physical education is to provide for the easy transfer of students to a less restrictive physical education class. Although some students are assigned to an adapted class permanently and some for a school year or a semester, there are many students in the school who need to be in the class only for a short period of time to recover from an injury or illness or to complete a program of rehabilitation that will prepare them for their return to a regular physical education section. Often, athletes injured during or between seasons can hasten their recovery with a special program of exercises and activities in an adapted class. In addition to the advantage of meeting the needs of all the students in the school more adequately, the provision of a system of easy transfer of students to and from the adapted class does much to erase the stigma sometimes attached to a class for students who have disabilities. When any student in the school may be assigned to this program for rehabilitation—the highly gifted as well as the disabled—there should be no stigma attached to such a transfer.

ROLES OF THE ADAPTED PHYSICAL EDUCATION TEACHER

The adapted physical educator's role in the social growth of the handicapped student has many facets. One of the major factors is helping disabled persons to understand their own feelings and the reactions of others. Handicapped students must be guided to make the most of their social assets—for example, improving appearance, manners, posture, and personal hygiene. Although desiring to withdraw from a potentially painful social situations, they should be encouraged to take part in group activities whenever possible. Also, it is particularly important that handicapped students learn many specific game and exercise skills as well as the joy of winning and the ability to lose gracefully.

Adapted physical education offers excellent opportunities for assisting handicapped students in self-understanding and in acquiring a more rewarding life-style. In addition to teaching the adapted physical educator must act as a counselor, a record keeper, and a motivator.

Counselor

In general, the function of a counselor is to provide the opportunity to increase self-understanding.[4] Although counseling and guidance in the school or clinical setting are normally carried out by special trained personnel, in many instances the adapted physical educator must assume this role. Some of the more common of these counseling situations can be categorized under five distinct headings: modulating energy output, reasonable goal setting, daily living practices, family adjustment, and social adjustment.

Modulating Energy Output

Persons who have problems of low vitality or who must limit energy expenditure must learn to carefully monitor their activity. Examples of conditions that demand careful monitoring are those affecting respiratory and cardiovascular systems. The adapted physical educator plays an integral part in helping these individuals stay within exercise and activity tolerances. Students who tend to rationalize their problems must be guided in fully understanding the nature of their problems and in accepting the limitations that they impose.

Reasonable Goal Setting

Instructional goals are set in the IEP planning conference by the parents, school personnel, and the student (when possible). Very often, persons who plan the goals either underestimate or overestimate the student's ability to learn. Therefore, goals may be set either too low or too high. Goals that are too low overprotect the individual, whereas goals that are too high indicate wishful thinking. This unrealistic attitude may be carried over to everyday living and to the selection of career or occupational goals.

Daily Living Practices

Handicapped persons often need to develop habits that will enrich their daily lives. The adapted physical educator is often in a position to counsel the student on important aspects of hygienic living, means of coping with or avoiding emotional stresses, ways to make life a little easier, and, most important, the selection of rewarding leisure time activities.[3]

Family Adjustment

Conducting the IEP often includes teacher involvement with the student's family. It is of the utmost importance that the adapted physical educator know the students' families and be available to them as a source of information and advice. The lines of communication must always be open between family and teacher.

An interview should take place between the family and teacher at the earliest possible time after the student is admitted to the program. It is highly desirable that the student and both parents be present when the interview takes place. The initial interview gives the teacher an opportunity to describe the program and, at the same time, discover the expectations of the parents. Moreover, it provides an opportunity for the teacher to determine home environmental factors that may enhance or deter the adapted physical education program.

Following the initial interview, periodic contacts with the family should be made as a means of providing feedback as to the child's progress. Such contacts give a continuous opportunity for exchanging ideas, clarifying procedures, and counseling as various problems arise. In essence, there should be a spirit of cooperation between the family and teacher for the betterment of the child.

Of major importance to the guidance of both the family and their handicapped child is the right of parents to know what is being done for their child and why. Too often, professionals keep parents in the dark about what services are being rendered to the young client. This attitude is unfortunate and usually stems from the fact that professionals think parents will not fully understand the procedures being employed. Careful communication with parents is provided through IEP conferences as a part of P.L. 94-142.

To further enhance the counseling and guidance of parents, several procedures might be tried. The first might be the planning of parent observation periods during the program, after which the teacher should be available to answer questions. A second possibility is the use of parents as aides for children other than their own. A third possibility requiring controlled conditions is that the parents extend activity in the home.

Social Adjustment

One of the most important—and sometimes most difficult—areas to deal with is the social adjustment of handicapped persons. Adapted physical education experiences provide major opportunities for helping the handicapped develop effective social skills.[4]

It is obvious that social acceptance or rejection cannot be entirely controlled by the handicapped person. For example, the public may be repulsed by the prospect of an epileptic having an unsightly seizure, or the drooling individual with cerebral palsy may not be considered esthetically desirable. The blind person's dependency and the deaf person's communicative problems may often make rewarding relationships difficult. The slowness of the mentally limited child and the uncommon speech quality of the individual with cleft palate may be factors that disallow typical social adjustment. The physical educator can, through interaction with the student, be a model to individuals who have difficulty accepting handicapped persons.

Record Keeper

Since most of the work of the adapted physical education teacher is related to the measured instruction progress on the IEP, it is essential that accurate, complete confidential records be maintained. These records should be filed in an orderly manner so that they can be located quickly. All records should be dated—for example, letters sent and received, examination information received or examination performed, photographs taken, and student or parent conferences held. Some of the types of records that should be retained are (1) medical examination card, (2) physical education progress record, (3) posture and body mechanics examinations, (4) letters to and from medical personnel, and (5) photographic records.

Motivator

Adapted physical education programs are most successful when they have the support of administrators, physicians, teachers, parents, and students and when the teachers are well qualified, dedicated, and able to highly motivate their students. We have observed programs in adjacent districts and schools having basically the same resources, with the exception of the qualifications of the adapted physical education teacher; one program proved to be excellent, the other extremely poor. A good teacher is the single most important factor in providing a quality program.

The superior teacher is able to motivate students in many ways. Each teacher must select the type of motivational techniques that prove successful for the particular situation.[2] Some of the motivation techniques and devices that work especially well in adapted physical education are the following:

1. Keeping students well informed about class rules and policies, including grading procedures
2. Maintaining teacher enthusiasm and interest in students
3. Using charts and graphs to record student progress (posture examination cards, weight charts)
4. Using photographs of students with posture or disability problems to show them their present problems and to indicate any improvement made
5. Using exercise cards to show day-by-day improvements
6. Employing esthetic considerations for students (firm figure, good posture, proper weight, etc.) and appropriate anthropometric measurements
7. Exercising to music
8. Using good equipment for exercises and testing
9. Maintaining interesting, informative bulletin boards[2]
10. Maintaining contact with the students in games and sports activities
11. Employing interesting adapted sports and games

Since organization and administration cut across the total adapted physical education program, topics relating to these areas are included in other chapters in this text. Chapters 2, 3, 6, 7, and 20 include detailed information about organization of students for adapted physical education, assignment of exercise routines, and procedures for teaching exercise and adapted sports programs.

SUMMARY

As early as 1951 guiding principles for adapted physical education programs were developed. Actual content areas for physical education were included in regulations of P.L. 94-142. Aims and objectives of an adapted physical education program should be consistent with the guiding principles and address the mandated content areas.

When attempting to establish an adapted physical education program it may be necessary to determine the number and type of handicapped children that need to be served, raise the level of administrators' awareness of physical education requirements, and secure agreement to begin long-range planning to provide an appropriate physical education program for students served by the school.

During the long-range planning for the adapted physical education program important factors to consider are selecting a supervisor with outstanding qualifications, appointing an advisory committee to help guide the program, surveying the school or district to determine specific needs, establishing goals for the adapted physical education program, and securing support for the program.

When the program is implemented specific student needs and appropriate activities must be determined through testing. Policies for classifying, scheduling, and transferring students should be established. In addition to teaching, the adapted physical education instructor counsels, keeps a complete set of records, and motivates students to perform to high standards of achievement.

REVIEW QUESTIONS

1. What skills, knowledge, and attitudes should an adapted physical education teacher have that are different from those of a teacher of the regular physical education program?
2. What types of information should be included in a physical education medical referral form?
3. When should adapted physical education classes be scheduled?
4. What types of information should be included on a comprehensive record card for handicapped students?

5. How can you identify children who need special assistance in physical education?
6. What are five motivation techniques that can keep adapted physical education students interested in improving their physical-motor skills?
7. What are the guiding principles of adapted physical education programs?
8. Who should be included on an adapted physical education advisory committee, and what should the responsibilities of the committee be?
9. What are three reasons a school might not have an adapted physical education program?
10. What are three important qualities a supervisor of adapted physical education should have?

STUDENT ACTIVITIES

1. Construct a letter describing an adapted physical education program that could be sent to a physician.
2. Develop an information sheet or brochure describing the adapted physical education program that would be suitable to send to parents.
3. Survey five parents of handicapped children. Inquire about what they believe an adapted physical education program is and what benefits they believe their children will realize from such a program.
4. Role play a discussion between a physician who is opposed to handicapped individuals' exercising and an adapted physical educator who is trying to communicate the value of an adapted physical education program for handicapped persons.
5. Role play a conference between parents who want their handicapped child excused from physical education and an adapted physical education teacher who has tested the child and found him or her in need of a special physical education program.

REFERENCES

1. Clarke, H.H., and Clarke, D.H.: Developmental and adapted physical education, ed. 2, Englewood Cliffs, N.J., 1978, Prentice-Hall Inc.
2. Crowe, W.C.: The use of audio-visual materials in developmental (corrective) physical education, Unpublished master's thesis, University of California, Los Angeles, 1950.
3. Daniels, A.S., and Davies, E.A.: Adapted physical education, ed. 3, New York, 1975, Harper & Row, Publishers Inc.
4. Hamilton, K.W.: Counseling the handicapped in the rehabilitation process, New York, 1950, Ronald Press Co.
5. Karpinos, B.D.: Health of children of school age, Washington, D.C., 1963, U.S. Department of Health, Education, and Welfare.
6. Schiffer, C.G., and Hunt, E.O.: Illness among children, Washington, D.C., 1963, U.S. Department of Health, Education, and Welfare.
7. U.S. Department of Health, Education, and Welfare: Education for All Handicapped Children Act, Fed. Reg. **42:**42474-42498, Aug. 23, 1977.
8. Vodola, T.M.: Individualized physical education program for the handicapped child, Englewood Cliffs, N.J., 1973, Prentice-Hall Inc.

SUGGESTED READINGS

Dexter, G.: Instruction of physically handicapped pupils: remedial physical education, Sacramento, Calif., 1973, California State Department of Education.
Drowatsky, J.N.: Physical education for the mentally retarded, Philadelphia, 1971, Lea & Febiger.
Fait, H.F.: Special physical education, ed. 5, Philadelphia, 1984, W.B. Saunders Co.
Geddes, D.: Physical activities for individuals with handicapping conditions, ed. 2, St. Louis, 1978, The C.V. Mosby Co.
Guide for programs in recreation and physical education for the mentally retarded, Washington, D.C., 1968, American Association for Health, Physical Education, and Recreation and the National Education Association.
Guidelines for adapted physical education, Harrisburg, Pa., 1966, Department of Public Instruction, Comonwealth of Pennsylvania.
Moore, C.A.: The handicapped can succeed, Phys. Educ. **24:**63-164, 1967.
Mosston, M.: Teaching physical education, Columbus, Ohio, 1966, Charles E. Merrill Publishing Co.
Physical activity programs and practices for the exceptional individual, Third National Conference, Long Beach, Calif., 1974, AAHPERD.
Physical activity programs and practices for the exceptional individual, Fourth National Conference, Los Angeles, 1975, AAHPERD.
Roice, G.R., and Stoner, W.: Administrative aspects of starting a remedial physical education program, Unpublished data, Los Angeles, 1975.
Slader, C.V.: A workable adaptive program, J. Health Phys. Educ. Rec. **39:**71-72, 1968.
Stein, J.: Sense and nonsense about mainstreaming, J. Health Phys. Educ. Rec. **47:**43, 1976.
Techniques and methods for handicapped youth, First National Conference, Los Angeles, 1973, Office of the Los Angeles County Superintendent of Schools, Division of Special Education.

CHAPTER 22

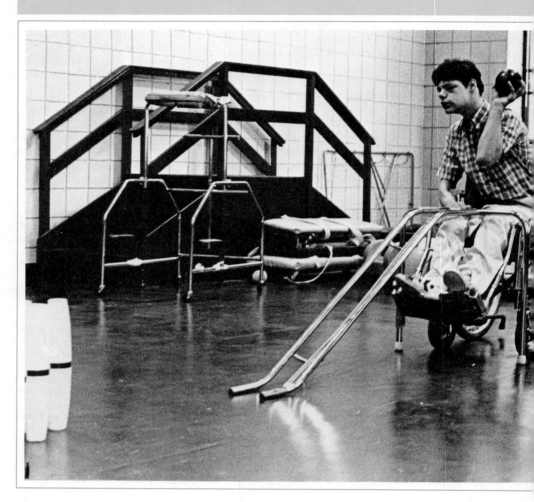

Facilities and Equipment

OBJECTIVES

♦ Know what types of equipment are needed for elementary level adapted physical education programs and for secondary and college level adapted physical education programs.

♦ Know how to arrange equipment for maximum use in the special physical education room.

♦ Be able to list inexpensive equipment that can be used in the adapted physical education room.

♦ Be able to identify ways in which special equipment can be used in the adapted physical education program.

Proper facilities and equipment are as important for classes in adapted physical education as they are for classes in regular physical education. They help the teacher of adapted physical education make the proper adjustment in the student's program of developmental exercise, perceptual-motor activities, modified sports, or rest and relaxation. The lack of such equipment, however, should never be an excuse for the failure to provide an adapted physical education program or for offering a poor program of exercises and activities for the handicapped student. A good teacher of adapted physical education can provide a quality program with minimum facilities and equipment by using some imagination and improvisation. However, good facilities and equipment make the teacher's job easier, make the program more meaningful, and provide motivation for the handicapped student.

The facility and equipment needs for adapted physical education programs may vary somewhat according to the type of students served. Factors such as whether the class is coeducational, ages and maturity levels of class members, and whether the students dress for activity all have an influence on facility and equipment needs. This chapter includes information about the kinds of facilities and equipment that should be provided for adapted physical education classes at the elementary, junior and senior high school, and college levels.

FACILITIES FOR ELEMENTARY SCHOOLS

Facilities for adapted physical education at the elementary school level vary extensively from district to district and from state to state. They may consist of nothing more than using the regular classroom for physical education or, under more desirable conditions, they may include other areas such as the cafeteria, the auditorium, grass or blacktop areas, a gymnasium, or a swimming pool.

As the importance of early intervention becomes increasingly apparent, many school districts are beginning to hire adapted physical educators for the elementary school level; however, in some areas of the country the adapted physical education program is woefully lacking. Elementary school classroom teachers may, under the best of conditions, have had only one or two courses designed to prepare them for all types of physical education instruction, including adapted physical education. It can readily be seen that an adapted program conducted under these conditions is severely restricted.

P.L. 94-142 mandates instructional programs for all children who qualify. Thus a qualified teacher on the faculty or a visiting teacher or supervisor must be provided or a contract with an adjacent school or school district must be made for such a special program. Some school districts have attempted to meet the needs of handicapped children at the elementary school level by providing special centers, located strategically in the district, where the students can be taken for this important part of their educational experience. Students from a number of schools in the district are transported to the center, where a specialist in adapted physical education, with a properly equipped facility, is able to offer them expert instruction with the assistance of specialists from the school district and other qualified personnel. Parents should be encouraged to attend these sessions so that the students will be able to engage in a special program of activities at home, in addition to the work done at the center. Some additional supervised work on these special exercises learned at the center may also be a part of the regular physical education program of the students' home school. The Los Angeles and Anaheim, California, schools have used visiting teachers and adapted physical education centers to meet the special needs of the children in their district. Hazleton, Pennsylvania, has provided a mobile unit especially designed for adapted physical education. It travels with two special teachers from school to school. Many rural school districts form special education cooperatives where specially trained teams, including adapted physical educators, are available for consultation. When requested, appropriate members of the team visit outlying schools to discuss specific children's problems, evaluate performance levels, and suggest appropriate intervention programs. This team then designs IEPs and serves as resource personnel to the teachers in schools throughout the area. In Kansas, several cooperatives have been formed that provide services to areas ranging from one to six counties.

Another possible arrangement that can be used to provide better facilities and equipment for elementary school children is to schedule children for a class at a nearby junior or senior high school where the adapted physical education room and equipment are available. Using this arrangement, classroom teachers of several elementary schools can bring their children to the nearby secondary school for an exercise and/or activity program conducted by a district specialist. Some modified equipment may be necessary for such a program, but the room and much of the equipment can be adapted for this type of class.

The minimum equipment needed for adapted physical education in an elementary school program includes six playground balls of various sizes, hoops, one low balance beam, a large mat, one small trampoline or rebound inner tube, three scooters, climbing apparatus, one plumb line or window pole (for assessing postural alignment), and towels. A towel can be substituted for an exercise mat and can be used by a student to perform a large number of special exercises for posture, fitness, and rehabilitation. Testing materials and sports and game equipment can be the same as those used for the regular classes. Individual exercise mats would be preferred to the towels because they are more comfortable, can be kept clean, and allow the students to use the towels for exercise programs while they are in the recumbent position on the mats. With some ingenuity, the teacher can provide an excellent adapted physical education program for students at the elementary school with minimum equipment.

Special exercises can be performed in the classroom, if sufficient space is provided, or on a blacktop or grass area outdoors. More extensive equipment for an elementary school program is desirable and may include many of the items described in greater detail in later portions of this chapter in connection with the secondary school and college level programs. Sports and game equipment for adapted physical education students at the elementary school level usually can be borrowed from the regular program, and a wide variety of excellent specialized equipment for use by persons of all ages and most types of disabilities has been developed by numerous manufacturers. Any adaptations to modify the activities in terms of size of the equipment, size of the court, and duration of the playing time can be worked out by the classroom teacher with the help of a district specialist.

FACILITIES FOR SECONDARY SCHOOLS AND COLLEGES

Facilities and equipment for adapted physical education in secondary schools and colleges are usually far more extensive than those found in the typical elementary school.

Special Exercise Room

At least one special room for adapted physical education should be provided for each school at the junior high school, senior high school, and college levels. If the school is large or if the number of students to be accommodated is greater that the number that can be handled in one room, traditionally separate facilities for girls and boys have been provided. Adapted classes should be coeducational.

The size of the adapted physical education room and related facilities adjacent to it is dependent on the philosophy of adapted physical education in each school and in each school district. The adapted physical education room is usually designed to handle a limited number of students. Since students in this program usually have individualized programs, fewer students can be han-

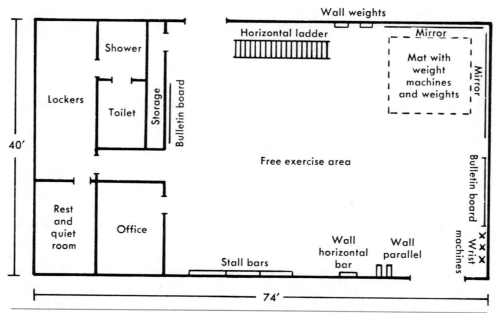

FIGURE 22-1
Self-contained adapted physical education room.

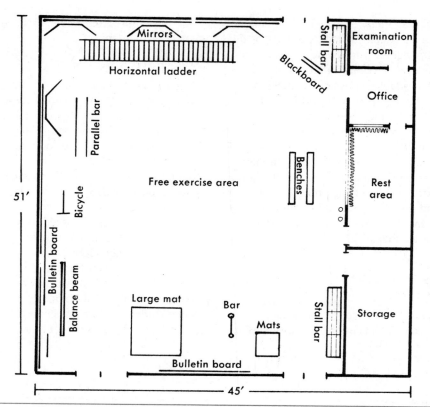

FIGURE 22-2
Secondary school adapted physical education room.

dled satisfactorily than in the regular physical education class. However, it must be remembered that this room must accommodate special equipment that occupies a considerable amount of floor, wall, and ceiling space. A clear area must also be provided for exercises and activities that do not involve the use of special equipment. The room therefore must be of sufficient size to meet these special needs comfortably. The minimum size of an adapted physical education room for a junior or senior high school would be 40 by 60 feet if the room is limited to use by adapted physical education classes.[14] If the room is used as a multipurpose facility accommodating regular physical education classes for special kinds of activities such as gymnastics or wrestling, additional space is necessary. This multipurpose arrangement has limitations, however, since much of the adapted equipment should be permanently installed on the floor, ceiling, and walls. An often-recommended 15-foot ceiling height is not sufficient if this room is also used for gymnastics or ball games, in which case the minimum height should be 20 to 25 feet.

A regular spring construction hardwood floor is preferred for this room, although parquet flooring has been used successfully in some facilities. The walls, at least to door height, should be of material that will withstand hard use (resistant to scarring and marking) and should provide for the mountings of special equipment. The ceiling may be of acoustical tile if ball games are not played

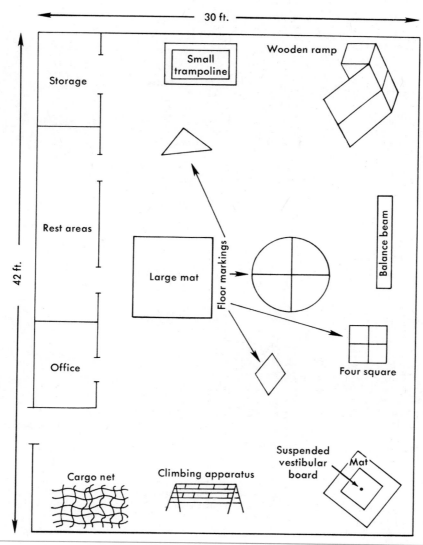

FIGURE 22-3
Elementary school adapted physical education room.

in the room. High windows are suggested for two sides of the room to allow for ample light and fresh air and to provide space for equipment on all four walls. Proper lighting and ventilation are important for a special exercise room. Doorways leading to this room from the locker area, hallways, and fields should be extra wide, with ramps leading to them. This arrangement allows for the easy movement of equipment and for the passing of students with wheelchairs or crutches. Bulletin boards and blackboards should be mounted on the walls (Figs. 22-1 and 22-2).

Considerable planning is required prior to the time that the equipment is located in the adapted physical education room. Efficient use should be made of the space available so that students who

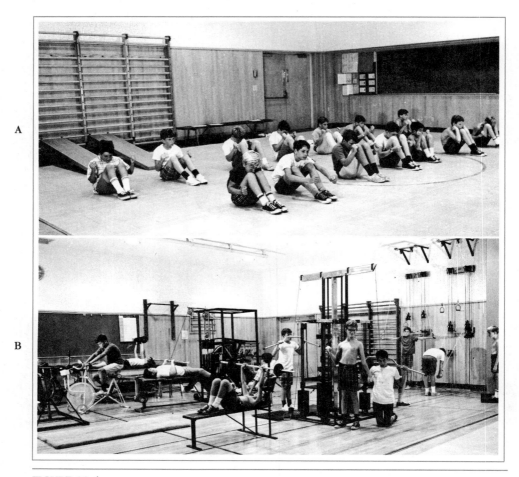

FIGURE 22-4
A, Use of the open space area in an adapted physical education room to conduct formal group exercises. **B,** An elementary school class uses a college facility. Each student performs an individual exercise on a piece of equipment.

are using special apparatus and equipment are able to use it effectively and so that hazards are not created while they use equipment such as barbells, the horizontal ladder, pulleys, and jump ropes (Figs. 22-3 and 22-4).

Instructor's Office and Student Rest Area

The instructor's office and a room suitable for a rest area and for quiet games should be located immediately adjacent to the adapted room. Observation windows on two sides of the office will allow the teacher to work at a desk and still su-

pervise both the adapted room and the rest area. Blinds on these windows provide privacy when needed. It is desirable that lavatories be located adjacent to these facilities.

Adapted Sports Area

An adapted sports area may be located immediately adjacent to the adapted physical education room. This area should consist of blacktop and grass for multipurpose use and space for special games. Activities that can be conducted on the blacktop include volleyball, paddle tennis, goal

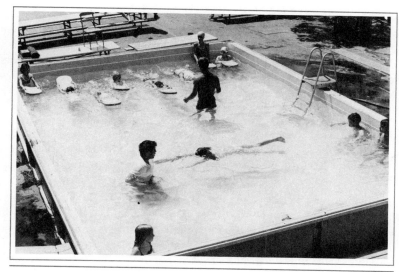

FIGURE 22-5
A portable pool.

hi, badminton, and deck tennis. A smooth concrete area provides space for shuffleboard, quoits, table tennis, and other adapted activities. A grass or dirt area provides space for horseshoes and croquet. The horseshoe-pitching area must be carefully laid out to ensure safety.

Other adapted sports activities can often be conducted between or adjacent to the regular physical education classes that are using a facility. They can also be conducted when an area such as that for archery, tennis, or swimming is not scheduled for other classes.

Students in the adapted program should have many opportunities to participate in activities that are similar to those engaged in by students in the regular physical education program so that they can be mainstreamed into regular classes at the earliest possible time. Instructors of regular physical education classes can accomplish this by making minor adaptations in the games, sports, and activities that are being conducted in the regular physical education curriculum.

There is a recent trend toward the use of community and private facilities by students in adapted physical education. Nearby recreation centers, private pools, bowling alleys, special ex-ercise facilities, and badminton, racquetball, golf, and archery facilities are often made available, and in some instances expert instruction is provided for handicapped persons by the personnel at the facility.

In many colleges swimming for students in the adapted classes is conducted during times when others are not using the pool. Sometimes it is possible to conduct an adapted swimming class while a small regular class is in session. Since swimming is such an important activity for handicapped persons, every effort must be made to provide pool experiences for as many of the students as possible. A small, warm, therapeutic pool would be an ideal facility for adapted physical education students, but in most schools both hydrotherapy activities and special swimming for handicapped students must be conducted in the regular pool. Some schools have successfully used a portable pool (Fig. 22-5), which is set up on a blacktop or grass area and then moved from school to school every 2 or 3 weeks so that all of the handicapped students in a district can participate in a swimming unit. This works especially well at the elementary school level, because a swimming pool is seldom included in the physical education facilities. One new practice for either a school or therapy unit for any age level is to use a portable pool built on a trailer. This type of pool can be drained and easily transported to different facilities for use without the expense of building a pool or the problems of labor and time required to take down, move, and set up a portable pool at each new locality.

USE OF THE ADAPTED ROOM AND EQUIPMENT

Orientation during the first week of school should include information on the rules that relate to the use of the adapted physical education room and its equipment. These rules include the following:

1. The room should be used only under proper supervision.
2. It is necessary to be instructed in the use of any specialized equipment before using it.
3. Exercises and activities should be performed only when they have been assigned or approved for use by the instructor; careful instruction in the execution of each exercise must precede its use.
4. It is necessary to be instructed in the proper use and care of barbells, dumbells, and other resistance equipment before beginning a progressive resistance program. Students should increase the number of repetitions and the amount of weight and the assigned number of repetitions.
5. All equipment must be returned to its proper place immediately after use.
6. Information about any faulty equipment must be reported immediately to an instructor.
7. Hazardous types of equipment (weights, horizontal ladders, Stegel, trampoline, ropes, cargo ladder, etc.) must be tested by the instructor before being used by students, and spotters should always be present to prevent accidents and injuries.
8. Students must stop their exercise or activity programs and report to an instructor immediately if they experience undue pain, dyspnea, or general discomfort.

9. Breath holding is discouraged during lifting activities and abdominal exercises, since this may cause an increase in intra-abdominal pressure and thus possible strain. This also causes the Valsalva effect, which constricts the carotid artery.

EQUIPMENT

The equipment needs of each of the special facilities just described are somewhat unique, depending on factors such as the number of students using each facility; whether the area is used for boys or girls or is coeducational; whether it is for elementary school, junior or senior high school, college, or community use; and whether minimum or ideal equipment is to be furnished.

Minimum Equipment

The minimum equipment needed in an adapted room in a secondary school or college level facility includes the following: sufficient individual 1-inch thick plastic-covered body mats to accommodate the peak class load plus five or six more, 2-inch thick mats of sufficient size to cover the floor under hazardous types of equipment such as the horizontal ladder or the horizontal bar, a platform or firm rubber mats to cover the floor where weight-training activities will take place, towels for use in the exercise program, a plumb line or posture screen for posture examinations, and miscellaneous inexpensive pieces of testing equipment such as measuring tapes and skin pencils. Ropes for skipping and school benches can usually be obtained from the maintenance department of the school. Since resistance exercises are desired in most programs, homemade weights can be constructed by the instructor or by the students. Thus with a minimum of expenditure sufficient equipment can be obtained to start a good adapted program. Special equipment for perceptual-motor training can be purchased or borrowed from regular classes or it can be improvised until funds are available. Equipment for most adapted sports can be borrowed from the regular physical education program.

Equipment for the instructor's office includes

desks, worktables, and filing equipment, with sufficient space remaining for the instructor to do small-group counseling. The rest and quiet game area should have bunks or cots to accommodate 2% of the boys and from 2% to 5% of the girls at the peak period of enrollment and tables and chairs for quiet game activities. A storeroom must be provided in which quiet game equipment, adapted sports equipment, and testing equipment can be stored.

Additional Equipment

Standard equipment for a remedial or adapted room includes the minimum equipment already described and, if possible, the following items:

1. A posture screen
2. Manufactured adjustable barbells and dumbbells and racks for their storage or resistive equipment constructed at the school
3. Stall bars
4. Pulley or chest weights (triplex preferred)
5. Iron boots or special knee exercise apparatus
6. A horizontal ladder
7. An incline board
8. A balance beam
9. Three-way mirrors
10. Special benches
11. Stall bar stools
12. A wall parallel bar
13. A wall horizontal bar
14. A trampoline or rebound inner tube

Equipment for special adapted sports should include the following:

1. Bowling ball with retractable handle
2. Goal ball
3. Beep baseball
4. Beep cones
5. Basketball standards with return nets

Elaborate Equipment

More elaborate equipment includes the following:

1. A multistation heavy resistance machine on which students can exercise a number of different areas of the body (this provides six to eight stations)
2. A stationary bicycle
3. Special wrist and forearm exercise machines
4. Shoulder wheels
5. Sound equipment for rhythmical training
6. Dynamometers
7. Tensiometers
8. Isokinetic exercise or testing equipment

Equipment for Perceptual-motor Activities

Special equipment for perceptual-motor activities should enhance the offerings of the adapted physical education program. Much of the equipment can be made by the teacher, the maintenance or industrial arts department at the school, or in some cases the students themselves.

Inexpensive Equipment

1. Pieces of rope and string of various diameters, composition, and length, to use for testing purposes and for many types of activities, including rope skipping, making shapes and forms, identifying size and texture, jumping over or climbing under, and typing knots (Fig. 22-6, A)
2. Cardboard boxes of various sizes and shapes to use as targets, to sit in, to climb through, to walk in, to catch with, and even to store other pieces of equipment
3. Masking tape to lay out test areas on the floor or walls, to mark boundaries of courts and play areas, to make identifying symbols (numbers, letters, triangles, squares, etc.), to mark special equipment, to mark a right arm or leg (to help a person identify right from left), and to tape things together
4. Chalk of different colors to mark items included in the previous lists to identify color, to draw on the blackboard (Fig. 22-6, B) or on paper (for all types of symbol and color identification), and for "draw-a-man" tests.
5. Plastic bottles or milk cartons of different sizes, shapes, and colors to use for identification; to fill with sand or other materials and serve as weights; to use for games (to run around, to knock over, to catch and throw, to float or sink in the swimming

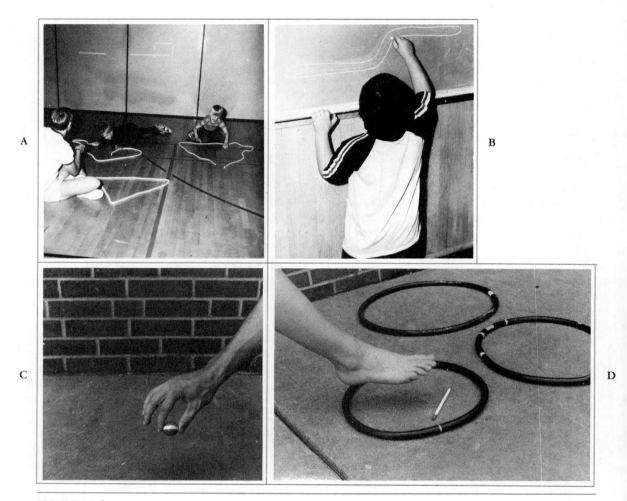

FIGURE 22-6
Inexpensive equipment for perceptual-motor activities. **A,** Rope or string. **B,** Chalk. **C,** Small ball.
D, Pencil and hoops.
*(**A** and **B** courtesy California State University, Audio Visual Center, Long Beach, Calif.)*

pool, to hang from strings, to be swung, to be hit, to be avoided, or be be blown)

6. Carpet squares to skate with, to slide on, and to use as targets
7. A household plunger to stick on the wall for jump and reach activities or to use to pull oneself along on a scooter[13]
8. A cardboard barrel to roll in, throw objects into, or store equipment
9. A truck innertube to walk on, roll in, or lie on
10. Hula hoops made out of garden hose to lay on the floor and curl the body around, form shapes over, or jump in and out of[13]
11. A ladder to crawl or step through
12. Traffic cones for boundary markers or obstacle courses
13. Beanbags to throw, catch, or balance on body parts while in motion
14. Balloons to hit, kick, or catch
15. Butcher paper or printer's paper for drawing

More Elaborate or Expensive Equipment

Equipment on which to bounce may include any of the following:

1. Trampoline (Fig. 22-7, *C*)
2. Minitrampoline
3. Truck tires or innertubes (or smaller sizes if desired) with canvas laced across the opening on one side to serve as a trampoline
4. Spring-O-Line bounce boards
5. Spring boards, jumping boards, and inner tubes

Protective and padded equipment may include the following:

1. Mats of various sizes, thicknesses, and consistencies for individual use and to protect the equipment
2. Bolsters to sit on, jump from, or roll on
3. Bataccas to wrestle with, to hit with, and to hit
4. Large padded boxing gloves and head guards
5. Boxers' heavy bag to hit, tackle, etc.
6. King-of-the-mountain pad

7. Jousting clubs
8. Specially shaped mats (inclined, round, square, cylindrical, and cone-shaped)
9. Large rubber balls with plastic covers

Special game equipment may include almost every item of equipment used in the regular physical education program, as almost all can be adapted for some use with selected students in the perceptual-motor program. Included would be the following:

1. All types of balls (large, small, light, and heavy; of different textures and air pressures; and special balls like the Whiffle ball, the Fleece ball, the Nerf ball, knitted balls)
2. Things with which to strike the balls, such as bats, rackets, paddles, and clubs
3. Nets of various sizes
4. Bases and goals
5. Standards to hold up nets, goals, and games (tetherball, basketball, volleyball, and goal hi)

Special Equipment

Special types of equipment for children's games, especially those requiring manipulation and allowing for identity of color, shape, texture, number, and letter concepts, may include the following:

1. Balance beams of various widths and heights (Figs. 22-7, *F*, and 22-8, *C* and *D*)
2. A Stegel for balancing and climbing activities (Fig. 22-7, *E*)
3. Stall bars (Fig. 22-11)
4. Incline boards (Fig. 22-7, *B*)
5. A horizontal ladder (Fig. 22-9)
6. Wall parallel and horizontal bars
7. Climbing ropes
8. Ladders
9. A cargo net (Fig. 22-7, *A*)
10. Pulley weights (Fig. 22-10)
11. Rocker boards
12. Scooter boards (Fig. 22-7, *B*)
13. Wheel toys
14. Stilts
15. Bongo boards
16. T stools

Text continued on p. 496.

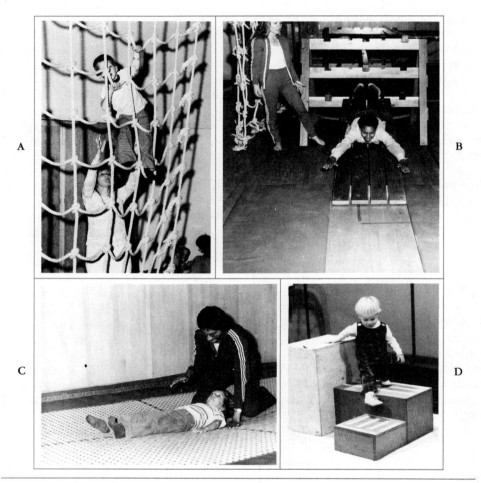

FIGURE 22-7
More elaborate equipment for perceptual-motor activities. **A,** Cargo net. **B,** Scooter on incline.
C, Trampoline. **D,** Wooden boxes. **E,** Stegel. **F,** Elevated scooter. **G,** Ball and plastic bowling pin.
*(**A** to **E** courtesy California State University, Audio Visual Center, Long Beach, Calif.; **F** courtesy
Verland Foundation, Inc.; **G** courtesy Children's Rehabilitation Center, Butler, Pa.)*

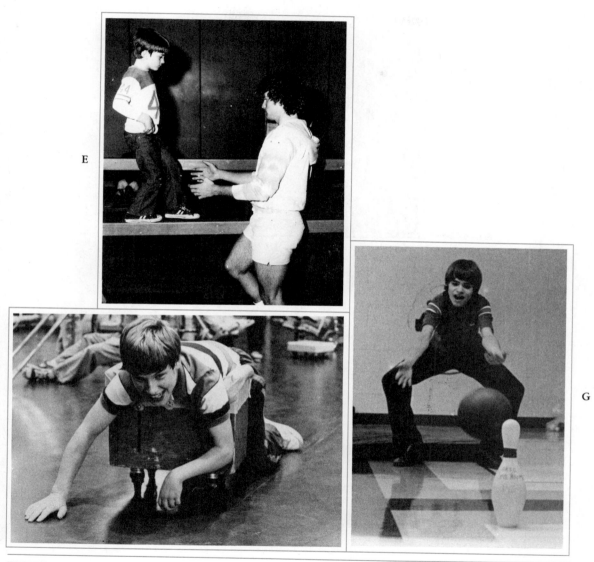

FIGURE 22-7
For legend see opposite page.

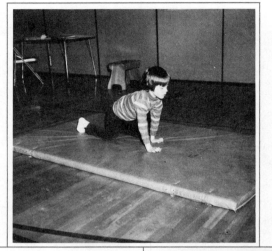

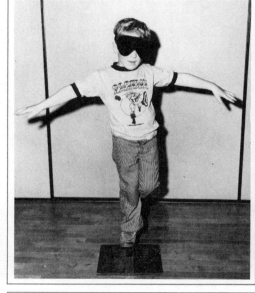

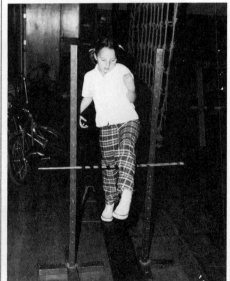

FIGURE 22-8

Activities using perceptual-motor testing equipment. **A,** Creeping. **B,** Static balance. **C,** Dynamic balance. **D,** Pincer grasp. **E,** Developing reflexes.
(A to C courtesy California State University, Audio Visual Center, Long Beach, Calif.; E courtesy Children's Rehabilitation Center, Butler, Pa.)

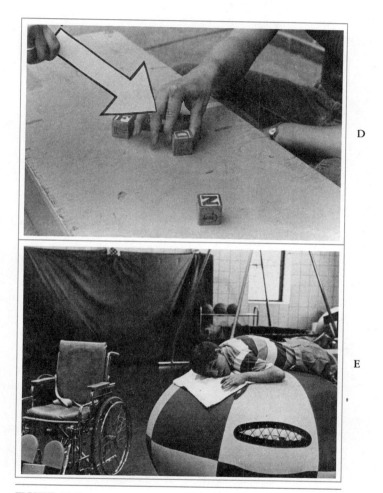

D

E

FIGURE 22-8
For legend see opposite page.

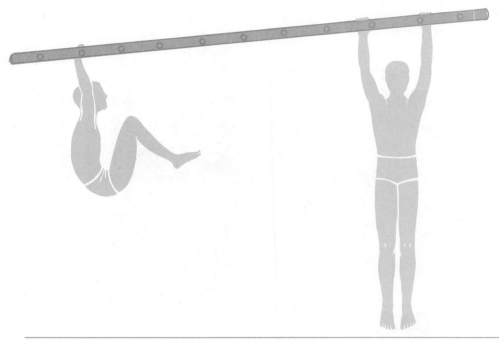

FIGURE 22-9
Horizontal ladder for abdominal exercise and asymmetrical hanging for scoliosis of low shoulder.

17. Wands
18. Three-way mirrors (Fig. 22-10)
19. Pitchbacks
20. Endurance equipment such as a treadmill and a bicycle ergometer

Rhythm equipment can provide an opportunity to meet motor development needs, but its use also involves creativity linked to a better self-concept and a broadened self-image. Rhythm equipment might include the following:

1. Lummi sticks
2. Poi-poi balls
3. A metronome
4. A recorder with tapes or records
5. Tambourines
6 Percussion instruments
7. Songbooks or song sheets

Outdoor play equipment such as slides, swings, teeter-totters, rings, sandboxes, tires, and jungle gyms provides opportunity for a variety of perceptual-motor activities in the fresh air and sunshine.

Testing equipment includes marked mats (or floor) stopwatches, yardsticks and metric tapes or sticks, targets, traffic cones, mats, ropes, hoops, beads, tapping board test equipment, and blocks (Fig. 22-8, *A* to *C*). Some standard tests and test kits that might be used include the following:

1. Purdue Perceptual Motor Survey[10]
2. Stott Motor Impairment Test[12]
3. Individual Motor Behavior Survey and Diagnostic Motor Ability Test[1]
4. Frostig Movement Skills Test[9]
5. Draw-a-Man Test[7]

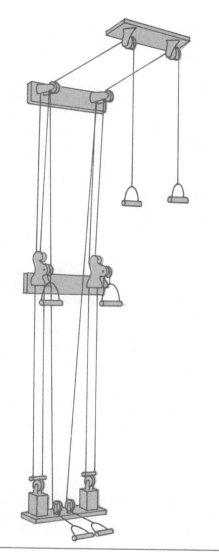

FIGURE 22-10
Triplex pulley weight.

6. Visual Perception Test[6]
7. Fiorentino Reflex Tests[5]
8. The Ayres Space Test, Figure-Ground Visual Perception Test, kinesthesia and tactual perception tests, and motor accuracy tests[2]
9. Physical fitness tests by the American Alli-

ance for Health, Physical Education, and Recreation[8,11,14]
10. Bruininks-Oseretsky Test of Motor Proficiency[3]

Construction of Equipment

Much of the equipment used in an adapted physical education program can be constructed by the instructor or by the maintenance or industrial arts department in a school. Homemade equipment will often suffice for a number of years until an adequate budget can be obtained to buy the more expensive manufactured equipment. Some items that can be constructed are the following: a three-way mirror (which can be mounted on the wall or placed on a rack or on wheels and moved around the room, with the wings on the sides of the mirror being held in place with piano hinges), posture screens, heel cord stretch boards, foot supinator boards, homemade barbells and dumbbells, pulleys for special types of exercises, balance beams, exercise benches, racks for weights, bicycle exercisers, and many items for the adapted sports and perceptual-motor programs.[4]

Description and Use of Equipment
Body Mats

Body mats are very useful in an adapted program. They are relatively small and light (usually 3 feet wide, 6 feet long, and 1 inch thick). They are plastic covered and therefore easy to clean, and some can be folded in half and stacked in a small space. They provide safety and comfort for the student during floor exercises. If they are always folded or stacked with the clean sides together, the surface always remains clean. If they are kept off the floor when not in actual use so that they are not walked on and are not used as crash pads underneath weight-lifting and similar types of equipment, they will prove quite durable.

Towels

A good, sturdy towel has many uses in the adapted program. If equipment is limited, the towels can be used instead of exercise mats, or if mats are old and soiled, towels can be used as covers for the mats during exercise. Many exercises can be performed with use of a towel. Almost every part of the body can be stretched or resistance can be applied by employing the towel in various ways. The towel can be folded three times lengthwise, then rolled into a tight cylinder and placed directly between the shoulder blades while the individual is resting on the back and can be used thus to stretch the anterior muscles of the chest and shoulder girdle. A folded towel can also be used instead of a headboard, and rolled or folded towels can be used for support in certain relaxation exercises (see Chapter 8).

Three-way Mirror

Some type of mirror is useful for adapted classes at all grade levels. A mirror with two side wings is preferable, since it allows the student to see three views of the body and thus to understand posture deviation problems better and to see when the body is in proper alignment. It also allows the student to watch movements during exercise and therefore to be more accurate in the execution of the exercise program. The instructor can use the mirror to point out to students the kinds of deviations in body mechanics observed while using the plumb line, the posture screen, and various other types of measuring devices. Students can check their body positions in relation to a gravity line if a plumb line is hung so that it drops straight in front of a section of the mirror. Mirrors can be mounted permanently on the wall in one section of the room or a three-way or one-way mirror can be mounted on wheels or on slides so that it can be moved to various areas of the adapted physical education room, thus increasing the flexibility of its use. Besides the upright mirror, overhead mirrors have been found to be beneficial for students performing in the reclined position.

Resistance Equipment

Each year many new types of resistance equipment are developed for use in adapted physical education and allied fields. Many of these devices are useful for equipping an adapted physic education room. In addition to the barbells, dumbbells, iron boots, and pulley weights that have been standard equipment for many years, a number of other kinds of special resistance equipment have been developed, consisting of springs, rubber tubing, and many other types of tension-producing or resistance-producing materials. Special exercise equipment has been designed for specific body parts. Recently, a number of very large and complex exercise machines have been developed for class use. These exercise machines provide 4 to 10 different exercise stations, each of which allows students to exercise a certain part of the body and all of which allow them to apply the principle of progressive resistance in the exercise program. The Universal Gym, the Nautilus, and several new types of isokinetic exercise equipment are examples of this type of machine. The instructor actually has a wide choice of resistance-producing devices, ranging from noncommercial equipment made of bags filled with sand and barbells and dumbbells made from tin cans, cement, and pipe to rather highly sophisticated manufactured resistance equipment, some of which actually creates a specific resistance related to the amount of force exerted by the subject. The types of resistance equipment selected by the instructor will depend on preference and on budget limitations.

Stall Bars

At least one set (three sections) of stall bars should be included in the equipment of the adapted room. The stall bar is a rather flexible piece of apparatus that allows students to perform many types of stretching and developmental exercises. One set of stall bars provides space for three students to exercise at one time and also can be used as a ladder for incline boards where space is at a premium. When wall space is severely limited, a set of pulley weights can be placed behind one section of the stall bars by the removal of one bar, and thus two pieces of apparatus can be placed in the space ordinarily occupied by one. A set of exercises for the stall bars is included in Appendix II.

Horizontal Ladder

The horizontal ladder should be placed so that one end is higher than the other. This provides more or less resistance for students as they climb from one end to the other and also allows certain kinds of asymmetrical hanging exercises to be done by students who have deviations in shoulder height and problems with lateral curvatures of the spine. The horizontal ladder has many uses, ranging from general conditioning exercises for the arms, shoulder girdle, and trunk to very specific stretching and developmental activities for posture and rehabilitation of other disabilities (Fig. 22-9).

Pulley Weights

Pulley weights have been a standard piece of apparatus in the adapted room for many years. There are several types, ranging from those with handles that are placed at the foot level, the chest level, or over the head to various combinations of these positions. The triplex pulley weight, which is a combination of the three just mentioned, provides for a good deal of flexibility in the assignment of exercises and takes a relatively small amount of space in the adapted room. It is also possible to purchase headstraps, footstraps, and handstraps so that specific exercises can be provided for special areas of the body that cannot be exercised with the standard pulley weight machine and so that students with paralysis or various types of disabilities can be accommodated (Fig. 22-10). A set of exercises for the pulley weights is included in Appendix III.

Balance Beam

The balance beam serves several purposes in the adapted room. It helps students improve their balance and coordination; it helps strengthen and develop the feet and legs; and, when it is constructed so that it acts as a supinator board, it can also help in the correction of certain foot, ankle, and knee deviations (Fig. 22-7, *E* and *F*).

Hand, Wrist, and Shoulder Machines

A number of wall-mounted commercial machines have been designed to help students develop the musculature in the hands, wrists, forearms, and upper arms. Most of these machines operate on a friction principle, with the amount of resistance adjustable. Muscles of the shoulder girdle, shoulder, elbow, wrist, and hand can be developed or stretched with properly assigned exercises on these pieces of apparatus (Fig. 22-12).

When budget limitations pose a problem, homemade equipment can often be substituted. For example, a hand, wrist, and forearm exerciser can be constructed by attaching a 2- to 4-foot length of clothesline with a weight on one end to a 10-inch long dowel. This simply constructed piece of equipment can be used to perform a whole set of progressive resistance exercises to develop the hand, forearm, and wrist.

Benches

Benches similar to regular playground benches can be very useful in the adapted room. They pro-

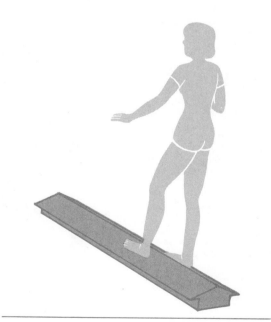

FIGURE 22-11
Supinator balance beam.

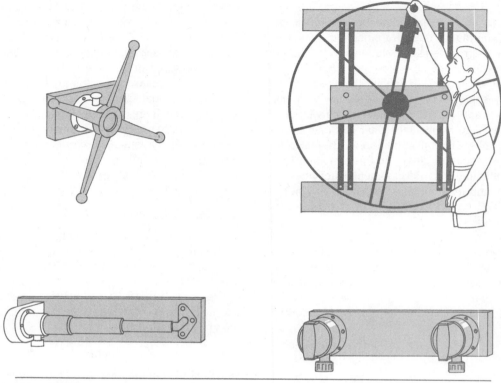

FIGURE 22-12
Various types of hand, wrist, forearm, and shoulder exercise devices.

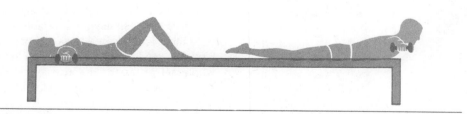

FIGURE 22-13
Narrow bench.

vide sitting stations for execution of foot and ankle exercises and are particularly useful for exercises performed in the prone and supine positions (Fig. 22-13).

Ropes

Rope skipping is an excellent activity for many students in the adapted physical education class. Because many exercise programs involve development of flexibility and strength, an endurance activity is often needed. Ropes can be purchased that have handles which facilitate turning the rope easily and rapidly. Jump ropes can also be made from clothesline. Rope ¼ or ⅜ inch in diameter makes a jump rope that is quite satisfactory for the adapted class. In addition to being used for various jumping routines, long and short ropes can also be used for many types of perceptual-motor tests and activities such as construction of geometric shapes and letters.

Heel Cord Stretch Apparatus

A number of devices can be used to stretch the heel cord, a desirable activity for certain deviations of the foot and ankle. The heel cord can be stretched while the student is standing on one of the lower rungs of the stall bar or standing with the forepart of the foot on a block 1½ or 2 inches thick and lowering the heel down over the edge of the block. Various pieces of apparatus can be constructed to provide a straight stretch in dorsiflexion of the ankle, or a stretch of the heel cord can be combined with a stretch of the foot everters by use of a supinator board tilted up at one end.

Bicycle Ergometer and Treadmill

The bicycle ergometer and the treadmill are especially useful for improving cardiovascular endurance under controlled conditions. Endurance programs can be carefully graded with these pieces of apparatus. Small portable treadmills are available if cost is a problem. A bicycle ergometer can be modified from any bicycle by persons in the industrial arts or maintenance department.

Bulletin Boards and Blackboards

Ample bulletin board and blackboard space is needed in the well-planned adapted physical education room. This space can be used for posting announcements, pictures, posters, bulletins, exercise cards, instructional information, and all types of material to interest students in the program. The boards should be attractive, posted material should be interesting and current, and students should be encouraged to contribute materials.

Rhythm Equipment

Many handicapped persons can profit from a variety of rhythmic activities. Equipment for these includes music tapes or records, which can be used for exercise programs, relaxation, rhythm training, and dance activities; percussion instruments; lummi sticks; a metronome; or various musical instruments to help establish a rhythm or beat. If special equipment is not available, the teacher or a student can lead rhythm programs by using such techniques as clapping, snapping fingers, marching, walking, running, and exercising to rhythmic patterns. The learners capture these beats and rhythms with the eyes and ears, by feeling the beat, or by various combinations of these senses.

Posture Screen

The instructor can use the posture screen to help objectify posture examinations of students in the standing position. The screen allows for a more accurate evaluation of the degree of posture deviation and a more meaningful follow-up examination (see Chapter 16). The screen should have an adjustable base so that it can be level, proper tension in the strings so that there is no sagging, and a center vertical line or gravity line of a different color so that it is easily identified. The screen should be light enough to be moved easily around the room and may even be constructed so that it can be folded and transported by a visiting teacher.

Plumb Line

A plumb line can be purchased from a hardware store, or the instructor can construct one easily by tying any weight such as a lead fishing sinker to the end of a piece of string. A plumb line is a very useful piece of equipment in the adapted program (see Chapter 16). It can be used as a gravity line against which both anteroposterior and lateral posture examinations can be taken; it can be used to check the alignment of the leg from the anterior, posterior, and lateral views; and it can be used to check the alignment of the spinal column, all in connection with various posture and body mechanics examinations. It also can be used to align such pieces of equipment as the posture screen before it is used to examine students.

SUMMARY

Facilities available for adapted physical education classes vary. Ideally one room in each school or district is designated and equipped for the adapted physical education program. More frequently the program is carried out in any room or space that is available. If a special room is provided, the room can be equipped with special pieces of equipment designed to meet specific needs of handicapped students. Neither special equipment nor a special room is necessary to carry out a successful adapted physical education room.

Inexpensive equipment can be purchased or built. Rope, boxes, masking tape, innertubes, milk cartons, carpet squares, rubber hose, cardboard barrels, and balloons are useful in the elementary adapted program. Homemade barbells, dumbbells, heel cord stretch boards, and posture screens can be used in the secondary adapted physical education program.

Expensive equipment such as balance beams, stall bars, vestibular boards, pulley weights, bicycle ergometers, and isokinetic exercise machines can be added when more money is available.

REVIEW QUESTIONS

1. What types of equipment would you find in an elementary adapted physical education room that you would not find in a secondary adapted physical education room?
2. What types of exercises can be done on the stall bars?
3. How can mirrors be used in an adapted physical education program?
4. What types of exercises can be done on a bench?
5. What are six inexpensive (or homemade) pieces of equipment that might be used in elementary physical education?

STUDENT ACTIVITIES

1. Observe a class being conducted in a special physical education room. List the equipment in the room and describe how it was being used.
2. Collect five inexpensive items (for example, milk cartons, boards, coat hangers, and hose) and construct equipment that could be used in an adapted physical education program.
3. Describe how three pieces of equipment used in a regular physical education program could be modified for use in an adapted physical education program.
4. Construct a posture screening tool that could be used to assess posture.
5. Design an adapted physical education room using only the equipment available in a regular physical education program. Tell how you would use each piece of equipment.
6. Make up a list of equipment you would buy for an elementary adapted physical education room if you had $50 to spend.

REFERENCES

1. Arnheim, D.D., and Sinclair, W.A.: The clumsy child: a program of motor therapy, ed. 2, St. Louis, 1979, The C.V. Mosby Co.
2. Ayres, A.J.: Southern California sensory integration tests, Los Angeles, 1972, Western Psychological Services.
3. Bruininks-Oseretsky Test of Motor Proficiency, Circle Pines, Minn., 1978, American Guidance Service.
4. Clarke, H.H., and Clarke, D.H.: Developmental and adapted physical education, Englewood Cliffs, N.J., 1978, Prentice-Hall Inc.
5. Fiorentino, M.R.: Reflex testing methods for evaluating C.N.S. development, ed. 2, Springfield, Ill., 1973, Charles C Thomas, Publisher.
6. Frostig, M.: Marianne Frostig Developmental Test of Visual Perception, Palo Alto, Calif., 1964, Consulting Psychologists Press.
7. Goodenough, R.L., and Harris, D.B.: Goodenough-Harris Drawing Test, New York, 1963, Harcourt Brace Jovanovich, Inc.
8. Health Related Physical Fitness Test, Reston, Va., 1980, American Alliance for Health, Physical Education, Recreation, and Dance.
9. Orpet, R.E.: Frostig movement skills tests battery, Los Angeles, 1972, Marianne Frostig Center of Educational Therapy.
10. Roach, E.G., and Kephart, N.C.: The Purdue Perceptual Motor Survey, Columbus, Ohio, 1966, Charles E. Merrill Publishing Co.
11. Special fitness test manual for mildly mentally retarded Persons, Reston, Va., 1976, American Alliance for Health, Physical Education, Recreation, and Dance.
12. Stott, D.H.: A general test of motor impairment for children, Dev. Med. Child. Neurol. **8:**523-531, 1966.
13. Werner, P., and Rini, L.: Perceptual motor equipment: inexpensive ideas and activities, New York, 1975, John Wiley & Sons Inc.
14. Youth fitness test manual, rev., Washington, D.C., 1961, The American Association for Health, Physical Education, and Recreation.

SUGGESTED READINGS

Dauer, V.P., and Pangrazi, R.P.: Dynamic physical education for elementary school children, ed. 7, Minneapolis, 1983, Burgess Publishing Co.
Geddes, D.: Physical activities for individuals with handicapping conditions, St. Louis, 1978, The C.V. Mosby Co.
Planning areas and facilities for health, physical education and recreation, Chicago, 1970, The Athletic Institute.
Safford, P.L.: Teaching young children with special needs, St. Louis, 1978, The C.V. Mosby Co.
Seaman, J., and DePauw, K.: The new adapted physical education: a developmental approach, Palo Alto, Calif., 1982, Mayfield Publishing Co.
Wood, M.A., editor: Developmental therapy sourcebook, vol. 1, Baltimore, 1981, University Park Press.

Selected Assessment Tests

A norm- and criterion-referenced developmental scale.

ADAPTATION OF THE DENVER DEVELOPMENTAL SCALE

STO: lifts head	Chin off table	1 month
STO: lifts head	Face 45° to surface	1½ months
STO: lifts head	Face 90° to surface	2 months
STO: arm support	Chest up, on forearms	3 months
Sit: head steady	Head upright for 10 seconds	3½ months
Rolls over	Completely two times or more	4 months
Pulls to sit	Head does not hang at any time	5 months
Weight on legs	Brief support of weight on legs	5½ months
Sits without support	5 seconds or more	5 months
Pulls self to stand	On a solid object	8 months
Gets to sitting	Without assistance	8½ months
Walks holding furniture	5 steps	10 months
Stands momentarily	2 or more seconds	11 months
Stoops and recovers	Pick and return without touching floor	12 months
Walks	Does not tip from side to side	13 months
Walks backward	Two or more steps	17 months
Walks up steps	Upright (assisted by rail)	18 months
Kicks ball	Without support	19 months
Throws ball overhand	3 feet	22 months
Balances on one foot	1 second two out of three times	26 months
Jumps in place	Both feet off floor at the same time	28 months
Broad jump	8½ inches, feet together	32 months
Balances on one foot	5 seconds	41 months
Balances on one foot	10 seconds	52 months
Hops on one foot	Two or more times	48 months
Heel-toe walk	Four or more steps, two out of three times	51 months
Catches bounced ball	3 feet, uses hands, two out of three times	52 months
Backward heel-toe walk	Four steps without falling off	60 months

Profile Chart for North Carolina Fitness Test

North Carolina Fitness Profile

Name_____ Age_____ Height_____ Weight_____
     (Last)   (First)

School_____ Grade_____ Sex_____

Percentiles

	0	5	10	15	20	25	30	35	40	45	50	55	60	65	70	75	80	85	90	95	100
Sit-ups																					
Side stepping																					
Standing broad jump																					
Pull-ups																					
Squat thrusts																					

Inferior	Poor	Average	Good	Excellent

Placed on obverse side of score card

Profile of a norm-referenced physical fitness test. (Redrawn from Barrow, H., and McGee, R.M.: Practical approach to measurement in physical education, Philadelphia, 1979, Lea & Febiger.)

RED CROSS PROGRESSIVE SWIMMING COURSES

BEGINNER SKILLS

1. Water adjustment skills
2. Hold breath—10 sec.
3. Rhythmic breathing—10 times
4. Prone float and recovery
5. Prone glide
6. Back glide and recovery
7. Survival float
8. Prone glide with kick
9. Back glide with kick
10. Beginner stroke or crawl stroke—15 yds.
11. Combined stroke on back—15 yds.
12. Leveling off and swimming
13. Jump (shallow water), swim
14. Jump (deep water), level, swim
15. Jump (deep water), level, turn over, swim on back
16. Changing directions
17. Turning over
18. Release of cramp
19. Assist nonswimmer to feet
20. Reaching and extension rescues
21. Use of personal flotation device (PFD)
22. Demonstration of artificial respiration
23. Safety information
24. Combined skills no. 1
25. Combined skills no. 2

ADVANCED BEGINNER SKILLS

1. Bobbing—deep water
2. Rhythmic breathing to side
3. Survival float—2 min.
4. Crawl stroke
5. Elementary backstroke
6. Survival stroke
7. Treading water—30 to 45 sec.
8. Changing positions and treading water—30 sec.
9. Standing front dive
10. Underwater swim—3 to 4 body lengths
11. PFD—swimming
12. PFD—jumping into water
13. Artificial respiration
14. Basic rescue skills
15. Personal safety skills

16. Safety information
17. Combined skills no. 1
18. Combined skills no. 2
19. Combined skills no. 3

INTERMEDIATE SKILLS

1. Sidestroke—arms
2. Sidestroke—scissors kick
3. Sidestroke—coordination
4. Breaststroke—arms
5. Breaststroke—kick
6. Breaststroke—coordination
7. Crawl stroke—improve
8. Elementary backstroke—improve
9. Survival float—3 min.
10. Survival stroke—3 min.
11. Back float—1 min.
12. Sculling on back—10 yds.
13. Open turns—front and side
14. Open turn—back
15. Tread water—1 min.
16. Swim underwater—15 to 20 ft.
17. Standing front dive
18. Use of backboard—demonstration only
19. Donning PFD—deep water
20. Basic rescues
21. Artificial respiration
22. Safety information
23. Combined skills no. 1
24. Combined skills no. 2
25. Combined skills no. 3
26. Combined skills no. 4
27. Combined skills no. 5

SWIMMER SKILLS

1. Sidestroke—review/improve
2. Back crawl
3. Breaststroke—review/improve
4. Crawl stroke—review/improve
5. Surface dives—pike, tuck
6. Feet-first surface dive
7. Long shallow dive
8. 1 meter board—jumping entry
9. 1 meter board—standing dive

10. Stride jump
11. Inverted scissors kick
12. Sculling—snail and canoe
13. Open turn—front
14. Open turn—back
15. Open turn—side
16. Survival float—review
17. Survival stroke—5 min.
18. Underwater swim—20 to 25 ft.
19. Basic rescues
20. Artificial respiration
21. Safety information
22. Combined skills no. 1
23. Combined skills no. 2
24. Combined skills no. 3
25. Combined skills no. 4
26. Combined skills no. 5
27. Combined skills no. 6

ADVANCED SWIMMER SKILLS
(must meet prerequisites)

1. Elementary backstroke—review
2. Back crawl—review/improve
3. Breaststroke—review/improve
4. Sidestroke—both sides, both kicks
5. Crawl stroke—review/improve
6. Overarm sidestroke
7. Inverted breaststroke
8. Trudgen stroke
9. Open turns—review/improve
10. Surface dives—review/improve
11. Survival float/survival stroke—fully clothed
12. Standing dives—review/improve
13. Jumping—1 meter board—review
14. Running front dive—1 meter board
15. Combined skills no. 1
16. Combined skills no. 2
17. Combined skills no. 3
18. Combined skills no. 4
19. Combined skills no. 5
20. Combined skills no. 6
21. Combined skills no. 7
22. Combined skills no. 8

CHECKLIST OF GYMNASTIC VAULTING TASKS

TEST ITEM 15 Difficulty	VAULT NO. 1 Skills
1.0	a. Knee mount
2.0	b. Squat mount
2.5	c. Straddle mount
3.0	d. Squat vault
3.5	e. Flank vault
4.0	f. Straddle vault
4.0	g. Wolf vault
4.5	h. Rear vault
5.0	i. Front vault
6.0	j. Thief vault
6.5	k. Headspring vault
7.0	l. Straddle half twist
9.0	m. Horizontal squat
9.5	n. Horizontal straddle
10.0	o. Horizontal stoop
11.0	p. Layout squat
11.5	q. Layout straddle
12.0	r. Layout stoop
13.0	s. Handspring vault
13.0	t. Giant cartwheel
14.0	u. Hecht vault
15.0	v. Yamashita
15.0	w. Handspring with half twist (on or off)

From Ellenbrand, D.A.: Gymnastics skills test for college women. In Baumgartner, T.A., and Jackson, A.S.: Measurement and evaluation in physical education, Dubuque, Iowa. Copyright 1980 by William C. Brown Publishers.

CHECKLIST OF SOCIAL TRAITS

Name _____ Date _____

Directions: Read each statement and think how it will describe your behavior. Put a check in the column that tells most nearly what statement is correct for you.

Always   Often   Seldom   Never   Self-Direction

———————————————— 1. I work diligently even though I am not supervised.

———————————————— 2. I practice to improve the skills I use with least success.

———————————————— 3. I follow carefully directions that have been given me.

———————————————— 4. I willingly accept constructive criticism and try to correct faults.

———————————————— 5. I play games as cheerfully as I can.

———————————————— 6. I appraise my progress in each of my endeavors to learn.

Social Adjustment

———————————————— 1. I am considerate of the rights of others.

———————————————— 2. I am courteous.

———————————————— 3. I am cooperative in group activities.

———————————————— 4. I accept gladly responsibility assigned me by a squad leader.

———————————————— 5. I accept disappointment without being unnecessarily disturbed.

———————————————— 6. I expect from the members of my group only the consideration to which I am entitled.

Always   Often   Seldom   Never   Participation

———————————————— 1. I am prompt in reporting for each class.

———————————————— 2. I dislike being absent from class.

———————————————— 3. I ask to be excused from an activity only when it is necessary.

———————————————— 4. I do the best I can regardless of the activity in which I am participating.

———————————————— 5. I give full attention to all instructions that are given in class.

———————————————— 6. I encourage others with whom I am participating in an activity.

Reprinted from Teachers' Guide to Physical Education for Girls in High School, compiled by Genevie Dexter, California State Department of Education. Sacramento, 1957, p. 318. Used by permission of the Department.

A checklist from a content analysis. There is no criterion for correctness. The list indicates what is incorrect, not what is correct.

CHECKLIST FOR RATING SOFTBALL BATTING SKILLS

Student's Name _____ Date _____

Rated by _____ Score _____

Directions: First check student's performance as good, fair, or poor on each item and then check deviations noted. Determine the student's score by assigning 1 point for poor, 2 for fair, and 3 for good, and totaling points.

	Rating	Deviations from Standard Performance
1. Grip	_____Good	_____Hands too far apart
	_____Fair	_____Wrong hand on top
	_____Poor	_____Hands too far from end of bat
2. Preliminary stance	_____Good	_____Stands too near the plate
	_____Fair	_____Stands too far from plate
	_____Poor	_____Stands too far forward toward pitcher
		_____Stands too far backward toward catcher
		_____Feet not parallel to line from pitcher to catcher
		_____Rests bat on shoulder
		_____Shoulders not horizontal
3. Stride or footwork	_____Good	_____Fails to step forward
	_____Fair	_____Fails to transfer weight
	_____Poor	_____Lifts back foot from ground before swing
4. Pivot or body twist	_____Good	_____Fails to "wind up"
	_____Fair	_____Fails to follow through with body
	_____Poor	_____Has less than 90° pivot
5. Arm movement or swing	_____Good	_____Arms held too close to body
	_____Fair	_____Rear elbow held too high
	_____Poor	_____Bat not held approximately parallel to ground
		_____Not enough wrist motion used
		_____Wrists not uncocked forcefully enough
6. General (eyes on ball, judgment of pitches, and the like)	_____Good	_____Body movements jerky
	_____Fair	_____Tries too hard; "presses"
	_____Poor	_____Fails to look at center of ball
		_____Poor judgment of pitches
		_____Appears to lack confidence
		_____Bat used not suitable

Reprinted from Teachers' Guide to Physical Education for Girls in High School, compiled by Genevie Dexter, California State Department of Education. Sacramento, 1957, p. 315. Used by permission of the Department.

The norm-referenced AAHPERD physical fitness test with percentiles and a classification system by letter grade and a rating. (From Kirkendall, D.R., Guber, J.J., and Johnson R.E.: Measurement and evaluation for physical education, Dubuque, Iowa. Copyright 1980 by William C. Brown Publishers.)

PHYSICAL FITNESS: SEMESTER PROFILE FOR _____ SEM. 1 2 19 ____

Rank In Group	INDEX	Letter Grade	T Score	AAHPERD Test Items						Alternate Items			Knowledge	Ratings
				Pull-Up or Flexed Arm Hang	Stand. Broad Jump	50-Yd. Dash (45.73 m)	No. of Sit-Ups In 60 Seconds	Shuttle Run	600-Yd. Run (548.78 m)	1-Mile Run Or 9 Min. Run	Step Test	Vertical Jump	Physical Fitness Knowledge Test Score	
99			80											
			78											
			76											Excellent
	6.5	A+	74											
			72											
98	6.0	A	70											
			68											
95			66											
	5.7	A−	64											Very Good
90	5.3	B+	62											
	5.0	B	60											
80	4.7	B−	58											
75			56											
70	4.3	C+												Above

				Average
60			54	Average
50	4.0	C	52	Below Average
40			50	
30		C−	48	
25	3.7		46	
20	3.3	D+	44	
	3.0	D	42	
			40	Poor
10	2.7	D−	38	
			36	
5			34	
			32	
	2.0	F	30	
			28	
2			26	
			24	Very Poor
			22	
1			20	

RECREATIONAL SPORT SKILLS ACQUIRED THIS SEMESTER _____

COMMENTS: _____

A content analysis of the breaststroke, with a subjective weighting of value of each component. Deficiencies are determined through study of the skill.

BREASTSTROKE WHIP KICK WEIGHTED CHECKLIST

Name _____ Evaluator _____

Date: pretest _____ posttest _____

	WEIGHTED VALUE	CHECK FAULT Pretest	CHECK FAULT Posttest
PHASE I. GLIDE PHASE			
1. Legs not fully extended	1	_____	_____
2. Ankles too far apart	1	_____	_____
3. Feet and ankles not in same plane as the body	2	_____	_____
4. Feet not plantar-flexed	2	_____	_____
PHASE II. RECOVERY PHASE			
1. Knees flexed too much or not enough	2	_____	_____
2. Hips flexed too much or not enough	2	_____	_____
3. Heels not brought close enough to the buttocks	2	_____	_____
4. Feet not pronated	2	_____	_____
5. Thighs not medially rotated at the hip joint	3	_____	_____
6. Feet not dorsiflexed	3	_____	_____
PHASE III. PROPULSIVE PHASE			
1. Legs are extended straight back instead of in a rounded or circular path	3	_____	_____
2. Feet travel laterally to an abducted leg position instead of in a rounded or circular path	3	_____	_____
3. Legs do not travel in the same or similar horizontal plane(s)	3	_____	_____
4. Legs travel in such a manner that the body is propelled toward or away from the surface of the water, instead of parallel to it	3	_____	_____
5. Vigorous action of the kick not sufficient to create an adequate propelling force	3	_____	_____
6. Legs actively squeezed together instead of coming together naturally	2	_____	_____
7. Feet not inverted as they come together	2	_____	_____
8. No inertial glide before the next kick is begun	2	_____	_____
SCORE		_____	_____

From Mansfield, J.R.: The effect of using videotape and loop films as aids in teaching the breaststroke whip kick. Master's thesis, Pennsylvania State University, 1972. Used by permission of the author.

GOLF SWING CLASSIFICATION

7. Excellent Full swing, coordination and timing consistently produce full speed at contact, flight of ball straight, trajectory appropriate to club.

6. Very good Does not achieve full swing, timing and coordination consistent.

5. Good Some inconsistency in swing, contact good most of the time, does not achieve full power.

4. Average Inconsistent in swing and contact, no major faults.

3. Fair Inconsistent in swing, some faults in form, does not maintain body relationship to ball, contact erratic.

2. Poor Several faults in swing, makes contact most of the time, but contact seldom produces proper flight.

1. Very poor Many faults in swing, frequently misses ball, contact usually poor.

Activities for Students with Specific Developmental Delays

VESTIBULAR STIMULATION ACTIVITIES

and ease movement up + down laterally up + down

Child who fail to demonstrate nystagmus after spinning are believed to have vestibular development delays and are in need of activities to facilitate development. *Concentrated activities to remediate balance problems that result from poor vestibular function should be administered by someone trained in observation of responses necessary by the child.* However, some activities can be done in fun, nonthreatening ways in a physical education class or on a playground with the supervision of parents or teachers.

CAUTION: Anyone who uses vestibular stimulation activities with children should observe closely for signs of sweating, paleness, flushing of the face, nausea, and loss of consciousness. These are all indications that the activities should be stopped immediately. Also, spinning activities should not be used with seizure-prone children.

Specific Activity Suggestions

1. Slow, safe, rhythm-inhibiting nonthreatening approach to the introduction and mastery of vestibular stimulation
2. No rapid spin can be disorganizing
3. Sitting in a net swing: different positions; push self, spin self
4. Rocking on a cage ball: prone, supine, sitting; ask child to respond (for instance, touch the floor, look at me)
5. Rolling in a barrel: log roll or on hands and knees
6. Tunnel roll: log roll inside a cloth tunnel
7. Blanket roll: lie on a blanket and roll self up and unroll
8. Log roll on a mat
9. Lying prone on a scooter and lifting head up
10. Lying prone on a scooter and holding rope while teacher spins and pulls child (head up, knees flexed, arms extended)
11. Spinning self prone on a scooter by crossing hand over hand
12. Swinging self on a tire swing
13. Bouncing self on trampoline: sitting, standing, kneeling, etc.
14. Teeter-totter
15. Moving self at varying speeds on a variety of surfaces: roll, turn, swing vigorously, lift head in prone position
16. Riding down ramp or incline on a scooter with head up, knees flexed, arms extended
17. Activities that give the child a sense of moving in space; movement or spinning should not be so fast as to be disorienting or disorganizing; for instance, letting the child spin *himself* on a scooter, swing himself, play on spinning playground equipment, go down on ramp prone on a scooter; activities must be nonthreatening and fun and give the child an opportunity to *respond* to changes of his position in space

Additional Notes

1. Obtain medical permission for participation in an adapted physical education program. On the permission form include a checklist for kinds of activities. Ask the physician to check the items that are allowed for the child. Include "spinning ac-

tivities," "rolling activities," or "vestibular activities" as items on the checklist.

2. Be trained in an adapted physical education program that includes vestibular stimulation and the precautions for and benefits to the child.

3. Do not spin a child who has a history of seizures, especially seizures that are triggered by light.

4. Let child move *himself* and spin *himself* as much as possible; then you can be more certain that the child is ready for the amount of stimulation in the activity.

5. In all spinning activities, watch for evidence of nystagmus (rapid lateral eye movements).

6. Allow child to respond and make adaptaive responses to position changes.

7. Slides, inclines, and bikes give the sensation of movement and gravity's effect on the body.

8. Merry-go-rounds, teeter-totters, and swings are good playground equipment to use.

9. Do not do spinning or jerky movements with children who have cerebral palsy; in fact, coordinate all movement activities for CP children with the child's physician and other therapists.

10. Take these precautions seriously!

BODY AWARENESS ACTIVITIES

1. Verbal commands to child: touch your knees, touch your ankles, touch your ears, touch your shoulders, etc.

2. Child stands with eyes open, teacher touches various body parts, and the child identifies them. Can be done in a variety of positions. Then have the child touch the same part that teacher touches and name it. Increase difficulty by blindfolding child.

3. Child touches teacher's body parts and teacher names them. Make a mistake every once in a while to see if the child can catch the mistake.

4. Trace child's outline on a large piece of paper or with chalk on the floor. Then have child get up and fill in all the details. Use front, back, and side drawings.
   a. Have child name all the body parts.
   b. Leave out a part and see if child notices it.
   c. Have child trace around teacher and name all parts; teacher can name parts and make mistakes.
   d. Have child trace certain body parts on the drawing with different colors, such as yellow for feet, blue for arms.

5. Place child under sheet; teacher touches certain body parts through the sheet and the child identifies them.

6. Angels-in-the-snow: give verbal commands or directions such as right arm, left leg, left arm; ask child to move one part or more parts simultaneously.

7. Have the child draw a picture of himself on the chalkboard and note how he sees himself. Does he forget any body parts? How detailed is he?

8. Teacher draws an incomplete picture of a person on the chalkboard and child fills in the missing parts.

9. Touch body parts to surroundings: ear to wall, hand to chair, elbow to door, etc.

10. Child imitates teacher's movements of specific body parts such as nodding head, shrugging shoulder, bending at the waist.
    a. Teacher gives verbal command and demonstrates.
    b. Teacher demonstrates.
    c. Teacher gives only verbal commands.

11. Teacher states the usage of a body part and the child demonstrates the usage and names the part.

515

I see and blink with my _____.
I wave with my _____.
I jump with my _____.

12. Direct child to move a designated body part in a specific direction.
13. Simon Says.
14. Imitate positions on cards.
15. Teacher draws a specific body part, such as a leg, and the child draws the body around it.
16. Child and teacher on beam; child imitates teacher's movements.
17. Ask child how many things there are alike about certain body parts such as hands and feet, knees and elbows, and then what are the differences. Then blindfold the child and repeat the tasks.
18. Have the child list as many things as possible about a certain body part, unblindfolded and blindfolded.
19. Ask child to bend or stretch different body parts.
20. Ask child to move around room by balancing on one, two, three, four, or five body parts.
21. Ask child to balance on different body parts.

OCULAR CONTROL ACTIVITIES

Fixation

1. Child is in a supine position, watching a spot high on the wall behind his head. The therapist then lifts the child up by his arms (standing over his stomach) while the child keeps his eyes on the spot.
2. Child sits and rocks back and forth while keeping his eyes on a tape on the wall directly in front of him.
3. Child is in a standing position, moving the body without moving the head. Eyes and head are directed at a fixation point.
4. a. Child is in a supine position with eyes on a fixation point on the wall. He then pushes up into a backbend position without moving his eyes from the point.

b. Begin in a standing position and fixate at a specific point as he bends backwards.
5. Child is in a standing position fixating on a point on the wall. He must jump and turn 180° and pick up a point on the opposite wall and fixate. (Points can be colored circles.)
6. Suspendible ball activities: Child is in a supine position. Have the child look at a fixation point on the ceiling. Swing the ball back and forth from left to right. Child keeps his eyes focused on the fixation point and uses his peripheral vision to track the ball.
7. Have the child focus on a fixation point on the ceiling and follow the ball with his finger as it swings from top to bottom.
8. Have the child focus on a fixation point on the ceiling and follow the ball with his finger as it swings in a clockwise direction.
9. a. Have the child focus on a fixation point on the ceiling and follow the ball with his finger as it swings in a diagonal direction from the upper left to lower right.

b. Same: upper right to lower left.

Convergence/Divergence

1. Child sits with arms extended and thumbs up. Have him look back and forth between thumbs. Note synchronization of eye movement or irregular movement.
2. Child sits at a table with hands folded in front of him, thumbs up. The child looks at his thumbs, then to an object placed at his right, then to an object at his left, and back to his thumbs. Repeat several times (maintain head position; only eyes should move.)
3. Draw two X's on the board (at shoulder height of a child) approximately 3 feet apart. Have the child stand centered about 2 inches in front of the board and track back and forth between the X's.
4. Have child sit at a table and look from an object on the table to an object on the wall directly ahead; continue back and forth 10 times. The table should be about 15 inches from the wall.

5. Have the child sit in a chair. Tie a rope to a small ball, swing the ball, and have the child follow it vertically, horizontally, diagonally, and at near and far distances. Head should not move. Note the following: (a) jerks at extremes, (b) if eyes jump ahead or lag behind, (c) if eyes cross smoothly when in the middle, (d) if eyes move together.

6. The child should be in a sitting position. Suspend a ball on a piece of string above his head. Rotate the ball so it goes all the way around his head. Notice if he anticipates the ball's appearance as it goes around. Note if eyes move together as they follow the ball.

7. The child should be in a sitting position. Using the suspendible ball, swing the ball in various directions. Have the child switch his focus from the fixation point on the ceiling to a fixation point on the ball. Have him try to see the fixation points on the ceiling and on the ball as clearly as he possibly can.

Visual Tracking

1. The child is on his back. Without moving his head, have him track lines, pipes, or lights on the ceiling (as far back as possible and as far forward).

2. Make a pattern on the wall with dots. Have the child stand in front of the wall and track the pattern (a) clockwise, (b) counterclockwise, and (c) diagonal positions.

3. A group of six children should be equally spaced and in a circle. One child sits in the middle and tracks each child as they come around. One child will be a different activity; that is, four jump, one hops. The child in the center of the circle claps his hands when he sees the odd activity.

4. The child is on his back. Attach a small ball to a string and swing the ball horizontally above the child's head. The child should track the swinging ball with his eyes, then point to it as it swings. (The ball should be hung the distance of the child's knuckles to elbow. Never closer than 8 inches).

5. Child assumes a supine or sitting position, then hits a suspended ball and tracks the movement with his eyes. He is responsible for tapping the ball to continue motion. (Ball should be at least 5 inches in diameter).

6. Child throws a ball up in the air and follows it with his eyes until it hits the floor. Let the ball bounce once or twice. (He should be able to follow ball movement with minimal head movement.)

7. Swing a jump rope in a large circle on the ground. Have the child stand so that he is facing the rope. At first have him follow the rope movements with his eyes and then try jumping as the rope comes around.

8. Swing the ball back and forth; catch the ball.
   a. Hit with a fist; hit hard and easy, but control direction.
   b. Use tips of fingers: right three times, left two times.
   c. Use side of hand (karate style: right and left)
   d. Use palm of hand: right and left.
   e. Hold both hands (interlock fingers).
   f. Use right elbow, left elbow.
   g. Keep shoulder easy and controlled.
   h. Use wrist front and back, right and left.
   i. Use side of arm.
   j. Control ball with knees.
   k. Keep in focus as head moves.
   l. Keep in focus as chin moves.

CROSS-LATERAL INTEGRATION ACTIVITIES

1. Rope or line on mat or floor; child crosses hands back and forth over line going forward, then crosses feet back and forth going forward.

2. Pick up dominoes (from right side of body) with right hand and place them in a can on the left side of the body. Repeat using left hand. Pick up only one domino at a time. Hold child's head still.

3. Connecting various dot patterns on the chalkboard.

4. Child prone and then supine on scooter. Pulls self along hand over hand with a rope strung overhead a few feet.

5. Place a straight tape line on the floor. Put red objects on the left side and blue objects on the right side. Have child crawl along line picking up red objects with right hand and placing them on the opposite side of the line and picking up the blue objects with his left hand and placing them on the opposite of the line.

6. Tracing tracks, mazes, or shapes on the chalkboard. Be sure the child is standing directly in front of the shape so he will have to cross the midline. Hold his shoulders to keep him from turning as he traces.

7. Play pat-a-cake.

8. Teacher and child join hands with arms crossed in front. Place a pillow on top of the crossed arms. Try to keep the pillow on the arms while swinging the arms back and forth and up high.

9. Using vibrator or any other brushing material put material in child's right hand and call out body parts for the child to rub or vibrate, such as left hand, left elbow, left knee, left thigh. Then change hands and the side of the body to be vibrated. Make sure child does not turn shoulder while crossing midline.

10. Using a low balance beam, have the child walk with a scissor gait across balance beam without stepping on it, forward and backward.

11. Put cardboard template on chalkboard and trace around shape crossing midline. Then teacher puts a pattern on a piece of paper and child copies it using the template on the board.

12. Consecutively smaller figures on chalkboard: draw large triangle or other shape on board, then draw the same shape again and again inside the large shape, getting progressively smaller and without touching the lines of the previous one. Teacher and child should each do one and see who can draw the most triangles within the large triangle.

13. Tracing templates on paper.

14. Child mirrors teacher's movements. Do things to make child cross midline, such as touch right hand to left shoulder, left hand to right foot, left elbow to right knee. Increase difficulty by doing movements on beam, trampoline, or barrel.

15. Tape line or rope on mat or floor. Child crosses hands back and forth over the line while going backward, then crosses feet back and forth over line while going backward, then feet and hands going forward, then feet and hands going backward.

16. Hang by hands on uneven bars; kick leg across midline to hit pillow target.

17. Negotiate stall bars from one end to the other crossing hands and feet.

18. Throw bean bags in tires or buckets; must use right hand when throwing to left target and left hand when throwing to right target.

19. Dropping colored foam bits from stage or table: child sits, picks up foam with right hand and drops it into can on left side on the floor. There are five cans glued on a board; he can drop it into any one of them. Increase difficulty by specifying can.

DYNAMIC BALANCE ACTIVITIES
Floor Activities

1. Four squares

2. Hopscotch

3. Various types of locomotor movements following patterns on the floor

4. Tape squares on mat or floor: jumping and turning, hopping

5. Various locomotor movements involving jumping and turning

6. Races: use different locomotor movements

7. Knee-ball races: walk on knees and bounce/dribble ball

8. Scales: stand on one foot/kneel on one

knee/stand on tip toe and extend other leg behind/in front/to side

9. Bunny hops: make bunny shape and jump and land on both feet simultaneously
10. Hopping through hoops: turning, two feet, one foot
11. Magpie hop game: bean bag between knees, hop to designated area
12. Hop tag: restricted area
13. Flag tag: children wear flag belts or handkerchiefs in pockets; other children try to pull flag without grabbing child's arm or tackling
14. Wood blocks on bottoms of feet: walk forward/backward/sideways
15. Stilts
16. Twister
17. Mother May I: using various locomotor movements
18. Walking forward heel to toe between a double line or on a single line
19. Walking backward heel to toe between a double line or on a single line
20. Walking on tiptoes: forward and backward
21. Walking on heels: forward and backward
22. Walking on knees: hold feet up off the floor
23. Balance tag: child is safe between bases if he balances on one foot (also safe on bases scattered throughout room)
24. Jump, hop, skip, gallop, leap (see animal walks section; activities to encourage each skill)

Long Jump Rope

1. Two people turning rope; child jumps in (front door or back door) and jumps on two feet
2. Child jumps rope while balancing bean bags on various body parts
3. "School": children run in and jump the number of times for each grade
4. Jump on one foot
5. Jump on alternating feet
6. Jump, squat, touch floor
7. Jump and do specified turns

8. Then combine jump, squat, touch floor, and turns
9. Jump individual rope inside of long rope
10. Jump with two long ropes together
11. Bounce ball while jumping
12. Count while jumping
13. Hot Peppers: double time, fast turning
14. Blue Bells: rope swings backward and forward without turning
15. Two or more people jumping at once
16. Play catch with self while jumping
17. Shoot baskets while jumping
18. Play catch with someone outside the rope while jumping
19. Play catch between two people while both are jumping
20. Throw bean bags at a target while jumping

Individual Jump Rope

1. Jump on two feet
2. Jump on one foot
3. Alternate left and right
4. Alternate two feet, one foot
5. Gallop, skip, walk, run while jumping rope
6. Turn while jumping
7. Count numbers while jumping
8. Balance bean bags on shoulder, head while jumping
9. Jump while blindfolded
10. Jump with weights on
11. Jump rope on tramp
12. Jump rope on balance beam
13. Click heels while jumping
14. Jump the shot
15. Jump and crisscross arms every other jump

Balance Beam

Start on floor without beam, then move to low beam, then high beam, then place low beam at an angle.

1. Walk forward
2. Walk backward
3. Walk sideways
4. Touch knee to beam
5. Walking over, under, through hoops
6. Use eraser or bean bags on various body parts while walking the beam

7. Place weights on the ankle
8. Place bean bags or weights in buckets; child holds buckets and walks beam; add more bean bags as he goes the length of the board
9. Hopping (low and short) on two feet while going forward and sideways
10. Hopping on one foot
11. Hopping around in a circle
12. Turns on two feet: quarter turns, half turns, three-quarter turns going right and left
13. Walking beam forward, backward, and sideways while playing catch
14. Balancing ball on back of hand while walking forward, backward, sideways
15. Turn on beam on one foot
16. Walk on heels
17. Walk on toes
18. Cat walk: hands and *feet*
19. Crawl on hands and *knees*
20. Walk stiff-legged on beam

STATIC BALANCE ACTIVITIES
Floor Activities

1. Freeze tag: play tag; child who is caught is "frozen" until a friend "unfreezes" by tagging; "It" tries to freeze everyone
2. Statues: each child spins himself around and then tries to make himself into a "statue" without falling first
3. Twister
4. Crouching on tiptoes
5. Standing heel to toe
6. Balance on one foot: other foot on supporting knee
7. Balance on one foot: other foot held up and behind body
8. Balance on one foot on tiptoe
9. Knee scales: child balances on one knee, keeping one or both hands on floor
10. Balance on one foot and then turn a complete circle and maintain balance
11. Balance on two feet: tiptoes
12. Jump into air, turn a full circle, and land on two feet and maintain balance
13. Jump into air, turn a full circle, and land on *tiptoes* and maintain balance

14. Jump into air, turn a full circle, and land on one foot and maintain balance
15. Egg sit: child wraps arms around knees to force egg shape and then rocks back to balance only on seat (feet off floor)
16. V-sit: child extends legs and arms to force V by leaning back
17. Heel slap: then land on both feet, tiptoes, one foot
18. Heel click: land on both feet, tiptoes, one foot
19. Toe slap or knee slap in front: land on both feet, tiptoes, one foot
20. Self kick (behind): land on both feet, tiptoes, one foot
21. Tripod: child balances by placing forehead and both hands on floor; knees balance on elbows to form tripod balance
22. Balancing bean bags on different parts of the body while performing balancing positions

Balance Beam and Balance Board

1. One foot scale: stand on one foot, extend other leg behind or in front of body
2. Squat down and touch beam or board
3. Step through a hula hoop held a few inches above a balance beam
4. Stand on two feet, balance on board and catch an object
5. Stand on one foot on balance beam and catch an object
6. While balancing on two feet stoop and pick up objects from the beam or from floor if on board (two feet)
7. Stand on beam and mirror arm and leg movements of another student or teacher
8. Barefoot, pick up marbles with toes and transfer to can
9. V-sit: child sits on beam or board and lifts both legs in extension; leans back to form a V
10. Standing and shooting baskets (two feet)
11. Standing and shooting baskets (one foot)
12. Points and patches on beam: on signal, child changes position

13. Balance object on body while on two feet
14. Balance object on body while on one foot
15. Balance object on body while doing points and patches
16. Balance and throw bean bags at target on wall
17. Balance on two knees
18. Balance on one knee

EYE-FOOT COORDINATION ACTIVITIES
Elementary Level

1. Soccer goalie standing in half circle
2. Foot wall-ball using one square
3. Nine squares/numbers hop
4. Hopscotch
5. Picking up marbles or other objects with toes and placing the objects in a can
6. Kicking ball into barrel on its side
7. Punting the ball
8. Place kicking
9. Kicking the ball for accuracy and distance
    a. Child and ball stationary
    b. Child moves toward stationary ball
    c. Child stationary, roll ball to him
    d. Child and ball moving, roll ball, child runs up and kicks ball
10. Hula hoops in a pattern on floor, child jumps from hoop to hoop with one or two feet
11. Child stands in front of an object and attempts to protect it from being hit with the ball; must use his feet to trap or kick the ball away from the object
12. Child tries to keep a balloon in the air by kicking it as he moves around the room
13. Sheets with lines or dots: child jumps out certain patterns
14. Child follows foot patterns on the floor
15. Jump the shot
16. Soccer
17. Foot wall-ball with two squares
18. Individual jump rope activities (see dynamic balance; jump rope activities)
19. Long jump rope activities (see dynamic balance; jump rope activities)
20. Child jumps rope forward and backward on trampoline
21. Scooter soccer: sitting on scooter and using feet to propel scooter and to kick ball
22. Soccer dribble ball around objects
23. Drop kicks: child holds ball, drops ball, and kicks ball before it hits floor
24. Set tires up in a pattern and have child move from tire to tire using a variety of moves and jumps
25. Child stands in front of two objects; must protect the objects from being hit with the ball; child must kick the ball

Games

1. Circle football: circle formation; children sit in crab position. The object of the game is to keep the football in the circle by kicking it. One half of the circle could be one team and the other side could be another team, with the object of the game being to kick the football out of the circle on the other side.
2. Boundary ball: teams line up on end lines of the court. The object of the game is to kick the cage ball over the opposite end line. The teams protect their own end line by kicking only.
3. Dribble tag: similar to tag, except all players are dribbling a ball with their feet. Cones may be set up to make obstacles.
4. Marching patterns and square dance foot rhythms: place tape on the floor to make a square. Each child steps inside, out, right, left into own taped square. Vary by asking for high/low steps, loud/soft, slow/fast. With square dancing music, do forward and backward kicking steps, leaps, gallops, jumps, hops, alternating steps.

EYE-HAND COORDINATION
Activities

1. Roll ball into barrel turned on its side
2. Roll ball between two objects
3. Roll ball under chair legs and into barrel
4. Pick up dominoes and place in coffee can; time for speed

5. Play catch in air or with bounce passes
6. Put child in tire on floor and throw ball to him
7. Child throws bean bag into barrel or stack of tires
8. Child dribbles ball while standing stationary
9. Child hits suspended tetherball back and forth and then every other time it goes around the circle
10. Play goalie: on hands and knees and then on knees only
11. Child stacks blocks as high as possible in front of him and then to the left and right
12. Two small buckets 12 inches apart; child, 6 feet away, throws bean bags into buckets with right and then left hand; increase distance as he improves
13. Child with back to wall: teacher throws ball against wall and child turns and hits the ball
14. Child throws ball at square marked on the wall: both hands, then right, and then left
15. Play two-square with child
16. Hot potato with the ball
17. Have child bat a balloon around in the air in an unrestricted space
18. Child tosses ball into air and catches it after one bounce and then after two bounces
19. Nerf ball: rolling, throwing, and catching
20. Child throws ball through hanging tire
21. Tire on floor, child bounces ball into tire and out to teacher
22. Dropping clothespins into a bottle
23. Child hits balloon in the air while standing within a restricted area such as within a tire
24. Child carries ball around waist and under and through legs, switching hands as he goes from side to side and around the body
25. Ball suspended from tetherball pole; child swings at it with bat

Games

1. Dribble: children play tag while dribbling a ball. Bases can be used as "safe" areas. The game can be modified so that the person who is "it" attempts to steal the ball from the dribblers.
2. Guard the castle: circle formation. One child is in the center of the circle, guarding a bowling pin (the castle). The other children attempt to knock down the castle by rolling or throwing a playground ball. Add additional balls to make the guarding more difficult.
3. Clean up your own backyard: use newspaper balls or nerf balls. Two teams stand on either side of a "fence" that divides their "yards." Each person has a ball to begin the game. On signal, everyone throws his ball across the fence and shouts "Clean up your own backyard!" When a ball lands in the yard, children pick up the ball and throw it back over the fence. On a whistle signal all children must stop throwing, and the teacher counts the number of balls in each yard. The team with the least amount of balls in its yard wins. This game is good for all skill levels and can be used to practice any kind of throw. (It is a good idea for the teacher to remind the children that this is only a game and that, really, trash should be put in trash cans, not just thrown back over into someone else's yard.)
4. Newspaper ball dodge ball: same rules as dodge ball games, but less threatening for wheelchair-bound children or young children.
5. Ball tag: similar to regular tag game, except the person who is "it" tries to throw a ball to catch a person. Place bases or mats on floor where children may stand to be "safe." Teacher can give children a signal to run to a new base.
6. Snatch ball basketball: divide class into two teams. Teams line up in two lines facing each other. Each child is given a number.

Place two basketballs in between the two lines. The teacher calls a number. The child on each team who is number 1, etc. runs and picks up a basketball and dribbles to a basket and shoots. Children are allowed to keep shooting until the teacher signals to stop. The score is the number of baskets the child makes in the allotted time. This game can also be played on scooters.

7. Hoop ball: each team is given many different kinds of balls to throw. A hoop can be suspended from a rope or placed on the ground. Each team aims at a different hoop. The class can be divided up into as many teams as possible. The score is the number of balls that go through the hoop or remain in the hoop on the floor.

accountability Acquisition of short-term instructional objectives of pupils over a specified time frame.

acute Condition having a quick onset and a short duration.

Adam's position Position to determine the extent to which a scoliosis is structural. The subject bends over from the waist with arms relaxed in a hanging position.

adapted physical education Modification of traditional physical activities to enable the handicapped to participate safely, successfully, and with satisfaction.

adapted physical educator A professional with specialized training in evaluating, designing, and implementing specialized physical education programs.

adaptive behavior The effectiveness of adapting to the natural and social demands of one's environment.

abdominal pumping An exercise to increase circulation of the blood through the pelvic region.

adult initiated activity Social activity that is initiated by another person.

aerobics A progressive conditioning program that stimulates circulorespiratory activity for a time sufficient to produce beneficial changes in the body.

aggression Offensive action or procedure.

agonist Muscle that is directly engaged in action.

allergy Hypersensitive reaction to certain foreign substances that are harmless in similar amounts to nonsensitive individuals.

anatomical task analysis Evaluation of the functional level of ability of specific muscles that contribute to a pattern of a skill.

anemia Condition of the blood in which there is a deficiency of hemoglobin.

angina pectoris Sense of suffocating contraction within the chest, usually associated with organic change in the heart.

ankle and foot pronation Abnormal turning of the ankle downward and medially (eversion and abduction).

ankle and foot supination Position of the foot when it is turned inward (inversion and adduction).

ankylosis Abnormal immobility of a joint (fusion).

antagonist Muscle that opposes the action of another muscle.

antigravity muscles Muscles that keep the body in an upright posture.

anxiety Uneasiness that is difficult to describe.

aphasia Impairment in use of words as symbols of ideas.

arteriosclerosis Hardening, thickening, and loss of elasticity of the walls of blood vessels.

arthritis Inflammation of a joint.

asocial Not knowing the expected normative behavior of the group.

asthma Labored breathing associated with a sense of constriction in the chest.

astigmatism Refractive error caused by an irregularity in the curvature of the cornea of the lens; vision may become blurred.

asymmetrical tonic neck reflex A reflex that causes extension of the arms on the face side and flexion of the arm on the skull side when the head is turned.

atrophy Wasting away of muscular tissue.

atonia Clinical type of cerebral palsy that is characterized by a lack of muscle tone.

athetoid Clinical type of cerebral palsy that is characterized by uncoordinated movements of the voluntary muscles, often accompanied by impaired muscle control of the hands and impaired speech and swallowing.

ataxia Clinical type of cerebral palsy that is characterized by a disturbance of equilibrium.

audible ball A ball that emits a beeping sound for easy location. It is used in activity for the blind.

audible goal locators Motor-driven noisemakers that enable the blind to position objects in space.

audiologist A specialist who measures hearing ability.

aura Warning preceding a seizure.

backward chaining The last of a series of steps is taught first.

barrel chest Abnormally rounded chest.

behavior modification Changing of behavioral characteristics through application of learning principles.

behavior training Anxiety reduction of problem situations for particular individuals.

behavioral objectives Objectives that contain an action, conditions, and criteria and that have not been mastered by the learner.

bilateral Pertaining to two sides.

blind Lacking the sense of sight.

BMR Basal metabolism rate; expenditure of energy of the body in a resting state.

body image System of ideas and feelings that a person has about his or her structure.

body righting Reflex that enables segmental rotation of the trunk and hips when the head is turned.

borderline retarded Mentally retarded persons who are usually capable of competing with most children in activities other than academic ones.

bronchial asthma Condition that affects the respiratory system and usually results from allergic states in which there is an obstruction of the bronchial tubes or lungs or a combination of both.

Bruininks-Oseretsky Test of Motor Proficiency A battery of tests that assesses motor proficiency of children between the ages 4 and 14 years.

cardiovascular disease Inclusive term that describes all diseases of the heart and blood vessels throughout the body.

cataract A condition in which the normally transparent lens of the eye becomes opaque.

central deafness Condition in which the receiving mechanism of hearing functions properly, but an abnormality in the central nervous system prevents one from hearing.

cephalocaudal control Gross motor control that starts with the head and progresses down the axial skeleton to the feet.

cerebral palsy Conditions in which damage is inflicted to the brain and is accompanied by motor involvement.

chaining Leading a person through a series of teachable components of a motor task.

chronic Condition having a gradual onset and a long duration.

chronologically age-appropriate skills Culturally appropriate skills performed by normal persons.

circumduction Moving a part in a manner that describes a cone.

classification assessment Instruments that classify learners according to homogeneous ability levels.

community-based programming Activities that enable acquisition of skills through habilitation/education and lead to independent living in the community.

competencies Predetermined standards of behavior.

competition Intense participation between performers using skills to their best advantage.

component building Pairing of a positive and a neutral event, then fading the positive in such a manner that there is transfer from the positive to the neutral to make the neutral positive.

conditions A description of *how* the learner is to perform an objective.

condition shifting program Program in which several conditions of behavioral objectives are altered to produce activities that are sequenced from lesser to greater difficulty.

conductive hearing loss Condition in which the inten-

sity of sound is reduced before reaching the inner ear, where the auditory nerve begins.

congenital Present at birth.

content analysis Breaking a task down into teachable components.

content-referenced assessment A process of determining where on a continuum or a hierarchy a person is performing.

contingency An agreement between the student and the teacher that indicates what the student must do to earn a specific reward.

contingency observation A technique in which an error is corrected by taking the person out of the activity to observe a peer doing the behavior correctly.

contracture (muscle) Abnormal contraction of a muscle.

cooperation The ability to work with others to achieve a common group goal.

cooperative learning Students work together on teams and carry out their responsibilities.

corrective physical education Activity designed to habilitate or rehabilitate deficiencies in posture or mechanical alignment of the body.

corrective therapy System of therapy using physical activities for the rehabilitation of a disability.

coronary heart disease Condition in which the coronary arteries become sclerotic or hardened and narrowed.

coxa plana Also known as Legg-Calvé-Perthes disease; avascular, necrotic flattening of the head of the femur.

coxa valga Increase in the angle of the neck of the head of the femur to more than 120 degrees.

coxa vara Decrease in the angle of the neck of the head of the femur to less than 120 degrees.

criterion Standard on which judgments may be made for task mastery.

criterion-referenced tests Arbitrarily established levels of mastery that represent educational goals. May also demonstrate levels of consistency of performance.

cross-lateral integration The ability to coordinate use of both sides of the body.

cycle constancy The continual recurrence of a specific motor task within similar time periods.

deaf Nonfunctional hearing for the ordinary purposes of life.

delay of gratification Ability to control emotional responses so one's social status in a group is not jeopardized.

development Proceeding from lower to higher; progression; process of growing to maturity.

developmental approach Matching instruction to the ability, as measured by developmental milestones.

developmental checklist A task list of chronologically sequenced behaviors in prerequisite order selected from developmental scales.

developmental disability Severe chronic disabilities, manifested before the age of 22, that result in substantial functional limitations in the capacity for independent living.

developmental period For practical purposes, from birth to approximately age 16 years.

deviant When some characteristic is judged different by others who consider the characteristic of importance and who value this difference negatively.

diabetes A chronic metabolic disorder in which the cells cannot use glucose.

diagnostic-prescriptive integrity A direct relationship between the assessment and the programming to remediate the assessed disabilities.

differentiation to integration Isolated movements of body parts become differentiated, and partial patterns emerge to permit purposive movement.

differential reinforcement of high rates Provision of reinforcement when high rates of desirable behavior are demonstrated.

differential reinforcement of low rates Reinforcing inappropriate behaviors as they are gradually decreased.

differential reinforcement of other behaviors A reinforcer is delivered after any response except the undesirable target response.

directionality Perception of direction in space.

direct service Such services as physical education that provide instruction in the curricula designed by the schools.

disability Physical or mental incapacity.

discrimination The cognitive ability to detect variations between sensory stimuli.

dislocation Abnormal displacement of a bone in relation to its position in a joint.

displacement Disguising of a particular goal by substituting another in its place.

distal A point away from an origin, as opposed to proximal.

domain-referenced assessment Tests a specific behavior to measure a general ability from which inference is made about a student's general capability.

domain-referenced test Represents a cluster of related behaviors.

dorsal Refers to back, back of hand, back of thoracic region, or top of foot.

dorsiflexion The act of bending the foot upward (flexion).

duration recording The length of time a behavior occurs.

dysmenorrhea Painful menstruation.

ECG Electrocardiogram, a record of heart muscle action potential.

ecological inventory A checklist of behaviors the learner should master to become self-sufficient in the natural environment.

educable mentally retarded Persons who are generally able to succeed in early school-related tasks (IQ 50 to 84).

electromyogram Recording of the action potential of skeletal muscles.

encephalitis An acute inflammatory condition of the brain.

epilepsy Disturbance in electrochemical activity of the brain that causes seizures and convulsions.

epiphysis Ossification center at the end of each developing long bone.

equal educational opportunity Compensatory education provided to handicapped children that enables opportunity for attainment of equal benefits or educational goals as compared with the nonhandicapped.

equally effective education Education that is not identical but that provides opportunity to achieve equal benefit or goals through the IEP in the least restrictive environment.

equilibrium reactions A reflex that helps a person maintain an upright position when the center of gravity is suddenly moved beyond the base of support.

esophoria A tendency for an eye to deviate laterally toward the nose.

esotropia A condition in which the eyes turn inward, such as cross-eyes.

event recording Noting the number of times a specifically defined behavior occurs within a time interval.

eversion Lifting the outer border of the foot upward.

etiology Study of the origin of disease (term often misused for "cause").

exercise intensity Amount of work load in relation to the functional capacity of the individual.

exophoria A tendency for an eye to deviate laterally away from the nose.

exotropia A condition wherein an eye deviates laterally away from the nose.

extension Movement of a part that increases a joint angle.

external evaluation Refers to a situation in which a person independent of the project evaluates the extent to which predetermined behaviors are acquired by pupils and the processes employed for achieving objectives.

extinction Removal of reinforcers that previously followed the behavior.

extrinsic Originating outside a part.

fading Gradually withdrawing help from a task.

fascial stretch An exercise designed to stretch the shortened fascial ligamentous bands that extend between the low back and anterior aspect of the pelvis and legs.

formative assessment Determination of whether a student's form or techniques replicate a defined model of performance.

forward chaining The first step of a series of tasks is taught first.

functional adaptation Modification by using assistive devices or by changing the demands of a task to permit participation.

fundamental motor patterns Motor patterns that are generic to the movement of normal individuals.

fundamental motor skills Motor skills that are generic to several specific sport skills, such as catching, striking, kicking, and throwing.

gait Walking pattern.

gallop A gait in which a leap is followed by a small step on the trailing foot, followed by another leap.

GAS General adaptation syndrome.

general abilities Prerequisites to performance of specific motor skills, such as strength, flexibility, and endurance.

general intellectual functioning Assessment of performance on an IQ test.

general to specific The progression of motor development from mass undifferentiated movements to specific voluntary motor control.

genu recurvatum Hyperextension at the knee joint.

genu valgum Knock-knee.

genu varum Bowleg.

geratrics Study of diseases of old age.

glaucoma A condition in which the pressure of the fluid inside the eye is too high, causing loss of vision.

goal A measurable, observable behavior achieved through attainment of several short-term instructional objectives.

goal ball A game for the blind in which gross motor movement is a response to auditory stimuli in a ball.

grand mal seizure Seizure that involves severe convulsions accompanied by stiffening, twisting, alternating contractions and relaxations, and unconsciousness.

gross motor to fine motor control The individual gains control over large muscles before small muscles.

growth Development of or increased size of a living organism.

handicap Any hindrance or difficulty imposed by a physical, mental, or emotional problem.

hallux valgus (pl. **halluces**) Displacement of the great toe toward the other toes as occurs with a bunion.

hard-of-hearing Conditions of hearing impairment or persons who have hearing impairments but who can function with or without a hearing aid.

heart murmurs Sounds that can be detected by a stethoscope that are caused by blood flowing past the valves of the heart.

hebephrenic Describing a condition that results in regression to childish behavior.

hemiplegia Neurological affliction of one half of the body or the limbs on one side of the body.

hernia Protrusion of an organ through an abnormal opening.

heterotropias Malalignments of the eyes in which one or both eyes consistently deviate from the central axis.

hierarchy A continuum of ordered activities in which a task of lower order and of lesser difficulty is prerequisite to acquisition of a related task of greater difficulty.

hopping Taking off from one foot into a flight phase and landing on the same foot.

hyperopia A condition in which the light rays focus behind the retina, causing an unclear image of objects closer than 20 feet from the eye.

hyperphoria A tendency for an eye to deviate in an upward direction.

hypertensive heart Commonly known as high blood pressure, which places a prolonged stress on the heart and major arteries.

hyperresponsiveness Overreaction to sensory stimuli.

hypertropia A condition in which one or both eyes swing upward.

hypophoria A tendency for an eye to deviate in a downward direction.

hyporesponsiveness Underreaction to sensory stimuli.

hypotropia A condition in which one or both eyes turn downward.

hysteria An involuntary loss of motor or sensory function in states of consciousness.

idiopathic Refers to disease of unknown cause.

incidental learning Learning that is unplanned.

Individual Education Program Specially designed instruction to meet the unique needs of a person for self-sufficient living.

inflammation Reaction of the tissue to trauma, heat and cold, chemicals, electricity, or microorganisms.

inhibition of primitive reflexes Overriding of primitive reflexes by higher control of the central nervous system to permit voluntary movement.

instruction Organized principles with established technical procedure involving action and practice.

interval measure A common unit of measure with no true zero point.

interval recording The occurrence or nonoccurrence of a behavior within a specific time interval.

intrinsic Originating within a part.

inventory assessment Checklists of tasks to be accomplished with little functional relationship that are usually not in sequential order.

inversion Turning upward of the medial border of the foot.

ischemia Local anemia caused by an obstruction of blood vessels to a part.

isometric muscle contraction Muscle contraction without any appreciable change in its length.

isotonic muscle contraction Muscle contraction whereby origin and insertion move toward one another.

jacksonian seizure Seizure characterized by local movements of some part of the body spreading to other parts of the body.

kinesthesis Awareness of the position of the limbs.

kyphosis Exaggerated thoracic spinal curve (humpback).

kypholordosis Exaggerated thoracic and lumbar spinal curves (round swayback).

laterality An awareness of the difference between both sides of the body.

leadership Provision of motivation for a group to achieve its goals.

leaping Taking off from one foot into a flight phase and then landing on the opposite foot.

least restrictive alternative The alternatives available for placement in least restrictive environments.

least restrictive environment A continuum of environments that curtail one's liberty and restrict free expression in a normal society. Placement should be least restrictive.

learning stations Areas in which activity is conducted to achieve specific objectives.

lordosis Exaggerated lumbar vertabral curve (swayback).

mainstreaming Placement of handicapped children in regular class with an IEP.

main task Of less difficulty than a skill and prerequisite to skills.

manualism Means by which the deaf communicate by use of hand signals (signing).

mastoiditis Chronic inflammation of the middle ear that spreads to the air cells of the mastoid process.

maturation The rate of sequential development of self-help skills of infancy, development of locomotor skills, and interaction with peers, which would occur irrespective of instructional intervention.

memory The length of time that information can be retained.

menarche Onset of menstruation.

meningitis Acute contagious disease characterized by inflammation of the meninges of the spinal cord.

menstruation The monthly loss of blood in mature females in response to hormonal cues.

mental retardation Subaverage intellectual functioning that originates during the developmental period and is associated with impairment in adaptive behavior.

MET Work metabolic rate divided by resting metabolic rate of a subject.

metatarsalgia Also known as Morton's toe; severe pain or cramp in metatarsus in the region of the fourth toe.

mobility training An adaptive technique that is applied to the blind and enhances the ability to travel.

modeling Demonstration of a task by the teacher or reinforcement by another student who performs a desirable behavior in the presence of the targeted student.

mononucleosis Disease of low virulence that affects the lymphocytes.

monoplegia Neurological affliction of one extremity of the body.

morbidity Number of disease cases in a calendar year per 100,000 population.

Moro reflex Startle reflex elicited by jarring or removing the supporting surface.

mortality Death rate.

most appropriate placement The placement in a least restrictive environment that is most appropriate for a specific person.

motor fitness Characteristics of movement that are essential to the efficient coordination of the body.

motor planning The ability to organize information in sequential segments and then carry out the plan in a smooth and integrated fashion.

motor skill Reasonably complex motor performance.

muscle setting Statically tensing a muscle without moving a part.

muscular dystrophy Chronic, progressive, degenerative, noncontagious disease of the muscular system, characterized by weakness and atrophy of muscles.

myocardial infarcts Limited function of the heart.

myopia A refractive condition in which the rays of the light focus in front of the retina when a person views an object 20 feet away or more.

narcotics Derivatives of opium used for sedative and analgesic actions.

negative reinforcer An event or stimulus that when terminated increases the frequency of the preceding response.

negative support A reflex in which there is flexion of the knees when pressure is removed from the feet.

neuromotor disorders Conditions in which damage is inflicted to the brain and is accompanied by motor involvement.

neuroses Mild aversions, phobias, and compulsions.

nominal measure A statement that represents a dichotomous value.

normalization Making available to the handicapped patterns and conditions of every day life that are as close as possible to the norms and patterns of the mainstream of society.

normative-referenced assessment Tests administered

under similar conditions in which the results can be classified according to percentiles.

nystagmus Rapid movement of the eyes from side to side, up and down, in a rotary motion, or in a combination of these movements.

objective Acceptance of events without distortion or prejudice; action toward which effort is directed for a purpose; to achieve goals that can be evaluated without prejudice.

obesity Pathological overweight in which a person is 20% or more above the normal weight (compare **overweight**).

occupational therapist Professionals who improve functional living and employment skills.

Office of Civil Rights A forum to address grievances resulting from the Rehabilitation Act of 1973 or P.L. 94-142.

ontogeny Historical development of an individual organism.

ophthalmologist Licensed physician who specializes in the treatment of eye disease and optical defects.

optical righting reaction A reflex that causes the head to move to an upright position when the body is suddenly tipped.

optician Technician who grinds lenses and makes up glasses.

optometrist Person who provides examination of the eye for defects and faults of refraction and the prescription of correctional lenses and exercises.

oralism Method of teaching the deaf by means of lip reading.

ordinal measure A unit of measure with a specialized order of rank that does not have a common unit of measure but can be hierarchically ordered.

organic brain injury Condition in which damage to the central nervous system exists.

orientation Obtaining the response and reinforcing the response.

orthopedics Branch of medicine primarily concerned with treatment of disorders of the musculoskeletal system.

orthoptic vision The ability to use the extraocular muscles of the eyes in unison.

orthoptist Person who provides eye exercises and orthoptic training as prescribed by medical personnel.

orthotics Construction of self-help devices to aid the patient in rehabilitation (braces, etc.).

Osgood-Schlatter disease Epiphysitis of the tibial tubercle.

osteoarthritis Chronic and degenerative disease of joints.

osteochondritis Inflammation of cartilage and bone.

osteoporosis Increased porosity of bone by the absorption of calcareous material.

otitis media Infection of the middle ear.

overweight Any deviation of 10% or more above the ideal weight for a person (compare **obese**).

parallel activity Play at the ability level of the individual in observable proximity of other play participants.

paralysis Permanent or temporary suspension of a motor function because of the loss of integrity of a motor nerve.

paranoia Characteristics of fear, distrust, and hostility toward others.

paraplegia Neurological affliction of both legs.

paresis Local paralysis.

pathology Study of disease (term often misused for diseased or "pathological conditions").

pattern analysis Study of sequential arrangement of movement behaviors to achieve a purpose.

peer-mediated reinforcement Reinforcement by peers of specific social or task behaviors.

peer isolation Removing an individual from a group setting.

peer tutoring Situation in which classmates learn material and assist peers who do not understand the material.

pelvic tilt Increase or decrease of pelvic inclination.

perceptive deafness Inability to hear caused by a defect of the inner ear or of the auditory nerve in transmitting the impulse to the brain.

perceptual-motor programming Use of activities believed to promote the development of balance, body image, spatial awareness, laterality, and directionality.

personality disorder Chronic maladaptive behavioral patterns that are culturally and socially unacceptable.

pes Refers to the foot.

pes cavus Exaggerated height of the longitudinal arch of the foot (hollow arch).

pes planus Extreme flatness of the longitudinal arch of the foot.

petit mal seizure Nonconvulsive seizure in which consciousness is lost for a few seconds.

phagocytosis Process of ingestion of injurious cells or particles by a phagocyte (white blood cell).

phenylketonuria (PKU) Physiological disturbance caused by an imbalance in the amino acids and resulting in mental limitations.

phobias Abnormal fears of specific objects, people, or situations.

phylogeny Development of a race or group of animals.

physiatrist Physician in physical medicine.

physical education Development of physical and motor fitness and fundamental motor patterns and skills.

physical fitness Refers to physical properties of muscular activity such as strength, flexibility, endurance, and cardiovascular endurance.

physical medicine Phase of medicine that uses various therapies to bring about a healing response.

physical priming Physically holding and moving the body parts of the learner through the activity.

physical therapist A professional who evaluates and treats physical impairments through the use of various physical modalities.

pigeon chest Abnormal prominence of the sternum.

plantar flexion Moving the foot toward its plantar surface at the ankle joint (extension).

pneumonia An infection of the air spaces of the lungs.

positive support A reflex that causes the legs to extend and the feet to plantar flex when one is standing.

posture Mechanical efficiency or inefficiency of body parts.

prerequisite analysis The analysis of a complex task to determine the ability prerequisites.

prescription Specification of action based on diagnosis prior to program implementation.

present level of educational performance The limits of capability in attainment of an unmet goal of the IEP; the base from which there is postulation of the short-term instructional objectives.

process Steps that lead to objectives in a particular manner; a progressive series of operations to be followed in a definite order that directs action toward achievement of objectives.

profoundly retarded Mentally retarded persons who require complete custodial care.

prognosis Prediction of the course of a disease.

program Sequential order of behavioral objectives that go from lesser to greater difficulty.

programmed instruction A set of hierarchical objectives that lead to a specific learning outcome. The outcome of each objective is used to make an instructional decision.

projection Disguising a conflict by excluding one's motives; blaming someone else.

progressive muscular dystrophy Progressive wasting and atrophy of muscles.

prompting Sensory or physical and to engage the participant in successful activity.

prone position Lying in a face-down position.

prosthesis Artificial limb or appliance.

protective extensor thrust A reflex that causes immediate extension of the arms when the head and upper body are tipped suddenly forward.

proximal Refers to a point nearest to the origin of an organ or body part, as opposed to distal.

proximal-distal Referring to body parts closest to the midline of the body, which develop first, followed by development of the shoulder, elbow, wrist, and then fingers.

protraction Forward movement of a part, for example, shoulder girdle.

psychogenic deafness Condition in which receptive organs are not impaired, but for emotional reasons the person does not respond to sound.

psychometrist A professional who administers and interprets cognitive achievement and behavioral tests.

psychomotor seizure Seizure in which one may lose contact with reality and manifest bizarre psychogenic behavior.

psychotomimetic agent Drugs, such as LSD, whose effects mimic the characteristics of psychosis.

ptosis Weakness and prolapse of an organ, for example, prominent abdomen.

punishment An aversive event that follows an undesirable behavior.

quadriplegia Neurological affliction of all four extremities.

ratio measure A common unit of measure between each score and a true zero point.

rationalization Resolution of a conflict by hiding a real motive and substituting another reasonable one.

reaction formation Disguised feeling in which a person acts opposite to the response toward which he or she may be motivated.

recreation therapy System of therapy using recreation as a means to rehabilitation.

reflexes Innate responses that all normal children develop.

regular class Public school class in which typical children are educated.

rehabilitation Restoration of a disabled person to greater efficiency and health.

reinforcer Any consequence that follows an action and strengthens that act.

reinforcement schedule The frequency with which reinforcers are given.

refractive vision The process by which light rays are bent as they enter the eyes.

Rehabilitation Act of 1973 Civil rights legislation for the handicapped which states that there is to be no exclusion or denial of benefits to the handicapped.

related services Services that help a person benefit from direct services.

relaxation Lessening of anxiety and muscle tension.

reliability The consistency with which one carries out assigned responsibility.

remedial physical education Activity designed to habilitate or rehabilitate functional motor movements and develop physical and motor prerequisites for functional skills.

repetitions The number of times the work interval is repeated under identical conditions.

repression Submerging distressing thoughts into the unconscious mind.

response cost The withdrawal of earned reinforcers or privileges following an inappropriate behavior.

rest interval The time between work intervals in progressive resistive exercise.

responsibility Carrying out a role that has been assigned by an authority figure of a social group.

retraction Backward movement of a part, for example, shoulder girdle.

rheumatic heart disease Condition caused by rheumatic fever, which damages the heart, its valves, and blood vessels by scar tissue.

rigidity Clinical classification of cerebral palsy characterized by rigid functional uncoordination of reciprocal muscle groups.

risk Used to describe persons who have a majority of factors pointing toward the potential development of coronary heart disease.

round shoulders Postural condition whereby the scapulae are abducted and the shoulders are forward.

salicylates Salt of salicylic acid used to reduce pain and temperature.

schizophrenia Abnormal behavior patterns and personality disorganization accompanied by less than adequate contact with reality.

scoliosis Lateral and rotation deviation of the vertebral column.

sedatives Drugs that induce sleep and have a calming effect.

self-evaluation Accurate interpretation of the consequences of instructional performance without the aid of outside information.

self-initiated activity Voluntary participation in activity that is initiated by the individual.

self-instruction Engaging in procedures to achieve one's objectives without personal and direct input from the instructor.

self-mutilating behavior Acts that injure oneself.

senility A physical and mental infirmity that sometimes accompanies old age.

sensory inputs Information received through the senses, such as vision, hearing, kinesthesis, and vestibular and tactile responses.

sensory integration Administration of activities believed to promote processing of sensory stimuli.

set The time between the work and the rest interval in progressive resistive exercise.

severely retarded Mentally retarded persons who can be trained to care for some of their bodily needs and to develop language but who have great difficulty in social and occupational areas.

shaping Reinforcement of small progressive steps that lead toward the desired behavior.

short-term instructional objectives A specific observable, and measurable behavior that functions as an intermediate step to extend present levels of educational performance toward the goals of the IEP.

skill Utilization of abilities to perform complex tasks competently as a result of reinforced practice.

slide A sideways gallop.

social interaction Interaction among persons who are engaged in common activities.

social worker A professional who is the link between the home and the school through work with intraprofessional specialties.

spatial relations The position of objects in space, particularly as the objects relate to the position of the body.

special class Class designed to give special educational help to mentally retarded, emotionally disturbed, deaf, or blind students or children with other handicaps.

special educator A professional involved directly or indirectly with the instruction of handicapped children.

speech therapist A professional who evaluates and provides intervention programs to children with speech deficiencies.

spina bifida Congenital separation or lack of union of the vertebral arches.

spasm Involuntary muscle contraction.

spastic Clinical type of cerebral palsy characterized by muscle contractures and jerky, uncertain movements of the muscles.

somatotype Certain body type (endomorphy, mesomorphy, or ectomorphy).

social adjustment Degree to which the individual is able to function independently in the community, achieve gainful employment, and conform to other personal and social responsibilities and standards set by the community.

standard teaching sequence A sequence of hierarchical potential short-term instructional objectives that enable the determination of a pupil's present level of educational performance, of short-term instructional objectives, and of learning gains made over a certain time period.

stenosis Incomplete opening of a valve that restricts blood flow.

stereotyped behavior Specific acts that are repeated over and over.

strabismus Crossed eyes resulting from inability of the eye muscles to coordinate.

stress Condition that causes the inability of an organism to maintain a constant internal environment.

sublimation Substitution of one activity for another, more accessible, activity.

submaximal intensity Below the functional level of maximum performance.

subtask Subdivision of a task; several subtasks compose the main task.

supination Rotation of the palm of the hand upward or adduction and inversion of the foot.

supine position Lying on the back and facing upward.

survey Assessment that provides broad guidelines for selection of instructional content.

symmetrical tonic neck reflex A reflex in which the

upper limbs tend to flex and the lower limbs extend when ventroflexing the head. If the head is dorsiflexed, the upper limbs extend and the lower limbs flex.

system Interdependent items that relate to a whole operation and function as a unit.

tactile sense Knowledge of where the body ends and the space begins and the ability to discriminate between pressure, texture, and size.

talipes equinus Walking on the toes or the anterior portion of the foot.

talipes valgus Walking on the inside of the foot (pronated).

talipes varus Walking on the outside of the foot (supinated).

target level Desired performance level of an individual while participating in activity.

task analysis Identification of prerequisite behaviors of tasks to be targets of instruction.

task-specific approach (top, down) Teaching a skill directly and generalizing it to a variety of environments. If it cannot be learned, teach the prerequisites.

tenotomy Surgical operation on the tendons.

tension State of being strained.

terminal objective Synthesis of all subobjectives that enable mastery of the main or general objective.

tetralogy of Fallot Abnormality of the opening of the septum between ventricles or positioning of the aorta to the right in such a manner that it lies over the defect of the septum of the left ventricle.

therapeutic modality Device designed to bring about a therapeutic response, for example, heat, cold, light, electrostimulation.

therapy Treatment of a disease or disability.

throwing Projection of an object through space with the arm.

tibial torsion Medial twisting of the lower leg on its long axis.

time out from reinforcement Withdrawal of reinforcement for a certain period of time.

token economy A form of contingency management in which tokens are earned for desirable behavior.

tonic labyrinthine reflexes Reflexes that are present when one maintains trunk extension when supine and trunk flexion when prone.

torticollis Also known as wryneck; contraction of neck muscles resulting in drawing the head to one side.

trainable mentally retarded Persons who are characterized by the general inability to succeed in problem-solving tasks and who do not have discernible, usable academic skills. They are frequently impaired in both maturation and social adjustment.

tranquilizers Drugs that reduce tension or anxiety. They affect the sympathetic nervous system by suppressing synaptic stimuli.

trauma Injury or wound.

travel vision Residual vision in the blind that enables travel.

treatment-referenced assessment Tests to determine which teaching strategy would be most successful with a given student.

tremor Clinical type of cerebral palsy evidenced by a rhythmic movement caused by alternating contractions between flexor and extensor muscles.

Trendelenburg sign Dropping of the pelvis on the unsupported side because of weakness or paralysis of hip abductor muscles.

tuberculosis A disease of the lungs caused by the tubercle bacillus.

unified process of development The conception of intellectual, physical, social, emotional development as a unified process.

uniformity of sequence The sequence of development is the same in all normal children.

unique need A behavior that is a target of instruction in the form of goals of the IEP; deficiencies are determined by a comparison of behaviors required for self-sufficiency in the community and present levels of performance.

valgus (valgum) Angling of a part in the direction away from the midline of the body (bent outward).

varus (varum) Angling of a part in the direction of the midline of the body (bent inward).

vestibular sense Response for balance; located in the nonauditory section of the inner ear.

visual motor control Ability to fixate on and visually track moving objects as well as the ability to match visual input with appropriate motor responses.

vocational counselors Professionals who guide disabled persons in seeking employment.

whiplash injury Deep-tissue neck injury resulting from the head being forcefully snapped forward and backward.

winged scapula Vertebral border of the scapula wings outward because of weakness of the serratus anterior or the middle and lower trapezius muscles.

Wolff's law of bone growth Bone alters its internal structure and external form according to the manner in which it is used.

work interval A prescribed number of repetitions of the same activity under identical conditions.

Author Index

Subject Index

A